# Channelopathies of the Nervous System

Commissioning Editor: Melanie Tait
Development Editor: Zoë Youd
Production Controller: Anthony Read
Desk Editor: Jackie Holding
Cover Designer: Fred Rose

# Channelopathies of the Nervous System

**Michael Rose BSc MD FRCP**
Consultant and Honorary Senior Lecturer in Neurology, King's Neurosciences Centre, King's College Hospital, and Guy's, St Thomas' and King's College School of Medicine and Dentistry, London UK

**Robert C. Griggs MD**
Chair, Department of Neurology, University of Rochester School of Medicine and Dentistry, Rochester, USA

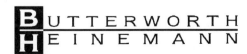

OXFORD   AUCKLAND   BOSTON   JOHANNESBURG   MELBOURNE   NEW DELHI

Butterworth-Heinemann
Linacre House, Jordan Hill, Oxford OX2 8DP
225 Wildwood Avenue, Woburn, MA 01801-2041
A division of Reed Educational and Professional Publishing Ltd

 A member of the Reed Elsevier plc group

First published 2001

**British Library Cataloguing in Publication Data**

Rose, Michael R. (Michael Robertson), 1955-
   Channelopathies of the nervous system
   1. Neurology  2. Nervous system – Diseases
   I. Title II.  Griggs, Robert C.
   616.8

**Library of Congress Cataloguing in Publication Data**

Channelopathies of the nervous system/[edited by] Michael Rose and Robert Griggs.
    p. ; cm.
   Includes index.
   ISBN 0-7506-4507-5
   1. Nervous system–Pathophysiology.   2. Ion channels.   3. Pathology, Molecular. I.
   Rose, Michael. II. Griggs, Robert C., 1939-
   [DNLM: 1. Nervous System Diseases–physiopathology.   2. Ion Channels–physiology.
   WL 140 C458 2001]
   RC347 .C475 2001
616.8'047–dc21
                                                2001025590

ISBN 0 7506 4507 5

www.bh.com/neurology

Typeset by Keytec Typesetting Ltd, Bridport, Dorset
Printed and bound in Great Britain by MPG Books Ltd, Bodmin, Cornwall

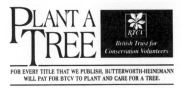

# Contents

# List of contributors

**Robert W. Baloh** MD
Professor of Neurology,
UCLA School of Medicine,
Los Angeles, CA, USA

**Jeffrey Balser** MD PhD
Associate Professor of Anesthesiology and
Pharmacology,
Associate Dean,
Physician-Scientist Development,
Vanderbilt University Medical Center,
Nashville, TN, USA

**Sam Berkovic** MD FRACP
Professor, Austin and Repatriation Medical Centre,
University of Melbourne,
Melbourne, Australia

**Kailash Bhatia** MBBS MD DM MRCP
Senior Lecurer/ Honorary Consultant Neurologist,
Institute of Neurology,
University College,
London, UK

**Peter Brown** MD FRCP
Consultant Neurologist,
National Hospital for Neurology and Neurosurgery,
London, UK

**Dennis Bulman** PhD
Senior Scientist,
Ottawa Hospital Research Institute,
Ottawa, ON, Canada

**Stephen C. Cannon** MD PhD
Associate Professor of Neurobiology,
Department of Neurobiology,
Harvard Medical School,
Boston, MA, USA

**Sam Chong** MD MRCP
Consultant Neurologist,
King's Neurosciences Centre,
King's College Hospital,
London, UK

**Andrew Engel** MD
McKnight-3M Professor of Neuroscience;
Consultant, Department of Neurology;
Director, Muscle Laboratory,
Mayo Clinic,
Rochester, NY, USA

**Paul A. Felts** PhD
Senior Research Fellow,
Department of Neuroimmunology,
Guy's, King's and St Thomas' School of Medicine,
London, UK

**Peter Fenner** MD(Lond) DRCOG FACTM FRCGP
National Medical Officer,
Surf Life Saving Australia,
Mackay,
Queensland, Australia

**Michel D. Ferrari** MD PhD
Associate Professor of Neurology,
Department of Neurology,
Leiden University Medical Centre,
Leiden, The Netherlands

**Alfred George** MD
Grant W. Liddle Professor of Medicine,
Director, Division of Genetic Medicine,
Vanderbilt University Medical Center,
Nashville, TN, USA

**Peter J. Goadsby** MD PhD DSc FRACP FRCP
Professor of Clinical Neurology/Wellcome Senior
Research Fellow,

University Department of Clinical Neurology,
Institute of Neurology,
The National Hospital for Neurology and Neurosurgery,
London, UK

**Ian Hart** PhD FRCP(G)
Senior Lecturer in Neurology,
University Department of Neurological Science,
Walton Centre for Neurology and Neurosurgery,
Liverpool, UK

**Lawrence J. Hayward** MD PhD
Assistant Professor,
Department of Neurology,
University of Massachusetts Medical Center,
Worcester, MA, USA

**Terry Heiman-Patterson** MD
Professor of Neurology,
MCP Hahnemann University,
Philadelphia, PA, USA

**John C. Hunter** PhD
Head, Department of Analgesia,
Center for Biological Research,
Neurobiology Unit,
Roche Bioscience,
Palo Alto, CA, USA

**Karin Jurkat-Rott** MD
Department of Applied Physiology,
University of Ulm,
Ulm, Germany

**Frank Lehmann-Horn** MD MS
Professor and Head of Department,
Department of Applied Physiology,
University of Ulm,
Ulm, Germany

**Richard Lewis** PhD
Principal Scientist,
Queensland Agricultural Biotechnology Centre (DPI),
Gehrmann Laboratories,
The University of Queensland,
Brisbane, Australia

**Kerry Mills** BSc PhD MB BS FRCP
Professor of Clinical Neurophysiology,
King's College and Guy's Hospitals,
London, UK

**Richard Moxley** III MD
Associate Chair for Academic Affairs,
Department of Neurology;
Director, Neuromuscular Disease Center,
University of Rochester,
Rochester, NY, USA

**Kinji Ohno** MD PhD
Assistant Professor,
Mayo Medical School;
Research Associate,
Mayo Clinic,
Rochester, NY, USA

**Reinhardt Rüdel** PhD
Professor,
Department of Physiology,
University of Ulm,
Ulm, Germany

**Valeria Sansone**
Assistant Professor of Neurology,
Department of Neurology,
University of Milan,
Instituto Policlinico San Donato,
Milan, Italy

**Kylie A. Scoggan** PhD
Post Doctoral Fellow,
Ottawa Hospital Research Institute,
Ottawa, ON, Canada

**Steven M. Sine** PhD
Associate Professor,
Mayo Graduate School,
Rochester, NY, USA

**Rabi Tawil** MD
Associate Professor of Neurology,
University of Rochester Medical Center,
Rochester, NY, USA

**Marina A. J. Tijssen** MD PhD
Neurologist,
Department of Neurology,
Academic Medical Centre,
University of Amsterdam,
Amsterdam, The Netherlands

**Enza Maria Valente** MD PhD
Research Fellow in Neurogenetics,
Institute of Neurology,
London, UK

**Angela Vincent** MB BS MSc FRCPath
University Lecturer in Clinical Neuroimmunology,
Institute of Molecular Medicine,
John Radcliffe Hospital,
Oxford, UK

**Stephen G. Waxman** MD PhD
Professor and Chairman,
Department of Neurology and PVA/EPVA Neuroscience
Research Center,
Yale University School of Medicine;
Director, Rehabilitation Research Center,
VA Hospital,
West Haven, CT, USA

# Foreword

Channelopathies of the Nervous System – just a few years ago, the very concept did not exist, and the book you now hold could not have been conceived. This volume documents a special time in our field, a time when the sometimes disparate threads of basic research and clinical investigation suddenly converge to generate totally new insight into the pathogenesis of human disease. Out of the intellectual explosion of that convergence emerges a new field, a new view, and a new approach to future research and clinical practice. This book surveys the new field of channelopathies, moving from an overview of channel structure, function, and expression, through a detailed discussion of channel abnormalities that are known to produce neurological disease, to end with a consideration of other areas ripe for research. But before the reader plunges into the rich details that follow, it is worth reflecting for a few moments on how we arrived at this special point in time.

Ion channels – highly specialized proteins that provide gated aqueous pathways for the movement of ions across cellular membranes – are relative newcomers in the history of science. When Hodgkin and Huxley published their landmark studies in 1952, describing the sodium and potassium currents responsible for action potentials in the giant squid axon, they conjectured that these currents might pass through discrete 'channels' or pathways in the cell surface membrane. The subsequent 20 years witnessed a tremendous amount of work on ionic currents in nerve and muscle, but the actual existence of such ion channels remained largely an article of faith in the scientific community. This situation changed dramatically in 1976 with the first recording of currents passing through single ion channels by Neher and Sachman, using

the newly developed patch clamp technique for which they would subsequently win the Nobel Prize. The 1980s witnessed the isolation and biochemical characterization of key ion channel proteins followed closely by the functional reconstitution of these purified proteins into artificial lipid bilayers, thus confirming their basic channel properties and completing the circle from mental construction to proof of concept. However, the sheer size of these proteins limited further progress using traditional biochemical and biophysical tools. Again, a quantal jump in technology – the advent of gene cloning – provided the substrate for the next major advances.

Numa and his colleagues blazed the trail in the early 1980s by cloning and sequencing several ion channels – an accomplishment that was at the time a technological tour de force. Within a few years sequences for many other important ion channels had been deduced. It became apparent that various ion channels with seemingly different biophysical properties shared fundamental similarities at the structural level. Families of channel genes were constructed; many of these families in turn showed evidence of common evolutionary origins. Methods for expressing cloned channel genes in cultured cells and oocytes then opened the way to the development of site-directed mutagenesis as a powerful tool for probing relationships between structure and function in these complex proteins.

Throughout this period of nearly 50 years, our concept of an ion channel looked like remaining a largely mental image; an image whose outlines were increasingly sharpened by experimentation, yet one still largely based on scientific intuition. Considerable early progress toward a true structural image was made with the acetylcholine receptor, but voltage-gated ion channels remained recalcitrant. That situation changed dramatically with the recent publication of the crystal structure for a primitive member of the potassium channel family. Overnight, a true picture of the guts of an ion channel was available, and the congruence of this image with our previous notions of channel structure surprised even the most optimistic in the field. As with each previous technological advance, however, this new and transformational information only served to raise more questions and accelerate the pace of discovery.

In parallel with this thread of basic research on ion channel structure and function, a complementary line of investigation was evolving in the clinical sciences, centered around an intriguing group of diseases characterized by abnormalities in membrane excitability. As in many areas of clinical research, the initial descriptions of these diseases and their distinguishing signs and symptoms had been in the medical literature for many decades. By the 1960s, evidence was accumulating that some of these disorders, at least in skeletal muscle, resulted from abnormalities in ion channel activity. The work of Bryant and his colleagues in the myotonic goat was particularly prescient in making this connection between clinical symptoms and abnormal channel function. However, progress was slow and ultimate proof of this hypothetical connection was lacking.

These lines of clinical and basic research converged explosively with the application of molecular biological techniques to both fields. Cloning of channel cDNA led rapidly to characterization of the chromosomal DNA encoding these primary sequences. Location of channel genes within the genome provided the basis for linkage analysis, and led to the first confirmation of a causal relationship between a channel gene mutation and the expression of a disease phenotype. Over a period of just a few years, the number of identified channel disorders and the number of known mutations in each key ion channel grew exponentially. A new field of clinical medicine was born, and a new descriptive term – channelopathy – was coined. Now, less than a decade after the first published report of a channel mutation causing an inherited neurological disorder, the body of knowledge in this area has grown to the point where separate texts are required to contain it.

Common themes are becoming apparent in this explosion of information. We now recognize that many different mutations can occur in a single channel gene. These different mutations may give rise to what appears clinically to be the same disorder, or may be expressed as completely different clinical phenotypes. Likewise, it is now clear that a particular clinical phenotype can be produced by mutations in unrelated genes encoding channels selective for different ions. Rational diagnosis and treatment of the channelopathies will require more than just clinical classification; genetic analysis and classification on the basis of the specific channel defect will ultimately be necessary.

Perhaps most important is the realization that our current knowledge in this area represents just the tip of the proverbial iceberg. The early focus of work in skeletal muscle reflects the homogeneity of the cell types and relatively uniform pattern of channel gene expression in this tissue, coupled with the compatibility of functional channel defects in skeletal muscle with survival. Ion channel defects in the central nervous system will be more difficult to recognize, reflecting the much larger number of channel isoforms expressed in the brain, the diversity of cell types in which they are expressed, and the complex regional organization of functionally related cells. However, as the later chapters in this book evidence, such neuronal channelopathies are beginning to be identified. Undoubtedly, the next ten years will see a flood of research in this area, and the second edition of this wonderful book may well run to several volumes.

Finally, in these challenging times for academic medicine and for clinical research, the advances described in this text provide ample evidence of the unique strength and importance of the academic medical center. It is in this special environment that clinician-scientists can make the sometimes serendipitous connections between the basic phenomena that they study in the laboratory and the clinical conditions that they treat in the hospital and the outpatient office. It is a very precious but delicate environment, and one that we must all work hard to maintain.

Robert Barchi
Office of the Provost
University of Pennsylvania
Philadelphia, PA

# Preface

In neurology, as in medicine, the recognition of a new mechanism of pathophysiology propels us forward in our understanding of diseases. Typically there is a wave of enthusiasm for such theories, which become fashionable for a while until they settle into their rightful perspective. Past examples of this principle include slow viruses, retroviruses, autoantibodies and mitochondrial disorders. A recent illustration of this principle is that of ion channel disorders: the so-called channelopathies. The essential basis for nervous system function is the ability to conduct electrical impulses along nerves, nerve/nerve junctions and nerve/muscle junctions, as well as within muscle itself. The propagation of such electrical impulses throughout the nervous system requires the rapid shifts of various electrolytes across cellular membranes. These shifts are conducted through ion-specific channels which use a variety of stimuli to trigger their opening, or so-called *gating* properties. Some channels are opened by changes in voltage, so-called *voltage-gated* channels, while others are opened by binding of a ligand to the channel, so-called *ligand-gated* channels. The fascinating mechanism by which this is achieved is detailed in this book by Cannon (Chapter 1). It therefore seems surprising, in retrospect, that proof that disorders of channels were a mechanism for neurological disease took so long.

The first disorders proven to be channelopathies were those of voltage-gated channels causing inherited muscle disease, the non-dystrophic myotonias and familial periodic paralyses. Soon afterwards, it was appreciated that channelopathies could also affect neuronal systems, with the discovery that episodic ataxia Type I was due to mutations in the potassium channel gene. Given the preponderance of excitable cells in the central and peripheral nervous system, all of which must rely on membrane ion channels for their essential function, there was expectation that disorders of such channels would be responsible for a large number of neurological diseases. Since the first discovery of the muscle, and then neuronal channelopathies described above, there has been a rapid expansion in the number of diseases that have been shown to result from ion channel abnormalities. While the initial recognition of channelopathies was in rare diseases, channelopathies have now been identified as a cause of many common diseases: epilepsy, migraine, myasthenia and the ataxias; as well as contributing to the pathophysiology of many more: multiple sclerosis, pain syndromes, myotonic dystrophies.

This book aims to inform both clinicians and neuroscientists as to the state of the art of neurological channelopathies, both clinically and scientifically. It will afford an appreciation of the commonalities and pathophysiology of channel disorders and define the important biomechanisms for a wide variety of neurological symptoms and diseases.

Chapters 1 to 3 concentrate on the basic science of ion channels: their physiology, molecular biology and pharmacology. Chapters 4 and 5 describe the assessment of ion channel function both in the laboratory and clinically. Chapters 6 to 8 highlight the plasticity of ion channel gene expression and distribution. This knowledge is having an important impact on our understanding of the mechanism underlying pain syndromes and demyelination, and the potential for pharmacological manipulation of these mal-adaptive responses. Chapters 9 to 19 consider the diseases known to be channelopathies. Some of these diseases, such as hyperekplexia, episodic ataxia and paroxymal movement disorders, are sufficiently unusual that details of their clinical manifestations are hard to find even in specialized neurological textbooks. At the other end of the clinical spectrum are familiar neurological diseases such as myasthenia, migraine and epilepsy in which the role of ion channel disorder is providing novel insights. For rare diseases we asked authors to concentrate on the clinical aspects, while for the more common diseases authors were asked to highlight the evidence for ion channel dysfunction and put it into the context of the wider knowledge of pathophysiology of those diseases. The diseases discussed span both genetic and acquired disorders of channel function affecting both central and peripheral nerve function. We have included a section on potential channelopathies – diseases in which it seems channel dysfunction is likely to be involved, but has yet to be definitively established. Finally, we conclude with our own thoughts regarding the common strands underlying the channelopathies and pose questions for future research in this exciting field.

Michael R. Rose
Consultant Neurologist
King's Neuroscience Centre
Department of Neurology
London
UK

Robert C. Griggs
Professor and Chair of Neurology
University of Rochester School of Medicine
New York
USA

# Acknowledgements

*Chapter 2:* This work was supported by a grant from the Medical Research Council of Canada. K. A. Scoggan is a Postdoctoral Fellow of the MRC and D. Bulman is a Research Scholar of the MRC.

*Chapter 3:* This work has been supported by the National Institutes of Health (NS32387, AR44506, GM56307) and American Heart Association (Established Investigator Award).

*Chapter 6:* Work in the author's laboratory has been supported, in part, by grants from the Rehabilitation Research Service and Medical Research Service, Department of Veterans Affairs; the National Multiple Sclerosis Society; the Paralyzed Veterans of America and the Eastern Paralyzed Veterans Association. I thank my many colleagues, especially D. Quick, R. Foster, J.A. Black, S. Dib-Hajj, T.R. Cummins, J.D. Kocsis, M. Rizzo, O. Honmou, J. Newcombe, D. Baker and M.L. Cuzner, and M. Tanaka, for permission to reproduce figures from studies carried out in collaboration with them.

*Chapter 8:* The author is supported by grants from the Multiple Sclerosis Society of Great Britain & Northern Ireland and the Guy's & St. Thomas' Charitable Foundation.

*Chapter 9:* The support by Interdisziplinüares Zentrum für Klinische Forschung (IZKF) of the University of Ulm and the European Community (TMR Programme on Excitation-contraction coupling) is gratefully acknowledged.

*Chapter 15:* This work was supported by National Institutes of Health grants AG09693 and DC02952.

*Chapter 19:* The work of P. Goadsby has been supported by the Wellcome Trust and the Migraine Trust. P. Goadsby is a Wellcome Senior Research Fellow.

# Basic science (physiology, molecular biology and pharmacology)

PART

1

# 1

# Physiology of ion channels

*Stephen C. Cannon*

## Introduction

The nervous system has evolved to conduct information rapidly over large distances of up to two metres. Diffusion is far too slow for this task. Instead, electrical signalling is used as a mechanism for propagating information along neurons and muscle fibres. Ion channels are crucial components of the molecular machinery to accomplish this signalling. These integral membrane proteins form water-filled pores in the cell membrane to allow the passage of ions. The movement of charged ions through channels is the source of electrical current that changes the potential difference (voltage) across the membrane. For biological signalling in excitable tissues, the membrane potential shifts by up to 100 millivolts (mV) within milliseconds (ms). These rapid voltage transients are possible because of the relatively high density of channels in the membrane (typically 10 to 1000 per square micron), the high throughput of an open channel (10 000 000 ions/s) and the ability of ion channels to convert between conducting (open) and non-conducting (shut) conformations within 1 ms or less. This chapter provides an introduction to the functional properties, protein structure–function relationships, and disease-associated defects of ion channels. Supplementary information is available from recent monographs on ion channel biophysics (Hille, 1992) and cellular electrophysiology (Aidley, 1998; Sperelakis, 1998).

## Functional properties of ion channels

The biophysical behaviour of ion channels is characterized by two properties: *permeation* and *gating*. Permeation refers to the ability of ions to pass through an open pore, from one side of the membrane to the other. Ions can traverse the pore in either direction. Under the influence of electrical and chemical (concentration) gradients across the membrane, there is a net flow of ions in one direction which can be detected as an electrical current. Under physiological conditions about $10^{-12}$ amperes of current flows through an open channel. This seemingly minute quantity represents an extremely high throughput. An ampere of current equals one coulomb of charge flowing per second. Thus, for a monovalent cation a one picoampere current represents:

$$(10^{-12} \text{coulomb/s})/(1.6 \times 10^{-19} \text{coulomb/ion})$$

$$= 6\,000\,000 \text{ions/s}.$$

This high throughput was one of the major pieces of experimental evidence that channels form aqueous pores in the membrane, rather than carriers or pumps.

For each permeant ion, flow across the membrane is driven by the concentration gradient and the membrane potential. There will be a net flux in one direction until the tendency for diffusion (net movement from the side with high concentration to low) is balanced by the electrical potential created by net transfer of charge across the membrane. When these two forces balance the system is in equilibrium because the inward movement of ions exactly balances the outward flow. The equilibrium or Nernst potential for ion X, $E_X$, can be computed from the electrochemical potential:

$$E_X = \frac{RT}{z_x F} \ln \left( \frac{[X^{+z}]_{out}}{[X^{+z}]_{in}} \right) \qquad (1.1)$$

where $T$ is absolute temperature (°K), $R$ is the gas constant (8.3 volt-coul °K$^{-1}$ mol$^{-1}$), $F$ is Faraday's constant ($9.6 \times 10^4$ coul mol$^{-1}$), $z_x$ is the valence and $[X^{+z}]$ is the concentration of permeant ion $X^{+z}$. At the normal body temperature of 37°C, $RT/F$ is 26.7 mV. Intracellular and extracellular ion concentrations and their corresponding equilibrium potential at 37°C are listed for a typical neuron in Table 1.1.

The permeability of most ion channels is highly selective, allowing the passage of one type of ion to the relative exclusion of others. Many ion channels are named for the ion that is preferentially conducted. Thus K channels are very permeable to K$^+$ ions, but not to Na$^+$, Ca$^{2+}$, or Cl$^-$. Selectivity is not perfect. On average, K$^+$ channels pass one Na$^+$ ion for every 100 K$^+$ ions that traverse the pore. The ability to achieve this degree of selectivity, while at the same time allowing ten million or more ions per second to flow through the pore, was a major question in channel biophysics. The definitive answer was gleaned from the crystal structure of a bacterial K$^+$ channel (Doyle *et al.*, 1998). An optimal fit is formed between an unhydrated K$^+$ ion and the carbonyl oxygens from the protein lining of the pore.

Energetically speaking, docking the K$^+$ ion in the pore is just as favourable as hydrating the ion with four water molecules in aqueous solution. Na$^+$ ions do not permeate as well, for although smaller in atomic radius than K$^+$ ions, they cannot interact simultaneously with four pore-lining carbonyl oxygens held rigidly and precisely in place by the scaffolding of the channel protein.

Ionic selectivity of channels is critical for bioelectrical signalling. Without it, cells could not shift their membrane potential in response to the opening and closing of specific ion channels. Working together, the selective permeability of an ion channel and the asymmetrical distribution of ions across the cell membrane determine $E_{rev}$, the membrane potential at which the direction of current flow through the channel reverses from inward to outward. If the membrane potential ($V_m$) does not equal $E_{rev}$, then net current will flow. The effect of this current is to bring the membrane potential toward $E_{rev}$. For membrane potentials less than $E_{rev}$, net inward current flow depolarizes the cell potential (makes $V_m$ more positive) toward $E_{rev}$. At potentials more positive than $E_{rev}$ net outward current flow hyperpolarizes the cell toward $E_{rev}$. By convention, positive current is defined as the outward flow of positively charged ions (cations).

The ionic selectivity varies widely among different types of channels. In general, voltage-gated channels have a higher ionic selectivity than ligand-gated ones. For example, K$^+$ channels conduct K$^+$ about 100 times more readily than Na$^+$, whereas the nicotinic acetylcholine receptor at the neuromuscular junction does not discriminate between Na$^+$ and K$^+$. The relative permeability of

| Ion | $[ion]_{out}$ mM | $[ion]_{in}$ mM | $\dfrac{[ion]_{out}}{[ion]_{in}}$ | $E_{rev}$ mV |
|---|---|---|---|---|
| Ca$^{2+}$ | 2 | <10$^{-4}$ | >20 000 | >+132 |
| Na$^+$ | 140 | 12 | 12 | +66 |
| K$^+$ | 4.2 | 140 | 0.03 | −94 |
| Cl$^-$ | 115 | 40 | 2.9 | −29 |

**Table 1.1 Ion concentrations and equilibrium potentials for a typical neuron**

two different ions, $P_X/P_Y$, can be quantified experimentally by measuring the reversal potential. $E_{rev}$ is measured by voltage-clamping at a series of test voltages to determine the potential at which the net current through the channel is zero. In general, when two permeant ions, $X^+$ and $Y^+$, are present on each side of the membrane:

$$E_{rev} = \frac{RT}{F} \ln \left( \frac{P_X[X^+]_{in} + P_Y[Y^+]_{in}}{P_X[X^+]_{out} + P_Y[Y^+]_{out}} \right) \quad (1.2)$$

Notice that equation 1.2 reduces to the Nernst equation (1.1) if only one permeant ion is present. Similarly, if a channel were highly selective for passing only X, then $P_X$ is much greater than $P_Y$ and $E_{rev}$ is approximately equal to the Nernst potential for X. In other words, if a channel's reversal potential is near the equilibrium potential for one of the ions in Table 1.1, then this channel is highly selective for that particular ion. Experimentally, the relative permeabilities can be determined more easily under bi-ionic conditions. In this type of experiment the only permeant ion on the inside is $X^+$ while the only permeant ion on the outside is $Y^+$. Moreover, the two concentrations are made equal. Under bi-ionic conditions $[X^+]_{out} = 0$ and $[Y^+]_{in} = 0$, the remaining concentration terms cancel and the relative permeability is given by:

$$P_X/P_Y = \exp \left( \frac{E_{rev}F}{RT} \right) \quad (1.3)$$

The reversal potential provides a measure of the *relative* permeabilities for the ions present during the experiment. The *absolute* permeability is usually determined by measuring the amplitude of the current when $V_m$ is held away from $E_{rev}$ (Hille, 1992).

Ion channels must be capable of being opened and shut in a precise fashion in order to generate action potentials or to encode biological signals as a change in membrane potential. The process of switching between the open (conducting) and shut (non-conducting) conformations of the channel is called *gating*. The term derives from the notion of a hypothetical gate that occludes the pore of the channel. Channels may be gated by membrane potential, ligand binding, mechanical stress, or intracellular signalling molecules such as $Ca^{2+}$ or cyclic nucleotides (cAMP, cGMP). In a quiescent

cell, the membrane potential is hyperpolarized to $-60$ or $-80\ mV$ and most channels are in a closed, resting state. Depolarization, ligand binding, or some other stimulus may cause channels to open. This process is termed *activation*. In the continued presence of the stimulus, most channels *inactivate* by spontaneously switching to a non-conducting state. Although neither resting nor inactivated channels can conduct ions, these two states have an important difference. Resting channels can be activated by application of the appropriate stimulus. Inactivated channels are closed and cannot be activated by further application of the stimulus. For inactivated channels, the stimulus must be removed (clearance of ligand or hyperpolarization of the membrane potential) to allow channels to recover to the resting state from which they can subsequently be activated.

An active channel opens and shuts randomly until it finally inactivates. Although the state of the channel (open or shut) at any one instant is random, the average behaviour of the channel is well defined. For example, the open probability, $P_{open}$, can be computed from the amount of time the channel is conducting divided by the total recording duration. The duration of individual open events is random, but the distribution of these open durations is exponential and the reciprocal of this time constant defines the rate of leaving the open state.

Figure 1.1 shows hypothetical recordings of channel activity to illustrate the properties of permeation and gating. In this voltage-clamp experiment, the membrane potential is controlled with a feedback circuit and the current conducted by a single channel isolated in this patch is recorded (see Chapter 3 for details on the voltage-clamp technique). Each trial starts at $-100\ mV$ where the channel is in a closed resting state. In response to depolarization at time 0, the channel opens and current flows either outward (positive) or inward (negative), depending on whether $V_m$ is greater than or less than $E_{rev}$, respectively. In response to larger depolarizations, a larger current flows, due to effects on both gating and permeation. First, the channel activates more rapidly, as shown by the shorter latency to the first opening. Second, the steady-state open probability is higher as can be seen late in the trial. Third, $V_m$ is farther

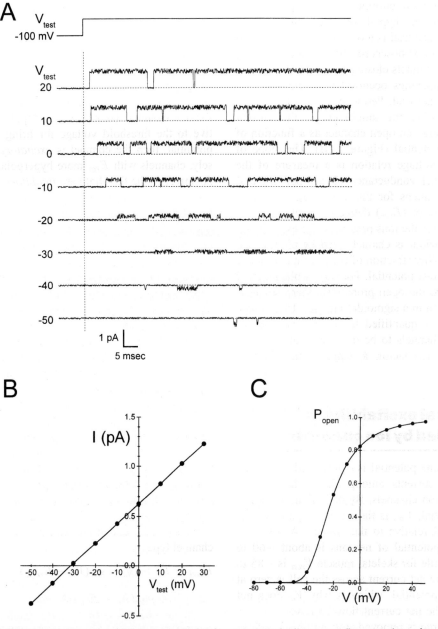

**Figure 1.1** Gating and permeation of single channels. (A) Simulated patch-clamp recordings are shown for a channel that activates upon membrane depolarization. Each trace shows current elicited in response to a voltage step from −100 mV to $V_{test}$. Trials are aligned with the onset of the voltage step (dotted vertical line). The channel is open during the pulse-like current fluctuations away from the zero-current baseline (dotted). With stronger depolarization (more positive $V_{test}$), the channel activates more quickly (latency to first opening is briefer) and the steady-state open probability is higher. (B) Permeability is quantified from the current amplitude measured while the channel is open. The current-voltage relation defines the reversal potential (−31.3 mV for this hypothetical $K^+$ channel with $[K^+]_{in} = 140$ mM and $[K^+]_{out} = 40$ mM) and the conductance (slope of 1pA/50 mV = 20 picosiemens). (C) The voltage dependence of gating is characterized by the steady-state open probability measured as a function of test potential.

from $E_{rev}$, so more current flows through an open channel. For this hypothetical $K^+$ channel, the duration of each trial is too short for the effects of inactivation to be observed. Inactivation would be manifest as channels closing to a state from which no further openings occurred throughout the remainder of that trial. Permeability can be quantified by plotting the amplitude of the current flowing through an open channel as a function of membrane potential (Figure 1.1B). The slope of the current voltage relation is a measure of the single channel conductance (2 pA per 100 mV, or 20 picoseimens for this example). The zero-current intercept ($E_{rev}$) defines the selectivity of the channel for the ions present in the experiment. Gating behaviour is characterized by plotting the open probability (fraction of time spent open) as a function of test potential. For most voltage-gated ion channels, the open probability increases with depolarization in a sigmoidal fashion. The voltage dependence is quantified by $V_{\frac{1}{2}}$, the voltage required for channels to be open 50% of the time, and a steepness factor, $k$, equal to the slope at $P_{open} = 0.5$.

## Electrical excitability is controlled by ion channels

The membrane potential is determined by the net balance of currents among all of the actively conducting ion channels. By definition, the membrane potential, $V_m$, is the electrical potential inside the cell relative to the outside. At rest, the membrane potential of neurons is about $-60$ to $-75$ mV, while for skeletal muscle $V_{rest}$ is $-85$ to $-95$ mV. The net current across the cell is zero at the resting potential, which is why $V_m$ does not change. If the net current flow becomes outward, positive charge is removed from the inside of the cell and the membrane potential will hyperpolarize. Conversely, when the net current flow is negative, the inside of the cell accumulates positive charge and the membrane potential will depolarize. The net current across the cell is simply the sum of the currents contributed by individual ion channels, and the direction of current flow through each type of channel is determined by the potential difference, $V_m - E_{rev}$. Recall, $E_{rev}$ is deter-

mined both by a channel's intrinsic selectivity properties and by the ionic composition of the intracellular and extracellular solutions (Eqn. 1.2).

The influence of an ion channel on the membrane potential can be viewed in terms of a weighted average. Current through a particular channel shifts the membrane potential toward $E_{rev}$ for that channel. Thus if $E_{rev}$ is depolarized relative to the threshold voltage for firing an action potential, then the channel is *excitatory*. Conversely, channels with $E_{rev}$ more hyperpolarized (i.e. negative) to the threshold are *inhibitory*. When all the channels in a cell are considered together, the membrane potential settles to a value equal to a weighted average of the reversal potentials. The relative weights depend on how much current flows through an open channel and how often it is open. Under physiological conditions, the current through most channels is proportional to the driving force, $V_m - E_{rev}$ (Figure 1.1B). The one notable exception is for Ca currents which are non-linear due to the huge concentration gradient for $Ca^{2+}$ of $\sim 1:10^7$ for inside:outside. For all other cases, the total current, I, through a particular type of channel is given by:

$$I = NP_{open}\gamma(V_m - E_{rev}) \qquad (1.4)$$

where $N$ is the number of channels in the cell, $P_{open}$ is the open probability (Figure 1.1C), $\gamma$ is the conductance for a single channel (slope in Figure 1.1B). Alternatively, the product $NP_{open}\gamma$ is often denoted as the macroscopic conductance, $g$. For a cell with $Na^+$ and $K^+$ channels, the total current is the sum of the currents through each channel type.

$$I_{total} = I_K + I_{Na} = g_K(V_m - E_{revK})$$
$$+ g_{Na}(V_m - E_{revNa}) \qquad (1.5)$$

Because $K^+$ channels are highly selective, their reversal potential, $E_{revK}$, equals the Nernst potential for $K^+$, $E_K$. The same approximation is true for $Na^+$ channels. The membrane potential, $V_m$, will shift until $I_{total} = 0$, at which point (1.5) can be rearranged as:

$$V_m = \frac{g_K}{g_K + g_{Na}}E_K + \frac{g_{Na}}{g_K + g_{Na}}E_{Na}. \qquad (1.6)$$

Equation (1.6) shows explicitly how $V_m$ can be

viewed as a weighted average of the reversal potentials for each type of channel, with the weight being a channel's conductance relative to the sum of all the conductances in the cell. The changes in $V_m$ during bioelectrical signalling are usually produced by changing the membrane conductance, $g$, for a particular ion, rather than altering its reversal potential (i.e. shifting the Nernst potential by changing the concentration gradient). The macroscopic conductance term, $g$, is often a function of voltage or agonist concentration and time. In the single-channel view of Eqn (1.4), these changes are embodied in the open probability. In a resting cell, $g_K$ dominates and $V_m$ is approximately equal to $E_K$. During the upstroke of the action potential, $g_{Na}$ becomes much larger than $g_K$, and so $V_m$ approaches $E_{Na}$. Inactivation of $Na^+$ channels and slow activation of $K^+$ channels cause $g_K$ to again be greater than $g_{Na}$ and the cell repolarizes toward $E_K$.

## Classes of ion channels

Historically, ion channels were named and categorized according to their electrophysiological and pharmacological properties. Thus, the voltage-gated $Na^+$ channel is activated by membrane depolarization and selectively conducts $Na^+$ ions. Subtypes were defined by further refinements in this scheme, for example, low-voltage activated (*t*hreshold) T-type $Ca^{2+}$ channels and high-voltage activated *l*ong-lasting L-type $Ca^{2+}$ channels. Once the first ion channel complementary DNAs were isolated by expression cloning, large families of related ion channel genes were identified by homology screens. Within each subclass, many more channel genes were cloned than had been identified by electrophysiological studies. Moreover, the genetic data revealed patterns of channel evolution and inter-relatedness among channels found to be functionally diverse. Although channel nomenclature is still debated, a general classification scheme, based on functional and genetic data, has emerged. In general, ion channels are still classified by the stimuli to which they respond: voltage-gated, ligand-gated, second-messenger gated, or specialized sensory (gated by stretch, osmolarity, heat, etc.).

Voltage-gated ion channels comprise a large diverse gene superfamily (Catterall, 1995). Most members of this family are steeply voltage dependent. For example $P_{open}$ typically increases 10-fold per $7-12$ mV of depolarization. The $Na^+$ and $K^+$ channels that generate action potentials in nerve and muscle are members of this class, as are the $Ca^{2+}$ channels in presynaptic terminals and in myocytes. In order to detect membrane potential, voltage-gated channel proteins must contain charged (basic or acidic) amino acid residues that reside within the transmembrane electric field. The amino acid sequences predicted by cDNAs coding for these channels each contain a cluster of four to eight positively-charged residues (lysine or arginine) at every third position in an otherwise hydrophobic segment that is predicted to form a membrane-spanning $\alpha$-helix (see Figure 1.2). This so-called S4 domain is the fourth of six predicted membrane-spanning segments that make up the primary subunit of $K^+$ channels or one of the internal homologous domains of $Na^+$ or $Ca^{2+}$ channels. Any channel with an S4 motif is classified as a member of the voltage-gated ion channel superfamily. Some S4-containing channels have very modest voltage dependence. For example, $Ca^{2+}$-activated $K^+$ channels open in response to internal $Ca^{2+}$ in the micromolar range, but have a much lower voltage sensitivity than other K channels. Cyclic nucleotide gated channels of the photoreceptors in the retina and of olfactory epithelium are potently modulated by intracellular cGMP and cAMP, respectively, but also contain S4 motifs and can be opened by depolarization. Both of these channel types probably evolved from a primordial voltage-gated $K^+$ channel. Not all voltage-gated ion channels contain an S4 motif. Several members of the Cl-C family of chloride selective anion channels are strongly voltage dependent and yet have no S4 motif.

Ligand-gated channels of fast chemical synapses contain the ligand-binding site and pore-forming channel within the same macromolecular structure. In these *ionotropic* channels, ligand binding to the receptor portion of the molecule is allosterically coupled to opening of the channel. The classical example is the nicotinic acetylcholine receptor in the post-synaptic membrane of the neuromuscular junction. Other members of this group include glutamate receptors (AMPA, kainate, and NMDA subtypes), a subtype of serotonin receptor ($5HT_3$), $\gamma$-aminobutyric acid receptors ($GABA_A$ type), and glycine receptors. Ligand-gated ion channels at excitatory synapses are cation-selective but do not discriminate between $Na^+$, $K^+$, or even $Ca^{2+}$, and so $E_{rev}$ is about 0 mV. In contrast, $GABA_A$ and glycine receptors at inhibitory synapses of the central nervous system are anion-selective and conduct predominantly $Cl^-$ ions.

Ligand-activated currents may also be regulated by *metabotropic* receptors. Ligand binding liberates an intermediary second messenger molecule which, in turn, modulates the activity of a separate pore-forming channel protein. Ligand binding to an extracellular domain of the receptor is coupled to activation of a heterotrimeric GTP-binding protein (G protein). Bound GDP is displaced by GTP and the G protein dissociates into $G_\alpha$ and $G_{\beta\gamma}$ subunits. The $G_\alpha$ or $G_{\beta\gamma}$ subunits may directly modulate the activity of an ion channel (Wickman and Clapham, 1995). In the heart for example, acetylcholine activates a muscarinic AChR which increases intracellular $G_{\beta\gamma}$ which in turn binds to a cytoplasmic domain on the $K_{Ach}$ channel and increases its open probability. The increased $K^+$ conductance hyperpolarizes the cell and slows the heart rate. G-protein coupled receptor signalling may also use an indirect pathway. The activated G-protein interacts with a membrane-associated enzyme (adenylate cyclase, phospholipase C, etc.) to generate cytoplasmic second messengers such as cAMP, $Ca^{2+}$ or $IP_3$. These second messenger molecules may directly activate an ion channel (e.g. $Ca^{2+}$-activated $K^+$ channel) or they may regulate additional enzymes that modulate channel activity, such as phosphorylation by protein kinase A. The G-protein coupled receptors constitute a large and diverse gene family which includes muscarinic ACh, $GABA_B$, metabotropic glutamatergic, aminergic (dopamine, histamine, norepinephrine, serotonin), and purineric (ATP, adenosine) receptors as well as receptors for neuroactive peptide modulators (enkephalin, somatostatin, substance P, etc.). The ion channels that mediate the responses for activated G-protein coupled receptors are classified as second messenger-gated or intracellular ligand-gated channels

and include: $Ca^{2+}$-activated $K^+$ or $Cl^-$ channels, cyclic-nucleotide gated non-selective cation channels, ATP-dependent $K^+$ channels, and $IP_3$-gated $Ca^{2+}$ release channels.

Finally, a diverse group of channels serve as specialized sensory transducers to detect membrane deformation, light, heat, odorants, salt, sweet, and sour. Mechanically-gated channels open within milliseconds, most likely due to direct coupling of mechanical force to the channel protein. Signalling in the visual, olfactory, and gustatory systems is much slower, with G-protein coupled cascade mechanisms used to amplify the sensitivity at the expense of speed.

# Channel architecture: structure–function relations

Over the past 15 years a combination of pharmacological, physiological and molecular genetic approaches has provided increasingly refined views of channel structure and function. The first conceptual models were based on electrophysiological approaches which defined the pore size and localized part of the inactivation gate machinery to the intracellular face of the channel. High-affinity ligands and toxins were used initially to map binding sites and then used as tools in the biochemical isolation of channel proteins from native tissues. Peptide digests and sequencing provided partial maps of a channel's primary amino acid structure. Full-length complementary DNAs coding for ion channels were then isolated using degenerate probes based on the peptide sequence or from expression cloning techniques. The primary amino acid sequences deduced from these cDNAs led to predictions of the channel topology in the membrane, consensus sites for glycosylation and phosphorylation, hydrophobic $\alpha$-helical segments likely to form membrane-spanning segments, and possible voltage-sensing elements. Much of the predicted structure has been supported by experimental data obtained from site-specific antibodies, alterations in glycosylation or phosphorylation pattern, and biochemical modification of the channel protein. The pore-region and some of the inactivation gates were mapped out by studying the functional consequences of site-directed mutations. Finally, the X-ray crystallographic structure of a 'minimalist' proto-$K^+$ channel from the bacterium *Streptomyces lividans* was resolved at 3.2 angstrom resolution (Doyle *et al.*, 1998). This landmark study showed how $K^+$ ions are passed single-file through a narrow selectivity filter. The KcsA channel has no voltage sensitivity and lacks many of the gating and regulatory behaviours found in eukaryotic channels. Consequently many fundamental structural questions remain. What is the detailed structure of the voltage sensor? Where are the gates and how do they move? How is movement of the voltage sensor or ligand binding allosterically coupled to channel opening?

Like most other proteins, ion channels are built from a concatenation of conserved structural motifs. This modular design of nature means that many structural and mechanistic features can be generalized across different channel types and that functional properties of channel behaviour can be attributed to specific domains within the channel protein. The prototypical structure of a voltage-gated ion channel is illustrated by the model for the *Shaker*-type $K^+$ channel in Figure 1.2. The channel is a tetramer of $\alpha$-subunits arranged symmetrically around a central ion-conducting pore. The $\alpha$-subunit is comprised of about 800 amino acids and has six hydrophobic stretches predicted to form membrane-crossing $\alpha$-helices (S1–S6). *Shaker* is the founding member of the six transmembrane (6TM) containing family of $K^+$ channels. The tetramerization domain (T) in the cytoplasmic amino-terminus determines the compatibility and assembly of $\alpha$-subunits into a homo- or heterotetramer. A 20-residue hydrophobic loop between the S5 and S6 segments forms the selectivity filter of the pore. This P-loop is highly conserved among all $K^+$-selective channels and contains the sequence [TS]-[MLQ]-T-T-[IV]-G-Y-G. This 'signature sequence' has been used to identify novel $K^+$ channel genes in genomic and expressed sequence tag databases. The S6 helix also contributes to the lining of the pore cavity.

Other regions of the channel protein are involved in gating. The S4 segment contains basic residues (arginine or lysine) at every third or fourth of its 26 amino acids. Mutational analyses

have demonstrated that these positively-charged residues contribute to the voltage sensitivity of channel gating. Moreover, the S4 segment has been shown to move outward in response to membrane depolarization (Yang *et al.*, 1996). These data convincingly establish the S4 segment as the sensor for voltage-dependent gating in $K^+$, $Na^+$, and $Ca^{2+}$ channels. The location of the activation gate and the mechanism by which movement of S4 controls the position of the gate remain to be elucidated. Recent data have implicated the 'bundle-crossing' of S6 segments at the cytoplasmic end of the pore as a likely candidate for the activation gate (Yellen, 1998). An inactivation gate has also been localized to the cytoplasmic face of the channel. *Shaker* $K^+$ channels inactivate within milliseconds after depolarization. Competition between inactivation and internal blocking agents, but not with impermeant external ones, demonstrated that the fast inactivation gate resides at the intracellular end of the pore. The fast inactivation gate or particle has been localized to the amino terminus, which is thought to occlude the open pore in a ball-and-chain like mechanism (Hoshi *et al.*, 1990).

Other classes of $K^+$-selective ion channels retain the conserved P-loop signature sequence, but have varying numbers of transmembrane segments (see Figure 1.2). The inwardly rectifying $K^+$ channels ($K_{IR}$) pass $K^+$ ions inward more readily than outward due to intracellular block of the pore by $Mg^{2+}$ or polyamines. $K_{IR}$ channels contain only two TM segments (homologous to S5 and S6) and are not gated by voltage. Another class of K channel contains four TM segments with P-loops between segments 1–2 and 3–4. These so-called two-pore $K^+$ channels probably assemble as dimers (a total of 4 P-loops) and form voltage-independent constitutively open 'leakage' channels that are thought to play a role in setting the resting potential.

Voltage-gated $Ca^{2+}$ and $Na^+$ channels are believed to have evolved from two duplications of a primordial 6TM $K^+$ channel. The resulting genes code for $Ca^{2+}$ or $Na^+$ channel $\alpha$ subunits with $2 \times 2 \times 6TM = 24TM$ segments. These proteins have four homologous internal repeats, termed domain I–IV, each of which has an S4 segment and P-loop (see Figure 1.2). The S4 segments

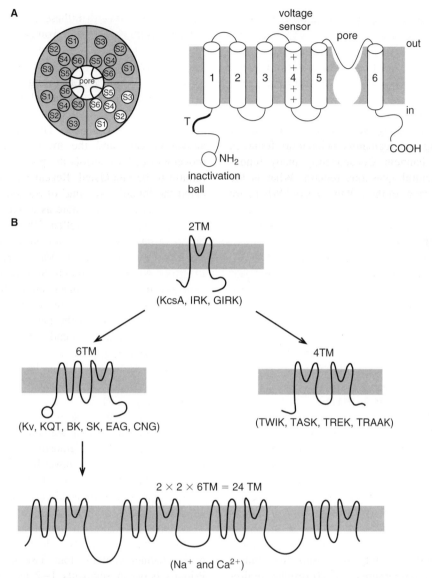

**Figure 1.2** Membrane topology of voltage-gated ion channels. (A) Top view looking down on the plane of the membrane (*left*) shows the four-fold symmetry of subunits (K$^+$ channels) or homologous repeats (Na$^+$ or Ca$^{2+}$ channels) about a central pore. Each subunit contains 6 transmembrane segments, shown opened into a linear membrane-folding diagram (*right*). The loop between S5 and S6 forms the pore and the voltage-sensor is denoted by the positive charges in S4. For K$^+$ channels, the cytoplasmic amino terminus acts as an 'inactivation ball' that plugs the pore in open channels, and the tetramerization domain (T) regulates which $\alpha$-subunits can assemble to form homo- or heteromeric channels. (B) Evolution of the voltage-gated ion channel superfamily is believed to have resulted from duplications of a primordial 2 transmembrane (TM) K$^+$ channel gene. The 2 TM group includes bacterial (KcsA) and inward rectifier K$^+$ channels (IRK, and G-protein coupled GIRK). A single duplication produced the 4TM group, with two pore-regions in each $\alpha$-subunit. These channels (TWIK, TASK, TREK, TRAAK) act as 'leakage' K$^+$-selective channels that are open at all membrane voltages and are thought to play a major role is setting the resting potential. Strong voltage-sensitivity first appears in the 6TM group, which includes voltage-gated (Kv, KQT, EAG), Ca$^{2+}$-activated (BK, SK), and cyclic-nucleotide gated (CNG) channels. CNG channels are non-selective cation channels while all other members of the 6TM group are highly K$^+$-selective. Two rounds of gene duplication gave rise to the 24TM group, which includes voltage-gated Na$^+$ and Ca$^{2+}$ channels. Each of the four internal repeats is homologous to a 6TM subunit of Kv channels, and a single $\alpha$-subunit is capable of forming a functional channel.

serve as voltage sensors for activation and the fast inactivation gate for $Na^+$ channels has been localized to the intracellular loop between domains III and IV (Stühmer *et al.*, 1989; West *et al.*, 1992). An inactivation gate has not yet been delineated for $Ca^{2+}$ channels.

In addition to the principal pore-forming $\alpha$-subunit, most if not all voltage-gated ion channels contain associated auxiliary subunits (Isom *et al.*, 1994). The auxiliary subunits may be transmembrane, intracellular, or even extracellular proteins that bind either non-covalently or by disulphide bonds to the $\alpha$-subunit. Auxiliary subunits are not capable of assembling into pore-forming channels, but when co-expressed with $\alpha$-subunits they modify the gating, expression level at the membrane, pharmacological properties and even the permeability of channels. Mutations in auxiliary subunits have been associated with neurological disorders in man, although less commonly than with $\alpha$-subunit mutations.

Ligand-gated channels of fast synapses also share many common structural features. Most are heteromeric complexes of five subunits arranged around a central pore. Each subunit contains four transmembrane segments (M1–M4). The amino and carboxy termini are extracellular, and the ligand binding site(s) is localized to the large amino terminus before the first transmembrane segment. The M2 segment plays a critical role in determining the permeability of the channel and is thought to form the pore. One notable exception to this topology is the ionotropic glutamate receptor. Both NMDA and AMPA receptors are tetrameric (Rosenmund *et al.*, 1998), and kainate receptors may be as well. The M2 segment in NMDA receptors makes a hairpin turn and therefore enters and leaves the membrane from the cytoplasmic side. Consequently the M3–M4 loop is extracellular and the carboxy terminus is intracellular.

## Functional defects in channelopathies

The functional consequences of disease-associated ion channel mutations have been identified for many disorders. In most cases, ion channel behaviour has been explored using heterologous expression systems, wherein the mutant channel cDNA is introduced into a fibroblast or mRNA is injected into a frog oocyte. Whole-cell and patch recordings enable investigators to characterize the permeation and gating properties of mutant channels at very high resolution. These techniques have led to the identification of several types of defects in channel function, some of which appear subtle but are known to cause dramatic alterations in cellular excitability (Cannon, 1997). The ability to compare mutant and wildtype channel behaviour with such precision, coupled with the known role(s) of most channels in setting electrical excitability, have given insights on the pathomechanism of the channelopathies that have not yet been attainable for most neurogenetic disorders. Moreover, the identification of specific alterations in mutant channel function provides a rational basis for the design of therapeutic interventions.

Many disease-associated mutations of ion channels cause gain-of-function defects. In other words, the mutation does not destroy the ability of the protein to form a channel in the membrane. Instead, the aberrant behaviour of mutant channels alters the electrical properties of the cell to produce a dominantly-expressed disease phenotype. For example, gating defects in the $\alpha$-subunit of the skeletal muscle $Na^+$ channel are a cause of periodic paralysis and myotonia (Figure 1.3). For over 20 identified mutations tested to date, inactivation is impaired (being either incomplete, too slow, or shifted to depolarized potentials) and for a subset of mutations activation is enhanced (less depolarization is required to fully open channels). Both gating defects result in a gain-of-function defect, more $Na^+$ current than occurs for wildtype channels. This aberrant inward current may generate bursts of repetitive discharges (myotonia) or may sufficiently depolarize the resting potential to produce flaccid electrically-inexcitable muscle by inactivation of $Na^+$ channels (Cannon, 1997). Gating defects in ligand-activated channels may also cause gain-of-function defects in neurological disorders. In the dominantly inherited slow-channel myasthenic syndromes, the post-synaptic responsiveness to acetylcholine release at the neuromuscular junction is increased. The increased response arises from mutations in the $\alpha$-, $\beta$-, $\delta$- or $\varepsilon$-subunits of the acetylcholine receptor that

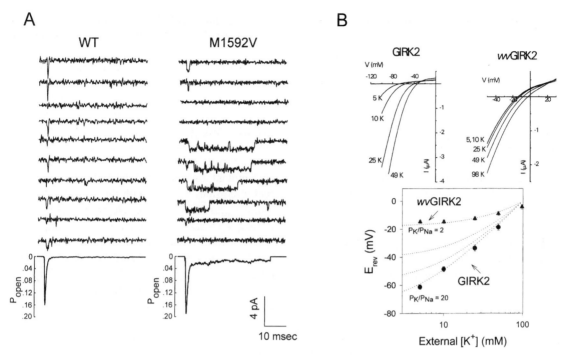

**Figure 1.3** Disease-associated mutations may alter channel gating or permeation. (A) Inactivation gating is disrupted by Na$^+$ channel mutations in hyperkalaemic periodic paralysis. Na$^+$ currents were recorded from cell-attached patches on cells transfected with wildtype or mutant (M1592V) cDNA. The latency to first opening (activation) and single-channel current amplitudes (permeation) are unchanged, but mutant channels have prolonged openings and reopenings due to impaired inactivation. (Adapted from Cannon and Strittmatter, 1993). (B) K$^+$-selectivity is impaired by the mouse *weaver* mutation (G156S) in the pore region of the G protein-coupled inwardly rectifying K$^+$ channel (GIRK2). E$_{rev}$ was determined by recording currents during slow voltage ramps in oocytes injected with GIRK2 or *wv*GIRK2 RNA (*top*). For mutant channels, E$_{rev}$ was more depolarized and much less sensitive to substituting extracellular Na$^+$ with K$^+$. The lower panel compares the observed variation in E$_{rev}$ with [K$^+$]$_0$ to values predicted by eqn (1.2) with P$_K$/P$_{Na}$ = 2, 5, 10, and 20. The relative K$^+$-selectivity is decreased approximately 10-fold by the *weaver* mutation. (Adapted from Kofuji *et al.*, 1996).

prolong the duration of individual channel openings (reduce the closing rate) or produce prolonged bursts of openings due to an increased affinity of the receptor for acetylcholine (Engel *et al.*, 1999). Gain-of-function defects may also arise from alterations in the permeability of mutant channels. The *weaver* mouse has ataxia, tremor and hyperactvitiy due to a failure of differentiation and migration of neurons into the granule cell layer of the cerebellum and the substantia nigra. The *weaver* phenotype is caused by a missense mutation (glycine to serine) in the pore-region of a G-protein coupled inwardly rectifying K$^+$ channel (GIRK2) (Patil *et al.*, 1995). Oocyte expression studies showed that the *weaver* mutant K$^+$ channel does not discriminate between monovalent cations (Figure 1.3). In addition, mu-

tant channels were constitutively open, without requiring the normal activation by G$_{\beta\gamma}$.

Loss-of-function changes may also occur with disease-associated mutations in ion channels. Missense mutations in KCNQ2 or KCNQ3 K$^+$ channel genes (both members of the voltage-gated 6TM family) cause benign familial neonatal convulsions. In oocyte studies, heteromeric co-expression of wildtype and mutant channels results in K$^+$ current amplitudes that are decreased by about 25% (Schroeder *et al.*, 1998). Apparently a loss of this magnitude is sufficient to enhance neuronal excitability enough to produce seizures. Mutations in a skeletal muscle Cl$^-$ channel, ClC-1, cause loss-of-function defects that may give rise to either dominant or recessive myotonia congenita. Heterologous expression studies have shown that most mutations associated with recessive inheritance result in truncated or non-functional proteins that are incapable of forming homomeric $Cl^-$ channels or of altering the behaviour of wildtype channels. Pharmacological studies in skeletal muscle have shown that a 50% reduction in $Cl^-$ conductance is not sufficient to cause myotonia, consistent with the molecular genetic data that heterozygotes carrying recessive mutations are asymptomatic. In contrast, $Cl^-$ channels containing mutations identified in dominant myotonia congenita do form functional channels, but a much larger depolarization is required for them to open (Pusch et al., 1995). Co-injection of wildtype and mutant RNA resulted in channels with a depolarized shift in the voltage dependence of opening. The interpretation is that wildtype and mutant subunits co-assemble to form channels that are reluctant to open. This dominant-negative effect reduces the $Cl^-$ conductance at the resting potential and thereby results in myotonia. Loss-of-function defects have also been identified for mutations in ligand-activated channels. A serine to phenylalanine mutation in the pore region (M2) of the $\alpha_4$ nicotinic acetylcholine receptor subunit causes autosomal dominant nocturnal frontal lobe epilepsy. This missense mutation reduces AChR function by altering both permeation and gating. In mutant channels, the single-channel conductance is reduced nearly two-fold, permeability to $Ca^{2+}$ is lost, desensitization occurs more rapidly and recovery from desensitization is prolonged (Kuryatov et al., 1997).

Elegant as they are, these electrophysiological studies are just the first step in elucidating the pathophysiology of these disorders. Channel behaviour is modulated by the cellular milieu, and it is likely that the functional consequences of a mutation will be different when the channel is expressed in its native tissue rather than a fibroblast or oocyte. In addition, these heterologous expression studies do not provide any information on transcriptional regulation, post-translational modification, subcellular localization, and endogenous modulation of channels. The cell biology of mutant channels, the link between disrupted cellular function to clinical phenotype, and the interplay between genetic predisposition and environmental influence on disease expression can best be explored in animal models. In recent years,

it has become feasible to produce genetically engineered mice with precisely introduced mutations on a large scale. These mice will undoubtedly provide an important tool in future studies of ion channelopathies.

# References

Aidley, D. J. (1998). The Physiology of Excitable Cells. Cambridge: Cambridge University Press.

Cannon, S. C. (1997). From mutation to myotonia in sodium channel disorders. Neuromusc Dis., 7, 241–249.

Cannon, S. C. and Strittmatter, S. M. (1993). Functional expression of sodium channel mutations identified in families with periodic paralysis. Neuron, 10, 317–26.

Catterall, W. A. (1995). Structure and function of voltage-gated ion channels. Ann Rev Biochem., 64, 493–531.

Doyle, D. A., Morais Cabral, J., Pfuetzner, R. A. et al. (1998). The structure of the potassium channel: molecular basis of $K^+$ conduction and selectivity. Science, 280, 69–77.

Engel, A. G., Ohno, K. and Sine, S. M. (1999). Congenital myasthenic syndromes: recent advances. Arch Neurol., 56, 163–7.

Hille, B. (1992) Ionic Channels of Excitable Membranes. Sunderland, MA: Sinauer.

Hoshi, T., Zagotta, W. N. and Aldrich, R. W. (1990). Biophysical and molecular mechanisms of Shaker potassium channel inactivation. Science, 250, 533–8.

Isom, L. L., De Jongh, K. S. and Catterall, W. A. (1994). Auxiliary subunits of voltage-gated ion channels. Neuron, 12, 1183–94.

Kofuji, P., Hofer, M., Millen, K. J. et al. (1996). Functional analysis of the weaver mutant GIRK2 K+ channel and rescue of weaver granule cells. Neuron, 16, 941–52.

Kuryatov, A., Gerzanich, V., Nelson, M., Olale, F. and Lindstrom, J. (1997). Mutation causing autosomal dominant nocturnal frontal lobe epilepsy alters $Ca^{2+}$ permeability, conductance, and gating of human alpha4beta2 nicotinic acetylcholine receptors. J Neurosci., 17, 9035–47.

Patil, N., Cox, D. R., Bhat, D., Faham, M., Myers, R. M. and Peterson, A. S. (1995). A potassium channel mutation in weaver mice implicates membrane excitability in granule cell differentiation. Nat Genet., 11, 126–9.

Pusch, M., Steinmeyer, K., Kock, M. C. and Jentsch, T. (1995). Mutations in dominant human myotonia congenita drastically alter the voltage dependence of the CLC-1 chloride channel. Neuron, 15, 1455–63.

Rosenmund, C., Stern-Bach, Y. and Stevens, C. F. (1998). The tetrameric structure of a glutamate receptor channel. Science, 280, 1596–9.

Schroeder, B. C., Kubisch, C., Stein, V. and Jentsch, T. J. (1998). Moderate loss of function of cyclic-AMP-modulated KCNQ2/KCNQ3 K+ channels causes epilepsy. *Nature, 396*, 687–90.

Sperelakis, N. (1998) *Cell Physiology Source Book.* London: Academic Press.

Stühmer, W., Conti, F., Suzuki, H. *et al.* (1989). Structural parts involved in activation and inactivation of the sodium channel. *Nature, 339*, 597–603.

West, J. W., Patton, D. E., Scheuer, T., Wang, Y., Goldin, A. L. and Catterall, W. A. (1992). A cluster of hydrophobic amino acid residues required for fast $Na^+$-channel inactivation. *Proc Natl Acad Sci USA, 89*, 10910–4.

Wickman, K. and Clapham, D. E. (1995). Ion channel regulation by G proteins. *Physiology Review, 75*, 865–85.

Yang, N., George, A. L., Jr and Horn, R. (1996). Molecular basis of charge movement in voltage-gated sodium channels. *Neuron, 16*, 113–22.

Yellen, G. (1998). The moving parts of voltage-gated ion channels. *Q Rev Biophys., 31*, 239–95.

# 2

# Molecular biology of ion channels

*Kylie A. Scoggan and Dennis E. Bulman*

## Introduction

Ion channels are regulated macromolecular pores in the cell membrane that allow particular ions to pass through. Ion movement can be regulated by having the channel in an open or closed state, while ion channels are controlled either by sensing changes in membrane potential or through the binding of ligands to channel proteins. The differing means of regulation have led to the classification of two large superfamilies of ion channels, the voltage-gated and the ligand- gated ion channels.

Biophysical methods were initially used to identify, distinguish and classify the properties of different ionic channels. The era of molecular genetics now dominates the field of ion channel biology through its approaches to determine the structure and the relatedness of the various ion channels. DNA sequencing has confirmed the biophysical findings that voltage-gated and ligand-gated ion channels comprise separate superfamilies of ion channels. In addition, DNA sequencing has revealed important information regarding amino acid sequence and structural similarities. Clearly, there are homologous channel proteins that would have evolved by processes of successive gene duplication, mutation, and selection from common ancestral channels. Molecular biological approaches have also revealed that the size of these superfamilies was strikingly underestimated. Surprisingly, there are many more genes and molecular subtypes of ionic channels than physiological and pharmacological experiments had previously suggested. This review will focus on the superfamily of voltage-gated ion channels. The structure of ligand-gated channels is mentioned in Chapters 1 and 13.

The voltage-gated $K^+$, $Na^+$ and $Ca^{2+}$ channels are part of a superfamily of evolutionarily related proteins, which share a fundamental design consisting of a set of six potentially membrane spanning segments (S1–S6) (Figure 2.1). These six segments comprise a domain which is repeated four times within the $\alpha_1$ subunit of the $Na^+$ and $Ca^{2+}$ channels, but is present only once in the $K^+$ channels. The region between S5 and S6 constitutes the P-loop which, when combined with the P-loops from the other domains, forms the pore of the channel. Containing basic residues at every third or fourth position, the S4 is suspected to function as the voltage sensor (Hille, 1991; Jan and Jan, 1994).

The amino acid sequence of individual channels is highly conserved across species, particularly S4 which demonstrates amino acid sequence conservation between humans and *Drosophila*. Such conserved regions are also observed between the different classes of voltage-gated ion channels. Overall, the high degree of amino acid sequence conservation has been interpreted as evidence of strong selective pressure on these channels. Such pressure could be due to the stringent criteria on these channels to maintain their structural conformation, ion selectivity, and gating abilities.

## $K^+$ channels

The family of $K^+$ channels can be divided into three main groups. The six transmembrane domain (TMD) family, which includes the voltage-gated and the $Ca^{2+}$-activated $K^+$ channels, the four TMD 'leak' $K^+$ channels and the two TMD inward rectifier $K^+$ channels. Based on amino acid

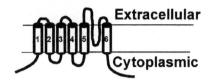

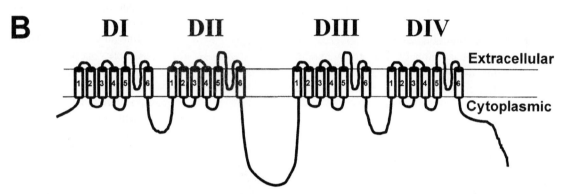

**Figure 2.1** (A) Schematic of the $\alpha$-subunit of a potassium channel. The six membrane spanning regions are numbered (S1–S6). The region between S5 and S6 is thought to line the pore of the channel. (B) Schematic of the $\alpha$-subunit of the voltage-gated sodium and calcium channel. The six transmembrane segments, corresponding to that of the $\alpha$-subunit of a potassium channel, comprise a single domain (DI–DIV). Within each domain the S4 represents the voltage sensor.

sequence similarities, the six TMD family has been subdivided into five subfamilies; eag, KQT, SK, slo and Kv. Crystallization and high-resolution structural analysis of a K$^+$ channel, the first natural membrane channel for which high-resolution real structural information is now available, revealed strong evidence of a tetrameric K$^+$ channel structure. Four independent $\alpha$-subunits form the infrastructure of a channel with a fourfold symmetry around a central pore. These $\alpha$-subunits consist of a single cluster of six transmembrane spanning segments with an analogous S4 segment which contains a series of positively charged amino acids every three residues and a P-loop between S5 and S6.

Biochemically purified Kv channels represent hetero-oligomers that contain Kv$\alpha$- and Kv$\beta$-subunits in a 1:1 ratio. Kv$\beta$-subunit sequences are consistent with the view that the $\beta$-subunit does not span the plasma membrane as suggested by hydropathy plots. In addition, glycosylated residues at potential N-glycosylation sites are absent, supported by the lack of evidence for attached carbohydrates on the native protein. Kv$\beta$-subunits are peripheral proteins that associate with a cytoplasmic domain of Kv$\alpha$-subunits (Pongs et al., 1999). Currently, three genes code for $\beta$-subunits and all three genes are known to undergo alternative splicing. A role for the $\beta$-subunits was proposed when it was demonstrated that in heterologous expression systems the $\beta$-subunits were shown to alter channel kinetics. A second role for the $\beta$-subunits is to act as chaperones during channel biosynthesis (Shi et al., 1996; Nagaya and Papazian, 1997). Structure–function analysis of Kv$\alpha$/Kv$\beta$-heteromultimers in heterologous expression systems have indicated a complex set of domains regulating the biochemical and functional interaction of Kv$\alpha$- and Kv$\beta$-subunits (Pongs *et al.*, 1999). It has been recently demonstrated that Kv$\beta$3 and KchAP appear to interact with Kv2 and enhance current levels without affecting channel kinetics or gating (Wible *et al.*, 1998).

There are more than 50 genes that encode for the principal subunit of mammalian K$^+$ channels. Many of these genes are subject to alternative splicing, which can result in multiple isoforms. Given that a functional channel can be a homo- or heteromultimeric unit, the number of possible functional channels is staggering. Currently, we have little understanding of the physiological significance of the enormous molecular diversity of K$^+$ channel protein subunits and their overall impact on the development and maintenance of life from the perspective of a single cell to the global perspective of the entire organism.

## Na$^+$ channels

Sodium and calcium channels are structurally similar. The major peptide of each channel contains a repeating motif, which is comprised of six predicted transmembrane regions with a distinguishable S4 segment. The hydrophilic loop between S5 and S6 is the pore-forming unit. These loops combine to form the pore through which ions pass. Since the hydropathy plots of the predicted $\alpha$-subunits do not start with a hydrophobic segment, there is no leading signal sequence and the NH$_2$-terminus of the chain would remain in the cytoplasm.

Sodium channels play a critical role in the initiation and generation of action potentials. The main functional unit of a sodium channel is the $\alpha$-subunit, which contains four repeated domains, designated D1 to D4. Each domain consists of approximately 300 to 400 amino acids with about 50% amino acid sequence similarity between each domain. A domain contains six membrane spanning $\alpha$-helical segments, S1 through S6, and together they contribute elements to form the structure surrounding the pore through which ions pass. The pore has selective permeability allowing a restricted class of small ions to flow passively down the electrochemical activity gradient of the

pore at a rate in excess of 10$^6$ ions per second (Hille, 1991). The channel is designed to open and close in response to an electrical potential change in the cell membrane ('voltage-gating') and the S4 segment of each domain probably acts as the voltage sensor for opening the gate. The pore of the channel is lined by the invagination into the plasma membrane of amino acids that join the S5 and S6 segments on the outer surface of the membrane (Stevens, 1991; Yellen *et al.*, 1991). The S4 segment is hydrophobic with every third amino acid being a positively charged lysine or arginine and opposing negative charges on the other transmembrane segments presumably balance the positively charged residues. Although our knowledge is still incomplete, occlusion of the voltage-gated sodium channel probably occurs on the inner membrane surface through folding of the cytoplasmic loop between the third and fourth domain into the pore, referred to as a 'hinged-lid' (Hille, 1991; Catterall, 1993). By contrast, the voltage-gated potassium channel is probably blocked by a 'ball and chain'-like structure tethered to the inner surface of the membrane at the amino end of the domain (Trimmer *et al.*, 1989; Miller, 1991).

Many mammalian sodium channel $\alpha$-subunits are associated with $\beta$-subunits. The skeletal muscle sodium channel is composed of an $\alpha$- and $\beta_1$-subunit, whereas the central nervous system sodium channel is composed of an $\alpha$-, $\beta_1$- and $\beta_2$-subunit. While the genes encoding the $\beta_1$- and $\beta_2$-subunits do not demonstrate a significant amino acid similarity score, both subunits contain a single transmembrane domain. Interestingly, the $\beta_2$ is covalently attached to the $\alpha$-subunit.

The family of mammalian sodium channel genes can be classified into three subgroups. The type 1 subgroup includes SCN1A, SCN2A, SCN3A, SCN4A, SCN5A, SCN8A, SCN9A and SCN10A and they share significant sequence similarity with each other (Goldin, 1999). The type 2 channels, which share approximately 50% sequence similarity with the type 1 channels, demonstrate sequence differences in regions responsible for channel function (George *et al.*, 1992). Members of this family include SCN6A and Na 2.3, the latter of which was identified in mouse (Felipe *et al.*, 1994). The third subgroup is composed of a single member, NaN which shows 50% sequence similarity to both the type 1 and type 2 sodium channel subgroups (Dib-Hajj *et al.*, 1998).

# Ca$^{2+}$ channels

Voltage-gated calcium channels regulate a number of biological functions, including the generation of action potentials in dendrites, allowing calcium entry into the cell thereby initiating neurotransmitter release and other intracellular regulatory processes. These channels play a pivotal role in the control of neuronal firing (Westenbroek *et al.*, 1992). Calcium channel types differ with respect to their voltage dependence, inactivation rate, ionic selectivity and pharmacology. The kinetics and the voltage dependence of inactivation define the specific channel subtype as L, N, P/Q, R or T. Each channel is composed of five subunits $\alpha_1$, $\alpha_2$, $\beta$, $\gamma$ and $\delta$, which are present stoichiometrically in a 1:1:1:1:1 ratio. Channel diversity is achieved in a number of ways. There are at least eight genes that encode for mammalian $\alpha_1$-subunits, while the $\beta$-subunits are encoded by one of four genes and the $\gamma$-subunit is encoded by one of two genes. The genes for $\alpha_{1C,D}$ or $\alpha_s$ can all form the 1,4-dihydropyridine sensitive L-type calcium channel, while $\alpha_{1B}$ (Fujita *et al.*, 1993), $\alpha_{1A}$ (Sather *et al.*, 1993; Gillard *et al.*, 1997) form the N and P/Q channels respectively. It appears that $\alpha_{1E}$, may code for the R-type channel (Randall and Tsien, 1995) which is a subtype of the low voltage-activated T-channel (Soong *et al.*, 1993). In 1998, two novel $\alpha_1$-subunits were identified. The gene encoding $\alpha_{1G}$ produces a product which represents a rapidly inactivating T-type channel (Perez-Reyes *et al.*, 1998) and the $\alpha_{1H}$ which represents another low voltage-activated T-channel (Cribbs *et al.*, 1998). Additional functional diversity has been achieved among the $\alpha_1$-subunits through extensive alternative splicing (Snutch *et al.*, 1991; Rettig *et al.*, 1996).

The $\alpha_2$-subunit, which is located extracellularly, is disulphide-linked to the $\delta$-subunit which itself is anchored into the membrane. There are at least five alternative splice variants of $\alpha_2$ which demonstrate a tissue specific distribution (Williams *et al.*, 1992). Co-expression studies of the $\alpha_2/\delta$ and the $\beta$-subunits show alterations in the voltage dependence of activation and inactivation and enhanced currents in *Xenopus* oocytes (Singer *et al.*, 1991). Recently it has been shown that the $\delta$-subunit is involved in the gating properties of the $\alpha_1$, while the $\alpha_2$ is related to the number of channels in the membrane (Felix *et al.*, 1997). Other than the $\alpha_{1S}$ and neuronal $\alpha_{1C}$ in which the co-expression of $\beta$-subunits had no effect on whole-cell currents (Tomlinson *et al.*, 1993), the $\beta$-subunits have major effects on every other $\alpha_1$ tested to date. The co-expression of the various $\beta$-subunits shows that these subunits can alter activation properties, steady state inactivation, inactivation kinetics, and peak current (Moreno, 1999). It has been recently proposed that $\beta$-subunits modify the interaction between calcium channel antagonists and the $\alpha_1$-subunit (Moreno, 1999).

The complex ramifications of mutations in any one subunit have not been fully appreciated, as the eight $\alpha_1$- and four $\beta$-subunits may form different combinations (Williams *et al.*, 1994; Tanaka *et al.*, 1995). The diversity of the channels is also enhanced by alternative splicing which can occur in all of the subunits.

# Origin of ion channels

Hille (1991) proposed that K$^+$ and Ca$^{2+}$ channel genes may have evolved from a common cation channel gene. The Na$^+$ channel gene probably evolved subsequently, via a gene duplication event, from the Ca$^{2+}$ channel gene. In support of this hypothesis is the observation that Ca$^{2+}$ channels and various K$^+$ channels appear to be prominent at an earlier stage of evolution than Na$^+$ channels (Hille, 1991). A common evolutionary pathway for the voltage-dependent ion channels is supported by amino acid sequence similarities among the family members. The extent of amino acid sequence conservation for both the sodium and calcium channel $\alpha$-subunits are shown in Figure 2.2. Clearly, the rate of evolutionary change among the family of ion channel genes has been at the slow end of the spectrum of observed rates of change (Hille, 1991).

A.

| | | | |
|---|---|---|---|
| Human Skeletal Muscle | VQGLSVLRSF | RLLRVFKLAK | SWPTLNML |
| Human Cardiac Muscle | msnLSVLRSF | RLLRVFKLAK | SWPTLNTL |
| Rat Skm Mus | VQGLSVLRSF | RLLRVFKLAK | SWPTLNML |
| Rat Brain I | VeGLSVLRSF | RLLRVFKLAK | SWPTLNML |
| Rat Brain II | VeGLSVLRSF | RLLRVFKLAK | SWPTLNML |
| Rat Brain III | VeGLSVLRSF | RLLRVFKLAK | SWPTLNML |
| E.electricus | mQGmSVLRSl | RLLRiFKLAK | SWPTLNiL |
| D.melanogaster | VQGLSVLRSF | RLLRVFKLAK | SWPTLNlL |

B.

| | | | |
|---|---|---|---|
| Human Skeletal Muscle | PLGISVLRCI | RLLRIFKITK | YWTSLSNL |
| Human Cardiac Muscle | PLGISVLRCv | RLLRIFKITr | YWnSLSNL |
| Rabbit Skeletal Muscle | PLGISVLRCI | RLLRLFKITK | YWTSLSNL |
| Mouse Skeletal Muscle | PLGISVLRCI | RLLRLFKITK | YWTSLSNL |
| Rabbit Cardiac Muscle | PLGISVLRCv | RLLRIFKITr | YWnSLSNL |
| Rat Brain | PLGISVLRCv | RLLRIFKITr | YWNSLSNL |

**Figure 2.2** Alignment of sodium channel (A) and DHP-sensitive calcium channel (B) amino acid sequences from various species. Highly conserved residues are represented by capital letters; non-conserved amino acids by lower case letters. Conservation of amino acid sequence is also observed between the sodium and calcium channels.

As stated previously, the voltage-gated $Na^+$ and $Ca^{2+}$ channels have four internal repeats, formed either by two rounds of duplication or by repeated duplication events of a single unit. Analysis of amino acid sequence changes suggests that the former mechanism occurred, as repeat I is most similar to repeat III while repeat II is most similar to repeat IV (Hille, 1991). Overall, the amino acid sequence of the voltage-gated $Ca^{2+}$ and $Na^+$ channels shows 29% amino acid identity (Tanabe et al., 1987). Following the formation of the four repeats, or domains, a third duplication event can be traced along the structural repeats of the $Na^+$ and $Ca^{2+}$ channels which represent the separation of these channel types and the expansion of the voltage-gated ion channel family. The establish-

ment of the mammalian sodium channel gene families probably occurred via another series of large DNA duplication events, which encompassed a number of genes, including members of the HOX gene family. This cluster of genes, which includes the sodium $\alpha$-subunit genes, maps to four chromosomal regions, 2q22, 3p21, 12q12 and 17q12. The conservation of intron–exon borders among the sodium $\alpha$-subunit genes has essentially been maintained with respect to the highly conserved transmembrane regions, however, substantial divergence has occurred with respect to the intron–exon structure among the large intracytoplasmic linkers (Spafford et al., 1998). Such divergence, however, is not indicative of the degree of amino acid sequence conservation which is extremely high when comparing humans and mice (Plummer *et al.*, 1998). Additional selective pressure has been applied to some channels through the development of resistance to various venoms. For more detail, the reader is encouraged to read an excellent review dealing with the evolution and diversity of mammalian sodium channel genes (Plummer and Meisler, 1999).

Molecular biology approaches have revealed a surprisingly large gene family as there are many more genes and molecular subtypes of ionic channels than were originally inferred by previous biophysical investigations. There are also important structural similarities between ion channels. The voltage-gated ion channel superfamily, which includes $Na^+$, $Ca^{2+}$, and $K^+$ channels, are all similar channel proteins. The repetitive units seem to group together to form the main part of the channel in which the ions pass through the cell membrane. The strict requirement for specific amino acid residues at given positions is strongly supported by the fact that amino acid substitutions can result in disease phenotypes (Bulman, 1997). Understanding the extensive diversity of these channels and the individual roles played by these isoforms will be key to our understanding of the complex neural network.

# References

Bulman, D. E. (1997). Phenotype variation and newcomers in ion channel disorders. *Hum Mol Genet.*, **6**, 1679–85.

Catterall, W. A. (1993). Structure and modulation of Na+ and $Ca^{2+}$ channels. *Ann N Y Acad Sci.*, **707**, 1–19.

Cribbs, L. L., Lee, K. H., Yang, J. *et al.* (1998). Cloning and characterization of alpha 1H from human heart, a member of the T-type $Ca^{2+}$ channel gene family. *Circ Res.*, **83**, 103–9.

Dib-Hajj, S. D., Tyrell, L., Black, J. A. and Waxman, S. G. (1998). NaN, a novel voltage-gated Na channel, is expressed preferentially in peripheral sensory neurons and down-regulated after axotomy. *Proc Natl Acad Sci USA*, **95**, 8963–8.

Felipe, A., Knittle, T. J., Doyle, K. L. and Tamkun, M. M. (1994). Primary structure and differential expression during development and pregnancy of a novel voltage-gated sodium channel in the mouse. *J Biol Chem.*, **269**, 30125–31.

Felix, R., Gurnett, C. A., De Waard, M. and Campbell, K. P. (1997). Dissection of functional domains of the voltage-dependent $Ca^{2+}$ channel alpha2delta subunit. *J Neurosci.*, **17**, 6884–91.

Fujita, Y., Mynlieff, M., Dirksen, R. T. *et al.* (1993). Primary structure and functional expression of the omega-conotoxin-sensitive N-type calcium channel from rabbit brain. *Neuron*, **10**, 585–98.

George, A. L. J., Knittle, T. J. and Tamkun, M. M. (1992). Molecular cloning of an atypical voltage-gated sodium channel expressed in human heart and uterus: evidence for a distinct gene family. *Proc Natl Acad Sci USA*, **89**, 4893–7.

Gillard, S. E., Volsen, S. G., Smith, W., Beattie, R. E., Bleakman, D. and Lodge, D. (1997). Identification of pore-forming subunit of P-type calcium channel: an antisense study on rat cerebellar Purkinje cells in culture. *Neuropharmacology*, **36**, 405–9.

Goldin, A.L. (1999). Diversity of mammalian voltage-gated sodium channels. *Ann N Y Acad Sci.*, **868**, 38–50.

Hille, B. (1991). *Ionic Channels of Excitable Membranes*. Sunderland, MA: Sinauer.

Jan, L. Y. and Jan, Y. N. (1994). Potassium channels and their evolving gates. *Nature*, **371**, 19–22.

Miller, C. (1991) 1990: Annus mirabilis of potassium channels. *Science*, **252**, 1092–6.

Moreno, D. (1999). Molecular and functional diversity of voltage-gated calcium channels. *Ann NY Acad Sci*, **868**, 102–17.

Nagaya, N. and Papazian, D. M. (1997). Potassium channel alpha and beta subunits assemble in the endoplasmic reticulum. *J Biol Chem.*, **272**, 3022–7.

Perez-Reyes, E., Cribbs, L. L., Daud, A. *et al.* (1998). Molecular characterization of a neuronal low-voltage-activated T-type calcium channel. *Nature*, **391**, 896–900.

Plummer, N. W. and Meisler, M. H. (1999). Evolution and diversity of mammalian sodium channel genes. *Genomics*, **57**, 323–31.

Plummer, N. W., Galt, J., Jones, J. M. *et al.* (1998). Exon organization, coding sequence, physical mapping and polymorphic intragenic markers for the human neuronal sodium channel gene SCN8A. *Genomics*, **54**, 287–96.

Pongs, O., Leicher, T., Berger, M. *et al.* (1999). Functional and molecular aspects of voltage-gated $K^+$ channel beta subunits. *Ann N Y Acad Sci.*, **868**, 344–55.

Randall, A. and Tsien, R. W. (1995). Pharmacological dissection of multiple types of $Ca^{2+}$ channel currents in rat cerebellar granule neurons. *J Neurosci.*, **15**, 2995–3012.

Rettig, J., Sheng, Z. H., Kim, D. K. *et al.* (1996). Isoform-specific interaction of the alpha 1A subunits of brain $Ca^{2+}$ channels with the presynaptic proteins syntaxin and SNAP-25. *Proc Natl Acad Sci USA*, **93**, 7363–8.

Sather, W. A., Tanabe, T., Zhang, J. F., Mori, Y., Adams, M. E. and Tsien, R. W. (1993). Distinctive biophysical and pharmacological properties of class A (BI) calcium channel alpha 1 subunits. *Neuron*, **11**, 291–303.

Shi, G., Nakahira, K., Hammond, S. *et al.* (1996). Beta subunits promote K$^+$ channel surface expression through effects early in biosynthesis. *Neuron*, **16**, 843–52.

Singer, D., Biel, M., Lotan, I. e*t al.* (1991). The role of the subunits in the function of the calcium channel. *Science*, **253**, 1553–7.

Snutch, T. P., Tomlinson, W. J., Leonard, J. P. and Gilbert, M. M. (1991). Distinct calcium channels are generated by alternative splicing and are differentially expressed in the mammalian CNS. *Neuron*, **7**, 45–57.

Soong, T. W., Stea, A., Hodson, C. D., Dubel, S. J., Vincent, S. R. and Snutch, T. P. (1993). Structure and functional expression of a member of the low voltage-activated calcium channel family. *Science*, **260**, 1133–6.

Spafford, J. D., Spencer, A. N. and Gallin, W. J. (1998). A putative voltage-gated sodium channel alpha subunit (PpSCN1) from the hydrozoan jellyfish, Polyorchis penicillatus: structural comparisons and evolutionary considerations. *Biochem Biophys Res Commun*, **244**, 772–80.

Stevens, C. F. (1991) Ion channels. Making a submicroscopic hole in one. *Nature*, **349**, 657–8.

Tanabe, T., Takeshima, H., Mikami, A. *et al.* (1987). Primary structure of the receptor for calcium channel blockers from skeletal muscle. *Naure*, **328**, 313–8.

Tanaka, O., Sakagami, H. and Kondo, H. (1995). Localization of mRNAs of voltage-dependent Ca(2+)-channels: four subtypes of alpha 1- and beta-subunits in developing and mature rat brain. *Brain Res Mol Brain Res*, **30**, 1–16.

Tomlinson, W. J., Stea, A., Bourinet, E. *et al.* (1993). Functional properties of a neuronal class C L-type calcium channel. *Neuropharmacology*, **32**, 1117–26.

Trimmer, J. S., Cooperman, S. S., Tomiko, S. A. *et al.* (1989). Primary structure and functional expression of a mammalian skeletal muscle sodium channel. *Neuron*, **3**, 33–49.

Westenbroek, R. E., Hell, J. W., Warner, C., Dubel, S. J., Snutch, T. P. and Catterall, W. A. (1992). Biochemical properties and subcellular distribution of an N-type calcium channel alpha 1 subunit. *Neuron*, **9**, 1099–115.

Wible, B. A., Yang, Q., Kuryshev, Y. A., Accili, E. A. and Brown, A. M. (1998). Cloning and expression of a novel K$^+$ channel regulatory protein, KChAP. *J Biol Chem.*, **273**, 11745–51.

Williams, M. E., Feldman, D. H., McCue, A. F. *et al.* (1992). Structure and functional expression of alpha 1, alpha 2 and beta subunits of a novel human neuronal calcium channel subtype. *Neuron*, **8**, 71–84.

Williams, M. E., Marubio, L. M., Deal, C. R. *et al.* (1994). Structure and functional characterization of neuronal alpha 1E calcium channel subtypes. *J Biol Chem*, **269**, 22347–57.

Yellen, G., Jurman, M. E., Abramson, T. and MacKinnon, R. (1991). Mutations affecting internal TEA blockade identify the probable pore-forming region of a K$^+$ channel. *Science*, **251**, 939–42.

# Pharmacology of ion channels

*Jeffrey R. Balser and Alfred L. George, Jr*

## Introduction

Ion channels are ubiquitous proteins that confer selective ionic permeability to the plasmalemma and to the membranes of intracellular compartments. They are critical participants in many diverse physiological processes including membrane excitability, synaptic transmission, signal transduction, cell volume regulation and ion transport. Virtually every living cell in every known species from the most primitive bacteria to humans utilizes ion channels to maintain electrochemical gradients, to generate cellular electricity, and to adapt to their environments. Ion channels also participate in a wide range of pathophysiological processes as illustrated by many of the chapters in this book. Finally, ion channels are important targets for an enormous variety of pharmacological agents and natural toxins.

This chapter on the pharmacology of ion channels will begin by presenting an overview on the classification of these proteins and general concepts about their structure and function. Next, fundamental mechanisms of ion channel modulation by drugs will be described with a particular focus on the mechanisms of ion channel block of voltage-gated Na and K channels. Finally, the chapter will provide more detailed descriptions on specific ion channels that are especially relevant to channelopathies of the nervous system.

## Classification and structure of ion channels

Ion channels may be broadly classified as either voltage-gated, ligand-gated, mechanosensitive,

and non-gated. This is not an entirely clean classification scheme, although it provides a convenient framework from which to discuss a broad topic such as pharmacology. Voltage-gated ion channels are opened and closed by abrupt changes in membrane potential. Most voltage-gated ion channels belong to a gene superfamily whose basic protein structure contains a positively charged transmembrane spanning segment known as an S4 helix that serves as a voltage-sensor. Notable exceptions to membership in the S4 family include inwardly rectifying potassium channels and Cl channels. Ligand-gated ion channels, such as neurotransmitter receptors, require binding of a specific molecule to open an ionic pore. Some ion channels are neither voltage nor ligand-gated. For example, the family of epithelial sodium channels, including various brain homologues, conduct ions with high probability and are rarely closed. Other ion channels with less well-defined structural characteristics are gated by mechanical forces that deform cell membranes. This chapter will primarily address the pharmacology of the voltage-gated ion channels.

The distinction between voltage-gated and ligand-gated ion channels can also be based on structural dissimilarities. The aforementioned S4 superfamily of voltage-gated cation channels is built from a common structural motif comprised of six transmembrane spanning segments (TM) and a single pore-forming loop (Figure 3.1). A single unit is represented by most voltage-gated potassium channels and the cyclic nucleotide-gated channels. This basic structural unit must be present in fourfold symmetry in order to form functional ion channels. This fourfold symmetry is achieved in potassium channels by the assembly

## Voltage-Gated Cation Channels

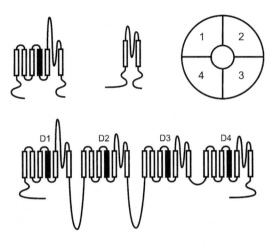

## Ligand-Gated Ion Channels

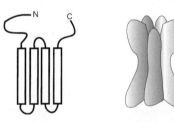

**Figure 3.1** General structural features of voltage-gated and ligand-gated ion channels. Representative transmembrane topology models are illustrated for voltage-gated K channels (6 TM and 2 TM families) and voltage-gated Na and Ca channels (24 TM). The S4 voltage-sensor is represented as a filled TM segment. Transmembrane topology for an acetylcholine receptor subunit and pentameric receptor complex are illustrated as representative ligand-gated ion channels.

of tetrameric complexes of four like subunits each consisting of one functional unit. A fourfold structure can also be achieved as in voltage-gated sodium and calcium channels by the incorporation of four repeat units into a single polypeptide chain. A fourfold symmetrical arrangement of calcium-release channel subunits and calcium-activated chloride channels is also known to occur. Ligand-gated neurotransmitter receptor ion channels are most commonly constructed as pentamers of a family of four TM proteins that assemble to

form a central ion pore. Exceptions to these two structural generalizations include the two TM domain channels: the inwardly rectifying potassium channels, P2X purinergic receptor family, and epithelial sodium channels. A twofold symmetrical quaternary structure has been postulated for ClC-type chloride channels that exhibit primary amino acid sequences unlike any of the other ion channel families.

The structural and functional diversity of ion channels provides many targets for pharmacological agents. Table 3.1 provides an overview of the classification and pharmacology of ion channels. This table lists three categories of pharmacological agents that interact with ion channels. Activators and agonists increase the activity of an ion channel either by substituting for its natural activating ligand or through other less direct mechanisms. Pore blockers are agents that impede the flow of the permeant ion through the channel, either by directly binding to residues within the pore region or through other mechanisms. Antagonists are typically molecules that compete with binding of the natural ligand, although in some cases binding may be non-competitive or uncompetitive. Finally, agents that modulate the function of ion channels without direct block of the ion pore or direct interference with binding of the natural ligand are referred to as allosteric modulators. Although not comprehensive, Table 3.1 attempts to present representative classes of compounds that interact with a diverse array of ion channels.

## General aspects of ion channel pharmacology

Ion channels are dynamic molecules that rapidly change their structural conformation in response to transmembrane electrical fields or bound ligands. In fact, the most unique feature of ion channel pharmacology is the striking sensitivity of the drug-receptor interaction to the 'motion' of the channel protein. Hence, advances in ion channel molecular pharmacology will require improved static information from crystallography and high-resolution spectroscopy, as well as complementary

**Table 3.1 Classification and pharmacology of ion channels**

| Ion channel family | Permeant ion(s) | Activators/agonists | Pore blockers/antagonists | Allosteric modulators |
|---|---|---|---|---|
| *Voltage-gated Na⁺ channels* | $Na^+$ | | Local anaesthetics Tetrodotoxin, saxitoxin, $\mu$-conotoxin | Local anaesthetics, batrachotoxin, scorpion toxins, veratridine |
| *Voltage-gated K⁺ channels* | | | | |
| $K_v$ channels | $K^+$ | | TEA, 4-aminopyridine, charybdotoxin, dendrotoxin, correolide ($K_v1.x$), methanesulfonilimides (HERG), chromanol 293B (KCNQ1) | |
| $K_{ir}$ channels | $K^+$ | | TEA, $Mg^{2+}$ | |
| $K_{ATP}$ channels | $K^+$ | pinacidil, cromakalim, diazoxide | sulphonylureas | |
| $K_{Ca}$ channels | $K^+$ | dehydrosoyasaponin | Apamin (SK), TEA (BK), charybdotoxin (BK), iberiotoxin (BK), clotrimazole (IK) | |
| *Voltage-gated Ca²⁺ channels* | | | | |
| L-type $Ca^{2+}$ channels | $Ca^{2+}$ | BayK 8644 | dihydropyridines, phenylalklamines, benzothiazepines | |
| N-type $Ca^{2+}$ channels | $Ca^{2+}$ | | $\omega$-conotoxin | |
| P/Q-type $Ca^{2+}$ channels | $Ca^{2+}$ | | $\omega$-agatoxin | |
| T-type $Ca^{2+}$ channels | $Ca^{2+}$ | | mibefradil | |
| *Epithelial Na⁺ channels* | $Na^+$ | | amiloride | |
| *Ca²⁺ release channels* | $Ca^{2+}$ | ryanodine, caffeine, halothane | local anaesthetics | dantrolene |

*continued overleaf*

**Table 3.1 (continued)**

| Ion channel family | Permeant ion(s) | Activators/agonists | Pore blockers/antagonists | Allosteric modulators |
|---|---|---|---|---|
| *Cl⁻ channels* | | | | |
| ClC-type Cl⁻ channels | $Cl^{-+}$ | | chlorotoxin, 9-AC, clofibrates, disulfonic stilbenes | |
| $Ca^{2+}$ activated Cl⁻ channels | $Cl^-$ | | niflumic acid, disulfonic stilbenes | |
| *Cyclic-nucleotide gated channels* | $Na^+$, $K^+$ | cGMP | pseudechetoxin, tetracaine, L-*cis*-diltiazem | tetracaine |
| *Ligand-gated ion channels* | | | | |
| Nicotinic acetylcholine receptors | $Na^+$, $Ca^{2+}$ | nicotine, carbachol succinylcholine | $\alpha$-bungarotoxin, curare alkaloids hexamethonium, trimethaphan | |
| GABA receptors | $Cl^-$ | muscimol, isoguvacine | bicuculline, picrotoxin | barbiturates, ethanol, benzodiazepines, general anaesthetics |
| Glycine receptors | $Cl^-$ | $\beta$-alanine, taurine | strychnine | glycine, ifenprodil |
| Glutamate receptors | $Na^+$, $Ca^{2+}$ | AMPA, NMDA, kainate, quisqualate | phencyclidine | |
| 5-HT₃ serotonin receptors | $Na^+$, $K^+$ | 2-methyl-5-hydroxytryptamine | ondansetron | |
| P2X purinergic receptors | non-selective cations | ATP | PPADS, suramin | ivermectin ($P_2X4$) |

dynamic information from patch-clamp studies in polarizable membranes.

## Ion channels as static receptors

### Bimolecular drug-receptor interactions

The basic elements of ion channel pharmacology follow the laws of mass action that apply generally to drug-receptor interactions. A. J. Clark (1885–1941) first observed that drugs combine with their receptors at a rate dependent upon the concentration of the drug and receptor. This suggested that drug-receptor interactions could be expressed in a quantitative manner identical to the method utilized by Michaelis and Menton for enzymes and their substrates. For one-to-one binding of a drug (D) to a receptor (R), the chemical equation is:

$$D + R \underset{k_2}{\overset{k_1}{\rightleftharpoons}} DR \qquad (3.1)$$

where, $k_1$ is a second order on-rate constant ($M^{-1}s^{-1}$), and $k_2$ is a first order off-rate constant ($s^{-1}$). At equilibrium, the on-rate of the drug-channel association equals the off-rate of dissociation, such that the fractional occupancy (F) of receptors occupied by drug is:

$$F = (1 + K_d/[D])^{-1} \qquad (3.2)$$

where $K_d$ is the drug dissociation constant ($k_2/k_1$) and [D] is the drug concentration.

For ion channel pharmacology, patch-clamp current measurements provide the most informative functional 'assay' of the drug-receptor interaction. However, because ion channels are quite dynamic, the relative time scale of the drug-receptor interaction and the ion channel gating kinetics must be considered when measuring drug block (Figure 3.2). This applies even in the simplest, static case where the affinity of the drug for the channel is independent of the gated conformational state. The first tracing (Figure 3.2A) illustrates current through a drug-free ion channel as it opens (in this example, passing outward current, an upward deflection) and closes (passing no current) over time. These stochastic conformational changes, known as gating, occur randomly but proceed at an average rate determined by the membrane potential (voltage-gated channels) or ligand concentration (ligand-gated channels). Hence, in drug-free conditions, the measured single-channel current is determined primarily by the intrinsic gating properties of the channel protein.

Conversely, when a pore-blocking drug is introduced, the channel opening events are modified by the action of the compound. Figures 3.2B–D schematically illustrate the effects of three different drugs on current recordings through a single ion channel, as might be seen in a patch-clamp experiment. For simplicity, we will assume that the on-rate for drug binding in all three cases (Fig 3.2B–D) is similar and very rapid (in fact, if the drug-binding is not limited by steric constraints, the on-rate $k_1$ may approach the diffusion limit, $10^8$ mole$^{-1}$ sec$^{-1}$). Hence, the observable differences in drug binding reflected in the current recordings often depend on how rapidly the drug dissociates ($k_2$) from the channel relative to the intrinsic rate of channel gating. Once bound to the channel, a drug that unbinds slowly relative to the rate at which channels normally open and close might eliminate channel openings entirely for a sustained period of time (Figure 3.2B). Conversely, individual blocking and unblocking events might be 'visible' when a drug dissociates from the channel with kinetics more similar to those of channel gating (Figure 3.2C). In this case, a direct assessment of the residence time of the drug on the channel may be possible. We assume that the drug binds and unbinds from the channel with on- and off-rates $k_1$ and $k_2$, in a manner quantitatively similar to Equation (3.1):

$$D + \underset{\text{channel}}{\text{unblocked}} \underset{k_2}{\overset{k_1}{\rightleftharpoons}} \underset{\text{channel}}{\text{blocked}} \qquad (3.3)$$

If $k_2$ is slightly more rapid than the intrinsic rate of channel opening and closing, then the individual blocking events create gaps in the individual opening events (Figure 3.2C, a pattern referred to as bursting). The gap length is described by an exponential distribution with a mean of $1/k_2$. In the simplest case, the average duration of these gaps in channel opening provides an estimate of the mean residence time of the drug on the channel (Colquhoun and Hawkes, 1983).

Finally, when a drug both binds and unbinds

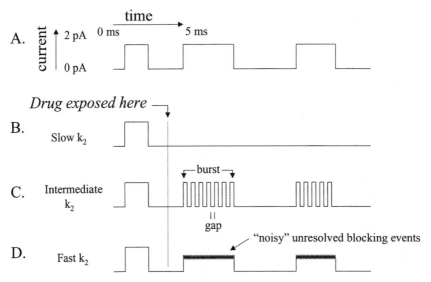

**Figure 3.2** Drug binding and unitary current records. (A) A typical unitary current record is illustrated, with stochastic opening events. An upward deflection in the current record signifies outward current is conducted by channel pore. The frequency of channel opening is dictated by the channel gating kinetics, a function of either the membrane potential (voltage-gated channels) or the ligand modulator (receptor-gated channel). (B, C, D) When exposed to a pore-blocker, the effect on the current records depends on the off-rate ($k_2$) of the drug-receptor interaction. In this example, the on-rate for drug binding is assumed to be diffusion limited ($\sim 10^8$ M$^{-1}$ s$^{-1}$). When $k_2$ is slow (B), channel openings are entirely eliminated for sustained periods. When $k_2$ has an 'intermediate' value, with a time scale similar to that of channel gating, 'bursting' behaviour is produced, where discrete blocking events are visible as gaps during a sustained channel opening. When $k_2$ greatly exceeds the time scale of channel gating (D), blocking events cannot be resolved, and the apparent unitary current is reduced. Adapted from Hille (1992).

much faster than the channels open or close, the rapid blocking reaction will produce an 'apparent' reduction in the single-channel current magnitude (Figure 3.2D). In this case, the individual blocking events are too rapid to measure, and the reduced unitary current amplitude is an artefact produced by the bandwidth limitations of the patch-clamp amplifier. A signature feature of this type of block is a 'noisy' open channel current that reflects incompletely resolved drug blocking events.

## Charged pore blockers bind within the transmembrane electric field

Many ion channel blockers are at least partially charged at physiological pH. If the drug binds within the ion pore, it follows that the charged moiety may pass partly through the membrane electric field. Hence, the kinetic features of the blocking reaction will be influenced directly by the membrane potential. Our first insights into ion channel block within the transmembrane electric field arose from studies of non-permeant cations. It has long been known that acid solutions lower the conductance through sodium channels. Woodhull (1973) proposed that extracellular protons bind to a site within the sodium channel pore that is partway (26%) across the electric field of the membrane, from outside to inside. Hence, the blocking effect of lowering pH is impeded by depolarization because depolarization of the cell membrane (making the inside more positive) opposes inward movement of positively charged protons.

The electrical distance to the blocking site in the membrane electrical field can only be loosely viewed as an actual physical distance, since the spatial distribution of the electrical field in the cell membrane and channel protein may not be defined. Moreover, the measurement is influenced by direct interactions between the charged ions that normally permeate the channel and the pore blocker (protons, drugs, etc.). Armstrong first showed that $K^+$ ions flowing through a K channel pore can actually expel a blocking drug (charged tetraethylammonium, $TEA^+$) from the pore (Armstrong, 1966). In some cases, coupled interactions between a blocker and permeating ions renders a voltage-dependence of block so steep that the apparent electrical distance is larger than 1.0 (that is, greater than the entire membrane electric field). Clearly, the distance to the blocking site cannot exceed 1.0, and models of ion channel block that allow many ions to occupy the pore simultaneously can account for this discrepancy by factoring in competition and electrostatic repulsion between permeating ions and the blocking species (Hille and Schwarz, 1978).

The gating conformational changes of ion channels are also voltage-dependent, and this may confound assessment of voltage-dependent block

when measurements are derived from currents through many ion channels at once (whole-cell currents). Although technically more challenging, resolving currents through a single ion channel using patch-clamp methods often allows an unambiguous assessment of the membrane electric field on the blocking reaction. Nonetheless, single-channel measurements of voltage-dependent block are susceptible to the issues of relative time scale illustrated in Figure 3.2. For example, $Cs^+$ ions block the inward rectifier K channel with intermediate kinetics, causing discrete interruptions in the measured current (Figure 3.3A, analogous to Figure 3.2C) (Fukushima, 1982). In this case, the frequency of blocking events increases markedly as the membrane potential is hyperpolarized. In contrast, $Cd^{2+}$ blocks voltage-gated Na channels with ultra-rapid kinetics, such that the individual blocking events cannot be resolved (Figure 3.3B, analogous to Figure 3.2D) (Backx et al., 1992). In this case, the apparent unitary current is reduced by $Cd^{2+}$ to a much greater extent during membrane hyperpolarization. Of note, this analysis of voltage-dependent block ignores entirely the effect that membrane potential may have on blocker

A

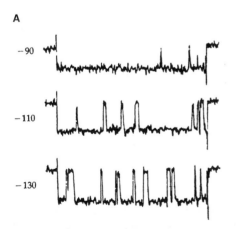

B

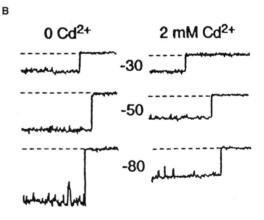

**Figure 3.3** Charged blockers bind with voltage-dependence. (A) Single inward-rectifier K channel recording from a tunicate egg exposed to 10 $\mu$M extracellular $Cs^+$. When the channel is open, the current is inward (downward), and the membrane potential during each recording is indicated (left). At −90 mV, $Cs^+$ rarely blocks the channel (only a few brief, upward current deflections are seen near the end of the recording). Conversely, at more negative membrane potentials brief, discrete interruptions in the current are frequently seen. From Fukushima (1992). (B) $Cd^{2+}$ block of rat skeletal muscle Na channels. The single-channel records were measured from *Xenopus* oocytes following cRNA injection. Channel openings are inward (downward current deflections) and are sustained due to fenvalerate treatment to remove fast inactivation. Cd reduced the current magnitude to a greater extent when the membrane potential was hyperpolarized (−80 mV versus −30 mV). In contrast to the discrete blocking events shown in panel (A), the kinetics of $Cd^{2+}$ block are rapid and manifest as an apparent reduction in the unitary current amplitude. From Backx et al., 1992.

affinity by virtue of changing the gated conformational state of the ion channel (see section Ion channels as dynamic receptors).

## The emerging view of a common static receptor

The ability to alter specific amino acid residues in recombinant ion channel proteins has revolutionized our approach to defining and characterizing drug receptor sites in ion channels. The first insights into the putative drug receptor in voltage-gated ion channels were provided by studies of triethyl ammonium ion (TEA$^+$) and larger quaternary ammonium derivatives (QA) on block of

delayed rectifier K channels in squid axons (Armstrong, 1975). These studies demonstrated that low concentrations of these compounds blocked the channel from the inside, and that the affinity increased as the hydrophobicity (length of the carbon tail; Figure 3.4A) of the blocking compound increased. In addition, internal blockade by TEA$^+$ suppressed outward current through the channel to a much greater degree than inward current, and increasing the inward flux of K$^+$ ions sped the rate of dissociation of the drug from its receptor. These directional effects were best explained by a hydrophobic drug receptor that lies within the pore, but in a vestibule on the internal side of the narrow cation selectivity 'filter'.

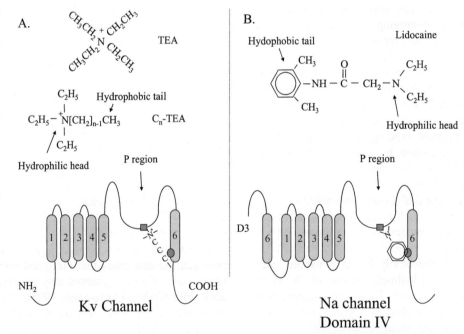

**Figure 3.4** Voltage-gated K and Na channels have analogous bidomain drug receptor motifs. (A, top) The structure of tetraethylammonium (TEA) and the longer-chain TEA derivatives (C$_n$-TEA) are shown. (A, bottom) Mutations at residue 469 in the S6 domain (shaded circle) of the *Shaker* K channel have prominent effects on the affinity of long-chain QA derivatives. Conversely, mutation of a threonine at position 441 in the P-region (shaded square) reduces binding of TEA and short-chain QA derivatives. (B, top) The structure of lidocaine, a local anaesthetic molecule, is shown with its hydrophobic aromatic tail and hydrophilic amino head group, separated by an amide linkage. (B, bottom) Mutation of residues that determine cation selectivity in the P region also modify local anaesthetic block. In addition, residues in the S6 segment of the fourth homologous domain critically determine local anaesthetic binding. In rat brain II Na channels, hydrophobic (aromatic) residues that modify local anaesthetic block in the domain IV S6 segment include F1764 and Y1771.

Empowered by the methods of molecular biology, later studies satisfied these predictions and mapped the locus of the K channel QA receptor to amino acid residues residing in the inner pore. Consistent with the two functional ends of QA compounds, two regions of the *Shaker* K channel influence drug binding from inside the cell (Figure 3.4A) (Choi *et al.*, 1993). The P region primarily influences TEA binding, but has less effect on longer (more hydrophobic) QA derivatives. Conversely, the binding affinity of long QA derivatives is determined by the hydrophobicity of amino acid residues lining the pore in the S6 segment. The picture that emerges is a bi-domain receptor, characterized by a hydrophilic binding interaction between the charged amino head of the QA compound with the P region, and hydrophobic interaction between the QA alkyl tail and amino acids in the S6 region. The importance of overlapping S6 regions in 4-aminopyridine (Kirsch *et al.*, 1993) and quinidine (Yeola *et al.*, 1996) binding to a number of other voltage-gated K channels has been demonstrated. For long chain QA derivatives, binding of the hydrophobic tail to S6 residues in *Shaker* seems to eliminate the interaction of the polar amino head with the P region, suggesting a 'tension' between binding at the two sites that might be modulated by changing the physical separation between the charged head and alkyl tail (Choi *et al.*, 1993).

A striking parallel exists between QA binding in K channels and binding of local anaesthetic (LA) molecules to their principal protein targets, voltage-gated Na channels. Local anaesthetics are characterized structurally by an ionizable amino head group and a hydrophobic tail, much like the QA compounds (Figure 3.4B). An intrapore binding site for LA molecules is well supported by evidence that the charged LA derivatives (e.g. QX-314) move deeply (50–70%) into the pore from the cytoplasmic side (Gingrich *et al.*, 1993; Strichartz, 1973). Specific hydrophobic residues in the S6 segment of domain IV line the inner pore of the channel, and are critical for the blocking action of virtually all local anaesthetics (Figure 3.4B) (Ragsdale *et al.*, 1994, 1996). Mutation of two particular S6 segment aromatic residues (F1764 and Y1771 in rat brain IIA Na channels) decreases the affinity of the channel for lidocaine,

etidocaine, and phenytoin by nearly 100-fold. At the same time, studies have also shown that the polar head of the local anaesthetic compound is repelled by residues in the ion selectivity filter (P-loop), suggesting that this region normally restricts extracellular access to (and escape from) the intrapore binding site (Sunami *et al.*, 1997). These qualitatively similar results for LA and QA binding locate the cation-selectivity domain in the P region adjacent to the S6 pore-lining segment in both Na and K channels. Analogous sites in domain IV, S6 of L-type Ca channels have been linked to both dihydropyridine and phenylalkylamine block of Ca current (Hockermann *et al.*, 1995; Schuster *et al.*, 1996). The S5 segments of both domains III and IV also appear to line the pore and are involved in dihydropyridine block of Ca channels (Peterson *et al.*, 1996; Ito *et al.*, 1997). The potential role of S5 residues and other pore-lining segments in Na and K channel pharmacology are subjects of active investigation.

## Ion channels as dynamic receptors

### Drug access and the gated conformational state

While the membrane potential directly influences the movement of a charged drug toward its receptor in the pore, a defining characteristic of ion channel pharmacology is the complex relationship between voltage-dependent conformational changes and drug-receptor interactions. Armstrong provided the first clues that the gated conformational state of an ion channel may directly influence drug binding (Armstrong, 1975). This work demonstrated that QA compounds block delayed rectifier K channels only after the channels are opened by membrane depolarization. Apparently, when the voltage-sensitive gates close the K channel at resting (hyperpolarized) membrane potentials, intracellular access of charged QA compounds to the drug receptor is prevented. At the same time, after the channel opens and the QA compound binds, closing the gate with hyperpolarization traps the QA compound inside the channel. Analogous studies have revealed that permanently charged derivatives of the local anaesthetic compounds (i.e. QX-314) are unable to bind from outside the cell, and only access their receptor from the inside when the channel is opened by a depolarization. For ionizable drugs such as the amine local anaesthetics that exist in both charged and neutral forms at physiological pH, the charged moiety interacts with its receptor from the intracellular side of the pore only when the channel assumes the open (ion conducting) conformational state (the hydrophilic pathway). At the same time, it is postulated that the uncharged moiety may approach its receptor through the membrane (the hydrophobic pathway), and may thus be less constrained by channel gates that control access to and egress from the aqueous pore (Hille, 1977). The existence of two pathways for drug binding is consistent with the complex, pH-sensitive block kinetics exhibited by many ionizable drugs.

## Drug binding modulates channel gating: the allosteric model

Changing the gated conformational state alters the access of a drug to its ion channel receptor and, conversely, drug binding alters the rate of ion channel conformational changes (Hille, 1992). This notion evolved primarily from the early observation that local anaesthetics seem to intensify Na channel inactivation. Na channels fluctuate between three putative conformational states, depending on the membrane potential, as follows (Hodgkin and Huxley, 1952):

$$\text{-----------------}\rightarrow \text{depolarization}$$
$$\textbf{Closed} \rightleftharpoons \textbf{Open} \rightleftharpoons \textbf{Inactivated} \qquad (3.4)$$
$$\text{hyperpolarization} \leftarrow\text{--------------}$$

When depolarized, Na channels open briefly, and then enter a stable, inactivated conformational state from which opening cannot occur. When the membrane is returned to a hyperpolarized (resting) potential, recovery to the closed state rapidly ensues, and the channel may open again. Surprisingly, low (but therapeutic) concentrations of LA do not suppress the Na current elicited by a single, brief depolarization, suggesting the drugs have low affinity for channel states occupied at the resting membrane potential (Closed, Equation 3.4). However, LAs evoke a cumulative reduction in Na current during a rapid train of depolarizing

stimuli, a classic pharmacological effect now appreciated for many drugs and ion channel targets, known as *use dependence* (Courtney, 1975). In many cases, use-dependent block seems to result from a high-affinity binding interaction with the inactivated conformational state (i.e. a state occupied when the channel is 'used'). A less obvious, but seminal feature of this state-dependent interaction is also observed; when drugs bind to non-inactivated states, this in turn augments the inactivation gating process (Hille, 1977; Cahalan and Almers, 1979). Hence, drug binding may be viewed as an 'effector' of ion channel gating, as follows:

$$
\begin{array}{ccc}
 & \overset{\alpha}{\underset{\beta}{\rightleftarrows}} & \\
\text{closed} & & \text{inactivated} \\
\text{drug} & & \text{drug} \\
\text{Low affinity} & & \text{High affinity} \\
(\text{high } K_d) & & (\text{low } K_d) \\
\text{drug-closed} & \overset{\alpha'}{\underset{\beta'}{\rightleftarrows}} & \text{inact-drug}
\end{array}
\qquad (3.5)
$$

$$\alpha'/\beta' > \alpha/\beta \text{ since } K_d \text{ (inactivated)} < K_d \text{ (closed)}$$

This model, known formally as the *modulated receptor model* (Hille, 1977), recapitulates the principles of state-dependent binding of substrates to allosteric enzymes (Monod *et al.*, 1965). The scheme implies that conformational transitions into states with high drug affinity (i.e. inactivated states) are enhanced by drug binding, and recovery from the drug-bound high-affinity states is delayed. Both of these kinetic effects promote use-dependent block. It is noteworthy that the reciprocal kinetic effect of drug binding on channel gating is predicted by the constraints imposed by microscopic reversibility (Equation 3.5). While the modulated receptor model was first proposed for LA block of Na channels, the model may apply equally well to K and Ca channels where complex relationships between drug binding and the channel conformational state are apparent (Hille, 1992).

Although the modulated receptor model provides a useful framework for examining the use-dependent properties of ion channel blocking agents, several deficiencies must be acknowledged. First, given that the open state is the only directly measured conducting state, unambiguous determination of the highest-affinity blocked state for many compounds has proven intractable. In fact, binding to pre-open closed states, and even open states, may exceed binding to the inactivated state for particular compounds. Second, most voltage-gated ion channels do not occupy a single inactivated state. Rather, channels undergo several distinct inactivation gating processes, each with unique conformational and kinetics signatures. Hence, the gated conformational states that truly underlie state-dependent drug receptor interactions are not fully understood or agreed upon. Some of the most recent studies that are enriching our understanding of these molecular mechanisms are discussed in later sections for particular drugs and ion channels.

# Pharmacology of specific ion channels

## Voltage-gated Na channels

Voltage-gated Na channels are heteromultimeric proteins belonging to the S4 superfamily of cation channels, and are extremely important for the electrical excitability of cells throughout the central and peripheral nervous system and striated muscles. They are critical mediators of the initial upstroke in the compound action potential and therefore have a primary role in the generation and propagation of electrical signals in the nervous system. There are currently 11 known isoforms of the principal pore-forming $\alpha$-subunit that arise from distinct genes. In addition, three types of accessory $\beta$-subunits ($\beta1$, $\beta2$, $\beta3$) that modulate Na channel function have been identified. Voltage-gated Na channels are important targets for local anaesthetics, anticonvulsants, and antiarrhythmic agents.

Local anaesthetics are a structurally diverse group of compounds that suppress excitability in both neuronal tissue and skeletal muscle by blocking current through Na channels. Our understanding of local anaesthetic action has been enriched over the last decade by studies that have exploited ion channel mutagenesis in an effort to link structure and function to molecular pharmacology. Early voltage-clamp studies of local anaesthetics revealed that Na channels rendered inactivation-deficient by internal exposure to proteases exhib-

ited marked resistance to use-dependent block by local anesthetics (Cahalan, 1978). More recent use of site-directed mutagenesis selectively to disable inactivation strengthened the hypothesis that inactivation gating is mechanistically linked to local anaesthetic action. Replacing a hydrophobic triplet of residues in the cytoplasmic III-IV linker with glutamines (IFM $\rightarrow$ QQQ) eliminates the most rapid component of inactivation (West et al., 1992) and markedly reduces use-dependent block by low (therapeutically relevant) concentrations of lidocaine (Bennett et al., 1995a). Experiments that disable the inactivation gate to varying degrees offer additional insight (Figure 3.5) (Balser et al., 1996). In the presence of lidocaine, Na channels with inactivation only partly disrupted (F $\rightarrow$ Q) seem to recover their more rapid inactivating character, while channels with a more severe disruption (IFM $\rightarrow$ QQQ) are resistant. Hence, greater disruption of the inactivation gating process incrementally disables the inactivation-enhancing effects of lidocaine, supporting the original postulate (Hille, 1977; Cahalan and Almers, 1979) that use-dependent LA action and inactivation gating are mechanistically linked. Surprisingly, recent covalent accessibility experiments have found that the III-IV linker is not directly 'trapped' by lidocaine during use-dependent block (Vedantham and Cannon, 1999), suggesting that the link between inactivation and LA block may be an indirect, or allosteric interaction. It is noteworthy that mutation of at least one of the residues implicated as part of the local anaesthetic receptor in domain IV, S6 (F1764; see Figure 3.4B) partially disrupts inactivation, and therefore may form part of the receptor for the rapid inactivation gate (McPhee et al., 1994). Hence, the same Na channel domains may influence both the static and dynamic (use-dependent) components of local anaesthetic action.

Mutant Na channels associated with dominant inherited disorders of striated muscle excitability may exhibit variable sensitivities to local anaesthetics. While Na channels normally open only briefly (and then inactivate), some mutant channels occasionally fail to inactivate. In the case of paramyotonia congenita, inherited mutations in the human skeletal muscle Na channel in the III-IV linker (T1313M) or in the S4 segment of

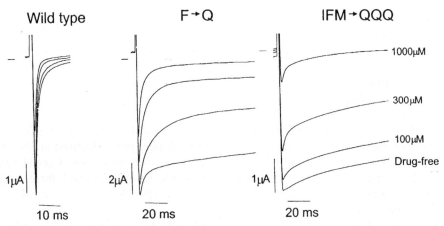

**Figure 3.5** Lidocaine block is modulated by mutations that alter inactivation. Whole-cell currents were recorded from *Xenopus* oocytes expressing wild-type and mutant rat skeletal muscle Na channels. Inactivation was damaged either partially (FQ) or severely (QQQ) by mutating residues in the III–IV interdomain linker. For wild-type and both mutant channels, currents were recorded in lidocaine concentrations of 0, 100, 300, and 1000 $\mu$M (right). Increasing the lidocaine concentration facilitates the inactivation of FQ channels to nearly resemble that of wild-type (1000 $\mu$M dose). The drug has less effect on the gating QQQ channels, but does reduce the overall current magnitude. Modified from Balser *et al.*, 1996.

domain IV (R1448C) predictably slow the fast inactivation gating process (Yang *et al.*, 1994). Analogous inactivation-disabling gating effects are seen with cardiac Na channel mutations linked to inherited forms of the long QT syndrome, a disorder that carries a high risk for fatal cardiac arrhythmias (Bennett *et al.*, 1995b). When exposed to low concentrations of LA agents (lidocaine, mexiletine), channels with inactivation-disabling mutations (Dumaine *et al.*, 1996; An *et al.*, 1996; Wang *et al.*, 1997; Kambouris *et al.*, 1998b) partially recover their wild-type inactivation phenotype. Lidocaine also normalizes the rate of recovery from inactivation in both F → Q mutant channels (Balser *et al.*, 1996) and the long QT mutants (An *et al.*, 1996). It is of particular interest that certain domain IV, S4 paramyotonia mutations (R1448C, R1448H) actually increase the sensitivity of the Na channel to lidocaine block (Fan *et al.*, 1996) or enhance use-dependent block by mexiletine (Weckbecker *et al.*, 2000). Studies suggest that while the S4 charge neutralization disrupts inactivation from the open state, inactivation from closed states is paradoxically enhanced (Ji *et al.*, 1996). It is postulated

that this peculiar gating feature is responsible for the augmented LA sensitivity of both the skeletal muscle (Nuss *et al.*, 2000) and cardiac (Kambouris *et al.*, 2000) Na channel mutants.

Certain local anaesthetic/antiarrhythmic agents have proven to be excellent treatments for non-dystrophic myotonias (myotonia congenita, paramyotonia congenita, and potassium-aggravated myotonia) caused by mutations in either the muscle Na channel (*SCN4A*) or chloride channel (*CLCN1*) genes. These drugs are effective in myotonia because of their ability to interrupt rapidly conducted trains of muscle action potentials through their use-dependent Na channel blocking action. Mexiletine and tocainide are widely used agents for the treatment of myotonia, although there are no large scale, randomized trials comparing these agents to either placebo or other treatments. The more potent Na channel blocker, flecainide, may also have utility in severe forms of myotonia that are resistant to mexiletine (Rosenfeld *et al.*, 1997). Phenytoin, carbamazepine and quinine are also effective antimyotonic agents, perhaps through their effects on Na channels. Adverse effects during long-term treatment of myotonia with Na channel blockers is the main limitation to their efficacy.

The relationship between the particular structural domains within LA molecules and the functional aspects of LA block are subjects of ongoing investigation. The hydrophobic residues that form the local anaesthetic receptor in domain IV, S6 (see Figure 3.4B) are a common molecular determinant for state-dependent binding of diverse Na channel blocking drugs. These include not only the traditional LA agents (lidocaine, etidocaine), but also anticonvulsants (phenytoin) and antiarrhythmic compounds (quinidine, flecainide) (Ragsdale et al., 1996). Like LA agents, QA compounds enhance the inactivation gating transitions in Na channels, and this effect increases as the size and hydrophobicity of the alkyl side chain increase (O'Leary et al., 1994). While this implies that the hydrophobic tail of the LA molecule interacts (directly or indirectly) with the inactivation gating structures, detailed local anaesthetic structure-activity relationships have not been evaluated in this regard. It has recently been shown that a substitution that increases the steric hindrance at the amino terminal end of the local anaesthetic molecule mexiletine increases the potency for blocking skeletal muscle Na channels, even when these channels are inactivation-disabled by toxins (Desaphy et al., 1999). Hence, in contrast to the hydrophobic tail, binding of the hydrophilic LA 'head' may depend less upon channel inactivation. Future studies that merge site-directed mutagenesis with a series of structural analogues should clarify the ideal structural arrangement of the LA molecule that will effectively suppress the pathological current through disease-causing mutant Na channels.

## Voltage-gated K channels

Voltage-gated K channels have critical roles in establishing and maintaining the resting membrane potential in most excitable cells, and participate in the repolarization phase of action potentials. An enormous variety of K channels within the nervous system provide for substantial functional heterogeneity relating to these two critical neurophysiological phenomena, and provide a wealth of pharmacological targets.

Voltage-gated K channels ($K_v$ channels) comprise an extensive family of S4 cation channels with more than 100 cloned isoforms. Based upon amino acid sequence comparisons, several distinct subfamilies have been defined and were originally clustered according to their homology with specific K channel genes identified in *Drosophila* (*shaker*, *shal*, *shab*, *shaw*, *eag*). Current nomenclature standards have reclassified these original *Drosophila* homology groups into less colourful alphanumeric symbols (ie: $K_v1.x$, $K_v2.x$, etc.). Additional K channel subfamilies that have been more recently characterized include the *eag*-related genes, and KCNQ channels.

Studies of the molecular pharmacology of $K_v$ channels have revealed important new concepts regarding use-dependent block of ion channels. The most accepted mechanism of use dependence is that a blocker binds to the channel with higher affinity to particular gated states when depolarized (or 'used'), and then dissociates slowly. In this context, 'modulated receptor' models (Hille, 1977) (Equation 3.5) have provided a framework for understanding the dynamic features of ion channel block for two decades. Recent studies in cloned (*Shaker*) K channels have unveiled a new mechanism for use-dependent block that links the dynamic features of channel gating with the fundamental permeation properties of the pore (Baukrowitz and Yellen, 1996). Yellen and Baukrowitz made the surprising observation that the QA compound binds to the intracellular side of the channel only briefly (1–10 ms), while recovery from use-dependent block is far slower (~ 10 seconds). During maintained depolarization, many K channels inactivate via structural rearrangements in the outer pore, so-called 'C-type' inactivation, that also recovers slowly (Liu et al., 1996). This gating process is inhibited by high $K^+$ occupancy in the outer pore. It was shown that even a brief period of block of the intracellular mouth of the pore by a QA compound is sufficient to reduce $K^+$ efflux, and thus deplete a $K^+$-occupied control site in the outer mouth of the pore that normally prevents C-type inactivation (Figure 3.6A) (Baukrowitz and Yellen, 1996). Hence, channels recover

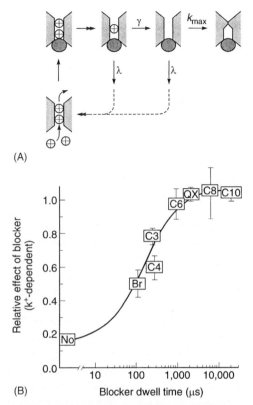

(A)

(B)

**Figure 3.6** Effects of K channel blockers on C-type inactivation correlate with dwell time. (A) Schematic model for use-dependent block that involves C-type inactivation. The pore of a conducting K channel (bottom) is filled with $K^+$ ions. When the intracellular blocker binds (filled circle), the K ions gradually evacuate the pore; the last ion leaves the pore with a rate $\gamma$. If the intracellular blocker unbinds at a rate $\lambda$, slower than the ion exit rate $\gamma$, then the pore becomes fully evacuated and C-type inactivation is allowed to proceed at its maximum rate ($k_{max}$). (B) The effects of various blockers on the rate of C-type inactivation correlate with the dwell time of the blocker on the channel. 'No' indicates the rate of C-type inactivation with no blocking agent, Br is bretylium, QX is QX-314, and the remaining compounds (C3...C10) are QA compounds of increasing chain length. From Baukrowitz and Yellen, 1996.

slowly from use-dependent block, not due to slow separation of drug from the channel, but due to the intrinsic slow recovery rate of C-type inactivation.

The effects of various blockers (including QA compounds, QX-314 and bretylium) to enhance

C-type inactivation correlate with their dwell-time in the channel pore (Figure 3.6B), suggesting that the release rate of $K^+$ from the outer-pore control site must be comparable to the blocker dwell time. Recall that binding of the long-chain QA derivatives in K channels is heavily determined by a hydrophobic site lining the pore in the S6 segment (see Figure 3.4A). Hence, the blocker dwell time on the channel, and consequent use-dependent blocking effects, may be heavily determined by the nature of the hydrophobic interaction between the 'tails' of various blocking compounds and the S6 segment. In addition, given the uncertainty surrounding the identity of the high-affinity state determining use-dependent LA block, it is useful to consider recent studies that postulate an analogous mechanism for use-dependent LA block in Na channels. Site-directed mutations, cation substitutions, and isoform differences that either enhance or antagonize a particular slowly-recovering inactivation process involving the Na channel outer pore all have parallel effects on use-dependent block by lidocaine (Kambouris *et al.*, 1998a; Nuss *et al.*, 2000; Chen *et al.*, 2000).

## Inward rectifying and ATP dependent K channels

The most structurally simple ion channels are those of the inwardly rectifying K channel family. These channels consist of a tetrameric arrangement of subunits each consisting of two TM domains and a single pore loop. Physiologically, inward rectifying K channels pass current only in a narrow range of membrane voltage and are thus important for setting the resting membrane potential and for regulating membrane excitability. Their degree of rectification is tightly controlled by intracellular molecules including magnesium ions and polyamines such as spermine and spermidine. A subset of this family of K channels are the ATP-dependent channels ($K_{ATP}$) (Ashcroft and Gribble, 1998). $K_{ATP}$ channels are comprised of four inwardly rectifying K channel subunits belonging to the $K_{IR}6.x$ family, and four sulphonylurea receptor (SUR) subunits (Aguilar-Bryan *et al.*, 1998). The SUR subunits are members of the ATP binding cassette superfamily of membrane proteins. These channels are capable of sensing the metabolic state of this cell by virtue of their ATP inhibition and thus enable coupling of metabolism to cellular excitibility. When energy stores are reduced, $K_{ATP}$ channels become activated causing membrane hyperpolarization and reduction in the energy consuming work of ion pumps that are needed to restore membrane voltage after an action potential. $K_{ATP}$ channels are best known for their role in insulin secretion by pancreatic islet cells (Aguilar-Bryan and Bryan, 1999). Recently, a bacterial inwardly rectifying K channel from *Streptomyces lividans* has provided the first opportunity to define the precise structure of a K channel pore at an atomic scale (Doyle *et al.*, 1998).

Inwardly rectifying K channels are sensitive to extracellular TEA and certain antiarrhythmic compounds such as quinidine. $K_{ATP}$ channels are the specific targets of two classes of pharmacological agents, the sulphonylureas and potassium channel openers. Sulphonylureas have been in use for many years as hypoglycaemic agents for the treatment of non-insulin dependent diabetes mellitus. These compounds bind specifically to the SUR subunit and can be considered allosteric modulators of the $K_{ATP}$ channel because they bind to the non-pore-forming subunit. High affinity binding sites for both classes of compounds are located within the TM13-16 region of SUR, and a single serine residue in SUR1 has been identified as a critical determinant of high sensitivity to tolbutamide, a prototype sulphonylurea (Ashfield *et al.*, 1999). $K_{ATP}$ channels bind one drug molecular per channel complex.

Potassium channel openers may have clinical utility in treating hypokalaemic periodic paralysis and may have other therapeutic uses (Lawson, 1996). Recent observations suggest that diminished activity of skeletal muscle $K_{ATP}$ may be important in the pathophysiology of episodic weakness in familial and acquired hypokalaemic periodic paralysis (Tricarico *et al.*, 1999). Cromakalim has been shown to improve the contractile force of muscle fibres excised from patients suffering from hypokalaemic periodic paralysis (Grafe *et al.*, 1990), but there have not been reports of the efficacy of these compounds in this clinical setting.

## Calcium-activated K channels

Calcium-activated K channels ($K_{Ca}$) are a physiologically and structurally diverse class of K channels that are important for neuronal excitability by participating in the repolarization and after-hyperpolarization of action potentials. These activities are important for controlling certain characteristics of the action potential firing pattern including interspike interval and a phenomenon known as spike-frequency adaptation. These channels derive their name from the observation that their open probability is increased by elevation of cytosolic calcium. They may also participate in modulating smooth muscle contraction, and the release of neurotransmitters and hormones.

Functionally, three classes of $K_{Ca}$ channels have been identified and categorized based on their single channel conductances (Vergara *et al.*, 1998). Large conductance or BK channels (also known as maxi-K channels) exhibit single channel conductances of up to 250 pS and are regulated by both intracellular calcium and membrane potential. BK channels are composed of two classes of subunits. The pore forming $\alpha$-subunit closely resembles the $K_v$ family of K channels with the exception that the amino terminus resides extracellularly and there is an additional TM segment. The $\alpha$-subunits associate in 1:1 stoichiometry with $\beta$-subunits that are two TM domain proteins. BK channels have an extended carboxy terminus that contains a 'calcium bowl' motif, a potential site involved in calcium activation. Alternative splicing appears to underlie the structural diversity of BK channels.

Small conductance $K_{Ca}$ channels (SK channels) exhibit single channel conductances of 5–20 pS and are relatively voltage-insensitive. This class of $K_{Ca}$ channels is probably responsible for the slow phase of neuronal after-hyperpolarization that serves to attenuate the firing frequency of repetitive action potentials in the nervous system. This phenomenon, known as spike-frequency adaptation, may help prevent the potentially injurious effects of rapid action potential conduction in neurons. Structurally, SK channels exhibit the characteristic transmembrane topology of $K_v$ channels with six transmembrane segments and a pore loop, although their overall amino acid sequence identity with $K_v$ channels is remote. Unlike BK channels, there is no identifiable calcium bowl or other calcium-binding motif present. The third class of $K_{Ca}$ channels exhibit an intermediate single channel conductance and are known as IK channels. The prototype IK channel is also referred to as the Gardos channel found in erythrocytes. At the molecular level, one IK channel has been identified that exhibits strong homology with SK channels, and Joiner *et al.* have also identified IK channels resulting from the heteromeric assembly of a BK channel with the *Slack* K channel in *C. elegans* (Joiner *et al.*, 1998).

BK channels are sensitive to low concentrations of TEA and charybdotoxin but are insensitive to apamin, a small peptide from the venom of honeybees (Vergara *et al.*, 1998). Most, but not all, SK channels are sensitive to apamin and insensitive to TEA. The pharmacology of IK channels is distinguished by apamin resistance and sensitivity to clotrimazole. Several additional pharmacological agents and natural products are known to block BK channels (Kaczorowski and Garcia, 1999). In addition to charybdotoxin, two other peptide inhibitors of BK channels have been isolated from scorpion venoms (iberiotoxin and limbatotoxin). These peptide inhibitors interact directly with residues within the external pore of the channel and depend on both electrostatic and hydrophobic interactions. A potent non-peptide class of BK channel blockers are the indole diterpenes, a family of fungal alkaloids. Compounds such as aflatrem and paxilline can block BK channels at nanomolar concentrations. Their mechanism of action appears state dependent as their activity is weaker when the channel open probability is high. Two natural product agonists of BK channels have also been identified. Dehydrosoyasaponin-1 and maxi-K diol increase the open probability of BK channels acting at the intracellular face by allosterically mediated effects on the channel pore. Certain substituted indole analogues, such as benzimidazolone compounds, also serve to activate the BK channels by shifting the voltage-dependence of activation toward the hyperpolarized direction. In most cases, antagonist and agonist of BK channels depend primarily on the $\alpha$-subunit. However, the $\beta$-subunit may contribute to charybdotoxin binding and has also recently been identi-

fied as the binding site of estradiol which activates BK channels from the extracellular side (Valverde *et al.*, 1999).

## Cyclic-nucleotide gated channels

A family of non-selective cation channels gated by direct interaction with cyclic nucleotides (CNG channels) are important for signal transduction especially in sensory neurons of the retina and olfactory system (Zagotta and Siegelbaum, 1996). A subset of structurally related ion channels has recently been identified as the hyperpolarization activated cyclic nucleotide gated channels (HCN channels) (Santoro *et al.*, 1998; Gauss *et al.*, 1998). HCN channels are important mediators of pacemaker functions within the sinoatrial node of the heart and spontaneously active neurons within the central nervous system. Pacemaker currents in both tissues have been referred to as $I_h$ or $I_f$. Structurally, all cyclic-nucleotide gated channels resemble the core structure of voltage-gated K channels including presence of an S4 helix and characteristic residues within the pore loop (GYG motif) (Zagotta and Siegelbaum, 1996). Despite the high conservation of residues within the pore that have generally been associated with high $K^+$ selectively, CNG and HCN channels are non-selective for the monovalent cations $Na^+$ and $K^+$. In addition to the core structural motif of K channels, CNG channels have an additional cyclic nucleotide-binding domain within their cytoplasmic carboxy terminus.

There are no highly specific pharmacological blockers of CNG or HCN channels. Certain analogues of cyclic GMP are capable of inhibiting channel function when applied intracellularly, but they also have concomitant effects on the activity of protein kinases. Similarly, tetracaine, L-*cis*-diltiazem, and pimozide are non-selective blockers of CNG channels. Tetracaine has been shown to block the pore of CNG channels (Fodor *et al.*, 1997). Recently, a snake venom toxin, pseudechetoxin, has been described that exhibits high affinity competitive blocking action on bovine rod CNG channels (Brown *et al.*, 1999). Other than the natural ligands cAMP and cGMP, there have not been any pharmacological agonists described for this class of ion channels.

## Voltage-gated Ca channels

Voltage-gated Ca channels mediate depolarization-induced $Ca^{2+}$ influx into excitable tissues such as muscle, heart and nerve (Catterall, 1996). They are involved in a wide variety of critical physiological functions such as excitation-contraction coupling, generation of action potentials, neurotransmitter release, and hormonal secretion. Calcium channels mediate the upstroke of the action potential in excitable tissues lacking voltage-gated Na channels, and are important for maintaining the action potential plateau in heart and certain neuronal tissues. Because of their pivotal roles in many physiological processes, Ca channels have become important targets for a variety of pharmacological agents designed to treat hypertension, cardiac arrhythmias, myocardial ischaemia, and migraine (Triggle, 1999).

The pore forming component of Ca channels, the $\alpha_1$ subunit, closely resembles the transmembrane topology of voltage-gated Na channels (Hofmann et al., 1999). In addition to the $\alpha_1$-subunit, Ca channels are composed of four other accessory subunits ($\alpha_2$, $\beta$, $\gamma$, $\delta$). Structural and functional diversity is achieved by the existence of at least seven identified mammalian $\alpha_1$ isoforms and multiple $\beta$-subunits that exhibit unique tissue distributions. Functionally, Ca channels have been characterized as either low-voltage threshold or high-voltage threshold. Additional categories of Ca channels are based on their detailed pharmacological and biophysical properties (Birnbaumer et al., 1994). The low-voltage activated T-type Ca channels help mediate pacemaker activity of cardiac and neuronal cells. The high-voltage threshold L-type Ca channels are important for excitation-contraction coupling, and smooth muscle contraction. N-type Ca channels contribute to neurotransmitter release from presynaptic nerve terminals. As described later in this book, both L-type and P/Q type Ca channels are responsible for a variety of ion channelopathies. There are three major classes of Ca channel blockers that bind to distinct sites on the $\alpha_1$-subunit. The dihydropyri-dines, phenylalkylamines, and benzothiazepines mediate high affinity block of L-type channels, whereas N-type, P/Q-type, and R-type channels are resistant to these compounds. Differences in drug sensitivity have been exploited in chimera studies to localize regions of the $\alpha_1$-subunit important for drug binding (Hockerman et al., 1997; Striessnig et al., 1998). This work has identified a short amino acid stretch in the fourth domain S6 segment that is important for dihydropyridine and phenylalkylamine binding. In addition, regions of the third domain pore region are needed for dihydropyridine binding. Certain polypeptide toxins are effective antagonists of N-type ($\omega$-conotoxin) and P/Q-type ($\omega$-agatoxin) channels. These peptide blockers block $Ca^{2+}$ permeation by interacting directly with extracellular regions of the pore, particularly in the third domain. Calcium channel antagonism can also be observed with transitional metal ions and therapeutic concentrations of aminoglycoside antibiotics (Pichler et al., 1996). BayK-8644 is a Ca channel agonist that acts by favouring very long channel openings without affecting the single channel conductance.

Clinically, Ca channel blockers are used for the treatment of hypertension and myocardial ischaemia through relaxation of vascular smooth muscle. They are also effective antiarrhythmic agents, particularly for the use in treating supraventricular tachycardias because of their action in slowing atrioventricular node conduction. These agents may also be effective in treating migraine, and the action of certain anticonvulsant agents may involve Ca channel blockade in the central nervous system (Stefani et al., 1997). At present there are no clinically available agonists.

## Ca-release channels

Two major classes of intracellular ion channels mediate the release of $Ca^{2+}$ from intracellular stores (ryanodine receptor, IP$_3$-receptor). In striated muscle, the predominant Ca-release channel is the ryanodine receptor (RyR), a massive tetrameric protein complex that represents the largest ion channel cloned to date (Zucchi and Ronca-Testoni, 1997). Each subunit of the ryanodine receptor consists of more than 5000 amino acids that is membrane-anchored to the terminal cisterna of the sarcoplasmic reticulum (SR) by four TM domains. The protein has an extensive extramembranous portion that occupies the narrow cytosolic space between the membranes of the transverse tubule and the SR. This large extramembranous domain can be observed by electron microscopy as the foot process in the triad junction. In this location, the RyR makes contact with the cytoplasmic face of L-type Ca channels, an association critical for mediating excitation-contraction coupling. The 12-kDa FK binding protein (FKBP12), the cytosolic receptor for the immunosuppressant FK-506, associates with the RyR and may modulate its function. This protein complex is responsible for releasing $Ca^{2+}$ from the SR, thus triggering other events that eventually lead to contraction. Calcium release is primarily triggered by cytosolic $Ca^{2+}$, and by coupled conformational changes in the L-type Ca channel. Release is also modulated by a variety of substances including ATP. Three RyR isoforms have been identified: RyR1 is expressed in skeletal muscle; RyR2 in heart and brain; RyR3 in epithelial tissues and some brain regions. Mutations in RyR1 underlie malignant hyperthermia susceptibility and central core disease (Mickelson and Louis, 1996; Hogan, 1998).

The pharmacology of ryanodine receptors has been extensively studied (Zucchi and Ronca-Testoni, 1997). The receptor is named for its ability to bind the plant alkaloid ryanodine, an agonist for SR $Ca^{2+}$ release (Sutko et al., 1997). The primary biophysical effect of ryanodine is to lock the channel in an open confirmation with a somewhat reduced single channel conductance. Methylxanthines, such as caffeine, also have an agonist affect on the RyR by shifting the relationship between channel activation and cytosolic $Ca^{2+}$ levels. Caffeine increases channel open probability at resting intracellular $Ca^{2+}$ concentrations, and can be used as a sensitive indicator for detecting mutant RyR1 in subjects at risk for malignant hyperthermia susceptibility (in vitro contraction assay). A wide variety of other agents belonging to the inhaled general anaesthetics also serve as agonists for SR $Ca^{2+}$ release by modulating open probability. Immunosuppressive agents, FK-506 and rapamycin, that exert their activity through FK binding proteins, modulate $Ca^{2+}$ release by affecting open probability of the channel. Similarly, cardiac glycosides and other ionotropic agents (e.g. milrinone) have a similar effect.

Calcium release from the SR can be antagonized by local anaesthetic agents and by the hydantoin derivative, dantrolene sodium. Dantrolene inhibits RyR-mediated SR $Ca^{2+}$ release and is the treatment of choice for malignant hyperthermia. Whether dantrolene exerts its effects on SR $Ca^{2+}$ release by a direct interaction with the RyR is unclear. Recent studies have demonstrated that dantrolene binding activity in SR membranes can be separated from ryanodine binding using sucrose density gradient centrifugation (Palnitkar et al., 1997). It is most likely that dantrolene interacts with another protein and exerts its effects indirectly on RyR activity.

## Cl channels

Chloride channels are a ubiquitous and structurally diverse class of ion channels. They mediate a wide range of physiological activities including stabilization of membrane potential, cell volume regulation, regulation of intracellular pH, signal transduction, modulation of neuronal excitability, and epithelial salt transport. There are many structurally dissimilar classes of proteins that mediate $Cl^-$ conductance, and this section will focus on two types: the ClC voltage-gated Cl channels, and the CLCA family of Ca-activated Cl channels.

Chloride channels belonging to the ClC family are composed of two identical subunits, each consisting of approximately 10 TM spanning regions (Jentsch, 1994). At least nine mammalian isoforms exist, and some are expressed in virtually all cells. ClC-1 is the predominant skeletal muscle isoform and mutations in this gene cause congenital myotonia. Skeletal muscle Cl channels are well characterized pharmacologically, although there are relatively few if any specific blockers available. The skeletal muscle Cl channel is blocked by 9-anthracene carboxylic acid (Furman and Barchi, 1978), and by clofibrate compounds (De Luca et al., 1992). The pharmacological interaction of clofibrates with skeletal muscle chloride channels may explain the occurrence of myotonia in some patients treated with these agents for hyperlipidaemia. Additional derivatives of clofibrates may have enhanced potency against ClC-1 and certain stereoisomers may exhibit agonist activity at low concentration (De Luca et al., 1992). To date there are no clinically available Cl channel openers that conceivably might be useful for treatment of myotonia congenita. Many, but not all ClC channels are inhibited by generic Cl channel antagonists such as disulphonic stilbenes (DIDS, SIDS). One polypeptide blocker, chlorotoxin may interact specifically with ClC chloride channels (DeBin et al., 1993; Lippens et al., 1995), and recent observations indicate that this peptide toxin may block a glioma-specific $Cl^-$ current possibly involved in enabling tumour invasiveness (Soroceanu et al., 1998, 1999).

Calcium-activated Cl channels are found in a wide variety of tissues especially in the central nervous system. These channels mediate $Cl^-$ flux in response to elevations in intracellular $Ca^{2+}$ and they appear to have a role in modulating neuronal excitability (Scott et al., 1995). Whether activation of Ca-activated Cl channels mediates inhibitory or excitatory influences depends upon the relative distribution of $Cl^-$ across the cell membrane and the Cl equilibrium potential. Lowering the intracellular $Cl^-$ concentration shifts the Cl equilibrium potential towards more hyperpolarized potentials and enables Ca-activated Cl channel activity to have an inhibitory effect on neuronal excitability. At least one class of Ca-activated Cl channels has been cloned. The CLCA family consists of proteins featuring four to five TM domains and 900–950 amino acids. This family of Cl channels was originally cloned from epithelial tissues (Cunningham et al., 1995), but other isoforms have been identified within the nervous system (Gruber and Pauli, 1999). These channels exhibit no sequence homology to ClC channels or other classes of $Cl^-$ conducting proteins. Studies of native tissues have long recognized that niflumic acid blocks Ca-activated chloride channels (White and Aylwin, 1990). Non-specific Cl channel blockers including disulphonic stilbenes and derivatives of benzoic acid also exhibit activity against Ca-activated Cl channels. None of these pharmacological agents exerts a specific effect on the channels, and high affinity blockers or agonists are not clinically available. There is little known about the structure-activity relationship between drug action in these channels but this should change soon with the availability of prototype cloned channels.

## Ligand-gated ion channels

Several classes of neurotransmitter receptors mediate their cellular effects by activating ionic currents when liganded by extracellular molecules. Ligand-gated ion channels are a diverse and important class of ion-conducting proteins that could be the subject of an entire book rather than a subsection of one chapter. Table 3.1 provides a summary of the major classes of ligand-gated ion channels and certain pharmacological characteristics, while Figure 3.1 illustrates prototype structures. Other than GABA and glycine receptors that mediate $Cl^-$ conductance, the other ligand-gated ion channels conduct cations in non-selective fashion. A variety of agonists, antagonists, and allosteric modulators have been well characterized for many of these ion channel families. Perhaps the most clinically useful agonist is succinylcholine, which directly activates nicotinic acetylcholine receptors in muscle and is useful as a neuromuscular blocking agent in anaesthesia. Antagonists that directly interfere with the binding of the natural ligand or block the ionic pore have been extensively characterized for many ligand-gated ion channels. Some of the more commonly deployed clinical agents are those that modulate the GABA receptor through allosteric mechanisms. This group of agents includes the barbiturates, benzodiazepines and general anaesthetics. Ethanol also modulates GABA receptors via allosteric mechanisms. A wide variety of agents that target glutamate receptors are currently in development as potential neuroprotective agents by virtue of their ability to impair the major excitatory neurotransmitter. Some of these agents may one day find utility in the treatment of ion channelopathies involving ligand-gated ion channels.

## Summary

Ion channels provide an extensive range of pharmacological targets within the nervous system and elsewhere in the body. The molecular basis for drug action has been accelerated greatly by the availability of cloned ion channels. Many suspect that many more members of the classes of ion channels listed in Table 3.1 will be identified shortly and these will no doubt provide new opportunities for identifying therapeutic compounds for treating disease of the nervous system.

# References

Aguilar-Bryan, L. and Bryan, J. (1999). Molecular biology of adenosine triphosphate-sensitive potassium channels. *Endocr Rev.,* **20,** 101–35.

Aguilar-Bryan, L., Clement, J. P., Gonzalez, G., Kunjilwar, K., Babenko, A., and Bryan, J. (1998). Toward understanding the assembly and structure of KATP channels. *Physiol Rev.,* **78,** 227–45.

An, R. H., Bangalore, R., Rosero, S. Z. and Kass, R. S. (1996). Lidocaine block of LQT-3 mutant human Na channels. *Circ Res.,* **79,** 103–8.

Armstrong, C. M. (1966). Time course of TEA-induced anomalous rectification in squid giant axons. *J Gen Physiol.,* **50,** 491–503.

Armstrong, C. M. (1975). Ionic pores, gates, and gating currents. *Q Rev Biophys.,* **7,** 179—210.

Ashcroft, F. M. and Gribble, F. M. (1998). Correlating structure and function in ATP-sensitive $K^+$ channels. *Trends Neurosci.,* **21,** 288–94.

Ashfield, R., Gribble, F. M., Ashcroft, S. J. and Ashcroft, F. M. (1999). Identification of the high-affinity tolbutamide site on the SUR1 subunit of the K(ATP) channel. *Diabetes,* **48,** 1341–47.

Backx, P. H., Yue, D. T., Lawrence, J., Marban, H. E. and. Tomaselli, G. F. (1992). Molecular localization of an ion-binding site within the pore of mammalian sodium channels. *Science,* **257,** 248–51.

Balser, J. R., Nuss, H. B., Orias, D. W. *et al.* (1996). Local anesthetics as effectors of allosteric gating: lidocaine effects on inactivation-deficient rat skeletal muscle Na channels. *J Clin Invest.,* **98,** 2874–86.

Baukrowitz, T., and. Yellen, G. (1996). Use-dependent blockers and exit rate of the last ion from the multi-ion pore of a K channel. *Science,* **271,** 653–6.

Bennett, P. B., Valenzuela, C., Li-Qiong, C. and Kallen, R. G. (1995a). On the molecular nature of the lidocaine receptor of cardiac $Na^+$ channels. *Circ Res.,* **77,** 584–92.

Bennett, P. B., Yazawa, K., Naomasa, M. and George, A. L. (1995b). Molecular mechanism for an inherited cardiac arrhythmia. *Nature,* **376,** 683–5.

Birnbaumer, L., Campbell, K. P., Catterall, W. A. *et al.* (1994). The naming of voltage-gated calcium channels. *Neuron,* **13,** 505–6.

Brown, R. L., Haley, T. L., West, K. A., and Crabb, J. W. (1999). Pseudechetoxin: a peptide blocker of cyclic nucleotide-gated ion channels. *Proc Natl Acad Sci USA,* **96,** 754–9.

Cahalan, M. D. (1978). Local anesthetic block of sodium channels in normal and pronase-treated squid axons. *Biophys J.,* **23,** 285–311.

Cahalan, M. D., and Almers, W. (1979). Interactions between quaternary lidocaine, the sodium channel gates, and tetrodotoxin. *Biophys J.,* **27,** 39–56.

Catterall, W. A. (1996). Molecular properties of sodium and calcium channels. *J Bioenerg Biomembr.,* **28,** 219–30.

Chen, Z., Ong, B.-H., Kambouris, N. G., Marban, E., Tomaselli, G. F. and Balser, J. R. (2000). Lidocaine induces a slow inactivated state in rat skeletal muscle sodium channels. *J Physiol.,* (Lond) **524,** 37–49.

Choi, K. L., Mossman, C., Aube, J. and Yellen, G. (1993). The internal quaternary ammonium receptor site of *Shaker* potassium channels. *Neuron,* **10,** 533–41.

Colquhoun, D., and Hawkes, A. G. (1983). The principles of the stochastic interpretation of ion-channel mechanisms. In *Single-Channel Recording* (eds Sakmann, E. and Neher, E.) p. 150. New York: Plenum Press.

Courtney, K. R. (1975). Mechanism of frequency-dependent inhibition of sodium currents in the frog myelinated nerve by the lidocaine derivative GEA 968. *J Pharmacol Exp Ther.,* **195,** 225–36.

Cunningham, S. A., Awayda, M. S., Bubien, J. K. *et al.* (1995). Cloning of an epithelial chloride channel from bovine trachea. *J Biol Chem.,* **270,** 31016–26.

De Luca, A., Tricarico, D., Wagner, R., Bryant, S. H., Tortorella, V. and Conte Camerino, D. (1992). Opposite effects of enantiomers of clofibric acid derivative on rat skeletal muscle chloride conductance: Antagonism studies and theoretical modeling of two different receptor site interactions. *J Pharm Exp Therap.,* **260,** 364–8.

DeBin, J. A., Maggio, J. E. and Strichartz, G. R. (1993). Purification and characterization of chlorotoxin, a chloride channel ligand from the venom of the scorpion. *Am J Physiol.,* **264,** C361–C369.

Desaphy, J. F., Camerino, D. C., Franchini, C., Lentini, G., Tortorella, V. and Luca, A. D. (1999). Increased hindrance on the chiral carbon atom of mexiletine enhances the block of rat skeletal muscle $Na^+$ channels in a model of myotonia induced by ATX. *Br J Pharmacol.,* **128,** 1165–74.

Doyle, D. A., Cabral, J. M., Pfuetzner, R. A. *et al.* (1998). The structure of the potassium channel: molecular basis of $K^+$ conduction and selectivity. *Science,* **280,** 69–77.

Dumaine, R., Wang, Q., Keating, M. T. *et al.* (1996). Multiple mechanisms of $Na^+$ channel-linked long-QT syndrome. *Circ Res.,* **78,** 916–24.

Fan, Z., George, A. L., Kyle, J. W. and Makielski, J. C.

(1996). Two human paramyotonia congenita mutations have opposite effects on lidocaine block of $Na^+$ channels expressed in a mammalian cell line. *J Physiol., 496,* 275–86.

Fodor, A. A., Gordon, S. E. and Zagotta, W. N. (1997). Mechanism of tetracaine block of cyclic nucleotide-gated channels. *J Gen Physiol, 109,* 3–14.

Fukushima, Y. (1982). Blocking kinetics of the anomalous potassium rectifier of tunicate egg studied by single channel recording. *J Physiol (Lond)., 331,* 311–31.

Furman, R. E. and Barchi, R. L. (1978). The pathophysiology of myotonia produced by aromatic carboxylic acids. *Ann Neurol., 4,* 357–65.

Gauss, R., Seifert, R. and Kaupp, U. B. (1998). Molecular identification of a hyperpolarization-activated channel in sea urchin sperm. *Nature, 393,* 583–7.

Gingrich, K. J., Beardsley, D. and Yue, D. T. (1993). Ultra-deep blockade of Na channels by a quaternary ammonium ion: catalysis by a transition-intermediate state? *J Physiol., 471,* 319–41.

Grafe, P., Quasthoff, S., Strupp, M. and Lehmann-Horn, F. (1990). Enhancement of $K^+$ conductance improves in vitro the contraction force of skeletal muscle in hypokalemic periodic paralysis. *Muscle Nerve, 13,* 451–7.

Gruber, A. D. and Pauli, B. U. (1999). Clustering of the human CLCA gene family on the short arm of chromosome 1 (1p22-31). *Genome, 42,* 1030–2.

Hille, B. (1977). Local anesthetics: hydrophilic and hydrophobic pathways for the drug-receptor reaction. *J Gen Physiol., 69,* 497–515.

Hille, B. (1992). Mechanisms of block. In *Ionic channels of excitable membranes* pp. 390–422. Sunderland, MA. Sinauer Associates, Inc.

Hille, B. and Schwarz, W. (1978). Potassium channels as multi-ion single-file pores. *J Gen Physiol., 72,* 409–42.

Hockermann, G. H., Johnson, B. D., Scheuer, T. and Catterall, W. A. (1995). Molecular determinants of high affinity phenylalkylamine block of L-type calcium channels. *J Biol Chem., 270,* 22119–22.

Hockerman, G. H., Peterson, B. Z., Johnson, B. D. and Catterall, W. A. (1997). Molecular determinants of drug binding and action on L-type calcium channels. *Annu Rev Pharmacol Toxicol., 37,* 361–96.

Hodgkin, A. L. and Huxley, A. F. (1952). A quantitative description of membrane current and its application to conduction and excitation in nerve. *J Physiol., 117,* 500–44.

Hofmann, F., Lacinova, L. and Klugbauer, N. (1999). Voltage-dependent calcium channels: from structure to function. *Rev Physiol Biochem Pharmacol., 139,* 33–87.

Hogan, K. (1998). The anesthetic myopathies and malignant hyperthermias. *Curr Opin Neurol., 11,* 469–76.

Ito, H., Klugbauer, N. and Hofmann, F. (1997). Transfer of the high affinity dihydropyridine sensitivity from L-type To non-L-type calcium channel. *Mol Pharmacol., 52,* 735–40.

Jentsch, T. J. (1994). Molecular biology of voltage-gated chloride channels. *Curr Top Membranes, 42,* 35–57.

Ji, S., George, A. L., Horn, R. and Barchi, R. L. (1996). Paramyotonia congenita mutations reveal different roles for segments S3 and S4 of domain D4 in hSkM1 sodium channel gating. *J Gen Physiol., 107,* 183–94.

Joiner, W. J., Tang, M. D., Wang, L. Y., Dworetzky, S. I., Boissard, C. G., Gan, L., Gribkoff, V. K. and Kaczmarek, L. K. (1998). Formation of intermediate-conductance calcium-activated potassium channels by interaction of Slack and Slo subunits. *Nat Neurosci., 1,* 462–9.

Kaczorowski, G. J. and Garcia, M. L. (1999). Pharmacology of voltage-gated and calcium-activated potassium channels. *Curr Opin Chem Biol., 3,* 448–58.

Kambouris, N., Hastings, L., Stepanovic, S., Marban, E., Tomaselli, G. F. and Balser, J. R (1998a). Mechanistic link between local anesthetic action and inactivation gating probed by outer pore mutations in the rat m1 sodium channel. *J Physiol., 512,* 693–705.

Kambouris, N. G., Nuss, H. B., Johns, D. C., Tomaselli, G. F., Marban, E. and Balser, J. R (1998b). Phenotypic characterization of a novel long QT syndrome mutation in the cardiac sodium channel. *Circulation, 97,* 640–4.

Kambouris N. G., Nuss, H. B., Johns, D. C., Marban, E., Tomaselli, G. F. and Balser, J. R. (2000). A revised view of cardiac sodium channel 'blockade' in the long-QT syndrome. *J Clin Invest., 105,* 1133–40.

Kirsch, G. E., Shieh, C. C., Drewe, J. A., Vener, D. F. and Brown, A. M. (1993). Segmental exchanges define 4-aminopyridine binding and the inner mouth of $K^+$ pores. *Neuron, 11,* 503–12.

Lawson, K. (1996). Potassium channel activation: a potential therapeutic approach? *Pharmacol Ther., 70,* 39–63.

Lippens, G., Najib, J., Wodak, S. J. and Tartar, A. (1995). NMR sequential assignments and solution structure of chlorotoxin, a small scorpion toxin that blocks chloride channels. *Biochemistry, 34,* 13–21.

Liu, Y., Jurman, M. E. and Yellen, G. (1996). Dynamic rearrangement of the outer mouth of a K channel during gating. *Neuron, 16,* 859–67.

McPhee, J. C., Ragsdale, D. S., Scheuer, T. and Catterall, W. A. (1994). A mutation in segment IVS6 disrupts fast inactivation of sodium channels. *Proc Natl Acad Sci., 91,* 12346–50.

Mickelson, J. R. and Louis, C. F. (1996). Malignant hyperthermia: excitation-contraction coupling, $Ca^{2+}$ release channel, and cell $Ca^{2+}$ regulation defects. *Physiol Rev., 76,* 537–92.

Monod, J., Wyman, J. and Changeux, J.-P. (1965). On the nature of allosteric transitions: a plausible model. *J Mol Biol., 12,* 88–118.

Nuss, H. B., Kambouris, N. G., Marban, E., Tomaselli,

G. F. and Balser, J. R. (2000). Isoform-specific lidocaine block of sodium channels explained by differences in gating. *Biophys J.,* **78**, 200–10.

O'Leary, M. E., Kallen, R. G. and Horn, R. (1994). Evidence for a direct interaction between internal tetra-alkylammonium cations and the inactivation gate of cardiac sodium channels. *J Gen Physiol.,* **104**, 523–39.

Palnitkar, S. S., Mickelson, J. R., Louis, C. F. and Parness, J. (1997). Pharmacological distinction between dantrolene and ryanodine binding sites: evidence from normal and malignant hyperthermia-susceptible porcine skeletal muscle. *Biochem J.,* **326** (Pt 3), 847–52.

Peterson, B. Z., Tanada, T. N. and Catterall, W. A. (1996). Molecular determinants of high affinity dihydropyridine binding in L-type calcium channels. *J Biol Chem.,* **271**, 5293–6.

Pichler, M., Wang, Z., Grabner-Weiss, C. *et al.* (1996). Block of P/Q-type calcium channels by therapeutic concentrations of aminoglycoside antibiotics. *Biochemistry,* **35**, 14659–64.

Ragsdale, D. S., McPhee, J. C., Scheuer, T. and Catterall, W. A. (1994). Molecular determinants of state-dependent block of $Na^+$ channels by local anesthetics. *Science,* **265**, 1724–8.

Ragsdale, D. S., McPhee, J. C., Scheuer, T. and Catterall, W. A. (1996). Common molecular determinants of local anesthetic, antiarrhythmic, and anticonvulsant block of voltage-gated $Na^+$ channels. *Proc. Natl. Acad. Sci USA,* **93**, 9270–5.

Rosenfeld, J., Sloan-Brown, K., and George, A. L., Jr (1997). A novel muscle sodium channel mutation causes painful congenital myotonia. *Ann Neurol.,* **42**, 811–4.

Santoro, B., Liu, D. T., Yao, H. *et al.* (1998). Identification of a gene encoding a hyperpolarization-activated pacemaker channel of brain. *Cell,* **93**, 717–29.

Schuster, A., Lacinova, L., Klugbauer, N., Ito, H., Birnbaumer, L. and Hofmann, F. (1996). The IVS6 segment of the L-type calcium channel is critical for the action of dihydropyridines and phenylalkylamines. *Embo J.,* **15**, 2365–70.

Scott, R. H., Sutton, K. G., Griffin, A., Stapleton, S. R., and Currie, K. P. (1995). Aspects of calcium-activated chloride currents: a neuronal perspective. *Pharmacol Ther.,* **66**, 535–65.

Soroceanu, L., Gillespie, Y., Khazaeli, M. B. and Sontheimer, H. (1998). Use of chlorotoxin for targeting of primary brain tumors. *Cancer Res.,* **58**, 4871–9.

Soroceanu, L., Manning, T. J., Jr. and Sontheimer, H. (1999). Modulation of glioma cell migration and invasion using Cl(−) and K(+) ion channel blockers. *J Neurosci.,* **19**, 5942–54.

Stefani, A., Spadoni, F. and Bernardi, G. (1997). Voltage-activated calcium channels: targets of antiepileptic drug therapy? *Epilepsia,* **38**, 959–65.

Strichartz, G. R. (1973). The inhibition of sodium currents in myelinated nerve by quarternary derivatives of lidocaine. *J Gen Physiol.,* **62**, 37–57.

Striessnig, J., Grabner, M., Mitterdorfer, J., Hering, S., Sinnegger, M. J. and Glossmann, H. (1998). Structural basis of drug binding to L $Ca^{2+}$ channels. *Trends Pharmacol Sci.,* **19**, 108–15.

Sunami, A., Dudley, S. C. Jr. and Fozzard, H. A. (1997). Sodium channel selectivity filter regulates antiarrhythmic drug binding. *Proc Natl Acad Sci U S A,* **94**, 14126–31.

Sutko, J. L., Airey, J. A., Welch, W. and Ruest, L. (1997). The pharmacology of ryanodine and related compounds. *Pharmacol Rev.,* **49**, 53–98.

Tricarico, D., Servidei, S., Tonali, P., Jurkat-Rott, K. and Camerino, D. C. (1999). Impairment of skeletal muscle adenosine triphosphate-sensitive $K^+$ channels in patients with hypokalemic periodic paralysis. *J Clin Invest.,* **103**, 675–82.

Triggle, D. J. (1999). The pharmacology of ion channels: with particular reference to voltage- gated $Ca^{2+}$ channels. *Eur J Pharmacol.,* **375**, 311–25.

Valverde, M. A., Rojas, P., Amigo, J., Cosmelli, D., Orio, P., Bahamonde, M. I., Mann, G. E., Vergara, C. and Latorre, R. (1999). Acute activation of Maxi-K channels (hSlo) by estradiol binding to the beta subunit. *Science,* **285**, 1929–31.

Vedantham, V. and Cannon, S. C. (1999). The position of the fast-inactivation gate during lidocaine block of voltage-gated $Na^+$ channels. *J Gen Physiol.,* **113**, 7–16.

Vergara, C., Latorre, R., Marrion, N. V., and Adelman, J. P. (1998). Calcium-activated potassium channels. *Curr Opin Neurobiol.,* **8**, 321–9.

Wang, D. W., Yazawa, K., Makita, N., George, A. L. and Bennett, P. B. (1997). Pharmacological targeting of long QT mutant sodium channels. *J Clin Invest.,* **99**, 1714–20.

Weckbecker, K., Wurz, A., Mohammadi, B. *et al.* (2000). Different effects of mexiletine on two mutant sodium channels causing paramyotonia congenita and hyperkalemic periodic paralysis. *Neuromuscul Disord.,* **10**, 31–9.

West, J., Patton, D., Scheuer, T.,. Wang, Y., Goldin, A. L. and Catterall, W. A. (1992). A cluster of hydrophobic amino acid residues required for fast $Na^+$-channel inactivation. *Proc Natl Acad Sci. USA,* **89**, 10910–4.

White, M. M. and Aylwin, M. (1990). Niflumic and flufenamic acids are potent reversible blockers of $Ca^{2+}$-activated Cl- channels in *Xenopus* oocytes. *Mol Pharmacol.,* **37**, 720–4.

Woodhull, A. M. (1973). Ionic blockage of sodium channels in nerve. *J Gen Physiol.,* **61**, 687–708.

Yang, N., Ji, S., Zhou, M., Ptacek, L. J., Barchi, R. L., Horn, R. and George, A. L. (1994). Sodium channel mutations in paramyotonia congenita exhibit similar biophysical phenotypes *in vitro. Proc Natl Acad Sci.,* **91**, 12785–9.

Yeola, S. W., Rich, T. C., Uebele, V. N., Tamkun, M. M. and Snyders, D. J. (1996). Molecular analysis of a binding site for quinidine in a human cardiac delayed rectifier K channel: role of S6 in antiarrhythmic drug binding. *Circ Res.,* **78**, 1105–14.

Zagotta, W. N. and Siegelbaum, S. A. (1996). Structure and function of cyclic nucleotide-gated channels. *Annu Rev Neurosci.,* **19**, 235–63.

Zucchi, R. and Ronca-Testoni, S. (1997). The sarcoplasmic reticulum $Ca^{2+}$ channel/ryanodine receptor: modulation by endogenous effectors, drugs and disease states. *Pharmacol Rev.,* **49**, 1–51.

# Assessment of channel function (*in vitro* and *in vivo*)

# Techniques for assessing ion channel function; *in vitro*

*Lawrence J. Hayward*

## Introduction

A major goal of electrophysiology, especially in relation to the channelopathies, has been to understand how ion channels operate from a molecular perspective. The occurrence of natural genetic mutations associated with ion channel diseases has highlighted channel variants likely to exhibit diverse functional consequences. A remarkable amount of information has been deduced by channel biophysicists despite the absence of structural data for membrane proteins. While emerging models based on X-ray crystal structures of some ion channels will undoubtedly clarify these mechanisms more precisely, *in vitro* electrophysiological approaches have revealed key insights regarding the dynamics of channel gating, modulation, and ion selectivity.

Advances in molecular genetics over the past decade have vastly expanded the known repertoire of unique ion channels while also defining complete sets of channel genes for some simple organisms. Molecular biological methods have enabled the engineering of specific ion channel modifications to test hypotheses regarding channel expression, structure, and function. A similar degree of progress in electrophysiological techniques, most notably the proliferation of the patch-clamp method and improved instrumentation for recording and data analysis, has increased the availability of these powerful tools and the range of problems that can be addressed.

This great variety of approaches can easily overwhelm those without practical experience who are interested in interpreting the channelopathy literature or in devising original experimental strategies. The goal of this chapter is to provide an introduction to *in vitro* electrophysiological methods, including a brief historical overview and a discussion of advantages and limitations for each technique. Further practical and theoretical aspects of electrophysiological recording have been thoroughly reviewed in several guides (Kettenmann and Grantyn, 1992; Rudy and Iverson, 1992; Sherman-Gold, 1993; Sakmann and Neher, 1995; Conn, 1998, 1999).

## Ions and excitability

Long before DNA encoding ion channels was envisioned, physiologists understood the importance of ionic fluxes in maintaining the excitability of nerve and muscle tissue. Sidney Ringer's experiments during the 1880s demonstrated that frog heart muscle must be perfused with a solution containing a particular balance of Na, K, and Ca salts in order to continue beating. In 1888, the physical chemist Walter Nernst used thermodynamic principles to explain the generation of electrical potentials by diffusion of an electrolyte in solution across a selectively permeable membrane. At equilibrium, net diffusion of the permeable ion down its concentration gradient was just balanced by the opposing electrical force produced by charge transfer of the ion across the membrane. Nernst formulated a simple expression to relate the concentration ratio and valence of a permeable ion, $X^{+z}$, to the voltage difference between the two solutions at equilibrium:

$$E_X = RT/zF \ln([X]_1/[X]_2),$$

where $E_X$ is the equilibrium potential, R is the gas constant, T is the absolute temperature, $z$ is the valence of the ion, and F is the Faraday constant. By the early 1900s, Julius Bernstein had proposed that excitable cells are composed of membranes that are selectively permeable to K ions at rest and that the membrane permeability to other ions increases during excitation. For a cell permeable only to ion $X^{+z}$, the Nernst equation simplifies, at 22 °C, to

$$E_X = 58/z \log_{10}([X]_o/[X]_i),$$

where $E_X$ is expressed in millivolts (mV) and $[X]_o/[X]_i$ is the ratio of the outside to inside ion concentrations. Bernstein's hypothesis predicted that a cell with an internal concentration of K, for example, that is 35-fold greater than the external concentration would have a resting membrane potential (inside minus outside) of about −90 mV if the membrane were selectively permeable to K ions alone. Subsequent determination of the ionic composition of the cytoplasm and the extracellular fluid for excitable cells revealed that the intracellular K ion concentration was indeed much greater than that of the blood, while the opposite was true for Na and Cl ions. In addition, the cytoplasm was shown to contain significant amounts of organic anions, primarily amino acids and proteins. These concentration gradients required for excitation were later shown to be maintained by ion pumps or coupled cotransport and exchange mechanisms.

According to Bernstein's idea, if the membrane somehow underwent 'breakdown' and became transiently permeable to other ions, the internal negativity would be lost. However, because some physiologists did not believe that cell membranes even existed, while others thought that nerve impulses resulted from chemical reactions, more information about the membrane impedance during excitation was clearly needed. Membrane impedance is determined by a combination of conductance (the ease of current flow) and capacitance (a measure of how much charge must be transferred from one conductor to another to produce a potential). Conductance, $g$, (measured in units of siemens, S) is the reciprocal of resistance and is defined by Ohm's law: $I = gE$, where I is the current flow through a conductor and E is the voltage difference across the conductor. Capacitance in biological membranes, which slows the

speed of membrane charging, arises from the insulating properties of thin lipid bilayers. A value for the cell capacitance of 1 $\mu F/cm^2$ is typically used to estimate the plasma membrane surface area from measured capacitive transients and thus to determine current densities.

## Current clamp recording

The development of hand-pulled glass capillary electrodes in the early 1900s set the stage for the first direct attempts to measure potentials across cellular membranes in the 1920s. Using the squid giant axon preparation and a Wheatstone impedance bridge circuit, Kenneth Cole and Howard Curtis later demonstrated that the membrane conductance increased about 40-fold during electrical activity without a significant change in membrane capacitance (Cole and Curtis, 1939). By 1949, the penetrating microelectrode was perfected with a tip diameter of about 0.5 $\mu m$, which was fine enough to impale fragile animal cells without causing appreciable damage. When filled with a strong electrolyte such as 3 M KCl, this type of electrode had a high resistance, usually between 5 and 40 MΩ, and was connected to an amplifier via a Ag/AgCl wire (Figure 4.1A). Advances in the design of recording amplifiers with input resistances much higher than the electrode resistance allowed intracellular recording of resting and action potentials from nerve and muscle cells.

In a current clamp experiment, a constant or time-varying current is applied to mimic a synaptic input, and the resulting change in membrane potential is recorded. Current clamp methods are useful today for cellular neurophysiologists interested in measuring properties of the action potential and electrical signalling in native tissues. Because a small change in ionic current can have a large effect on the action potential, this technique is highly sensitive to detect functionally important perturbations, such as an increased susceptibility to myotonia in muscle fibres.

Figure 4.1A illustrates a basic current clamp recording configuration used to measure the resting potential or the membrane voltage response to current injection. A standard current clamp employs a unity gain buffer amplifier, also called a

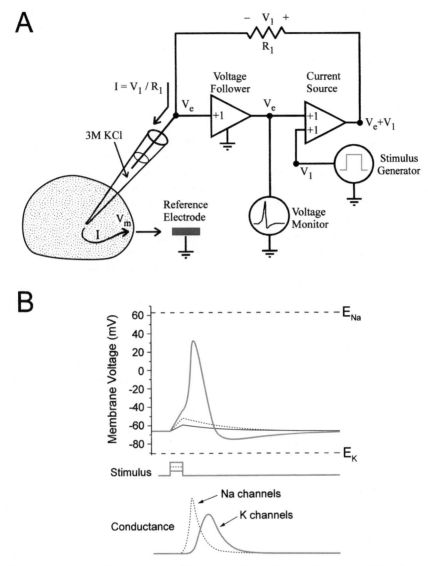

**Figure 4.1** A current clamp amplifier may be used to measure the resting membrane potential or the response of the membrane voltage to an injection of current. (A) A microelectrode filled with 3M KCl is connected by a wire to a unity gain (+1) voltage follower to measure the voltage at the electrode, $V_e$, with respect to a reference electrode in the recording solution. The voltage follower ideally draws no input current and effectively isolates the voltage monitor from the cell. A second amplifier acts as a current source by adding to $V_e$ the signal defined by the output of a stimulus generator, $V_1$, and then directing the resulting current flow into the microelectrode. The amount of injected current, $I = V_1/R_1$, is independent of $V_e$ and can be clamped to a desired value. When $I = 0$, the resting potential is measured. A compensating circuit known as a bridge balance (not shown) subtracts the voltage drop across the pipette from $V_e$ to yield the true membrane voltage, $V_m$. (B) Injection of subthreshold current stimuli into an excitable cell elicits only passive electrotonic responses of the membrane voltage (thin lines). A slightly larger current injection triggers the production of an action potential (thick lines). During an action potential, voltage-dependent Na channels open rapidly, which shifts $V_m$ toward the equilibrium potential for Na($E_{Na}$). The response is terminated by rapid inactivation of the Na conductance and delayed opening of K channels, which both repolarize the membrane (lower traces). The underlying Na and K conductances (lower traces) cannot be measured using the current clamp but, instead, were derived from voltage clamp measurements by Hodgkin and Huxley.

voltage follower, that compares the potential difference between a microelectrode inserted into a cell and a reference electrode in the bath solution. A second amplifier can superimpose the waveform from a stimulus generator to direct a user-defined current pulse into the preparation. Figure 4.1B shows possible responses of the membrane voltage ($V_m$) to an injection of positive current into the cell. Prior to current injection, the clamp measures the resting potential, which is mainly influenced by the resting conductances for K and Na. A small injected current (thin lines) produces only passive depolarization of $V_m$, known as an electrotonic potential, that remains below the threshold for opening an appreciable number of voltage-gated Na channels. In contrast, a larger injected current (thick line) depolarizes the membrane to open enough Na channels to trigger an action potential. The action potential occurs in an all-or-none fashion because the Na conductance eventually produces an inward Na current that overcomes the stabilizing outward K and leakage currents. This causes a further depolarization toward the equilibrium potential for Na (+60 mV), which quickly opens many more Na channels (Figure 4.1B). Termination of the action potential is produced by both the inactivation of Na channels, which rapidly progress to a non-conducting refractory state, and by the repolarizing influence of voltage-dependent K channels, which activate more slowly than Na channels and bring $V_m$ toward the equilibrium potential for K. The essential changes in membrane permeability for Na and K channels that were used to simulate the action potential appear at the bottom of Figure 4.1B, but their derivation as a function of voltage required a method in which ion currents could be directly measured while the membrane was held at fixed voltages defined by the investigator.

## Voltage clamp recording

In the late 1940s, Alan Hodgkin and Andrew Huxley further developed the voltage clamp technique invented by Marmont and Cole and applied it to the squid giant axon preparation. By 1952, well before ion channel proteins were identified, they provided the first complete account of voltage-dependent ionic mechanisms that underlie the action potential. Their quantitative mathematical model to describe the temporal and voltage dependence of the membrane conductance changes for Na and K ions during an action potential (Hodgkin and Huxley, 1952) is still very useful today.

A voltage clamp amplifier regulates the membrane potential at a command voltage, $V_c$, by using a negative feedback loop to measure and inject an amount of current equal and opposite to the ionic current that flows through open channels (Figure 4.2A). In a two-electrode voltage clamp, one electrode measures the membrane potential and another passes current. The constant membrane voltage minimizes transient capacitive currents and prevents regenerative effects such as the production of action potentials. Moreover, by preventing current flow from changing the voltage, the voltage clamp isolates the time-dependent phenomena from the voltage-dependent effects. By using one of several pulse protocols and recording configurations to apply step changes in voltage to the preparation (Figure 4.3), the magnitude and time course of the ionic currents elicited can be examined quantitatively to characterize normal and mutant ion channel function.

Certain imperfections of the voltage clamp should always be considered. First, it is difficult to clamp the voltage uniformly for cells that are elongated in shape, contain fine processes, or are in contact with neighbours. Second, errors introduced by the series resistance of recording pipettes can severely distort current records and can slow the clamp speed. These errors can be reduced by series resistance compensation, which employs positive feedback to overshoot the applied voltage, but this can also introduce ringing. Third, liquid junction potentials at the electrode tip caused by charge separation upon diffusion of anions and cations of different mobilities can result in a voltage offset error, which must be taken into account.

A typical voltage clamp measurement of a Na current elicited by a step depolarization is shown in Figure 4.2B. In this case, a very brief current flows during the voltage shifts, caused by charging of the membrane capacitance (arrows). An inward (negative) ionic Na current follows the transient

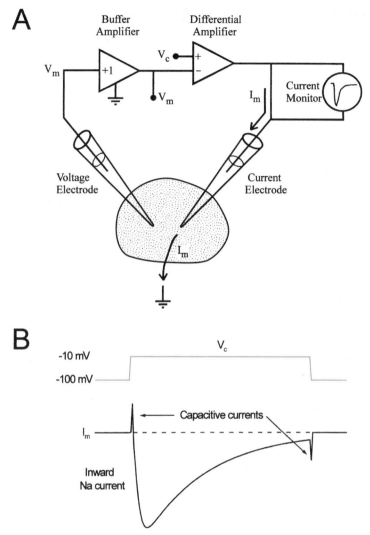

**Figure 4.2** The voltage clamp is very useful for studying the behaviour of many ion channels because it provides experimental control over the membrane voltage that underlies channel gating. A simplified two-microelectrode configuration is depicted in (A). One electrode records the membrane voltage, $V_m$, while the other electrode injects current. A differential amplifier compares $V_m$ to the command voltage, $V_c$, and injects a current proportional to their difference. This current acts to hold $V_m$ equal to $V_c$ and is of the same magnitude, but opposite sign, as the current that flows across the cell membrane, $I_m$. (B) The membrane current, $I_m$, contains both capacitive and ionic components. The capacitive currents appear as brief transients (arrows) that indicate the time needed to charge the membrane upon a shift of $V_c$. The speed of the transient depends on the membrane capacitance and the series resistance of the current electrode. Ionic current flow, proportional to the membrane conductance, can be either inward (downward) or outward (upward).

and reflects the sum of currents through all open channels in the cell membrane. This superimposition of thousands of discrete channel openings is referred to as a 'macroscopic' current to distin-

guish it from a single-channel current. Important aspects of channel gating and permeation can be measured by observing the dependence of macroscopic currents upon membrane voltage.

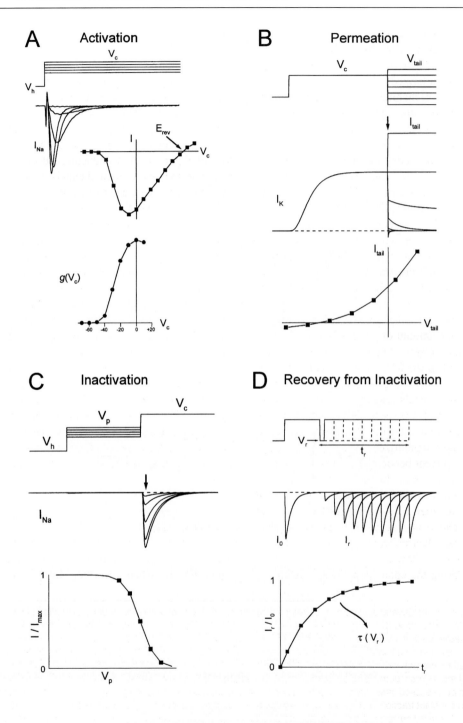

Figure 4.3 (A–D) illustrates some of the more commonly used voltage clamp pulse sequences, typical macroscopic current responses, and standard formats for summarizing voltage-dependent properties.

## Activation gating

The simplest pulse protocol measures voltage-dependent opening, or activation gating, of ion channels. Because many channels are opened by depolarization, activation is usually characterized by measuring current flow for a series of voltage shifts from a constant negative holding voltage, $V_h$, to more depolarized command potentials, $V_c$ (Figure 4.3A). For channels that do not inactivate, the extent of activation can be measured as the plateau current amplitude at a fixed time after depolarization to $V_c$ (isochronal activation). The peak current amplitude, on the other hand, is typically measured for currents that inactivate, such as the Na currents in Figure 4.3A. With stronger depolarizations, the activation process occurs faster and the peak current occurs earlier. The time required to reach half of the peak current or the rise time between 10% and 90% of the peak may be obtained from the raw current traces to describe the speed of activation as a function of voltage.

A plot of the current-voltage relationship, I(V), summarizes the amount of current flow for a given depolarization voltage (Figure 4.3A). It is important to realize that the I(V) measurement combines the effects of channel gating and current flow through open channels. For the I(V) plot of a Na current, note that the peak inward current approaches zero and then becomes outward (positive) at strongly depolarized voltages. The voltage at which the current becomes zero is known as the reversal potential, $E_{rev}$. In this case, if Na is the only permeant ion and is present at physiological concentrations, then $E_{rev} = E_{Na} \approx +60$ mV. Even though Na channels may be open at the reversal potential, the electrochemical driving force is zero, so no current flows.

In considering the channelopathies, it is conve- nient to remove the effect of the driving force to compare whether mutations alter the voltage-de- pendent activation gating properties of a channel. A simple representation of channel activation is the conductance as a function of voltage, g(V), which is defined by Ohm's law as the current amplitude, I(V), divided by the electrochemical driving potential ($V - E_{rev}$), as shown at the bot- tom of Figure 4.3A. Conductance differences be- tween normal and mutant channels are quantitated in terms of the voltage at which the conductance is half-maximal and the steepness, with respect to $V_c$, of the transition from closed to maximally open channels. These parameters are usually re- ported by fitting the normalized conductance curve to a sigmoidal Boltzmann function. In this example, a small fraction of Na channels open after a depolarization to $-40$ mV, half of the maximal fraction of channels open at $-25$ mV, while the largest fraction will open at $0$ mV or greater (Figure 4.3A, bottom graph). Note that because all channels are not necessarily open at the time of the peak current, the g(V) curve yields only a relative measure of the extent of channel opening. One would need to know the total num- ber of channels in the membrane and the single- channel conductance to determine the absolute fraction of open channels, $p_{open}(V)$, from the g(V) data.

## Permeation

The macroscopic current that is measured over time, I(V, t), when recording from a set of *n*

**Figure 4.3** (opposite) Several voltage clamp protocols can be employed to measure ion channel activation (A), relative permeation (B), inactivation (C), and recovery from inactivation (D). (A) To measure voltage-dependent activation of Na currents, for example, the membrane voltage is depolarized from a holding potential, $V_h$, to a range of command potentials, $V_c$, and the resulting current is recorded. The peak current as a function of $V_c$ can be displayed as an I(V) plot and compared for normal and mutant channels. The relative conductance, $g(V) = I(V)/(V - E_{rev})$, can be calculated from the I(V) plot if the reversal potential, $E_{rev}$, is known (bottom graph). (B) The relative amount of current flow through open channels can be assessed independent of gating conformational changes by measuring tail currents. For this example of a K current, a constant fraction of channels is opened by an initial depolarization to $V_c$. By then shifting the voltage to $V_{tail}$ and recording the initial currents, the ease of current flow with respect to the driving force can be assessed. In this case, the response is highly non-linear, and inward currents are strongly disfavoured. (C) Inactivation can be measured in terms of channel availability following a depolarizing prepulse, $V_p$. Availability is assessed after the prepulse by stepping the voltage to a fixed $V_c$ and comparing the peak current elicited to that obtained in the absence of a prepulse. (D) Recovery from inactivation is determined using a double-pulse protocol in which the first pulse inactivates channels, a variable time is allowed for recovery at $V_r$, and the second pulse assesses the degree of recovery attained. For each $V_r$, a recovery rate, $\tau(V_r)$, can be obtained by fitting the recovery curve to one or more exponential functions.

identical ion channels in a membrane depends on both gating (opening and closing over time) and permeation (ease of current flow for a particular ion through an open channel), both of which may be voltage-dependent. This can be expressed as:

$$I(V, t) = n \times p_{open}(V, t) \times i(V),$$

where $p_{open}(V, t)$ represents the channel open probability over time (gating) and $i(V)$ represents the current that would flow through a single open channel (time-independent permeation) at a voltage, V. One way to distinguish experimentally between gating and permeation is to perform single-channel patch-clamp recording (see below). Thousands of records will yield detailed statistical information about open times, shut times, and the amount of current that flows through a single open channel or possible subconductance states. However, certain voltage clamp protocols for macroscopic currents can also provide data to separate the contributions of gating and permeation to the total ionic current.

Permeation can be examined in the absence of gating changes by measuring tail currents that reflect $i(V)$, also known as the instantaneous current vs. voltage curve. For the example of a K current in Figure 4.3B, channels are activated by a depolarizing voltage pulse, $V_c$, of fixed voltage and duration. At the end of the pulse, the voltage is then stepped to a series of different values, $V_{tail}$, which shifts the driving force for current flow immediately but does not allow time for any conformational changes in conductance of the channel proteins to occur. The tail current measured immediately following the voltage shift to $V_{tail}$ (Figure 4.3B, arrow) is proportional to $i(V_{tail})$, since $p_{open}(V_c, t)$ and $n$ remain constant for all trials. An advantage of this measurement is that it requires no assumptions about whether permeation is ohmic (linear with voltage) or non-linear, which is usually the case when the ionic concentration gradient across the membrane is asymmetrical (Figure 4.3B, bottom).

A given ion channel may be permeable to more than one type of ion. Even highly selective voltage-gated channels cannot completely exclude other physiological ions from passage. Other channels, such as the nicotinic acetylcholine re-

ceptor of the muscle endplate, discriminate poorly among small cations but can effectively exclude anions. The ionic selectivity, or relative permeability of a particular channel to ion A vs. ion B, can be calculated by measuring the change in reversal potential, $\Delta E_{rev}$, of the current upon substituting ion B for ion A in the recording bath. Under conditions in which the cytoplasmic ion concentrations remain constant and the ions A and B have the same charge, it can be shown that:

$$\Delta E_{rev} = \Delta E_{rev,B} - \Delta E_{rev,A} = RT/zF$$

$$\times \ln\{(P_B \times [B]_o)/(P_A \times [A]_o)\},$$

from which the permeability ratio, $(P_B/P_A)$, can be found given the extracellular concentrations of ion A and B. This method was used to show that Na channels are typically 10–20 times more permeable to Na than to K, while certain K channels allow K ions to pass > 100-fold more easily than Na ions.

## Gating currents

Voltage-gated channels sense changes in the membrane potential and respond by moving charged components of the channel to open or close the ion-conducting pore. This concept predicts that even before the pore opens, a small current should be detected arising from the movement of these gating charges within the electric field. Hodgkin and Huxley predicted that such gating currents should be detectable using the voltage clamp, but they were not actually measured until the 1970s (Armstrong and Bezanilla, 1973; Schneider and Chandler, 1973). Because gating currents are very fast and very small compared to ionic currents, they are best measured in the presence of ionic current blockers in preparations with high channel densities. Gating currents have provided useful data to interpret transitions that occur among nonconducting states and may also be important for certain physiological processes such as the coupling of excitation to contraction in muscle. For example, Armstrong and Bezanilla (1977) used gating current measurements to show that the return of Na channel voltage sensors to their fully 'closed' position (deactivation) upon repolarization required the relief of the inactivation process. This supported their hypothesis that Na channel fast inactivation represented a conformational change distinct from the reversal of activation gating.

## Separation of currents

When a cell membrane contains more than one type of channel, several approaches can be used to isolate the desired current. For instance, reversible blocking agents that act from the outside or inside of the membrane may be added to the recording solutions to remove specific interfering currents. Several useful inhibitors include tetraethylammonium (TEA), which blocks many different types of K channels with different affinities, tetrodotoxin (TTX), which binds to some voltage-sensitive Na channels with high affinity, and a variety of marine snail conotoxins that can block certain Na or Ca channels. (For a review of toxins and drugs relevant to ion channel electrophysiology, see Narahashi and Herman, 1992.) Some channels are effectively blocked by ions such as $Ba^{2+}$, $Co^{2+}$, $Cs^+$, $Mn^{2+}$, or $Zn^{2+}$ or by small metabolites, such as adenosine triphosphate (ATP). For instance, the impermeable $Cs^+$ ion is frequently substituted for $K^+$ in the recording solution to eliminate K currents. Another approach to reveal a current in isolation is to subtract currents obtained in the presence from those obtained in the absence of a specific inhibitor to the channel of interest.

Other methods to separate currents do not require pharmacological intervention or solution changes. For example, it is sometimes possible to manipulate the holding voltage to induce inactivation of interfering channels. In other cases, tail currents for the channel of interest may be measured at the reversal potential of the interfering current, where no flow for that ion occurs. The voltage protocol is designed such that either $V_c$ or the pulse duration, t, is variable and $V_{tail} = E_{rev}$ remains constant. Under these conditions, $i(V_{tail})$ is also constant, and the initial value of the tail current is proportional to $p_{open}(V_c, t)$.

## Inactivation gating

In addition to affecting activation, mutations associated with channelopathies may perturb inactivation gating of certain channels. The voltage dependence of macroscopic current decay is a very useful measurement and is easily obtained by fitting the declining phase to one or more exponential functions. In some cases, mutations can produce dramatic changes in the decay rate and have clarified the role of channel structural components in activation and inactivation gating processes. However, it should be remembered that macroscopic currents alone generally do not provide enough information to specify uniquely the component activation and inactivation rates. The decay of macroscopic Na currents, for instance, depends on both the rate of channel activation and the rate of progression of open channels to inactivated (refractory) states. A channel with rapid activation and relatively slow inactivation can produce a macroscopic current profile almost indistinguishable from a channel with slow activation and fast inactivation (Hille, 1992). Supplementary data obtained from other methods, such as measurement of single channel kinetics or gating currents may be required to specify more completely rates between different kinetic states in functional gating models.

Because the number of available channels in a tissue can have dramatic effects on excitability, electrophysiologists studying the channelopathies are very interested in the mechanisms by which channels may be recruited when needed or temporarily sidelined when present in excess. Na channels, for instance, normally inactivate and become unavailable to open when the membrane is held at depolarized potentials. This helps produce the refractory period and can affect the firing rate of action potentials. On the other hand, at strongly hyperpolarized potentials, more Na channels become available to open upon a subsequent depolarization. The degree of inactivation is sharply voltage dependent, so that for normal Na channels, even small changes in the resting potential can have a large effect upon channel availability. To measure whether mutations associated with disease alter the availability of channels to open, a prepulse to varying voltages ($V_p$) is applied for a fixed duration, and the peak current that is available following the prepulse is assayed by an activation pulse to a fixed $V_c$, as shown in Figure 4.3C. A plot of the relative peak currents vs. $V_p$ reflects channel availability and corresponds to the steady-state value of the Hodgkin-Huxley $h$ parameter ($h_\infty$).

Once a channel is inactivated, time is required upon return to hyperpolarized potentials for the channel to recover to an available, but closed, state. The conformational changes that permit recovery from inactivation appear to be strongly voltage dependent. If the inactivated state is destabilized by a mutation, for instance, one might expect a more rapid rate of recovery away from that state at a given voltage. To measure recovery from inactivation, a double-pulse protocol is generally employed (see Figure 4.3D). In the case of Na channels, an initial depolarizing pulse is applied to inactivate the channels, which is followed by hyperpolarization at a constant voltage ($V_r$) to allow partial recovery. The degree of recovery for a given duration at the recovery voltage is assayed by measuring the peak available current during a second depolarizing pulse. The rate of recovery at a given voltage can typically be fit by one or more exponential functions, and the rates at several voltages can then be compared for normal and mutant channels.

## Single-channel and patch-clamp recording

The development of patch-clamp recording methods in the late 1970s by Erwin Neher and Bert Sakmann (Neher and Sakmann, 1976) vastly extended the experimental options available to electrophysiologists and permitted the analysis of currents through single ion channels (for a comprehensive review, see Sakmann and Neher, 1995). This was accomplished by measuring minute ionic currents, in the picoampere (pA) range, from channels present in a small patch of membrane attached to the tip of a glass pipette. An extremely low-noise recording was obtained by tightly apposing the pipette against the cell membrane such that a seal resistance of $> 10^9\ \Omega$ was formed. This 'gigaseal' minimized background electrical noise that would otherwise swamp the signal and also prevented voltage division of the stimulus, so that the full command voltage was transmitted to the patch membrane. Resolution of individual channel opening and closing events over time allowed the complete separation of gating and permeation effects and the identification of channel species based on their single-channel conductance. In addition, the patch clamp enabled electrophysiologists to analyse mechanisms of channel gating and modulation in statistical terms and to refine kinetic models that describe distinct channel states.

The original 'cell-attached' gigaseal technique was quickly adapted to allow recording from several different membrane configurations (Hamill et al., 1981), including 'inside-out,' 'outside-out,' and 'whole-cell' arrangements (Figure 4.4). The

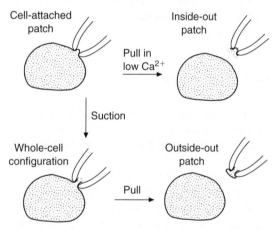

**Figure 4.4** Patch-clamp recording generally refers to the use of 'gigaseal' electrodes for measuring ion currents using any of these configurations (Hamill et al., 1981, and adapted from Hille, 1992, p. 89). In practice, a polished glass pipette filled with recording solution is gently applied to the surface of the cell using a micromanipulator, and suction is applied until a high resistance seal forms between the cell membrane and the glass tip. Small currents between the pipette and cytoplasm can be recorded from such cell-attached patches. After careful suction to the pipette, the membrane patch separating the cell from the pipette interior bursts, and cellular solutes exchange with the pipette solution. This whole-cell configuration allows currents to be recorded through channels residing in the large remaining area of membrane. Withdrawal of the pipette away from the intact cell in the presence of low $Ca^{2+}$ or from the whole-cell configuration forms an inside-out or an outside-out patch, respectively.

popular whole-cell voltage clamp method allows recording of macroscopic currents from small cells using a single electrode, which generally has a low electrode series resistance and allows the cell to be perfused or dialysed intracellularly with drugs or toxins. After recording whole-cell currents, it is possible to obtain mRNA or DNA from the same cell for molecular genetic analysis. A variant of the cell-attached technique, known as perforated patch recording, employs pore-forming substances such as nystatin in the pipette to gain low-resistance access to the cell while preventing diffusion of cellular macromolecules (Horn and Marty, 1988). This allows recording from the whole cell while minimizing the washout of cellular constituents into the pipette that could alter channel function. Disadvantages of this method include a worsened electrode resistance with greater noise, less control of the cytosolic environment, and a significant time lag until access to the cell is achieved.

## Noise analysis

Before single-channel currents could be measured directly, the presence of macroscopic current fluctuations in excess of the background noise provided evidence for the existence of discrete channels. Though individual channel events could not be distinguished once superimposed within macroscopic current records, the analysis of current fluctuations, also known as noise analysis, provided reliable estimates of the single-channel conductance and the peak open probability.

For a homogeneous population of $n$ statistically independent channels that can be either open or closed, $\sigma^2 = i\,I - I^2/n$, where I is the mean macroscopic current at corresponding time points in response to many identical stimulations, $\sigma^2$ is the current variance, and $i$ is the single-channel current amplitude (Sigworth, 1980). Since $\sigma^2$ and I can be extracted from repetitive macroscopic current records containing a range of open probabilities, a plot of $\sigma^2$ vs. I yields a parabola with an initial slope equal to $i$ (since $I^2/n$ can be ignored for very small open probabilities) and a zero-crossing at the maximal current, when $I = i\,n$, from which the number of channels can be

calculated. Given $i$ and $n$, the peak open probability can be determined from the peak macroscopic current.

Noise analysis is still useful today in cases where the patch clamp is not sensitive enough to measure a particular single-channel current (e.g. some Cl channels) or where kinetics may be very fast (e.g. Na channels at physiological temperatures). In addition, the technique is very helpful to estimate the number of channels present in a patch during macropatch recording (see below). However, the existence of a homogeneous channel population with a single conducting state, as assumed for noise analysis, may not always hold true. (For further review of the theory and practical implementation of this method, see Heinemann and Conti, 1992.)

## Native cell preparations

The underlying abnormal currents responsible for some channelopathies were identified through detailed electrophysiological analyses of diseased tissue samples, sometimes well before isolation and characterization of the corresponding ion channels. For example, Shirley Bryant performed studies of membrane conductance in the 1960s using excised intercostal muscle from a strain of congenitally myotonic goats (Bryant, 1969). His results clearly implicated an abnormally reduced Cl conductance as the cause for myotonia of resting muscle fibres in this animal model for myotonia congenita. The same preparation clarified the importance of the T-tubular system in producing repetitive action potentials (Adrian and Bryant, 1974). Another electrophysiological analysis performed by Frank Lehmann-Horn, Reinhardt Rüdel, and Kenneth Ricker (Lehmann-Horn *et al.*, 1987a, b) identified defective inactivation of Na currents in excised muscle samples from patients with hyperkalaemic periodic paralysis and paramyotonia congenita prior to the cloning of the human skeletal muscle Na channel.

Electrophysiological recording from *in vitro* preparations avoids some of the practical difficulties associated with *in vivo* methods that rely on the use of intact invertebrates or mammals. Advantages include direct access to cells, stability of recording, and experimental control of the bath solutions with respect to ionic composition, temperature, oxygenation, and absence of anaesthetics. In some cases, native cells are desirable compared to heterologous expression systems (described below) because they are more likely to contain intact modulatory systems or accessory components that may be required for normal channel function. On the other hand, because a variety of unrelated ion channels may be expressed in native cells at high levels, it is frequently necessary to alter the ionic composition of the bath solution in non-physiological ways or to add channel-blocking toxins to isolate the current of interest. Even under these conditions, one cannot be sure that the observed currents derive from a single type of ion channel or that the physiology of interest has not been perturbed.

Native cell systems can be employed using either intact preparations or cultured dissociated cells. Intact preparations retain some degree of normal cytoarchitecture and neuronal connectivity, which may be critical for experiments that address the role of ion channels in neuronal signalling and synaptic transmission. Intact slice preparations, used for physiological investigations since the early 1970s (Andersen and Langmoen, 1980), can be obtained from a variety of rodent structures, including the hippocampus, neocortex, and cerebellum. Preservation of the laminar organization and synaptic contacts within slices permits selection of well-defined stimulation and recording sites for investigating specific pathways within complex neural circuits. For example, tetanic stimulation of distinct inputs in hippocampal slices has helped to clarify mechanisms of long-term potentiation (LTP) in memory storage (reviewed in Kandel *et al.*, 2000).

To prepare neuronal slices, freshly dissected brain or spinal cord tissue is cut with a vibratome into sections, roughly 0.15–0.50 mm thick, incubated in an oxygenated bath solution for at least 30 minutes, and then transferred to an oxygenated recording chamber. Bipolar extracellular electrodes or micropipettes deliver stimulus pulses from an isolation unit to a specific location in the slice, and patch-clamp methods may be used to record responses from diverse cell types. Organotypic cultures, in which thin neural tissue sections are maintained in culture for up to several weeks, allow preservation of synaptic morphology and many pharmacological phenotypes. The roller tube method (Gahwiler, 1981) results in a flattening of the slice to 1–3 cell diameters over the first week or two *in vitro*, allowing visualization and access to single cells for electrophysiological recording. One advantage of such co-cultures is that multiple cell types present may provide critical influences to direct differentiation or survival of the cells of interest.

Primary cell cultures derived from dissociated tissues allow growth of diverse cell types expressing specific types of channels. Dissociated cultures offer some advantages and disadvantages compared to intact tissues. The elongated geometry of muscle fibres, for instance, prevents synchronous voltage clamping because of the time required for membrane charging along the length of the muscle fibre, while small dissociated myoblasts can be more readily studied. Also, because dissociated cell systems offer excellent accessibility and control of growth conditions over time, the effects of trophic factors or drugs upon ion channel properties can be examined. On the other hand, propagation in culture may alter cellular differentiation or modulation of ion channel function and thereby introduce artefacts. Normal interactions or connections between different cell types may also be disrupted in dissociated cultures. Sometimes mitotic inhibitors, such as cytosine arabinoside (Ara-C) must be added to prevent highly proliferative cells such as fibroblasts from outgrowing the terminally differentiated cells of interest.

## Expression and mutagenesis of ion channels

A variety of heterologous expression systems allow electrophysiologists to study specific ion channels or combinations of channel subunits in the absence of unrelated background activity. Rapidly expanding DNA sequence databases and libraries have accelerated the discovery of new channels and increased the availability of ion channel cDNA clones. Once identified, unique cDNAs may be easily stored, amplified, sequenced, and shared among investigators. Full-length cDNAs may be subcloned into expression plasmids for high-level transcription of mRNA, suitable for microinjection into *Xenopus* oocytes for translation into functional ion channels (see below). Alternatively, the DNA construct itself can be transfected into cultured cell lines to obtain transient expression over several days. Conditions can be established to select for stable integration of the DNA into the genome of the host cell, which may yield clonal cell lines that continuously express high levels of the desired channel.

Site-directed mutagenesis refers to the design of specific mutations within a DNA sequence, often to alter a single amino acid or to modify a restriction enzyme site marker. Mutations are usually chosen based on a structural hypothesis or the location of known mutations correlated to disease states. A number of mutagenesis procedures are commonly employed using custom oligonucleotide primers to generate mutagenic DNA fragments that can be subcloned into an ion channel expression construct (Ling and Robinson, 1997). It is important to verify the presence of a desired mutation and the absence of spurious mutations by sequencing the final DNA construct.

Several additional methods exist to modify ion channels. A powerful strategy to relate channel structure and function involves the substitution of individual residues with the reactive amino acid, cysteine. Ionic currents from these channels can be characterized before and after chemical modification of cysteine residues by agents that introduce charged or bulky groups (Horn, 1998; Karlin and Akabas, 1998). The accessibility of the mutant residues to modifying agents can be probed by following the kinetics of the current change. Related to site-directed mutagenesis is the technique known as epitope tagging, in which a short antigenic amino acid sequence is inserted to allow localization of the channel protein using a specific antibody. Epitope tags may also help to estimate the accessibility of the channel region under various conditions or to assign the topology of specific channel loops. In addition, chimeric channels, which replace a portion of one channel with sequence from another, can delineate functionally important channel domains.

# Expression in *Xenopus* oocytes

Oocytes from *Xenopus laevis*, the South African clawed frog, were shown to translate injected foreign mRNA efficiently into proteins in the early 1970s (Gurdon *et al.*, 1971). The versatility of the oocyte system for expression of ion channels, receptors and transporter proteins from the nervous system was demonstrated in the early 1980s (Gundersen *et al.*, 1983; Miledi *et al.*, 1983). The large diameter of these cells, up to 1.3 mm, allows straightforward injection of mRNA or drugs and electrode penetration for two-electrode voltage clamp recording of expressed channels. In addition, both macropatch recording of currents at high density (see below) or single-channel recording can be achieved using this system. A major advantage of oocytes is the presence of only low-amplitude endogenous channels (the largest being a Ca-activated Cl channel), which allows study of exogenous channels in almost complete isolation. In addition, the cells survive well *in vitro* and can be surgically removed from a donor frog in large numbers without sacrificing the animal.

For two-electrode recording, the advantages of large oocyte size must be weighed against the kinetic limitation of a long time constant for charging of the membrane during voltage clamping. Because the cell membrane is extensively invaginated, the cell capacitance is high, and realistic time resolutions fall in the range of 200 to 1000 $\mu$s. Even with fast amplifier circuitry and capacitive transient compensation, this means that several milliseconds pass before the voltage fully responds to the desired clamp value, so it is difficult to obtain meaningful measurements of fast ion channel kinetics using this configuration. For example, the inactivation of Na currents, which occurs on a millisecond time scale, appears artefactually slowed.

To overcome the limitation of slow membrane charging, the macropatch technique can be used to decrease the effective membrane surface (Stühmer *et al.*, 1987). In this approach, voltage clamping occurs and ionic current flows only across a patch of membrane at the electrode tip, so the time resolution improves to 50–200 $\mu$s. After removal of the thick vitelline envelope, a polished glass pipette, with a tip opening diameter of 1–8 $\mu$m, is placed against the oocyte membrane. Gentle suction is applied to allow giga-ohm seal formation, and a patch recording configuration is chosen. Once formed, patches can be very stable and contain high current densities from expressed channels. Care must be taken to avoid the formation of omega-shaped patches, which limit solution accessibility and voltage control of the membrane surface.

Additional limitations should be considered regarding the oocyte system. For example, expressed channels may not be distributed uniformly over the oocyte membrane surface, and channel densities can be quite variable from patch to patch. The amount and purity of mRNA injected can also introduce variability of channel expression, while seasonal changes can make it more difficult to obtain tight seals in the summer months. Moreover, post-translational modifications may differ in the oocyte compared to mammalian cells, and other channel subunits or modulatory systems required for normal channel function may be absent.

## Transfection of mammalian cells

Expression of cloned ion channels in mammalian cell lines for electrophysiological analysis offers some advantages over the oocyte system. *In vitro* transcription of mRNA is unnecessary, for example, because the DNA construct is directly transfected into the cells. Moreover, the smaller size of the cells allows rapid membrane charging so that whole-cell voltage clamp methods may be employed to resolve fast kinetic events. In the whole-cell configuration, both pipette (internal) and bath (external) recording solutions can be defined, and complete exchange of the intracellular solutes with that of the pipette solution occurs very rapidly. Agonist or inhibitor drugs may be applied quickly to the cell.

Transformed embryonic kidney cells (HEK-293) are commonly used for ion channel expression because they contain low levels of endogenous currents. These cells divide rapidly in serum-fortified media, are fairly easy to maintain in a humidified $CO_2$ incubator, and can be stored frozen for years as low-passage stocks under liquid nitrogen. HEK-293 cells can be transfected with DNA using the simple $CaPO_4$ procedure (Sambrook *et al.*, 1989) or electroporation. High amplitude ionic currents usually appear within 24–48 hours after transient transfection and can persist for about 2–3 days. Even under ideal conditions, the transfection is often less than 50% efficient, so it is very helpful to co-transfect a marker DNA to allow visual identification of successfully transfected cells. For example, a cDNA for the cell surface protein CD8 may be used to allow tagging of transfected cells with small anti-CD8 coated beads (Jurman *et al.*, 1994).

Transfected cells may produce more authentic mammalian currents in some cases compared to oocytes. For example, expression of rat or human Na channel alpha subunits in oocytes without co-expression of the beta subunit yields currents that inactivate abnormally slowly. In contrast, transfection of the alpha subunit alone in HEK-293 cells reveals currents with normal kinetics, although the current density increases about fivefold upon co-transfection of the beta subunit. An endogenous Na channel current of less than 100 pA is present in untransfected cells, while the expressed currents are typically 1–20 nA.

The limitations of heterologous expression systems should be borne in mind. As noted above, some channels require co-expression of accessory subunits or other factors, which may be missing in the chosen expression system. Certain Ca channels, for instance, require co-expression of multiple subunits to produce a characteristic current, and this must often be determined empirically. There is also no guarantee that a mutant DNA construct will encode a functional ion channel that will be correctly targeted to the membrane surface. Moreover, other factors in addition to isolated channel behaviour, such as the cellular architecture, intracellular trafficking, or association with other channels or proteins may contribute to the observed channelopathy phenotype. In such cases, it may be informative to observe channel behaviour in native tissues or to consider computational models in order to appreciate the functional consequences of known electrophysiological defects.

# References

Adrian, R. H. and Bryant, S. H. (1974). On the repetitive discharge in myotonic muscle fibres. *J Physiol.,* **240**, 505–15.

Andersen, P. and Langmoen, I. A. (1980). Intracellular studies on transmitter effects on neurones in isolated brain slices. *Q Rev Biophys.,* **13**, 1–18.

Armstrong, C. M. and Bezanilla, F. (1973). Currents related to movement of the gating particles of the sodium channels. *Nature,* **242**, 459–61.

Armstrong, C. M. and Bezanilla, F. (1977). Inactivation of the sodium channel. II. Gating current experiments. *J Gen Physiol.,* **70**, 567–90.

Bryant, S. H. (1969). Cable properties of external intercostal muscle fibres from myotonic and nonmyotonic goats. *J Physiol.,* **204**, 539–50.

Cole, K. S. and Curtis, H. J. (1939). Electrical impedance of the squid giant axon during activity. *J Gen Physiol.,* **22**, 649–70.

Conn, P. M. (ed.) (1998). Ion Channels Part B. In *Methods in Enzymology,* **293**, pp. 1–805, Academic Press, San Diego, CA.

Conn, P. M. (ed.) (1999). Ion Channels Part C. In *Methods in Enzymology* **294**, pp. 1–788, Academic Press, San Diego, CA.

Gahwiler, B. H. (1981). Organotypic monolayer cultures of nervous tissue. *J Neurosci Methods,* **4**, 329–42.

Gundersen, C. B., Miledi, R. and Parker, I. (1983). Voltage-operated channels induced by foreign messenger RNA in Xenopus oocytes. *Proc R Soc Lond., B* **220**, 131–40.

Gurdon, J. B., Lane, C. D., Woodland, H. R. and Marbaix, G. (1971). Use of frog eggs and oocytes for the study of messenger RNA and its translation in living cells. *Nature,* **233**, 177–82.

Hamill, O. P., Marty, A., Neher, E., Sakmann, B. and Sigworth, F. J. (1981). Improved patch-clamp techniques for high-resolution current recording from cells and cell-free membrane patches. *Pflügers Arch.,* **391**, 85–100.

Heinemann, S. H. and Conti, F. (1992). Nonstationary noise analysis and application to patch clamp recordings. *Methods in Enzymology,* **207**, 131–48.

Hille, B. (1992). In *Ionic channels of excitable membranes*, pp. 490–491, Sinauer, Sunderland, MA.

Hodgkin, A. L. and Huxley, A. F. (1952). A quantitative description of membrane current and its application to conduction and excitation in nerve. *J Physiol.,* **117**, 500–44.

Horn, R. (1998). Explorations of voltage-dependent conformational changes using cysteine scanning. *Methods in Enzymology,* **293**, 145–5.

Horn, R. and Marty, A. (1988). Muscarinic activation of ionic currents measured by a new whole-cell recording method. *J Gen Physiol.,* **92**, 145–59.

Jurman, M. E., Boland, L. M., Liu, Y. and Yellen, G. (1994). Visual identification of individual transfected cells for electrophysiology using antibody-coated beads. *Biotechniques,* **17**, 876–81.

Kandel, E. R., Schwartz, J. H. and Jessell, T. M. (eds). (2000). In *Principles of Neural Science*, pp. 1254–67, McGraw-Hill, New York, NY.

Karlin, A. and Akabas, M. H. (1998). Substituted-cysteine accessibility method. *Methods in Enzymology,* **293**, 123–45.

Kettenmann, H. and Grantyn, R. (eds). (1992). In *Practical Electrophysiological Methods*, pp. 1–449, Wiley-Liss, New York, NY.

Lehmann-Horn, F., Kuther, G., Ricker, K., Grafe, P., Ballanyi, K. and Rüdel, R. (1987a). Adynamia episodica hereditaria with myotonia: a non-inactivating sodium current and the effect of extracellular pH. *Muscle Nerve,* **10**, 363–74.

Lehmann-Horn, F., Rüdel, R. and Ricker, K. (1987b). Membrane defects in paramyotonia congenita (Eulenburg). *Muscle Nerve,* **10**, 633–41.

Ling, M. M. and Robinson, B. H. (1997). Approaches to DNA mutagenesis: an overview. *Anal Biochem.,* **254**, 157–78.

Miledi, R., Parker, I. and Sumikawa, K. (1983). Recording of single gamma-aminobutyrate- and acetylcholine-activated receptor channels translated by exogenous mRNA in Xenopus oocytes. *Proc R Soc Lond., B* **218**, 481–4.

Narahashi, T. and Herman, M. D. (1992). Overview of toxins and drugs as tools to study excitable membrane ion channels: I. Voltage-activated channels. *Methods in Enzymology,* **207**, 620–43.

Neher, E. and Sakmann, B. (1976). Single-channel currents recorded from membrane of denervated frog muscle fibres. *Nature,* **260**, 799–802.

Rudy, B. and Iverson, L. (eds). (1992). Ion Channels. In *Methods in Enzymology,* **207**, pp. 1–917, Academic Press, San Deigo, CA.

Sakmann, B. and Neher, E. (eds). (1995). In *Single-Channel Recording*, pp. 1–700, Plenum Press, New York, NY.

Sambrook, J., Fritsch, E. F. and Maniatis, T. (1989). In *Molecular Cloning: A Laboratory Manual*, Cold Spring Harbor Press, Cold Springs Harbor, NY.

Schneider, M. F. and Chandler, W. K. (1973). Voltage dependent charge movement of skeletal muscle: a possible step in excitation-contraction coupling. *Nature,* **242**, 244–6.

Sherman-Gold, R. (ed.) (1993). In *The Axon guide for electrophysiology and biophysics laboratory techniques*, pp. 1–282, Axon Instruments, Inc, Foster City, CA.

Sigworth, F. J. (1980). The variance of sodium current fluctuations at the node of Ranvier. *J Physiol.,* **307**, 97–129.

Sumer, W., Methfessel, C., Sakmann, B., Noda, M. and Numa, S. (1987). Patch clamp characterization of sodium channels expressed from rat brain cDNA. *Eur Biophys J.,* **14**, 131–8.

# Neurophysiological investigation of channelopathies *in vivo*

*Kerry Mills*

## Introduction

It is now established that the primary abnormality in several human diseases affecting nerve and muscle is dysfunction of ion channels. This chapter is concerned with electrophysiological investigations of these abnormalities *in vivo*. We will consider disorders of peripheral nerve, for example neuromyotonia, now shown to be caused by dysfunction of axonal potassium channels, disorders of the neuromuscular junction such as myasthenia gravis and the Lambert Eaton myasthenic syndrome, and disorders of muscle, for example the periodic paralyses. Although methods for investigation of neuromuscular junction function are well established, newer methods for investigating axonal excitability and hence making inferences about ion channel function in diseases of peripheral nerve will also be described.

## Measurements of axonal excitability *in vivo*

It should be noted from the outset that the measures of axonal excitability to be described refer only to the nerve membrane under the point of stimulation and are therefore applicable only when there is a generalized abnormality of excitability. Conditions such as mulifocal motoneuropathy with conduction block may well be normal unless tested over the focal area of abnormality. This introduces another complication; stimuli applied over a relatively inexcitable region of nerve membrane (e.g. due to demyelination) will preferentially excite adjoining normal nerve segments.

Nevertheless, despite these limitations, progress has recently been made in assessing motor and sensory axon excitability *in vivo*.

## Post impulse excitability changes

When a nerve impulse traverses a myelinated axon, it leaves in its wake a sequence of changes of excitability of the axon membrane. The changes occur both at the nodes of Ranvier and at the internodes and reflect the activity of ion channels. It is well known, for instance, that if a nerve is excited electrically, it becomes, for a short time, inexcitable no matter how intense is the stimulus – the absolute refractory period. Following this, the nerve again becomes excitable but only if the stimulus is more intense than the initial stimulus – the relative refractory period. By using this test paradigm, in which a conditioning stimulus is followed by a test stimulus, it is known that the axon becomes first inexcitable, then is subnormally excitable, then becomes super-excitable, before a final late subexcitability (Figure 5.1). All these changes are highly dependent on the membrane potential of the axon and absolute values can be used as indirect measures of membrane potential. The early subexcitable phase or relative refractory period is due to the voltage dependence of sodium channel inactivation and can be measured as an increase in threshold for 2–3 ms after a nerve impulse. Super-excitability is due to long-lasting passive depolarization of the internodal membrane. The late sub-excitable phase is due to the slow inactivation of slow potassium channels (Bostock *et al.*, 1998).

## Excitability

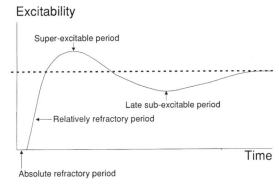

**Figure 5.1** Post impulse excitability changes. Following the passage of a nerve impulse, the axon goes through phases of reduced and increased excitability. Within the first 1–2 ms after the impulse, the axon is inexcitable no matter how strong the stimulus. Excitability then increases and becomes supernormal, the peak of supra-excitability being at about 6 ms. There then follows a longer subexcitable period.

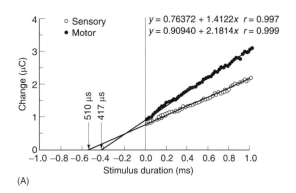

(A)

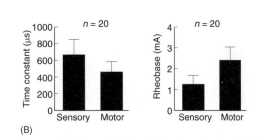

(B)

**Figure 5.2** The calculation of the strength-duration time constants. In A, data from a single subject are plotted as stimulus charge (current × duration) against stimulus duration. The relationship is linear with the intercept on the duration axis indicating the strength-duration time constant and the rheobase being the slope of the regression lines. Data from motor fibres are indicated by closed circles and from sensory fibres by open circles. In B, the mean (±SD) strength-duration time constants from 20 normal subjects in sensory and motor axons are shown as are their rheobases. Strength-duration time constants of sensory fibres are significantly longer than those of motor fibres. (Reproduced from Mogyoros *et al.*, 1996, *Brain*, **119**, 439–447 by permission of Oxford University Press.)

## Strength-duration measurements

The intensity of a stimulus required to activate a single axon or to evoke a defined fraction of the surface recorded compound muscle or sensory action potential depends on its duration. The longer the stimulus then the lower is the required intensity. The relationship between intensity and duration for threshold excitation is very well described empirically by Weiss's law: the stimulus charge (Q), i.e. the multiple of stimulus current (I) and duration (t) is directly proportional to stimulus duration (Figure 5.2). The slope of this linear relationship defines the rheobase and the intercept on the time axis the strength-duration time constant (SDTC), equivalent to the old term, 'chronaxie'. SDTC and rheobase are different in motor and sensory axons, probably because the latter have more prominent persistent nodal sodium channels. SDTC is sensitive to membrane potential being increased by depolarization, but is also influenced by demyelination of the axon.

## Threshold electrotonus

When current of insufficient intensity to initiate an action potential is applied to the nerve, changes in membrane conductance are nevertheless still evident. This is called the local response or electrotonus (Figure 5.3). It can be detected by using a test stimulus to measure the threshold for axon excitation at various times after the start of subthreshold current applications. The resulting plots of threshold change as a function of time after the start of the current application document threshold electrotonus (Figure 5.4). At the onset of current flow, there is a fast reduction in threshold due to rapid depolarization of the nodes of Ranvier. This is followed by a further but slower reduction in threshold due to current flow in the internodal membrane. Threshold reduction is maximal after

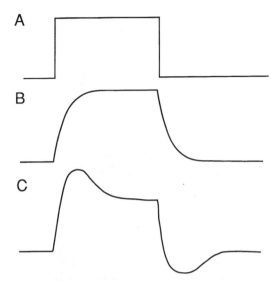

**Figure 5.3** The local response of a nerve fibre. A, a depolarizing current pulse of rectangular waveform applied to a nerve fibre. B, the predicted waveform of current through the nerve membrane assuming the nerve fibre was acting as a passive core conductor. C, the actual current passage through the nerve membrane illustrating the adaptive responses consequent on the interaction of current flow with ion channels.

fully automated (Bostock *et al.*, 1991, 1994; Mogyoros *et al.*, 1997b). For tracking of motor axon excitability, for example, a compound muscle action potential (CMAP) amplitude of say, 30% of the maximum is chosen as a target level and then as successive trials are given, the test stimulus intensity is automatically adjusted to produce the required CMAP amplitude. Using these techniques, the effects on threshold of interleaved depolarizing and hyperpolarizing conditioning currents of various levels can be continuously tracked (Figure 5.5).

## Clinical application of axonal excitability measurements

Measurements of axonal excitability have been made *in vivo* in a number of conditions, e.g. diabetes (Weigl *et al.*, 1989; Horn *et al.*, 1996), amyotrophic lateral sclerosis (ALS) (Bostock *et al.*, 1995; Mogyoros *et al.*, 1998a, b), toxic neuropathies (Schilling *et al.*, 1997), demyelinating neuropathies (Kaji, 1997), carpal tunnel syndrome (Mogyoros *et al.*, 1997a) and neuromyotonia (Maddison *et al.*, 1999).

Horn *et al.* (1996) found abnormalities in diabetic patients, especially those with a peripheral neuropathy; threshold electrotonus to depolarization was indistinguishable from normal but the response to a hyperpolarizing pulse was slower to recover. This difference resembles the difference between normal motor and sensory axons leading to the suggestion that it was due to an abnormality of the inward rectifier channel. Impaired inward rectification might allow hyperpolarization by the sodium pump to develop during high frequency nerve discharge and may be responsible for some of the sensory loss in diabetic neuropathy.

Axonal excitability changes have also been measured in amyotrophic lateral sclerosis since a membrane abnormality was postulated as a cause for fasciculations (a manifestation of motor axon hyperexcitability). However, fasciculations are thought to originate in the distal nerve terminals which may not be amenable to axon excitability measurements. Rather conflicting results have been obtained in ALS. However, in many patients, threshold electrotonus to a depolarizing pulse has

about 20 ms after which a second slow change brings threshold back towards its initial values; this is due to the operation of slow potassium channels, predominately located at the nodes.

Events are slightly different if a hyperpolarizing current is applied. The second slow reduction in threshold is larger and more prolonged and is eventually reversed by a third slow component due to activation of an inward rectifier channel by the hyperpolarization. This is permeable to both potassium and sodium ions, is blocked by calcium ions and is present widely in excitable cells. This channel is also expressed differently in motor and sensory axons and may account for differences in the behaviour of these fibres, to ischaemia, for example. Like the other measures of axon excitability mentioned above, threshold electrotonus is predominantly governed by membrane potential for which it can also act as an indirect measure.

Documentation of threshold electrotonus has been greatly facilitated by the development, by Hugh Bostock, of a tracking protocol which is

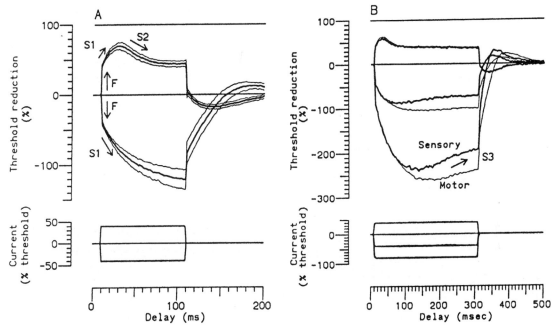

**Figure 5.4** Normal threshold electrotonus waveforms. In A, average motor responses to 100 ms polarizing currents at 40% above and below threshold for 38 subjects are seen. Thick lines indicate the mean, thin lines the mean ±SD. The fast and slow (S1 and S2) components are indicated. In B, a comparison is made between mean motor and sensory responses to a 300 ms current pulse at 40% above and 80% below threshold from 8 subjects showing the additional component of threshold electrotonus (S3) due to inward rectification activated by hyperpolarization. The different behaviour of motor and sensory axons to hyperpolarizing pulses can be seen. (Reproduced from Bostock *et al.*, 1998, *Muscle & Nerve,* **21**, 137–158, by permission of John Wiley & Sons Inc.)

been found to be exaggerated (Figure 5.5), described as 'fanning out' of the threshold electrotonus wave forms (Bostock, 1997).

## Neuromyotonia

Neuromyotonia (NMT) is a condition of spontaneous continuous muscle activity of peripheral nerve origin. Clinically, this is characterized by muscle twitching at rest (myokymia), cramps, which can be triggered by voluntary muscle contraction, and muscle stiffness. The clinical features are described in detail in Chapter 14. The syndrome, originally described as continuous muscle fibre activity (Isaacs, 1961), is now referred to as acquired neuromyotonia (Newsom-Davis and Mills, 1993). The peripheral nerve origin of neuromyotonia is established by:

1. Its persistence after proximal nerve block
2. No change during general anaesthesia, and
3. Complete block by a neuromuscular blocking agent such as curare.

Acquired neuromyotonia is an autoimmune disorder with antibodies to voltage-gated potassium channels detected by immunoprecipition in some 50% of patients and by an improved method in 100% (Hart *et al.*, 1997). The antibodies interfere with the function of the neuronal voltage-gated potassium channels allowing the nerve fibres to discharge repetitively and produce the symptoms of neuromyotonia.

The strength-duration time constants of motor and sensory nerve fibres have been measured in nine patients with acquired neuromyotonia (Maddison *et al.*, 1999). In contrast to healthy controls, four patients had motor SDTCs greater

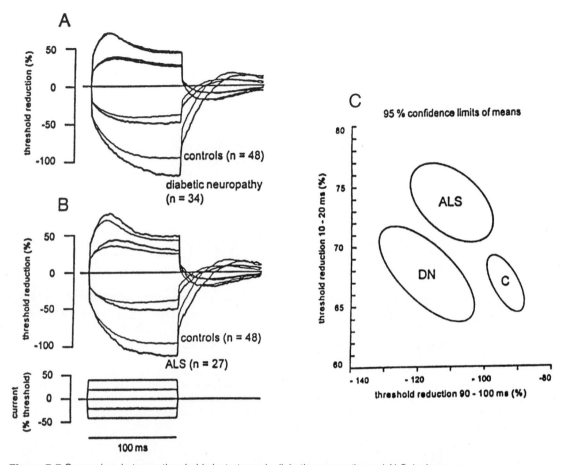

**Figure 5.5** Comparison between threshold electrotonus in diabetic neuropathy and ALS. In A are seen mean responses from 34 patients with diabetic neuropathy compared with 48 controls. In B, are the mean responses from 27 patients with definite ALS compared with the same controls. In C, threshold reduction 90–100 ms after the start of a 40% hyperpolarizing current are plotted against threshold reduction 10–20ms after the start of a 40% depolarizing current with ellipses corresponding to 95% confidence limits for the group means. (Reprinted from Horn *et al.*, 1996, *Muscle & Nerve*, **19**, 1268–1275, with permission from John Wiley & Sons Inc.)

than sensory, and the mean motor SDTC constant was significantly longer than normal (Figure 5.6). As we have seen in the above, prolongation of SDTC can occur as a consequence of a relative axonal depolarization, greater persistent sodium conductance at the node, or as a result of paranodal demyelination. Antibodies against voltage-gated potassium channels (VGKCs) appear to be specific for the fast A-type VGKCs which are predominately situated at paranodal sites and would be protected from immune attack by the myelin sheath. Therefore anti-VGKCs would only be capable of prolonging SDTCs if they resulted in pronounced axonal depolarization, segmental paranodal demyelination or if they are capable of binding to sites affecting the function of the slow delayed rectified type VGKCs present mostly at the node. As the determinant of fast A-type and slow delayed rectifier potassium channels may only differ by a single subunit, it seems plausible that antibodies may be capable of binding to and down regulating the slow potassium channels at the node (Maddison *et al.*, 1999).

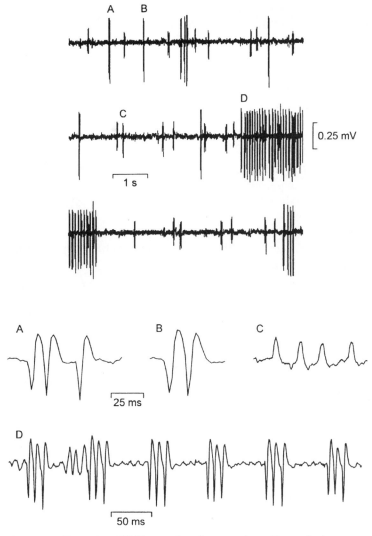

**Figure 5.6** Examples of EMG recordings from a patient with acquired autoimmune neuromyotonia. Recordings were made from the first dorsal interosseous muscle and above is shown a continuous recording with several spontaneous discharges. These are identified by letters which are seen below at higher time resolution and are seen to consist of doublet, triplet or mulitplet discharges. In D, a triplet motor unit discharge is repeated in a rhythmic fashion.

# Investigation of the neuromuscular junction

## Myasthenia gravis

Myasthenia gravis (MG) usually presents as fatiguable muscle weakness, i.e. weakness which is provoked by muscular exercise and reversed by rest. MG is the prototypical immune-mediated channelopathy affecting the nervous system. The existence of antibodies against acetylcholine receptors (ACHR) at the neuromuscular junction and the passive transfer of these antibodies from affected patients to animals represent the classic mode of proof of immune mediation (Drachman, 1983). The effect of ACHR antibodies is to interfere with the structure and function of acetylcholine receptors. The consequence of malfunction of acetylcholine receptors is impairment of neuromuscular transmission, the detection of which *in vivo* is the subject of this section.

If recordings are made of the membrane potential across the post-synaptic membrane (i.e. of the muscle fibre) and stimuli are applied to the nerve then, in a suitable preparation, a large change in potential is recorded, the endplate potential (EPP), reflecting the depolarization produced by a large number of released vesicles of acetylcholine. If repetitive stimuli are applied to the nerve, then the size of successive EPPs declines somewhat; this is a normal phenomenon and reflects diminishing numbers of available acetylcholine vesicles. The threshold for excitation of the post-synaptic membrane is much lower than the size of the EPP and so, under normal circumstances, every EPP, even though its amplitude may be reduced, is able to cause propagation of a muscle fibre action potential. This difference between EPP amplitude and the threshold of the post-synaptic membrane is described as the 'safety factor' for transmission. It is the ratio of the EPP size to the value of the threshold and usually has a value of four or more. Transmission will fail under two circumstances:

1. If the size of the EPP falls, e.g. if the number or size of ACh vesicles is reduced
2. If the threshold of post-synaptic membrane rises, e.g. if acetylcholine (ACH) receptors are blocked.

In the first situation the defect is described as presynaptic and in the second as post-synaptic (Figure 5.7).

In MG, AChR antibodies interfere with the structure and function of the post-synaptic membrane, effectively increasing the threshold for excitation of the muscle fibre and reducing the safety factor. Thus the normal reduction of EPP amplitude during repeated nerve stimulation now becomes critical and transmission may fail on the third or fourth endplate potential.

Two basic methods are available for investigating these phenomena *in vivo*; repetitive nerve stimulation (RNS) with surface recordings of mus-

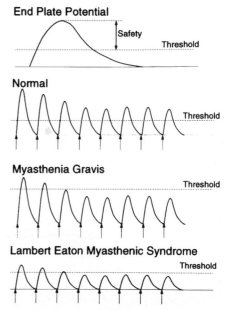

**Figure 5.7** A diagram to illustrate the changes in EPP. In the upper trace, a single EPP is illustrated. In a normal neuromuscular junction, repetitive stimulation of the nerve results in a decreasing EPP over the first few stimuli which then plateaus. EPP amplitude, however, remains well above threshold and transmission is secure. In myasthenia gravis the threshold for activating the post-synaptic membrane is raised and the normal decreasing response to repetitive stimulation now results in EPPs below threshold resulting in neuromuscular block. In the Lambert Eaton myasthenic syndrome, EPPs are smaller than normal and if threshold remains normal, the decreasing response to repetitive stimulation again take EPP amplitude below threshold.

cle responses and single fibre electromyography (SFEMG). What has been described above is the effect of impaired transmission at a single neuromuscular junction. Surface recordings from a muscle in which large (e.g. 1 cm diameter) electrodes are taped over the muscle belly reflect the function of all neuromuscular junctions in the muscle. The compound muscle action potential (CMAP), evoked by a supramaximal nerve stimulus, is the summation of all single fibre muscle action potential in the muscle. The safety factor at each neuromuscular junction will vary throughout the muscle: at some neuromuscular junctions, the safety factor will be critically compromised, at others, transmission will be secure. Only if a significant number of neuromuscular junctions in the muscle are close to failure will repetitive nerve stimulation result in the reduction of the amplitude of the evoked CMAP. It is therefore not surprising that repetitive nerve stimulation tests are relatively insensitive to junction impairment.

Techniques for performing RNS have been described for a number of different muscles: intrinsic hand muscles (Slomic *et al.*, 1968), anconeus (Kennett *et al.*, 1993), biceps (Krarup *et al.*, 1979), deltoid and trapezius (Schady *et al.*, 1992). RNS can also be used with facial muscles (Crespi *et al.*, 1976). It appears that the more proximal the muscle the more sensitive is RNS in detecting a defect in neuromuscular transmission. Conversely, the more proximal the muscle, the more technically difficult is the RNS study and therefore the more prone to artefact and misinterpretation.

In approximately 40% of patients with generalized MG the response to RNS in intrinsic hand muscles is abnormal. Usually, supramaximal stimuli are applied at frequencies of 1 and 3 Hz. Little is to be gained by using higher frequencies. In hand muscles, a reduction of CMAP amplitude of more than 10% is regarded as abnormal.

A slightly greater diagnostic sensitivity can be achieved by examining the response to RNS after exercise. A common protocol is to ask the patient to perform maximum contraction of the muscle for 15 s and then to repeat RNS at 3 Hz at 1-minute intervals for 2–3 minutes. In MG, the decrement to RNS is maximal at about 2 minutes after such an exercise (Figure 5.8). Immediately after exercise the CMAP might be slightly larger than before (but not as large as the increment found in Lambert Eaton myasthenia syndrome) and decrement is minimal. If RNS is performed on a more proximal muscle, e.g. trapezius, abnormalities are detectable in generalized MG in up to 60% of the cases. For trapezius, the patient is examined sitting and the spinal accessory nerve is stimulated supramaximally in the posterior triangle. Again a decrement of more than 10% is considered abnormal.

While RNS techniques examine the whole of the muscle and allow an assessment of all neuromuscular junctions, single fibre electromyography examines the transmission of a single or a pair of neuromuscular junctions. A specialized needle with a small exposed area is used to record the discharge of a single muscle fibre: this can be recognized because the waveform is identical with each firing. Two methods are available. The original method, described by Stalberg (Stalberg *et al.*, 1994), demands the isolation of two muscle fibres

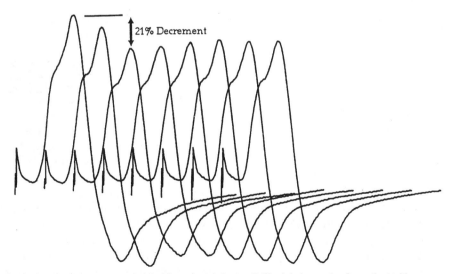

**Figure 5.8** Responses recorded from the abductor digiti minimi muscle of a patient with generalized myasthenia gravis during 3/s supramaximal stimulation of the ulnar nerve at the wrist. CMAPs decrease in amplitude showing a maximum decrement of 21% on the third response.

belonging to the same motor unit within the pick-up area of the electrode. The second uses electrical stimulation of the fine intramuscular nerve fibres and the selective recording of just a single muscle fibre potential (Trontelj *et al.*, 1986.). The second method is faster to perform, does not depend on the ability of the patient to drive just a few motor units voluntarily, but has greater potential technical pitfalls. In particular, submaximal stimulations resulting in the fibre only firing on a fraction of trials leads to an artefactual increase in jitter. In both methods, the difference in timing of fibre discharge on each trial (either in relation to another muscle fibre with the first method or in relation to the stimulus in the second method) are measured and expressed as jitter. To eliminate trends in the recording, jitter is best calculated as the mean difference between successive trials, termed the mean consecutive difference (Stalberg *et al.*, 1994).

Neuromuscular jitter arises because of the shape of the EPP and because of noise in post-synaptic membrane potential. In normal muscle, the sharp rising phase of the EPP cuts through the threshold level at almost the same point with each trial and consequently the variability is very low. Jitter in the normal EDC muscle amounts, for example, to no more than about 40 $\mu$s. In MG the EPP has a slower rise time and is smaller in amplitude and therefore the region of the EPP which could potentially exceed threshold is longer giving rise to increased jitter (Figure 5.9). Normal values for jitter (Gilchrist, 1992) are available for a number of limb muscles but, even in patients with generalized symptoms, the facial muscles around the eye give the greatest chance of demonstrating an abnormality. SFEMG is the most sensitive test for neuromuscular junction abnormality exceeding that of RNS, acetylcholine receptor antibody estimation and the tensilon test (Oh *et al.*, 1992).

## Lambert Eaton myasthenic syndrome

The Lambert Eaton myasthenic syndrome (LEMS) usually presents as fatiguable proximal limb weakness, the legs being affected more than the arms (O'Neill *et al.*, 1988). The tendon reflexes in relaxed muscle are often absent and reappear after

## Origin of single fibre jitter

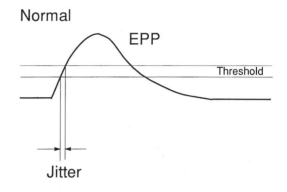

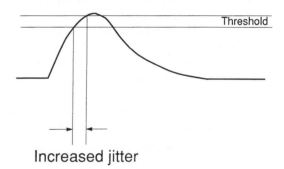

**Figure 5.9** Origin of single fibre jitter. In the normal situation, the rising phase of the EPP cuts through threshold which is indicated as a band to represent the noise which may be present over a very limited time period. In contrast, below, in myasthenia gravis, the peak of the EPP now falls within the threshold region giving rise to increased jitter.

a short period of voluntary exercise. This is termed post-tetanic potentiation and is the clinical correlate of the increment in CMAP found after exercise neurophysiologically. Autonomic features may also be prominent, especially a dry mouth. Approximately 50% of LEMS cases are associated with an underlying carcinoma, usually small cell carcinoma of the lung (O'Neill *et al.*, 1988). The tumour itself is usually evident within 2 years of presentation but, if the duration of the condition exceeds 4–5 years, then it is unlikely that a carcinoma will be found. The remaining 50% of cases have an autoimmune aetiology: antibodies are directed against voltage-gated calcium channels in the presynaptic terminal and impede the release of acetylcholine and hence reduce the size of endplate potentials at the junction. The cardinal features (Figure 5.10) neurophysiologically of the Lambert Eaton myasthenic syndrome are:

1. Small CMAPs (less than 5 mV) recorded in intrinsic hand muscles after supramaximal nerve stimulation.
2. An increase in size of the compound muscle action potential of at least 50% after a short period of exercise or after high frequency (20 Hz) RNS of the nerve. Despite the fact that weakness is often proximal, intrinsic hand muscles offer the best opportunity for detecting this increment (Maddison *et al.*, 1998).
3. Frequency-dependent increased jitter on single fibre EMG in which a higher frequency of stimulation leads to a reduced degree of jitter

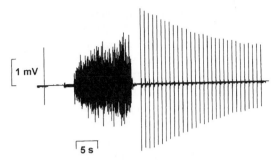

**Figure 5.10** The CMAP from the abductor digiti minimi muscle following supramaximal ulnar nerve stimulation is seen in the resting state. There then follows a period of maximal exercise during which the EMG envelope is seen to increase in size. Immediately following the exercise, the CMAP is considerably increased in size and then decreases towards normal over a period of about 1 minute.

(Chaudhry *et al.*, 1991; Tim and Sanders, 1994).

Conventional EMG of proximal muscles in LEMS cases often appears 'myopathic' with

## SLOW CHANNEL SYNDROME

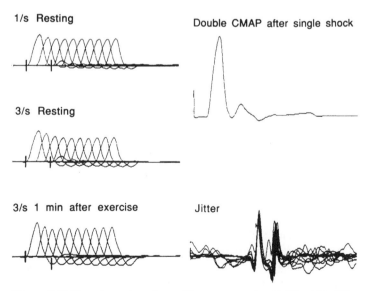

**Figure 5.11** Slow channel syndrome. The responses to repetitive stimulation show a decrement in response to 1 and 3/s stimulation which is also present 1 minute after 15 s maximal exercise. The CMAP recorded from an intrinsic hand muscle following a single supramaximal nerve shock shows a double peak and single fibre jitter is increased.

spikey and small polyphasic motor unit potentials. As exercise progresses, the EMG may become more normal. The myopathic features are due to many neuromuscular junctions being blocked at the start of the contraction: they become progressively unblocked as exercise continues. It is for this reason that any patient with proximal muscle weakness with small spikey motor unit potentials on EMG should have a motor nerve conduction study with measurement of the CMAP from an intrinsic hand muscle before and after exercise.

## Slow channel syndrome

A number of congenital disorders of the neuromuscular junction have been described. In the slow channel syndrome, in which at least eight point mutations in the alpha or beta subunits have been described, the receptor-gated ACH channel is opened for longer than normal. This results in prolonged duration miniature EPPs and EPPs. Clinically, this syndrome presents as fatiguable weakness in a young individual with predominately limb and hand muscle weakness rather than bulbar weakness. Neurophysiologically, a mild to modest decrement is found on RNS and SFEMG confirming the defect in neuromuscular transmission. In addition, single stimuli to a peripheral nerve evokes repetitive muscle discharges recognizable as a double peak in the compound muscle action potential (Figure 5.11).

## Investigation of muscle fibre membrane channelopathies

For muscles to contract normally, the action potentials evoked in muscle fibres must be transmitted along the fibre membrane and into the T-tubular system to activate contractile proteins. Hyperexcitability of the fibre membrane may lead to repetitive discharge, manifest clinically as a persistent contraction (myotonia). Reduced excitability of the fibre membrane may lead to failure of propagation of action potentials and paralysis. Sodium channel dysfunction of muscle fibre membrane can lead to both myotonia (due to repetitive discharge) and inexcitability due to depolarization in periodic paralysis. Chloride channel mutations cause a reduction in resting conductance, which enhances excitability and gives rise to myotonia. In contrast, missense mutations of the L-type calcium channel reduce membrane excitability and give rise to hypokalaemic periodic paralysis. Hypokalaemic periodic paralysis, paramyotonia congenita and potassium aggravated myotonias are all caused by point mutations of the alpha subunit of the sodium channel.

A number of neurophysiological investigations are available to investigate these phenomena. It should be pointed out, however, that myotonia from whatever cause has similar electrical manifestations and it is currently not possible to differentiate the various causes of myotonia neurophysiologically. Similarly, since it is not possible to stimulate muscle fibre membrane directly, depolarization block of muscle fibres is difficult to prove. Excitability of nerve fibres is always higher than that of the muscle fibre and electrical stimuli applied over a muscle will inevitably excite the intramuscular nerve twigs and hence recordings will reflect both nerve conduction and neuromuscular transmission.

## Muscle fibre conduction velocity

One consequence of reduced muscle fibre membrane excitability, short of complete block, is a reduction in the velocity of propagation of the action potential along the fibre membrane. Two methods are available for measuring this parameter. First, since muscle fibres run along a large fraction of the length of the muscle, surface recordings over two points, separated by a given interval, will contain components from the same fibres. By mathematically cross-correlating the two EMG signals, common components can be isolated and knowing the distance between the two sites and the times between the arrival of common activity at the two electrodes, an estimate of muscle fibre conduction velocity can be made (Sadoyama et al., 1985; Nishizono et al., 1995; Arendt-Nielsen et al., 1998) (Figure 5.12). Using this technique, it has been shown that

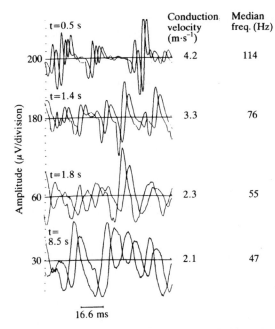

**Figure 5.12** Examples of EMG signals recorded from the brachial radialis muscle of a patient with myotonia congenita. Surface electrodes were 10 mm apart and similar components in the two EMG signals are easily recognized. From above down, the conduction velocity calculated during a short fatiguing contraction is seen to decline from 4.2 to 2.1 m/s. (Reproduced from Schwartz and Van Wierden, 1989, *Brain*, **112**, 665–680 by permission of Oxford University Press.)

transient weakness suffered by patients with recessive myotonia congentia is associated with a dramatic fall in muscle fibre conduction velocity (Zwarts and van Weerden., 1989). In contrast, patients with dystrophia myotonica showed no such change in muscle fibre conduction velocity. Similarly, muscle fibre conduction velocity in hypokalaemic periodic paralysis has been shown to be reduced (Links *et al.*, 1994) and, furthermore, is also less than normal in proven gene carriers (van der Hoeven *et al.*, 1994). A second method of measuring muscle fibre conduction velocity is more invasive and involves inserting a multichannel needle electrode into the muscle which is manipulated so that two channels can record from the same muscle fibre. Knowing the distance between the recording surfaces, and the time difference between same muscle fibre action

potential, then velocity can be calculated (Stalberg and Trontelj, 1994).

## Short exercise test

The transient weakness experienced by some patients with myotonia on resting the muscle after exercise can be demonstrated using a short exercise test (Subramony and Wee, 1986). Recordings are made from the intrinsic muscles of the hand and, prior to testing, the hand should be rested for at least 5–10 minutes. Following this, at one-minute intervals supramaximal stimuli are applied to the nerve and the amplitude of CMAPs is measured. Maximum voluntary isometric exercise for 10 s is then followed by supramaximal nerve stimuli at 10-s intervals for one minute. In many cases of myotonia, compound muscle action potential is reduced after exercise and recovers over a time course of many minutes (Streib, 1987a) (Figure 5.13).

A prolonged exercise test has also been used to investigate patients with paramyotonia congenita and hyperkalaemic periodic paralysis. In this test, the patient performs repeated maximum contractions of the fingers for 15–20 s followed by a short rest with the exercise being continued for at least 4–5 minutes. In patients with periodic paralysis, the CMAP progressively declines during the 20–40 minutes following exercise (McManis *et al.*, 1986; Kuntzer *et al.*, 2000).

## Potassium challenge

These tests are potentially hazardous and should be conducted only in a controlled situation where plasma potassium can be monitored regularly and there are facilities for dealing with untoward events such as cardiac arrhythmias. Potassium challenge is contraindicated in patients with renal or cardiac disease. The electrocardiogram should be monitored throughout the procedure and CMAP amplitudes from supramaximal nerve stimuli to the ulnar nerve, say, should be monitored at 15-minute intervals. Patients' responses to oral potassium vary considerably and plasma potassium levels should be monitored at 15-minute

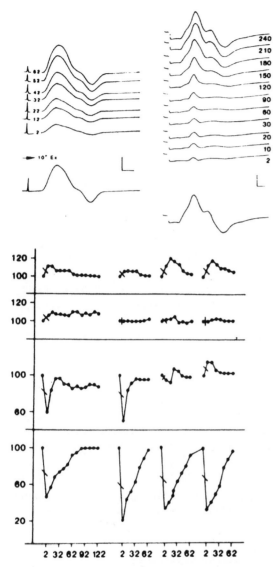

**Figure 5.13** On the left are CMAPs in a patient with a recessive generalized myotonia at intervals after a period of 5 s maximal isometric exercise. On the right side are, from above down, the results of short exercise test in which CMAP amplitude is provoked against time in first a control subject, secondly a patient with myasthenia gravis, thirdly a patient with myotonic dystrophy and at the bottom a patient with a recessive generalized myotonia.
(Reproduced from Streib, 1987, *Muscle & Nerve*, **10**, 603–315 with permission from John Wiley & Sons Inc.)

intervals also. Weakness induced by potassium can be measured clinically or by myometry, but the best quantitation is measurement of the CMAP amplitude.

## Muscle cooling

Myotonia in general becomes worse if the muscle is cooled. This is particularly the case of course, in paramyotonia congenita. Cooling the muscle sufficiently is not a trivial exercise; because blood at body temperature is continuously supplied to the muscle, cooling should be done over a period of 20–30 minutes with the aim of getting skin temperature down to at least 20–25°C. This may be achieved by using ice packs. Again CMAP amplitudes should be monitored throughout. In patients with paramyotonia congenita, a short period of exercise in the cooled muscle often leads to a dramatic fall in the amplitude of the CMAP correlating with clinical evidence of weakness.

## References

Arendt-Nielsen, L. and Mills, K. R. (1998). Muscle fibre conduction velocity, mean power frequency, mean EMG voltage and force during submaximal fatiguing contractions of human quadriceps. *Eur J Appl Physiol.*, **58**, 20–5.

Bostock, H. (1997). Abnormal excitability of motor axons in ALS. In *Physiology of ALS and Related Diseases*, (ed. J. Kimura and R. Kaji), pp. 133–43. Amsterdam: Elsevier.

Bostock, H., Baker, M., Grafe, P. and Reid, G. (1991). Changes in excitability and accommodation of human motor axons follwing brief periods of ischaemia. *J Physiol (Lond.)*, **441**, 513–35.

Bostock, H., Burke, D. and Hales, J. P. (1994). Differences in behaviour of sensory and motor axons following release of ischaemia. *Brain*, **117**, 225–34.

Bostock, H., Cikurel, K. and Burke, D. (1998). Threshold tracking techniques in the study of human peripheral nerve. *Muscle Nerve*, **21**, 137–58.

Bostock, H., Sharief, M. K., Reid, G and Murray, N. M. (1995). Axonal ion channel dysfunction in amyotrophic lateral sclerosis. *Brain*, **118**, 217–25.

Chaudhry, V., Watson, D. F., Bird, S. J. and Cornblath, D. R. (1991). Stimulated single-fiber electromyography in Lambert-Eaton myasthenic syndrome. *Muscle Nerve*, **14**, 1227–30.

Crespi, V., Paserini, D., Bassi, S. and Albizzati, M. G. (1976). Repetitive stimulation of the facial nerve in myasthenic and normal subjects. *Electromyogr Clin Neurophysiol.*, **16**, 433–8.

Drachman, D. (1983). Myasthenia gravis: immunobiology of a receptor disorder. *Trends Neurosci.*, **6**, 446–51.

Gilchrist, J. C.-O. (1992). Single fiber EMG reference values: a collaborative effort. Ad Hoc Committee of the AAEM Special Interest Group on Single Fiber EMG. *Muscle Nerve*, **15**, 151–61.

Hart, I. K., Waters, C., Vincent, A. *et al.* (1997). Autoantibodies detected to expressed K$^+$ channels are implicated in neuromyotonia. *Ann Neurol.*, **41**, 238–46.

Horn, S., Quasthoff, S., Grafe, P., Bostock, H., Renner, R. and Schrank, B. (1996). Abnormal axonal inward rectification in diabetic neuropathy. *Muscle Nerve*, **19**, 1268–75.

Isaacs, H. (1961). A syndrome of continuous muscle fibre activity. *J Neurol Neurosurg Psychiatr.*, **24**, 319–25.

Kaji, R. (1997). Pathophysiology and clinical variants of multifocal motor neuropathy. In *Physiology of ALS and Related Diseases*, (ed. J. Kimura and R. Kaji), pp. 85–98. Amsterdam: Elsevier.

Kennett, R. P. and Fawcett, P. R. (1993). Repetitive nerve stimulation of anconeus in the assessment of neuromuscular transmission disorders. *Electroencephalor Clin Neurophysiol.*, **89**, 170–6.

Krarup, C. and Horowitz, S. H. (1979). Evoked responses of the elbow flexors in control subjects and in myopathy patients. *Muscle Nerve*, **2**, 465–77.

Links, T. P., van der Hoeven, J. H. and Zwarts, M. J. (1994). Surface EMG and muscle fibre conduction during attacks of hyperkalaemic periodic paralysis. *J Neurol Neurosurg Psychiatr.*, **57**, 632–4.

Maddison, P., Newsom-Davis, J. and Mills, K. R. (1998). Distribution of electrophysiological abnormality in Lambert-Eaton myasthenic syndrome. *J Neurol Neurosurg Psychiatr.*, **65**, 213–7.

Maddison, P., Newsom-Davis, J. and Mills, K. R. (1999). Strengh-duration properties of peripheral nerve in acquired neuromyotonia. *Muscle Nerve*, **22**, 823–30.

McManis, P. G., Lambert, E. H. and Daube, J. R. (1986). The exercise test in periodic paralysis. *Muscle Nerve*, **9**, 704–10.

Mogyoros, I., Kiernan, M. C. and Burke, D, (1997a). Strength-duration properties of sensory and motor axons in carpal tunnel syndrome. *Muscle Nerve*, **20**, 508–10.

Mogyoros, I., Kiernan, M. C., Burke, D. and Bostock, H. (1997b). Excitability changes in human sensory and motor axons during hyperventilation and ischaemia. *Brain*, **120**, 317–25.

Mogyoros, I., Kiernan, M. C., Burke, D. and Bostock, H. (1998a). Ischemic resistance of cutaneous afferents and motor axons in patients with amyotrophic lateral sclerosis. *Muscle Nerve*, **21**, 1692–700.

Mogyoros, I., Kiernan, M. C., Burke, D. and Bostock, H. (1998b). Strength-duration properties of sensory and motor axons in amyotrophic lateral sclerosis. *Brain*, **121**, 851–9.

Newsom-Davis, J. and Mills, K. R. (1993). Immunological associations of acquired neuromyotonia (Isaacs'

syndrome). Report of five cases and literature review. *Brain*, **116**, 453–69.

Nishizono, H., Fujimoto, T., Kurata, H. and Shibayama, H. (1995). Non-invasive method to detect motor unit contractile properties and conduction velocity in human vastus lateralis muscle. *Med Biol Eng Comput.*, **33**, 558–62.

O'Neill, J. H., Murray, N. M. and Newsom-Davis, J. (1998). The Lambert-Eaton myasthenic syndrome. A review of 50 cases. *Brain*, **111**, 577–96.

Oh, S. J., Kim, D. E., Kuruoglu, R., Bradley, R. J. and Dwyer, D. (1992). Diagnostic sensitivity of the laboratory tests in myasthenia gravis. *Muscle Nerve*, **15**, 720–4.

Sadoyama, T., Masuda, T. and Miyano, H. (1985). Optimal conditions for the measurement of muscle fibre conduction velocity using surface electrode arrays. *Med Biol Eng Comput.*, **23**, 339–42.

Schady, W. and MacDermott, N. (1992). On the choice of muscle in the electrophysiological assessment of myasthenia gravis. *Electormyogra Clin Neurophysiol.*, **32**, 99–102.

Schilling, T., Heinrich, B., Kau, R. *et al.* (1997). Paclitaxel administered over 3 h followed by cisplatin in patients with advanced head and neck squamous cell carcinoma: a clinical phase I study. *Oncology*, **54**, 89–95.

Slomic, A., Rosenfalck, A. and Buchthal, F. (1968). Electrical and mechanical responses of normal and myasthenic muscle. *Brain Res.*, **10**, 1–78.

Stalberg, E. and Trontelj, J. (1994). Single fibre electromyography. In *Studies in healthy and diseased muscle*, 2nd edn. New York: Raven Press.

Streib, E. W. (1987). AAEE minimonograph no. 27: differential diagnosis of myotonic syndromes. *Muscle Nerve*, **10**, 603–15.

Subramony, S. H. and Wee, A. S. (1986). Exercise and rest in hyperkalemic periodic paralysis. *Neurology*, **36**, 173–7.

Tim, R. W. and Sanders, D. B. (1994). Repetitive nerve stimulation studies in the Lambert-Eaton myasthenic syndrome. *Muscle Nerve*, **17**, 995–1001.

Trontelj, J., Mihelin, M., Fernandez, J. and Stalberg, E. (1986). Axonal stimulation for end-plate jitter studies. *J Neurol Neurosurg Psychiatr.*, **49**, 677–85.

van der Hoeven, J. H., Links, T. P., Zwarts, m. J. and van Weerden, T. W. (1994). Muscle fiber conduction velocity in the diagnosis of familial hypokalemic periodic paralysis-invasive versus surface determination. *Muscle Nerve*, **17**, 898–905.

Weigl, P., Bostock, H., Granz, P., Martius, P., Muller, W. and Grafe, P. (1989). Threshold tracking provides a rapid indication of ischaemic resistance in motor axons of diabetic subjects. *Electroencephalogr Clin Neurophysiol.*, **73**, 369–71.

Zwarts, M. J. and van Weerden, T. W. (1989). Transient paresis in myotonic syndromes. A surface EMG study. *Brain*, **112**, 665–80.

# Channel gene expression, distribution and its relationship to disease and normal development

PART

**3**

# Plasticity of ion channel gene expression as a substrate for channelopathies

*Stephen G. Waxman*

## Introduction

The channelopathies include disorders in which structural changes within ion channels (e.g. due to mutations which alter the amino acid sequence of the channel protein itself) produce changes in function. But dysfunction at the clinical level can also occur in settings in which the amino acid sequence of channels is unaltered, but channel function is abnormal as a result of changes in the expression, i.e. of alterations in the synthesis and deployment, of channels. As a result of this, it is important to understand the ways in which channel expression can change, i.e. dynamic aspects of channel expression, in various disease states. Pathological alterations in channel expression, however, do not necessarily occur in the context of a quiescent baseline of fixed or constant channel expression in normal cells. It has recently become clear that ion channel expression within the normal nervous system (even the mature nervous system) is dynamic, and this provides a complex substrate for disease-induced or injury-triggered changes. This chapter will summarize recent progress in understanding plasticity of channel expression in the normal and pathological nervous system, using sodium channels as a model.

In most neurons within the mammalian central nervous system, voltage-gated sodium channels are responsible for the inward transmembrane currents which produce the regenerative depolarization that underlies the action potential. This pivotal role of sodium channels in electrogenic activity is reflected, for example, by their clustering within the neuronal cell membrane at critical regions such as the axon initial segment (Waxman and Quick, 1978) which functions as an action potential trigger zone in most neurons (Coombs *et al.*, 1957; Fatt, 1957; Fuortes *et al.*, 1957; Dodge and Cooley, 1973) and by the aggregation of sodium channels in high densities within the axon membrane at the nodes of Ranvier, which serve as way-stations for saltatory conduction along myelinated axons (Ritchie and Rogart, 1977; Waxman, 1977; Shrager, 1989).

Although classical neurophysiological doctrine referred to 'the' sodium channel, it has become clear that multiple sodium channel genes encode molecular distinct sodium channels (see, e.g. Noda *et al.*, 1986a; Black *et al.*, 1996). At least eight of these genes are expressed in the nervous system and, as a result of this, a relatively rich repertoire of multiple sodium channels with different functional characteristics is available for deployment within neurons.

## The distribution of neuronal sodium channels is non-uniform and dynamic

The non-uniform spatial pattern of distribution of sodium channels within the healthy nervous system is illustrated in myelinated axons where there are sharp gradients of sodium channel density. Sodium channels are aggregated in high densities ($> 10^3/\mu m^2$) within the axon membrane at the node of Ranvier, where they support saltatory conduction via their voltage-dependent actions. In contrast, the density of sodium channels falls rapidly outside of the nodes and is much lower ($< 25/\mu m^2$) in the internodal axon membrane beneath the myelin sheath (Ritchie and Rogart,

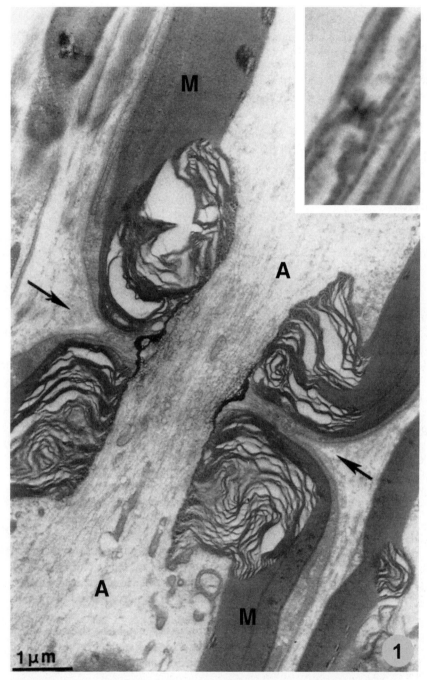

**Figure 6.1** Non-uniform distribution of sodium channels in the axon membrane. This electron micrograph shows cytochemical staining of a normal myelinated fibre from guinea-pig sciatic nerve with ferric ion and ferrocyanide. There is selective staining of the axon membrane at a node of Ranvier (arrows), while the internodal axon membrane remains unstained. This stain provides a marker for regions of the axon membrane expressing a high density of sodium channels. A = axoplasm; M = myelin. × 16 000. Modified from Quick and Waxman (1976).

1977; Waxman, 1977; Shrager, 1989). This non-uniform distribution of sodium channels in normal myelinated axons is illustrated in Figure 6.1.

Although there is a stereotyped pattern of sodium channel localization in mature, uninjured myelinated axons, the pattern of sodium channel distribution is not immutable. It changes markedly, in fact, both during development and in response to pathological insults. Maturation of peripheral nerves and white matter tracts, for example, involves a distinct phylogenetic sequence, whereby premyelinated axons initially display a uniform membrane structure and, at a later stage of development, clusters of sodium channels develop at the precursors of nodes close to the time when myelin is first laid down (Waxman and Foster, 1980; Wiley-Livingston and Ellisman, 1980; Waxman et

al., 1982; Vabnik et al., 1996). Later in myelination, there is a molecular remodelling of the internodal part of the axon membrane. Sodium channel expression in axon regions destined to become myelinated is maintained at a nearly constant level which can support electrogenesis (Waxman et al., 1989) until the formation of compact myelin, which provides capacitative and resistive shielding; following myelination there is a suppression of sodium channel expression in the underlying internodal axon membrane (Waxman, 1987).

Despite its highly differentiated structure, the internodal axon membrane retains the capability for significant molecular plasticity. Cytochemical (Weiner et al., 1980) and saxitoxin (STX)-binding studies (Ritchie, 1982) suggest that sodium channels aggregate at the newly formed nodes along

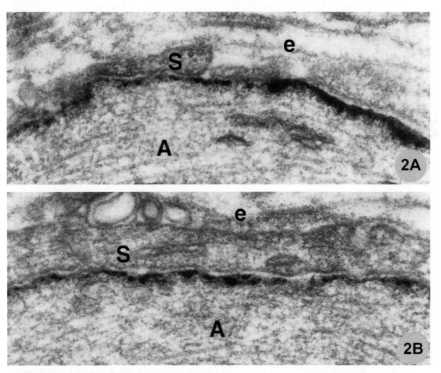

**Figure 6.2** Plasticity of ion channel expression in the demyelinated axon membrane. These electron micrographs illustrate the acquisition, by chronically demyelinated (formerly internodal) axon membrane, of node-like staining with ferric ion and ferrocyanide (compare to Figure 6.1). The development of higher-than-normal sodium channel densities in the demyelinated axon membrane permits it to support action potential conduction in the absence of myelin, thus providing a basis for restoration of impulse conduction that contributes to clinical remissions in disorders such as multiple sclerosis. A = demyelinated axon. S = Schwann cell. e = extracellular space. × 65,000 Modified from Foster *et al.* (1980).

remyelinated axons, which are more closely spaced than normal, and immunocytochemical studies with sodium channel-specific antibodies (Dugandzija-Novakovic et al., 1995) confirm this. In chronically demyelinated axons the formerly internodal axon membrane can reorganize, so as to acquire a density of sodium channels that is much higher than normal (Foster et al., 1980; England et al., 1990, 1991). Figure 6.2 illustrates this in an experimentally demyelinated axon from sciatic nerve. The acquisition of increased numbers of sodium channels within the demyelinated axon membrane is functionally important because it endows the bared membrane with the capability to conduct action potentials, in the absence of myelin (Bostock and Sears, 1976, 1978; Waxman and Brill, 1978). The demonstration of increased saxitoxin (STX) binding in demyelinated white matter from multiple sclerosis patients (Moll et al., 1991) supports the idea that axons express a higher than normal number of sodium channels in this disorder. This plasticity of sodium channel deployment within the axon membrane, and the resultant recovery of axon potential conduction in chronically demyelinated axons, appear to contribute to the clinical recovery that occurs during remissions in disorders such as multiple sclerosis (Waxman, 1998). Little is known about the transcriptional events involved in this plasticity, however, and the identity of the sodium channel subtypes (see below) that are inserted into the membrane of the demyelinated axon has not been determined. Moreover, plasticity in ion channel expression can be adaptive or non-adaptive. While the insertion of sodium channels along demyelinated axons appears to provide a substrate for restoration of impulse conduction, there is also evidence, as noted below, for dysregulation of sodium channel transcription, i.e. a channelopathy, in multiple sclerosis.

## Multiple sodium channels within neurons

Building upon the molecular cloning of the first three sodium channels from the brain by Numa and his colleagues (Noda et al., 1986a), it has become clear that nearly a dozen, molecularly distinct voltage-gated sodium channels are encoded by different genes (see Noda et al., 1986b; Kayano et al., 1988; Auld et al., 1988; Suzuki et al., 1988; Schaller et al., 1995). At least eight putative sodium channel genes are expressed within neurons in the mammalian nervous system. It is now apparent that multiple sodium channels are expressed within even morphologically homogeneous groups of neurons (although, as noted below, the presence of different types of sodium channels confers physiological heterogeneity on these cells).

Dorsal root ganglion (DRG) neurons (Figure 6.3) provide an excellent example of this. These primary sensory neurons express the mRNAs for at least six sodium channels. The sodium channel transcripts expressed within DRG neurons include high levels of mRNAs for the $\alpha$-I and Na6 sodium channels, which are also present at high levels within many other neuronal cell types in the CNS (Black et al., 1996). DRG neurons also express high levels of three primary sensory neuron-specific sodium channel mRNAs and a fourth putative sodium channel mRNA, which are not detectable at significant levels, or are present at only low levels, in other neuronal cell types:

1. PN1/hNE is a sodium channel that is expressed preferentially in DRG neurons (Toledo-Aral et al., 1997). It produces a fast transient tetrodotoxin (TTX)-sensitive current in response to sudden depolarizations and a smaller persistent current that is evoked by slow depolarizations close to resting potential (Cummins, et al., 1998).
2. SNS/PN3 is expressed preferentially in small DRG and trigeminal ganglion neurons (but not in other types of neurons). It encodes a slowly inactivating TTX-resistant sodium current when expressed in oocytes (Akopian et al., 1996, 1999; Sangameswaran et al., 1996).
3. NaN is expressed preferentially in C-type and trigeminal neurons and exhibits an amino acid sequence that, while only 47% similar to SNS-PN3, predicts that it encodes a distinct TTX-resistant sodium channel (Dib-Hajj, 1998a). Patch-clamp studies have demonstrated that it produces a persistent TTX-resistant current with relatively hyperpolarized voltage-dependence (Cummins et al., 1999).

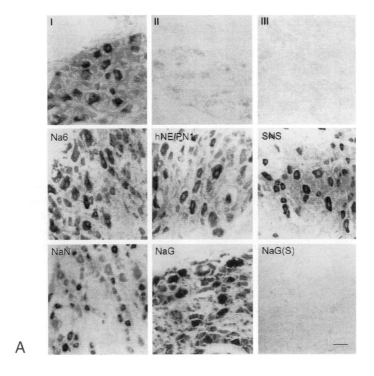

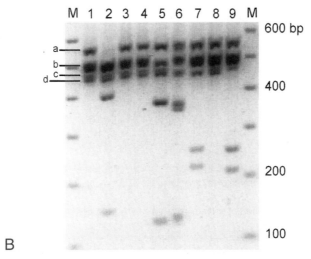

**Figure 6.3** (A) Dorsal root ganglion neurons express multiple sodium channel transcripts. The micrographs illustrate sodium channel $\alpha$-subunit mRNAs visualized in sections from adult rat DRG by *in situ* hybridization with subtype-specific antisense riboprobes. mRNAs for $\alpha$-I, Na6, hNE/PN1, SNS, NaN and NaG are present at moderate-to-high levels in DRG neurons. Hybridization signal is not present with sense riboprobes, e.g., for NaG (S). Bar indicates 40 $\mu$m. Modified from Black *et al.* (1996) and Dib-Hajj *et al.* (1998a). (B) Restriction enzyme analysis confirms the expression of multiple Na channels in DRG neurons. 'M' lanes contain 100-bp ladder marker. Lane 1 contains amplification products (bands a–d) from domain 1 in DRG cDNA. Lanes 2–9 show the result of cutting this DNA with EcoRV, EcoN1, Aval, SphI, BamH1, AflII, XbaI, and EcoR1, which are specific to subunits $\alpha$-I, -II, -III, Na6, PN1, SNS, NaG, and NaN, respectively. Reproduced with permission from Dib-Hajj *et al.* (1998a).

4. NaG was originally cloned from astrocytes and initially considered to be a glial cell-specific sodium channel (Gautron *et al.*, 1992). However, it is also expressed at high levels within DRG neurons (Black *et al.*, 1996) and at low levels within some neurons of neural crest origin (Felts *et al.*, 1997a). However, since NaG mRNA is also present in lung, pituitary and bladder and because it encodes relatively few positively charged amino acid residues in

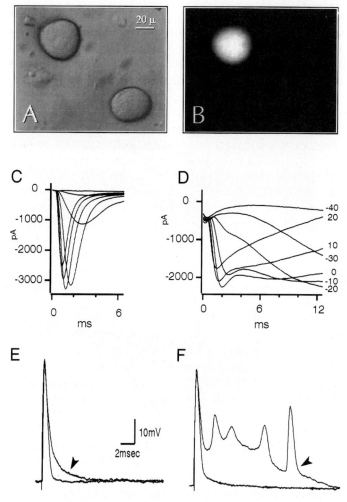

**Figure 6.4** Different sodium currents can be recorded by patch clamp in functionally different types of DRG neurons. (A) DRG neurons in cell culture. (B) Fluorescence microscopy following intracutaneous injection of Fluorogold facilitates identification of cutaneous afferent neurons which are brightly labelled. (C, D) Whole-cell patch-clamp records demonstrate kinetically distinct Na$^+$ currents in muscle (C) as compared to cutaneous afferent (D) DRG neurons. Deployment of different ensembles of sodium channels in these different types of neurons endows them with different electrogenic properties which can be seen following blockade of potassium channels with 4-aminopyridine; note the different action potential characteristics (arrow heads) following potassium channel blockade in muscle afferent axons (E) compared to cutaneous afferents (F). Modified from Honmou *et al.* (1994).

the putative voltage sensor region, there are doubts as to whether NaG does function as a voltage-dependent sodium channel (Akopian *et al.*, 1997).

Analysis of the physiological signature and function of each of these channels is complicated by the co-expression of different channel types within single cells (see Rizzo *et al.*, 1996; Schild and Kunze, 1997). Nevertheless, electrophysiological methods can be used to record the currents produced by the different types of sodium channels, and indicate that there are functionally important differences in the currents produced by different channels. 'Top-down' analyses indicate that there is selective expression of different channel subtypes within DRG neurons with different sensory functions, which endows them with different transductive and/or encoding properties. Figure 6.4 shows, for example, whole-cell patch-clamp recordings of sodium currents from a cutaneous afferent DRG neuron and a muscle afferent DRG neuron (Honmou *et al.*, 1994). The sodium currents in these two subtypes of DRG neurons display different kinetics and voltage-dependence (Figure 6.4C, D); these contribute to the different action potential characteristics that are displayed by these cells (Figure 6.4E, F).

The top-down analysis has been complemented by a 'bottom-up' approach for some of the sodium channel transcripts that are expressed in DRG neuron, such as the PN1/hNE channel. One way to carry out this 'bottom-up' approach is to study channels expressed in mammalian cell lines that do not express high levels of other sodium channels, so that the channel under study can be examined nearly in isolation. When studied by patch clamp in the expression system provided by HEK 293 cells, PN1/hNE can be seen to encode a sodium channel characterized by slow closed-state inactivation. As a result of this property and their voltage-dependence, PN1/hNE channels can be activated by slow depolarizations close to resting potential, a property that poises them to respond to, and amplify, small depolarizing stimuli such as generator potentials (Cummins *et al.*, 1998). The distribution of PN1/hNE channels is consistent with their subserving this function within DRG neurons (possibly together with other sodium

channel subtypes such as Na6 channels which, as described below, can also activate in response to slow, small depolarizations; Vega-Saenz de Miera *et al.*, 1997; Raman *et al.*, 1997; Tanaka *et al.*, 1999). PN1/hNE channels are localized at the distal tips of terminals arising from sensory neurons *in vitro* (Toledo-Aral *et al.*, 1997); a distal localization at the sensory terminals *in situ* would locate PN1/hNE channels close to the trigger zones which produce trains of action potentials, where they could amplify slow depolarizing inputs (Cummins *et al.*, 1998).

## Dynamic aspects of sodium channel gene expression

Sodium channel expression in neurons is not a static process. On the contrary, it is highly dynamic. During development of the mammalian nervous system, the level of expression of some sodium channels increases, while expression of others (e.g. $\alpha$-III) concomitantly decreases in most parts of the nervous system (Beckh *et al.*, 1989; Brysch *et al.*, 1991; Waxman *et al.*, 1994; Felts *et al.*, 1997b).

Some of these developmental changes appear to reflect regulatory effects of neurotrophins and other growth factors on transcription of various sodium channel genes. These effects are highly specific. For example, nerve growth factor (NGF) has opposing actions on expression of the $\alpha$-SNS and $\alpha$-III sodium channel genes, up regulating the former and down regulating the latter in mature DRG neurons (Black *et al.*, 1997; Dib-Hajj *et al.*, 1998b). Although some of the effects of NGF on sodium channel expression involve intracellular pathways involving protein kinase A (Kalman *et al.*, 1990), there is evidence indicating that NGF modulates the expression of different types of sodium channels via several distinct signal transduction pathways, some of which are protein kinase A-independent (D'Arcangelo *et al.*, 1993).

The specific action of neurotrophin effects on sodium channel expression is further illustrated by observations, indicating that brain-derived growth factor (BDNF) increases sodium channel mRNA and sodium current expression in PC12 sublines engineered to express trkC receptors (Fanger *et al.*, 1995), but does not significantly alter sodium current expression in DRG neurons, although it has significant effects on GABA receptor expression in these cells (Oyelese *et al.*, 1997). Glial-derived growth factor (GDNF) strongly up regulates the expression of sodium channel NaN in IB4+ DRG neurons, which are known to express the ret receptor (Fjell *et al.*, 1999); consistent with this, intrathecal administration of GNDF partially protects against the reduction in conduction velocity that occurs in c-fibres following axotomy (Bennett *et al.*, 1998). Although more research is needed, multiple neurotrophins and growth factors appear to have effects on DRG neurons, probably via multiple signalling pathways, and it is possible that sodium channel expression in these cells reflects combinatorial effects of multiple factors.

Electrical activity itself may modulate the expression of sodium channels within excitable cells. Catterall and colleagues (Sherman *et al.*, 1985; Offord and Catterall, 1989) have shown that electrical activity, cAMP levels, and intracellular calcium can modulate the expression of sodium channels in muscle cells; elevation of intracellular calcium has also been shown to modulate sodium channel mRNA and sodium current expression in neuroblastoma cells (Hirsh and Quandt, 1996). Deafferentation of the olfactory bulb, via surgical transection of the olfactory nerve, results in a down regulation of $\alpha$-II sodium channel mRNA in tufted and mitral cells (Sashihara *et al.*, 1996). This effect is not due to denervation *per se*, but rather appears to be due to a change in the level of synaptic activity since similar changes occur following cauterization of the naris of newborn rats, which abolishes access to olfactory stimuli without interrupting the innervation of the olfactory bulb (Sashihara *et al.*, 1997). A hint that the effects of neurotrophins on expression of sodium channels may be time-dependent and possibly activity-dependent is provided by the results of Toledo-Aral *et al.* (1995) who demonstrated that pulsed administration of NGF (for periods as short as 1 minute) can induce the selective expression of the PN1 sodium channel subunit (but not the $\alpha$-II subunit) in PC12 cells via a signalling pathway requiring immediate early genes.

# Dynamic aspects of sodium channel expression in uninjured neurons

The changes in sodium channel expression described above occur during development. However, the electrophysiological state of neurons can change in the mature nervous system, as these cells pass from one functional state to another, e.g. from a relatively quiescent state (generating action potentials at low frequencies) to a bursting (high frequency discharge) state. This raises the question: when a neuron passes from one state of activity to another, does it utilize a fixed repertoire of pre-existing sodium channels in different ways? Or does it remodel itself by deploying a different ensemble of sodium channels so as to re-tune its electrogenic machinery? In a more general sense, the question is: Is the expression of various types of sodium channel fixed at steady-state levels in uninjured neurons, or is it dynamic?

Evidence that sodium channel expression is dynamic has been provided by studies on the magnocellular neurosecretory neurons within the supraoptic nucleus of the hypothalamus (Tanaka *et al.*, 1999). These neurons project their axons to the neural lobe of the pituitary. In their basal state these cells are relatively quiescent, firing at low frequencies (< 3 impulses/s) and irregularly but, in response to changes in osmotic state, they generate bursts of action potentials which trigger the release of vasopressin (Walters and Hatton, 1974; Mason, 1980). The magnocellular neurons possess an intrinsic regenerative mechanism (Hatton, 1990; Andrew and Dudek, 1983) which can be triggered by endogenous mechanosensitive channels (Ollet and Borque, 1993) and by synaptic inputs from other osmosensitive neurons in circumventricular regions (Richard and Borque, 1992). Action potential activity in magnocellular neurons is sodium-dependent and TTX-sensitive, indicating that it is mediated by sodium channels (Andrew and Dudek, 1983; Inenaga *et al.*, 1993; Li and Hatton, 1996). To determine whether the membranes of these cells contain the same, or a different, ensemble of channels in the quiescent and bursting states, magnocellular neurons were studied (Tanaka *et al.*, 1999) under normal conditions and following salt-loading, a manoeuvre which is known to expose supraoptic neurons to a milieu of elevated extracellular osmolality which triggers bursting (Jones and Pickering, 1969; Balment *et al.*, 1980).

*In situ* hybridization of the supraoptic nuclei of control adult rats (which had not been salt-loaded) revealed that low levels of the mRNA for the α-II and Na6 sodium channel α-subunits were present within magnocellular neurons. α-I and α-III mRNA could not be detected at significant levels in these cells. In salt-loaded animals, there was a significant up regulation of the α-II and Na6 mRNAs (Figure 6.5). These experiments thus showed that in response to salt-loading, expression of α-II and Na6 sodium channels is up-regulated at the transcriptional level, i.e. the expression of the α-II and Na6 sodium channel genes is increased (Tanaka *et al.*, 1999).

Because ion channel and receptor expression within the cell membrane are subject to control at transcriptional, translational, and post-translational levels (Ginty *et al.*, 1992; Sharma *et al.*, 1993; Sucher *et al.*, 1993; Hales and Tyndale, 1994; Black *et al.*, 1998), it was next necessary to determine whether these changes in sodium channel gene transcription were paralleled by increases in sodium channel protein. Immunocytochemical and immunoblotting methods utilizing antibody SP20, directed against a conserved region of sodium channels (Westenbroek *et al.*, 1989, 1992), demonstrated a distinct increase in sodium channel immunoreactivity following salt-loading in these neurons (Figure 6.6A, B), and there was an increase in the density of the 230 kDa immunoreactive band characteristic of sodium channels (see Westenbroek *et al.*, 1989) in membrane preparations from the supraoptic nucleus of salt-loaded rats (Figure 6.6C).

These observations demonstrated an up-regulation transcription of α-II and Na6 sodium channel mRNA in magnocellular neurons in response to osmotic changes, and further showed that this results in an increased level of sodium channel protein, a change which could support functional changes in these cells. Demonstration that these channels were inserted into the cell membrane, where they could alter the electrogenic properties of these cells, however, required patch-clamp

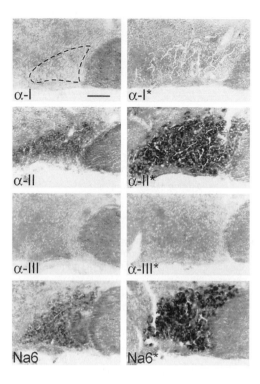

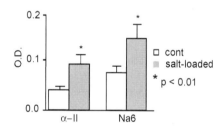

**Figure 6.5** Channel expression is dynamic even in the normal mature nervous system. α-II and Na6 sodium channel mRNA are up-regulated in supraoptic magnocellular neurons following salt-loading, which causes a transition from a quiescent to a bursting state. The micrographs, from control (left column) and salt-loaded (right column) rats, were digitally enhanced to show *in situ* hybridization with subtype-specific riboprobes for Na channel subunits α-I, α-II, α-III and Na6. α-I and α-III mRNA are not detectable, and low levels of α-II and Na6 mRNA are present in the control supraoptic nucleus (no asterisks). Expression of the α-II and Na6 transcript is up-regulated following salt-loading (asterisks). Optical densities from unenhanced micrographs (graph) provide a quantitative measure of mRNA levels and show a significant increase in α-II and Na6 mRNA following salt-loading. * $= P < 0.01$. Bar $= 100$ $\mu$m. Modified from Tanaka *et al.* (1999).

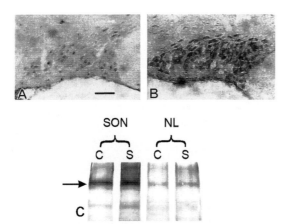

**Figure 6.6** Na channel immunoreactivity with SP20 antibody is increased in the supraoptic nucleus following salt-loading (B) compared to controls (A). Immunoblotting (C) shows a 230 kD band (arrow) that is denser in the salt-loaded (S) supraoptic nucleus (SON) than in the control (C). There is a less pronounced increase in density of this band in the salt-loaded pituitary neural lobe (NL), which contains the terminals of the axons of the supraoptic neurons. Bar = 100 $\mu$m. Modified from Tanaka *et al.* (1999).

recording (Tanaka *et al.*, 1999). These recordings demonstrated the presence of two distinct sodium currents in control magnocellular neurons, corresponding to the two channels. First, there was a fast transient sodium current which contributes to the rapid upstroke of the action potential. Second, these cells generate TTX-sensitive 'ramp' sodium currents, which are activated by slow depolarizations close to resting potential. Both of the currents, the fast transient current and the slow ramp current, are increased in salt-loaded magnocellular neurons, but they are increased to different degrees (Tanaka *et al.*, 1999). Density of the fast transient sodium current is 20% higher in salt-loaded rats. In contrast, the ramp current density is approximately 50% larger in salt-loaded neurons (Figure 6.7).

The presence of two sodium currents correlates well with the expression of $\alpha$-II and Na6 sodium channels in the magnocellular neurons. Studies in other neuronal cell types, such as Purkinje cells, have demonstrated that the Na6 sodium channel can produce a persistent or ramp current (Vega-Saenz de Miera *et al.*, 1997; Raman *et al.*, 1997). The $\alpha$-II channel, in contrast, has been shown to

produce a fast transient current (Noda *et al.*, 1986b; Auld *et al.*, 1988). As a result of the different voltage-dependence and kinetics of these two channels, they collaborate in electrogenesis, the Na6 current being evoked by small, slow depolarizations close to threshold and thereby boosting depolarizing inputs, and the $\alpha$-II current underlying the rapid depolarizing upstroke of the action potential. The larger increase in expression of the Na6 channels in salt-loaded rats would be expected to lower the threshold for action potential generation. Changes in sodium channel expression thus re-tune the electrogenic membrane of these neurons, facilitating the generation of impulse bursts, as they pass from the quiescent to the bursty state.

These changes demonstrate that sodium channel deployment within neurons, even in the absence of disease states, is subject to modulation. The molecular and functional plasticity of sodium channel expression in normal neurons provides a dynamic baseline, on which pathological changes are superimposed.

# Changes in sodium channel expression in injured neurons: sometimes adaptive, sometimes maladaptive

As noted above, redistribution of sodium channels appears to support the restoration of conduction in demyelinated axons. This is an example of an adaptive charge in sodium expression after damage to the nervous system. But, in some cases, plasticity of sodium channel expression can be maladaptive. An especially well-studied example is provided by the changes in sodium channel expression that occur in neurons whose axons have been transected by nerve injury. Eccles and his colleagues (1958) demonstrated in early experiments on motor neurons that, following axonal transection, there were changes in somatodendritic excitability which appeared to represent the deployment of increased numbers of sodium channels within the neuronal membrane. More recent electrophysiological studies have confirmed these findings (Kuno and Llinas, 1970) and have shown

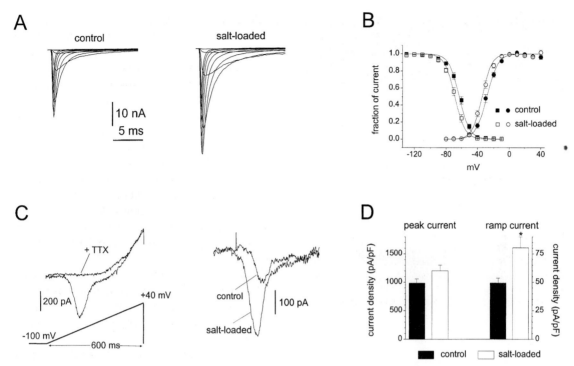

**Figure 6.7** Two distinct sodium currents are differentially increased in supraoptic neurons following salt-loading. (A) Families of traces are shown from representative supraoptic neurons acutely isolated from control (left panel) or salt-loaded (right panel) rats. The currents were elicited by 40 ms test pulses to various potentials from −60 to 30 mV. Cells were held at −100 mV. (B) Normalized activation (circles) and steady-state inactivation (squares) curves show only small differences between control (filled symbols) and salt-loaded (open symbols) neurons. Curves are fits to Boltzmann functions. Steady-state inactivation was measured with 500 ms inactivating prepulses, in cells held at prepulse potentials ranging from −130 to −10 mV prior to a test pulse to 0 mV for 20 ms. Error bars indicate s.e. (C) Ramp currents are elicited in supraoptic neurons by slow voltage ramps (600 ms ramp extending from −100 to +40 mV). The left panel shows that TTX (250 nM) blocks the ramp current in salt-loaded supraoptic neurons, thus demonstrating that this current is produced by sodium channels. The right panel shows the TTX-sensitive ramp currents in representative control and salt-loaded supraoptic neurons. Leak currents recorded after application of 250 nM TTX were subtracted. Note the larger ramp current in salt-loaded neurons (D) The peak and ramp current densities (estimated by dividing the maximum currents by the cell capacitance) are larger following salt-loading; the increase is proportionately greater for the ramp currents. Error bars indicate s.e., and the $^*$ indicates $P < 0.005$. From Tanaka *et al.* (1999).

that the abnormal somatodendritic excitability is sodium-dependent (Sernagor *et al.*, 1986; Titmus and Faber, 1986), providing additional evidence for alterations in sodium channel deployment in neurons following axonal injury. Other studies have demonstrated increased sodium channel immunoreactivity within the injured axonal tips of neuromas (Devor *et al.*, 1989; England *et al.*, 1994, 1996).

New research techniques have recently made it possible to examine the molecular basis for these changes. It has become possible to ask whether, in addition to accumulation of abnormally large numbers of sodium channels following injury, different types of sodium channels are deployed and, if so whether this is due to changes in gene transcription. These studies have shown that, following axonal transection, there is an up regulation of several sodium channel genes in adult DRG neurons, including a striking up regulation of the previously silent $\alpha$-III sodium channel gene (Waxman *et al.*, 1994). These changes are not due to an overall increase in protein synthesis but they are paralleled by an increase in the level of type

III sodium channel protein, which is localized both in DRG neuron cell bodies and in the tips of transected axons within experimental neuromas (Black *et al.*, 1999a). Using *in situ* hybridization and RT-PCR, we have also shown (Dib-Hajj *et al.*, 1996, 1998a) that there is a down regulation of the

$\alpha$-SNS and NaN sodium channel genes in axotomized DRG neurons (Figure 6.8). These changes in sodium channel expression can persist for months following injury (Dib-Hajj *et al.*, 1996; Cummins and Waxman, 1997).

These injury-induced changes in sodium chan-

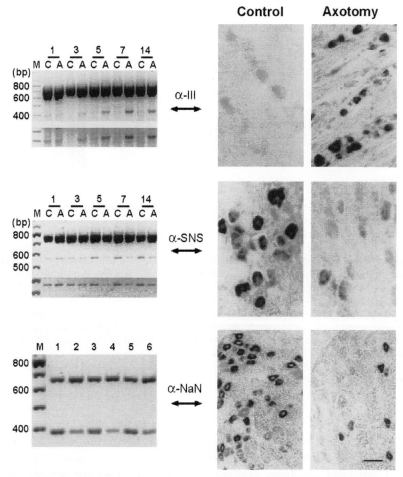

**Figure 6.8** Sodium channels $\alpha$-III (top) are up regulated, and SNS (middle) and NaN (bottom) are down regulated, in DRG neurons following axotomy within the sciatic nerve. The *in situ* hybridizations (right side) show $\alpha$-III, SNS/PN3, and NaN mRNA in control DRG, and at 5–7 days post-axotomy. RT-PCR (left side) shows products of co-amplification of $\alpha$-III and SNS together with $\beta$-actin transcripts in control (C) and axotomized (A) DRG (days post-axotomy indicated above gels), with computer-enhanced images of amplification products shown below gels. Co-amplification of NaN (392 bp) and GAPDH (6076 bp) shows decreased expression of NaN mRNA at 7 days post-axotomy (lanes 2,4,6) compared to controls (lanes 1,3,5). Top, middle panels modified from Dib-Hajj *et al.* (1996), bottom panel modified from Dib-Hajj *et al.* (1998a).

nel gene expression are accompanied by physiological changes in the voltage-sensitive sodium currents that can be recorded in injured neurons. Following axonal transection, there is a change in the properties of the fast, TTX-sensitive sodium current in DRG neurons (Figure 6.9); specifically, axotomy triggers a switch from a slowly repriming current (i.e. a current which recovers slowly from inactivation; $\tau \approx 60$ ms), to a more rapidly-repriming current ($\tau \approx 15$ ms) (Cummins and Waxman,1997). We have suggested that the emergence of the rapidly repriming current is due to the up regulation of $\alpha$-III channels (Cummins and Waxman, 1997). Axotomy also triggers a down regulation of TTX-resistant sodium currents in DRG neurons (Rizzo *et al.*, 1995; Cummins and Waxman, 1997), consistent with the down-regulation of SNS/PN3 and NaN sodium channel transcripts (Figure 6.10).

A number of lines of evidence suggest that

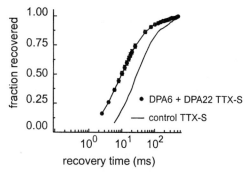

**Figure 6.9** A rapidly-repriming sodium current, not detectable in normal DRG neurons, emerges in these cells following transection of their axons within the sciatic nerve. The graph shows recovery of TTX-sensitive sodium current from inactivation as a function of time, for DRG neurons following axonal transection (6 and 22 days post-axotomy [DPA], results pooled) and for control, uninjured controls. Note the leftward shift in the recovery curve which is due to the emergence of a rapidly-repriming sodium current in the axotomized neurons. Modified from Cummins and Waxman (1997).

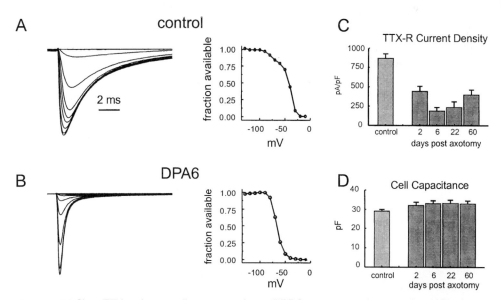

**Figure 6.10** Slow, TTX-resistant sodium currents in small DRG neurons are down-regulated following axotomy. (A, B) (left side): whole-cell patch-clamp recordings from representative control (A) and axotomized (B, 6 days post-axotomy [DPA]) DRG neurons. Note the loss of the TTX-resistant, slowly-inactivating component of sodium current following axotomy. Steady-state inactivation curves (A, B, right side) show loss of a component characteristic of TTX-resistant currents. (C) Attenuation of TTX-resistant sodium current persists for at least 60 days post-axotomy. (D) Cell capacitance, which provides a measure of cell size, does not change significantly following axotomy. Modified from Cummins and Waxman (1997).

these changes in sodium channel expression should predispose DRG neurons to fire spontaneously, or at inappropriately high frequencies, following injury. First, increased numbers of sodium channels at sites of action potential generation, in themselves, should lower threshold (Waxman and Brill, 1978; Matzner and Devor, 1992). Second, there is overlap between steady-state activation and inactivation curves of different types of sodium channels in some axotomized DRG neurons and this, together with weak voltage-dependence of TTX-resistant sodium channels, would be predicted to permit subthreshold oscillations in voltage, supported by TTX-resistant channels, to activate other sodium channels, thus producing abnormal spontaneous activity (Rizzo et al., 1996). Third, because TTX-sensitive sodium current in DRG neurons following axotomy reprimes more rapidly than normal TTX-sensitive sodium currents in these cells (Cummins and Waxman, 1997), injured DRG neurons would be expected to display a reduced refractory period, and to fire at higher-than-normal frequencies. Fourth, low-threshold, persistent sodium currents, which appear to be partially activated close to resting potential, are present in DRG neurons (Baker and Bostock, 1997; Cummins et al., 1999). Persistent sodium channels are known to contribute to resting potential in optic nerve axons (Stys et al., 1993). Loss of the channels responsible for persistent currents in DRG neurons and their axons following axonal injury could produce a hyperpolarizing shift in resting potential which, by relieving resting inactivation, might increase the availability of TTX-sensitive sodium current for electrogenesis in response to rapid depolarizations (Cummins and Waxman, 1997). Additionally, altered sodium channel expression in injured DRG neurons may be accompanied by changes in expression of other ion channels, which also modulate excitability. For example, there is evidence for a down regulation of potassium channel expression in DRG neurons following axotomy (Everill and Kocsis, 1999; Ishikawa et al., 1998).

Although most of the studies on plasticity in sodium channel expression after neuronal injury to date have focused on axotomized DRG neurons, observations in a number of experimental models indicate that changes in neuronal excitability can

occur as a result of altered sodium channel expression following other types of insult, and in other types of neurons following injury. It is now clear that sodium channel densities can increase in DRG neurons as a response to inflammation in their projection fields (Tanaka et al., 1998; Gould et al., 1998), and it has been demonstrated that this is due, at least in part, to changes in sodium channel gene expression (Tanaka et al., 1998).

There is now also evidence for an acquired channelopathy both in animal models or demyelination in multiple sclerosis. Within the normal nervous system sensory neuron specific sodium channel SNS (Akopian et al., 1996; Sangamaswaran et al., 1996) is expressed in a highly specific manner within primary sensory neurons within DRG and trigeminal ganglion. As noted above, SNS is not present within neurons within the uninjured brain. The SNS sodium channel displays slow activation and inactivation kinetics and a relatively depolarized voltage-dependence (Akopian et al., 1996; Sangameswaran et al., 1996), and more rapid recovery from inactivation (Elliott and Elliott, 1993; Dib-Hajj et al., 1997) than traditional 'fast' sodium channels. As a result of these characteristics, the presence of SNS-type channels can alter the firing properties of neurons (Schild and Kunze, 1997; Akopian et al., 1999).

Multiple sclerosis has classically been viewed as a demyelinating disease. Recent studies, however, have demonstrated abnormal SNS expression in experimental models of demyelination and in multiple sclerosis. In studies on the taiep rat, a mutant model in which myelin is initally formed normally, but then lost due to an oligodendrocyte abnormality, SNS sodium channel mRNA and protein are expressed in cerebellar Purkinje cells following loss of myelin (Black et al., 1999b). More recent studies have demonstrated that SNS mRNA and protein, which are not detectable in normal Purkinje cells, are expressed within Purkinje cells in chronic relapsing experimental allergic encephalomyelitis, a mouse model of multiple sclerosis (Black et al., 2000). SNS mRNA (Figure 6.11a, b) and protein (Figure 6.11e, f) are also expressed within cerebellar Purkinje cells from human brain tissue obtained post-mortem from MS patients, but not in controls with no neuro-

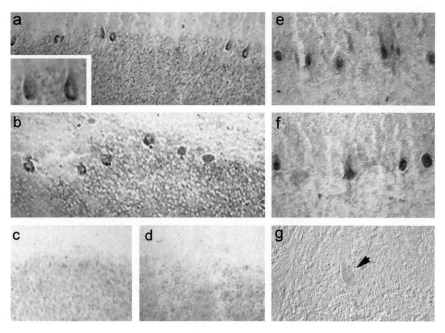

**Figure 6.11** Sensory neuron specific sodium channel (SNS) is not expressed within the normal cerebellum, but is expressed in Purkinje cells within brains obtained at post-mortem from MS patients. Panels on left, which show *in situ* hybridization with SNS-specific antisense riboprobes, demonstrate the absence of SNS mRNA in control cerebellum (a) and its presence in Purkinje cells in post-mortem tissue from two patients with MS (b, c). SNS signal is not present following hybridization with sense riboprobe (d). Panels on right demonstrate immunostaining of Purkinje cells in MS brains with an antibody directed against SNS, (e, f) and illustrate the absence of SNS protein in control cerebellum (g, arrow indicates Purkinje cell). Modified from Black *et al.* (2000).

logical disease (Figure 6.11c, g) (Black *et al.*, 2000).

The abnormal expression of SNS sodium channels within Purkinje cells in experimental and human 'demyelinating' disorders may have important functional consequences. Normal cerebellar functioning depends on precise timing of impulses. Multiple sodium currents interact within Purkinje cells to shape the firing properties of these cells (Llinas and Sugimori, 1980; Raman and Bean, 1997). Mutations of the sodium channels that are normally expressed in Purkinje cells result in altered patterns of firing which appear to produce cerebellar ataxia in mutant models such as jolting mice (Kohrman *et al.*, 1996; Raman *et al.*, 1997). The dysregulated expression of SNS sodium channels within Purkinje cells in the de-

myelinating disorders is likely to change the firing pattern of these neurons. This molecular mis-tuning might be expected to contribute to clinical abnormalities such as ataxia.

There are hints in the literature which suggest that abnormalities of sodium channel transcription may contribute to other neurological disorders. Sashihara *et al.* (1992) observed the production of larger-than-normal numbers of sodium channels in the brains of genetically seizure-susceptible mice. Bartolomei *et al.* (1997) and Gastaldi *et al.* (1997) observed transient changes in neuronal sodium channel mRNA expression that persisted for approximately 24 hours following kainate-induced seizures in a rat model of epilepsy, and suggested that these changes could lead to alterations in excitability. Vreugdenhil *et al.* (1998) observed a shift in voltage-dependence in sodium currents within hippocampal neurons in a model of epileptic kindling, consistent with the idea that there is a switch in the pattern of expression of sodium channel genes. There is evidence that persistent sodium channels constitute a particularly important substrate for the sustained depolarizations associated with epileptiform activity (Segal, 1994; Segal and Douglas, 1997). Thus, even in the absence of a global change in sodium channel expression, changes in expression of sodium channels producing persistent sodium currents could increase neuronal excitability and contribute to epileptogenesis.

As noted above, it is well established that sodium channel gene expression changes in DRG neurons following injury to their axons (Waxman et al., 1994; Dib-Hajj et al., 1996, 1998a). Similar changes have been observed in facial motor neurons following axonal transection (Iwahashi et al., 1994). It thus seems reasonable to ask whether sodium channel expression is altered in corticospinal neurons following damage to their axons. If this occurs, excitability of these cells might be altered following spinal cord injury. It has been demonstrated that there are changes in the relative densities of TTX-sensitive and resistant sodium currents in afferent neurons innervating the urinary bladder following experimental spinal cord injury (Yoshimura and de Groat, 1997). Changes of this type in axotomized corticospinal neurons could alter their excitability and might at least in part explain the post-traumatic epilepsy seen in some patients following spinal cord injury.

## Dynamic channel expression and the channelopathies

As discussed in this chapter, channel expression – in normal as well as injured neurons – is a dynamic process. Moreover, changes in the pattern of ion channel expression can have significant effects on neuronal electrogenic properties and, when channels are expressed in abnormal patterns, this can have profound effects on neuronal function. In cell compartments, such as dendrites or thin axonal branches where input impedance is high, even small changes in conductance, and thus in channel density, can have large effects on neuronal function (Jack et al., 1983; Miller et al., 1985; Perkel and Perkel et al., 1985). Observations on neuronal cell bodies, which are the site of recordings in most patch-clamp studies, thus may underestimate the functional consequences of plasticity of ion channel expression.

Although changes in ion channel gene expression have been most extensively studied after axonal transection, they also occur in demyelinating disorders. This may present some therapeutic opportunities. As we learn more about the regulatory mechanisms that control channel expression and about the effects of changes in channel expression and function on neuronal behaviour, and as subtype-specific channel-modifying drugs are developed, it should become possible to understand more fully the contribution of abnormal patterns of channel expression to the channelopathies and to devise therapeutic strategies that correct at least some of the abnormalities caused by abnormal channel expression and function.

## References

Akopian, A. N., Sivilotti, L. and Wood, J. N. (1996). A tetrodotoxin-resistant voltage-gated sodium channel expressed by sensory neurons. *J Biol Chem.*, **271**, 953–6.

Akopian, A. N., Souslova, V., Sivilotti, L. and Wood, J. N. (1997). Structure and distribution of broadly expressed atypical sodium channel. *FEBS Letts,* **400**, 183–7.

Akopian, A. N., Souslova, V., England, S. *et al.* (1999). The tetrodotoxin-resistant sodium channel SNS has a specialized function in pain pathways. *Nature Neurosci.,* **2**, 541–8.

Andrew, R. D. and Dudek, F. E. (1983). Burst discharge in mammalian neuroendocrine cells involves an intrinsic regenerative mechanism. *Science,* **221**, 1050–2.

Auld, V. J., Goldin, A. L., Krafte, D. S. *et al.* (1988). A rat brain $Na^+$ channel $\alpha$ subunit with novel gating properties. *Neuron,* **1**, 449–61.

Baker, M. D. and Bostock, H. (1997). Low-threshold, persistent sodium current in rat large dorsal root ganglion neurons in culture. *J Neurophys.,* **77**, 1503–13.

Balment, R. J., Brimble, M. J. and Forsling, M. L. (1980). Release of oxytocin induced by salt loading and its influence on renal excretion in the male rat. *J Physiol Lond.,* **308**, 439.

Bartolomei, F., Gastaldi, M., Massacrier, A. *et al.* (1997) Changes in the mRNAs encoding subtypes I, II and III sodium channel alpha subunits following kainate-induced seizures in rat brain. *J Neurocytol.,* **26**, 667–8.

Beckh, S., Noda, M., Lubbert, H. and Numa, S. (1989). Differential regulation of three sodium channel messenger RNAs in the rat central nervous system during development. *EMBO J.,* **8**, 3611–16.

Bennett, D. L., Michael, G. J., Ramachandran, N. *et al.* (1998). A distinct subgroup of small DRG cells express GDNF receptor components and GDNF is protective for these neurons after nerve injury. *J Neurosci.,* **18**, 3059–72.

Black, J. A., Dib-Hajj, S., McNabola, K. *et al.* (1996). Spinal sensory neurons express multiple sodium channel α-subunit MRNAs. *Molec Brain Res.,* **43**,117–32.

Black, J. A., Langworthy, K., Hinson, A. W., Dib-Hajj, S. D. and Waxman, S. G. (1997). NGF has opposing effects on Na⁺ channel III and SNS gene expression in spinal sensory neurons. *NeuroReport,* **8**, 2331–5.

Black, J. A., Dib-Hajj, S., Cohen, S., Hinson, A. W. and Waxman, S. G. (1998). Glial cells have heart: rH1 Na⁺ channel mRNA and protein in spinal cord astrocytes. *Glia,* **23**, 200–8.

Black, J. A., Cummins, T. R., Plumpton, C. *et al.* (1999a). Upregulation of a silent sodium channel following peripheral, but not central, nerve injury in DRG neurons. *J Neurophysiol.,* **82**, 2776–85.

Black, J. A., Fjell, J., Dib-Hajj, S. *et al.* (1999b) Abnormal expression of SNS/PN3 sodium channel in cerebellar Purkinje cells following loss of myelin in the taiep rat. *NeuroReport,* **10**, 913-918.

Black, J. A., Dib-Hajj, S., Baker, D., Newcombe, J. Cuzner, M. L. and Waxman, S. G. (2000). Sensory Neuron Specific sodium channel SNS is abnormally expressed in the brains of mice with experimental allergic encephalomyelitis and humans with multiple sclerosis. *Proc Natl Acad Sci.,* **97**, 11598.

Bostock, H. and Sears, T. A. (1976). Continuous conduction in demyelinated mammalian nerve fibres. *Nature, Lond.,* **263**, 786–7.

Bostock, H. and Sears, T. A. (1978). The internodal axon membrane: Electrical excitability and continuous conduction in segmental demyelination. *J Physiol (Lond.),* **280**, 273–301.

Brysch, W., Creutzfeldt, O. W., Luno, K., Schlingensiepen, R. and Schlingensiepen, K.-H. (1991). Regional and temporal expression of sodium channel messenger RNAs in the rat brain during development. *Exp. Brain Res.,* **86**, 562–7.

Coombs, J. S., Curtis, D. R. and Eccles, J. C. (1957). The generation of impulses in motoneurons. *J. Physiol. (Lond.),* **139**, 232–49.

Cummins, T. R. and Waxman, S. G. (1997). Down-regulation of tetrodotoxin-resistant sodium currents and upregulation of a rapidly repriming tetrodotoxin-sensitive sodium current in small spinal sensory neurons after nerve injury. *J Neurosci.,* **17**, 3503–14.

Cummins, T. R., Howe, J. R. and Waxman, S. G. (1998). Slow closed-state inactivation: A novel mechanism underlying ramp currents in cells expressing the hNE/PN1 sodium channel. *J Neurosci.,* **18**, 9607–19.

Cummins, T. R., Dib-Hajj, S. D., Black, J. A. *et al.* (1999). A novel persistent tetrodotoxin-resistant sodium current in SNS-null and wild type small primary sensory neurons. *J Neurosci.,* **19**, 1–6.

D'Arcangelo, G., Pardiso, K., Shepherd, D., Brehm, P., Halegoua, S. and Mandel, G. (1993). Neuronal growth factor regulation of two different sodium channel types through distinct signal transduction pathways. *J Cell Biol.,* **122**, 915–921.

Devor, M., Keller, C. H., Deerinck, T. J. and Ellisman, M. H. (1989). Na⁺ channel accumulation on axolemma of afferent endings in nerve end neuromas in Apteronotus. *Neurosci Lett.,* **102**,149–54.

Dib-Hajj, S., Black, J. A., Felts, P. and Waxman, S. G. (1996). Down-regulation of transcripts for Na channel α-SNS in spinal sensory neurons following axotomy. *Proc Natl Acad Sci USA,* **93**,14950–4.

Dib-Hajj, S. D., Black, J. A., Cummins, T. R., Kenney, A. M., Kocsis, J. D. and Waxman, S. G. (1998b). Rescue of α-SNS sodium channel expression in small dorsal root ganglion neurons after axotomy by nerve growth factor in vivo. *J Neurophysiol.,* **79**, 2668–78.

Dib-Hajj, S. D., Tyrrell, L., Black, J. A. and Waxman, S. G. (1998a). NaN, a novel voltage-gated Na channel, is expressed preferentially in peripheral sensory neurons and down-regulated after axotomy. *Proc Natl Acad Sci.,* **95**, 8963–9.

Dib-Hajj, S. D., Ishikawa, I. Cummins, T. R. and Waxman S. G. (1997). Insertion of a SNS-specific tetrapeptide in the S3-S4 linker of D4 accelerates recovery from inactivation of skeletal muscle voltage-gated Na channel μ1 in HEK293 cells. *FEBS Letts,* **416**, 11–14.

Dodge, F. A., Jr. and Cooley, J. W. (1973). Action potential of the motoneuron. *IBM J. Res. Dev.,* **17**, 219–29.

Dugandzija-Novakovic, S., Koszowski, A. G., Levinson, S. R. and Shrager, P. (1995). Clustering of Na⁺ channels and node of Ranvier formation in remyelinating axons. *J Neurosci.,* **15**, 492–503.

Eccles, J. C., Libet, B. and Young, R. R. (1958). The behavior of chromatolysed motoneurons studied by intracellular recording. *J Physiol.,* **143**, 11–40.

Elliott, A. A. and Elliot, J. R. (1993). Characterization of TTX-sensitive and TTX-resistant sodium currents in small cells from adult rat dorsal root ganglia. *J Physiol Lond.,* **463**, 39–56.

England, J. D., Gamboni, F., Levinson, S. R. and Finger, E. (1990). Changed distribution of sodium channels along demyelinated axons. *Proc Natl Acad Sci USA,* **87**, 6777–86.

England, J. D., Gamboni, F. and Levinson, S. R. (1991). Increased numbers of sodium channels form along demyelinated axons. *Brain Res.*, **548**, 334–347.

England, J. D., Gamboni, F., Ferguson, M. A. and Levinson, S. R. (1994). Sodium channels accumulate at the tips of injured axons. *Muscle Nerve*, **17**, 593–598.

England, J. D., Happel, L. T., Kline, D. G. *et al.* (1996). Sodium channel accumulation in humans with painful neuromas. *Neurology*, **47**, 272–6.

Everill, B. and Kocsis, J. D. (1999). Reduction in potassium currents in identified cutaneous afferent dorsal root ganglion neurons after axotomy. *J Neurophysiol.*, **82**, 700–8.

Fanger, G. R., Jones, J. R. and Maue, R. A. (1995). Differential regulation of neuronal sodium channel expression by endogenous and exogenous tyrosine kinase receptors expressed in rat pheochromocytoma cells. *J Neurosci.*, **15**, 202–13.

Fatt, P. (1957). Sequence of events in synaptic activation of a motoneurone. *J Neurophysiol.*, **20**, 61–80.

Felts, P. A., Black, J. A., Dib-Hajj, S. D. and Waxman, S. G. (1997a). NaG: A sodium channel-like mRNA shared by Schwann cells and other neural crest derivatives. *Glia*, **21**, 269–77.

Felts, P. A., Yokoyama, S., Dib-Hajj, S., Black, J. A. and Waxman, S. G. (1997b). Sodium channel α-subunit mRNAs I, II, III, NaG, Na6 and hNE: Different expression patterns in developing rat nervous system. *Molec Brain Res.*, **45**, 71–83.

Fjell, J., Cummins, T. R., Dib-Hajj, S. D., Fried, K., Black, J. A. and Waxman, S. G. (1999). Differential role of GDNF and NGF in the maintenance of two TTX-resistant sodium channels in adult DRG neurons. *Molec Brain Res.*, **67**, 267–82.

Foster, R. E., Whalen, C. C. and Waxman, S. G. (1980). Reorganization of the axonal membrane of demyelinated nerve fibers: morphological evidence. *Science*, **210**, 661–3.

Fuortes, M. G. F., Frank, K. and Becker, M. C. (1957). Steps in the production of motoneuron spikes. *J Gen Physiol.*, **40**, 735–52.

Gastaldi, M., Bartolomei, F., Massacrier, A., Planells, R., Robaglia-Schlupp, A. and Cau P. (1997). Increase in mRNAs encoding neonatal II and III sodium channel alpha-isoforms during kainate-induced seizures in adult rat hippocampus. *Mol Brain Res.*, **44**, 179–90.

Gautron, S., Dos Santos, G., Pinto-Henrique, D., Koulkoff, A., Gros, F. and Berwald-Netter, Y. (1992). The glial voltage-gated sodium channel: cell- and tissue-specific mRNA expression. *Proc Natl Acad Sci USA*, **89**, 7272–6.

Ginty, D. D., Fanger, G. R., Wagner, J. A. and Maue, R. A. (1992). The activity of cAMP-dependent protein kinase is required at a posttranslational level for the induction of voltage-dependent sodium channels by

peptide growth factors in PC12 cells. *Cell Biol.*, **116**, 1465–73.

Gould, H. J. III, England, J. D., Liu, Z. P. and Levinson, S. R. (1998). Rapid sodium channel augmentation in response to inflammation induced by complete Freund's adjuvant. *Brain Res.*, **802**, 69–74.

Hales, T. G. and Tyndale, R. G. (1994). Few cell lines with GABA$_A$ mRNA have functional receptors. *J Neurosci.*, **14**, 5429–36.

Hatton, G. I. (1990). Emerging concepts of structure-function dynamics in adult brain: The hypothalamo-neurohypophysial system. *Progr Neurobiol.* **34**, 437–504.

Hirsh, J. K. and Quandt, F. N. (1996). Down-regulation of Na channel expression by A23187 in N1E-115 neuroblastoma cells. *Brain Res.*, **706**, 343–6.

Honmou, O., Utzschneider, D. A., Rizzo, M. A., Bowe, C. M., Waxman, S. G. and Kocsis, J. D. (1994). Delayed depolarization and slow sodium currents in cutaneous afferents. *J Neurophysiol.*, **71**, 1627–38.

Inenaga, K., Nagamoto, T., Kannan, H. and Yamashita, H. (1993). Inward sodium current involvement in regenerative bursting activity of rat magnocellular supraoptic neurones in vitro. *J Physiol Lond.*, **465**, 289–301.

Ishikawa, K., Tanaka, M., Black, J. A. and Waxman, S. G. (1998). Changes in expression of voltage-gated potassium channels in dorsal root ganglion neurons following axotomy. *Muscle Nerve*, **22**, 502–7.

Iwahashi, Y., Furuyama, T., Inagaki, S., Morita, Y. and Takagi, H. (1994). Distinct regulation of sodium channel types I, II and III following nerve transection. *Molec Brain Res.*, **22**, 341–5.

Jack, J. J. B., Noble, D. and Tsien, R. W. (1983). *Electrical Current Flow in Excitable Cells*. Oxford: Oxford University Press.

Jones, C. W. and Pickering, B. T. (1969). Comparison of the effects of water deprivation and sodium chloride inhibition on the hormone content of the neurohypophysis of the rat. *J Physiol Lond.*, **203**, 449–58.

Kalman, D., Wong, B., Horvai, A. E., Cline, M. J. and O'Lague, P. H. (1990). Nerve growth factor acts through cAMP-dependent protein kinase to increase the number of sodium channels in PC12 cell. *Neuron*, **2**, 355–66.

Kayano, T., Noda, M., Flockerzi, V., Takahashi, H. and Numa, S. (1988). Primary structure of rat brain sodium channel III deduced from the cDNA sequence. *FEBS Lett.*, **228**, 187–94.

Kohrman, D. C., Smith, M. R., Goldin, A. L., Harris, J. and Meisler, N. H. (1996). A missense mutation in the sodium channel scn8a is responsible for cerebellar ataxia in the mouse mutant jolting. *J Neurosci.*, **16**, 5993–9.

Kuno, M. and Llinas, R. (1970). Enhancement of synaptic transmission by dendritic potentials in chromatolysed motoneurons of the cat. *J Physiol Lond.*, **210**, 807–21.

Li, Z. and Hatton, G. I. (1996). Oscillatory bursting of phasically firing rat supraoptic neurones in low-$Ca^{2+}$ medium: $Na^+$ influx, cytosolic $Ca^{2+}$ and gap junctions. *J Physiol Lond.*, **496**, 379–94.

Llinas, R. and Sugimori, M. (1980). Electrophysiological properties of in vitro Purkinje cell somata in mammalian cerebellar slice. *J Physiol.*, **305**, 171–96.

Mason, W. T. (1980). Supraoptic neurones of rat hypothalamus are osmosensitive. *Nature,* **287**, 154–7.

Matzner, O. and Devor, M. (1992). $Na^+$ conductance and the threshold for repetitive neuronal firing. *Brain Res.,* **597**, 92–8.

Miller, J. P., Rall, W. and Rinzel, J. (1985). Synaptic amplification by active membrane in dendritic spines. *Brain Res.*, **325**, 325–30.

Moll, C., Mourre, C., Lazdunski, M. and Ulrich, J. (1991). Increase of sodium channels in demyelinated lesions of multiple sclerosis. *Brain Res.*, **556**, 311–16.

Noda, M., Ikeda, T., Kayano, T. *et al.* (1986a). Existence of distinct sodium channel messenger RNAs in rat brain. *Nature*, **320**, 188–92.

Noda, M., Ikeda, T., Suzuki, H. *et al.* (1986b). Expression of functional sodium channels from cloned cDNA. *Nature*, **322**, 826–8.

Novakovic, S. D., Tzoumaka, E., McGivern, J. G. *et al.* (1988). Distribution of the tetrodotoxon-resistant sodium channel PN3 in rat sensory neurons in normal and neuropathic conditions. *J Neurosci.*, **18**, 2174–87.

Offord, J. and Catterall, W. A. (1989). Electrical activity, cAMP, and cytosolic calcium regulate mRNA encoding sodium channel $\alpha$ subunits in rat muscle cells. *Neuron,* **2**, 1447–52.

Ollet, S. H. R. and Bourque, C. W. (1993). Mechanosensitive channels transduce osmosensitivity in supraoptic neurons. *Nature*, **364**, 341–3.

Oyelese, A. A., Rizzo, M. A., Waxman, S. G. and Kocsis, J. D. (1997). Differential effects of NGF and BDNF on axotomy-induced changes in $GABA_A$-receptor-mediated conductance and sodium currents in cutaneous afferent neurons. *J Neurophysiol.*, **78**, 31–42.

Perkel, D. H. and Perkel, D. J. (1985). Dendritic spines: role of active membrane in modulating synaptic efficacy. *Brain Res.*, **325**, 331–5.

Quick, D. C. and Waxman, S. G. (1977). Specific staining of the axon membrane at nodes of Ranvier with ferric ion and ferrocyanide. *J Neurol Sci.*, **31**, 1–11.

Raman, I. M. and Bean, B. P. (1997). Resurgent sodium current and action potential formation in dissociated cerebellar purkinje neurons. *J Neurosci.*, **17**, 4157–4166.

Raman, I. M., Sprunger, L. K., Meisler, M. H. and Bean, B. P. (1997). Altered subthreshold sodium currents and disrupted firing patterns in Purkinje neurons of Scn8a mutant mice. *Neuron*, **19**, 881–91.

Richard, D. and Bourque, C. W. (1992). Synaptic activation of rat supraoptic neurons by osmotic stimulation of the organum vasculosum lamina terminalis. *Neuroendocrinology,* **55**, 609–11.

Ritchie, J. M. and Rogart, R. B. (1977). The density of sodium channels in mammalian myelinated nerve fibers and the nature of the axonal membrane under the myelin sheath. *Proc Natl. Acad Sci USA*, **74**, 211–5.

Ritchie, J. M. (1982). Sodium and potassium channels in regenerating and developing mammalian myelinated nerves. *Proc R Soc.*, **B215**, 273–87.

Rizzo, M. A., Kocsis, J. D. and Waxman, S. G. (1995). Selective loss of slow and enhancement of fast $Na^+$ currents in cutaneous afferent dorsal root ganglion neurones following axotomy. *Neurobiol. Dis.*, **2**, 87–96.

Rizzo, M. A., Kocsis, J. D. and Waxman, S. G. (1996). Mechanisms of paresthesiae, dysesthesiae, and hyperesthesiae: Role of $Na^+$ channel heterogeneity. *Eur Neurol.*, **36**, 3–12.

Sangameswaran, L., Delgado, S. G., Fish, L. M. *et al.* (1996). Structure and function of a novel voltage-gated tetrodotoxin-resistant sodium channel specific to sensory neurons. *J Biol Chem.*, **271**, 5953–6.

Sashihara, S., Yanagihara, N., Kobayashi, H. *et al.* (1992). Overproduction of voltage-dependent $Na^+$-channels in the developing brain of genetically seizure-susceptible E1 mice. *Neuroscience*, **48**, 285–91.

Sashihara, S., Greer, C. A., Oh, Y. and Waxman, S. G. (1996). Cell-specific differential expression of $Na^+$-channel $\beta$1 subunit mRNA in the olfactory system during postnatal development and following denervation. *J Neurosci.,* **16**, 702–14.

Sashihara, S., Waxman, S. G. and Greer, C. A. (1997). Down-regulation of $Na^+$ channel mRNA following sensory deprivation of tufted cells in the neonatal rat olfactory bulb. *NeuroReport*, **8**, 1289–93.

Schaller, K. L., Krzemien, D. M., Yarowsky, P. J., Krueger, B. K. and Caldwell, J. H. (1995). A novel, abundant sodium channel expressed in neurons and glia. *J Neurosci.*, **15**, 3231–42.

Schild, J. H. and Kunze D. L. (1997). Experimental and modeling study of $Na^+$ current heterogeneity in rat nodose neurons and its impact on neuronal discharge. *J Neurophysiol.*, **79**, 3198–209.

Segal, M. M. (1994). Endogenous bursts underlie seizurelike activity in solitary excitatory hippocampal neurons in microcultures. *J Neurophysiol.*, **72**, 1874–84.

Segal, M. M. and Douglas, A. F. (1995). Late sodium channel openings underlying epileptiform activity are preferentially diminished by the anticonvulsant phenytoin. *Neuron,* **77**, 3021–34.

Sernagor, E., Yarom, Y. and Werman, R. (1986).

Sodium-dependent regenerative responses in dendrites of axotomized motoneurons in the cat. *Proc Natl Acad Sci USA,* **83**, 7966–70.

Sharma, N., D'Arcangelo, G., Kleinhaus, A., Halegous, S. and Trimmer, J. S. (1993). Nerve growth factor regulates the abundance and distribution of $K^+$ channels in PC12 cells. *J Cell Biol.,* **123**, 1835–45.

Sherman, S. J., Chrivia, J. and Catterall, W. A. (1985). Cyclic adenosine 3′,5′-monophosphate and cytosolic calcium exert opposing effects on biosynthesis of tetrodotoxin-sensitive sodium channels in rat muscle cells. *J Neurosci.,* **5**, 1570–6.

Shrager, P. (1989). Sodium channels in single demyelinated mammalian axons. *Brain Res.,* **483**, 149–54.

Stys, P. K., Sontheimer, H., Ransom, B. R. and Waxman, S. G. (1993). Non-inactivating, TTX-sensitive $Na^+$ conductance in rat optic nerve axons. *Proc Natl Acad Sci.,* **90**, 6976–80.

Sucher, N. J., Brose, N., Deitcher, D. L. *et al.* (1993). Expression of endogenous NMDAR1 transcripts without receptor protein suggests post-transcriptional control in PC12 cells. *J Biol Chem.,* **268**, 22299–304.

Suzuki, H., Beckh, S., Kubo, M. *et al.* (1988). Functional expression of cloned cDNA encoding sodium channel III. *FEBS Lett.,* **228**, 195–200.

Tanaka, M., Cummins, T. R., Ishikawa, K., Black, J. A., Ibata, Y. and Waxman, S. G. (1999). Molecular and functional remodeling of electrogenic membrane of hypothalamic neurons in response to changes in their input. *Proc Natl Acad Sci USA,* **96**, 1088–94.

Tanaka, M., Cummins, T. R., Ishikawa, K., Dib-Hajj, S. D., Black, J. A. and Waxman, S. G. (1998). SNS $Na^+$ channel expression increases in dorsal root ganglion neurons in the carageenan inflammatory pain model. *NeuroReport,* **9**, 967–72.

Titmus, M. J. and Faber, D. S. (1986). Altered excitability of goldfish Mauthner cell following axotomy. II. Localization and ionic basis. *J Neurophysiol.,* **55**, 1440–54.

Toledo-Aral, J. J., Brehm, P., Halegoua, S. and Mandel, G. (1995). A single pulse of nerve growth factor triggers long-term neuronal excitability through sodium channel gene induction. *Neuron,* **14**, 607–11.

Toledo-Aral, J. J., Moss, B. L., He, Z.-J. *et al.* (1997). Identification of PN1, a predominant voltage-dependent sodium channel expressed principally in peripheral neurons. *Proc Natl Acad Sci.,* **94**, 1527–32.

Vabnick, I., Novakovic, S. D., Levinson, S. R., Schachner, M. and Shrager, P. (1996). The clustering of axonal sodium channels during development of the peripheral nervous system. *J Neurosci.,* **16b**, 4914–22.

Vega-Saenz de Miera, E., Rudy, B., Sugimori, M. and Llinas R. (1997). Molecular characterization of the sodium channel subunits expressed in mammalian cerebellar Purkinje cells. *Proc Natl Acad Sci USA,* **94**, 7059–64.

Vreugdenhill, M., Faas, G. C. and Wadman, W. J. (1998). Sodium currents in isolated rat CA1 neurons after kindling epileptogenesis. *Neuroscience,* **86**, 99–107.

Walters, J. K. and Hatton, G. I. (1974). Supraoptic neuronal activity in rats during five days of water deprivation. *Physiol Behav.,* **13**, 661–7.

Waxman, S. G. (1977). Conduction in myelinated, unmyelinated, and demyelinated fibers. *Arch Neurol.,* **34**, 585–90.

Waxman, S. G. and Brill, M. H. (1978). Conduction through demyelinated plaques in multiple sclerosis: computer simulations of facilitation by short internodes. *J Neurol Neurosurg Psychiatr.,* **41**, 408–17.

Waxman, S. G. and Quick, D. C. (1978). Functional architecture of the initial segment. In *Physiology and Pathobiology of Axons* (ed. Waxman, S.G.), pp. 125–130. New York: Raven Press.

Waxman, S. G. and Foster, R. E. (1980). Development of the axon membrane during differentiation of myelinated fibres in spinal nerve roots. *Proc Roy Soc Lond.,* **209**, 441–6.

Waxman, S. G., Black, J. A. and Foster, R. E. (1982). Freeze-fracture heterogeneity of the axolemma of premyelinated fibers in the CNS. *Neurology,* **32**, 418–21.

Waxman, S. G. (1987). Rules governing membrane reorganization and axon-glial interactions during the development of myelinated fibers. In *Progress in Brain Research*, Vol. 71 (ed. Seil, F.J., Herbert, E. and Carlson, B.), Elsevier, Amsterdam, pp. 121–142.

Waxman, S. G., Black, J. A., Kocsis, J. D. and Ritchie, J. M. (1989). Low density of sodium channels supports action potential conduction in axons of neonatal rat optic nerve. *Proc Natl Acad Sci.,* **86**, 1406–10.

Waxman, S. G., Kocsis, J. D. and Black, J. A. (1994). Type III sodium channel mRNA is expressed in embryonic but not adult spinal sensory neurons, and is re-expressed following axotomy *J Neurophysiol.,* **72**, 466–71.

Waxman, S. G. (1998). Demyelinating diseases: New pathological insights, new therapeutic targets. *New Eng J Med.,* **338**, 323–5.

Weiner, L. P., Waxman, S. G., Stohlman, S. A. and Kwan, A. (1980). Remyelination following viral-induced demyelination: Ferric ion-ferrocyanide staining of nodes of Ranvier within the CSN. *Ann Neurol.,* **8**, 580–3.

Westenbroek, R. R., Merrick, D. K. and Catterall, W. A. (1989). Differential subcellular localization of the RI and RII $Na^+$ channel subtypes in central axons. *Neuron,* **3**, 695–704.

Westenbroek, R. R., Noebels, J. L. and Catterall, W. A. (1992). Elevated expression of type II $Na^+$ channels in hypomyelinated axons of shiverer mouse brain. *J Neurosci.,* **12**, 2259–67.

Wiley-Livingston, C. A. and Ellisman, M. H. (1980). Development of axonal membrane specializations defines nodes of Ranvier and precedes Schwann cell myelin elaboration. *Dev Biol.*, **79**, 334–55.

Yoshimura, N. and de Groat, W. C. (1997). Plasticity of $Na^+$ channels in afferent neurones innervating rat urinary bladder following spinal cord injury. *J Physiol.*, **503**, 269–76.

# CHAPTER 7

# The role and consequences of ion channel distribution and dysfunction in pain

*Sam Chong and John C Hunter*

## Introduction

In the mammalian peripheral and central (CNS) nervous systems, sodium, calcium and potassium voltage-gated ion channels are crucial for controlling neuronal excitability. Each of these voltage-gated ion channels is made up of different subunits encoded by multiple genes. Different combinations of these subunits make up different subtypes

of voltage-gated channels with diverse biophysical and pharmacological properties (for reviews see Catterall, 1992, 1995; Pongs, 1992; Kallen *et al.*, 1993; Reuter, 1996). The selective expression of combinations of channel subtypes determines the heterogeneity and functional specialization of many types of cells, particularly the neurons. The importance of voltage-gated ion channels to normal cell physiology can be gauged by the large

## PATHOPHYSIOLOGY OF THE SENSORY NEURON

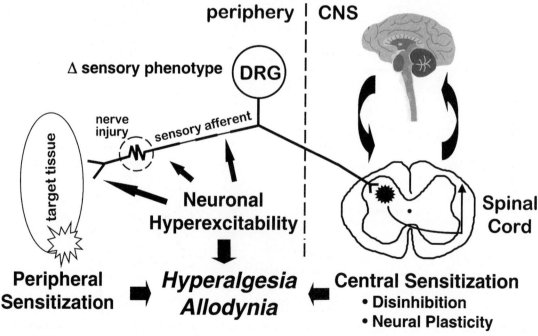

**Figure 7.1** Peripheral nociceptive input causing secondary changes in multiple levels of the neuroaxis is fundamental to the development and persistence of chronic pain.

variety of clinical syndromes, some quite debilitating and even fatal, that is caused by ion channel dysfunction (Ackerman and Clapham, 1997).

The possibility that voltage-gated channels are altered after nerve injury was suggested by initial work on motor neurons (Eccles *et al.*, 1958). Their importance for the sensory system was highlighted by the experiments of Wall and Gutnick (1974) and Kirk (1974). Spontaneous electrical excitability was reported in primary afferent nerve fibres that originate from a neuroma. We now know that changes in the expression and function of voltage-gated channels contribute to the ongoing abnormal repetitive discharge from ectopic sites established within primary afferent neurons following injury (reviewed by Devor, 1994). It is this barrage of spontaneous and/or evoked afferent impulses that set up the process of central sensitization involving increased neuronal excitability and synaptic

reorganization within the spinal dorsal horn (Devor, 1994; Woolf and Doubell, 1994). Furthermore, voltage-gated ion channels may have a role in influencing the system of descending inhibitory control and alter the rostral transmission of nociceptive signals. Such changes in the peripheral and central neuronal function are believed to underlie the paraesthesias, dysaesthesias and pain associated with nerve injury.

In everyday clinical practice, the role of voltage-gated ion channels in the pathogenesis of chronic pain is supported by the efficacy of agents that act primarily through a common, use-dependent block of sodium channels. Local anaesthetics, antiarrhythmics and anticonvulsants (Catterall, 1987) are reported to relieve many types of chronic, especially neuropathic, pain (Backonja, 1994; Tanelian and Victory, 1995). Similarly, drugs like ziconotide that act on calcium channels

## SOMATOSENSORY TARGETS FOR THE TREATMENT OF ACUTE/CHRONIC PAIN

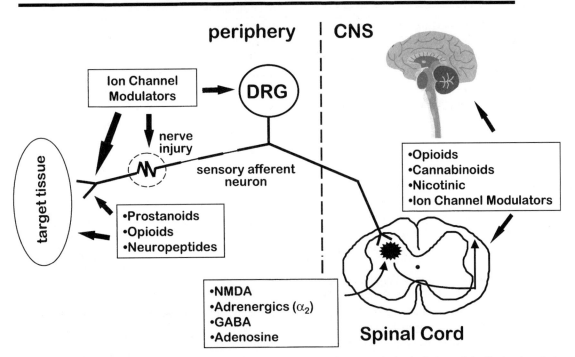

**Figure 7.2** These are potential targets for intervention to alter nociceptive transmission in the search for the treatment of acute and chronic pain. It is likely that a combination of different medications with different modes and sites of action are necessary for the successful alleviation of pain.

are reported to be effective for treating neuropathic pain (see below). At present, there is no licensed drug that acts specifically on the voltage-gated potassium channel. Therefore we know far less about the role of voltage-gated potassium channels in nociception. Nevertheless, it can be argued that membrane events that play a role in the redistribution of sodium channels can also cause alterations in the localization and distribution of membrane-bound voltage-gated potassium channels. Consequently, they could contribute to the establishment and maintenance of the neuronal hyperexcitability (Devor, 1994). It has been reported that a large reduction in some subtypes of voltage-gated potassium channels occur in DRG neurons after axotomy (Ishikawa et al., 1999) and this may be responsible for neuronal hyperexcitability after nerve damage. Therefore, modulation of the function or distribution of potassium channels has the potential for providing novel agents for the treatment of chronic pain.

## Sodium channels

In excitable tissue such as nerve and muscle, voltage-gated sodium channels (VGSCs) located in the plasma membrane permit entry of sodium ions into the cell causing depolarization and generation of the action potential (Catterall, 1992; Kallen et al., 1993). This control of membrane excitability is mediated by the tissue-dependent expression of distinct genes encoding individual VGSC subtypes that have been distinguished on the basis of primary structure, but can also be differentiated by their biophysical properties and sensitivity to the neurotoxin tetrodotoxin (TTX). Most VGSCs like the rat brain types I, IIA and III, skeletal muscle type I (Catterall, 1992; Kallen et al., 1993) and the recently described channels, Sodium Channel Protein 6 (SCP6; Schaller et al., 1995), the closely homologous Peripheral Nerve 4 (PN4; Dietrich et al., 1998) and Peripheral Nerve 1 (PN1; Sangameswaran et al., 1997; Toledo-Aral et al., 1997) are characterized by rapid inactivation kinetics and low, nanomolar sensitivity to TTX. However, more persistent sodium currents with slower inactivation kinetics have also been described, specifically in heart and sensory gang-

lia. The cardiac channel H1 (Catterall, 1992; Kallen et al., 1993) exhibits low, micromolar (1–5 $\mu$M) sensitivity to TTX, while the recently described channel termed either Peripheral Nerve 3 (PN3; Sangameswaran et al., 1996) or Sensory Nerve Specific (SNS; Akopian et al., 1996), is TTX-resistant ($\sim$ 100 $\mu$M).

Dorsal root ganglia (DRG) neurons express at least six types of VGSCs. High levels of Na6 and $\alpha$-1 found in DRG cells are also seen in other neurons. They are responsible for TTX-sensitive currents. There is another TTX-sensitive VGSC that seems to be found exclusively in DRG cells, the PN1/hNE channel. As mentioned above, two TTX-resistant VGSCs have now been described in DRG neurons, the SNS/PN3 and NaN channels. The other VGSC subtype that is reported to be expressed by DRG neurons is NaG. This channel is also described in tissue of neural crest origin but not found in other types of neurons (see Chapter 6).

The initial discovery of spontaneous discharges and hypersensitivity in damaged axons prompted a search for the underlying pathophysiology. It is now clear that a major contributing factor to this initiation and maintenance of ectopic, repetitive firing of primary afferent fibres following injury is the redistribution of sodium channels along injured or regenerating axons. The end result of post-injury changes is an abnormal accumulation and increased membrane density of sodium channels at focal sites of injury like in neuroma end bulbs or at demyelinated sites (Devor et al., 1993; England et al., 1996). This membrane remodelling contributes to a lower threshold for action potential generation at these sites and consequently precipitates ectopic impulse generation in chronically injured nerves (Wall and Devor, 1983; Matzner and Devor, 1994; Devor, 1994). This immunocytochemical and neurophysiological evidence was further strengthened by mathematical modelling performed by Devor and colleagues. It is now clear that changes in membrane hyperexcitability could be solely accounted for by the increase in sodium channel density (Matzner and Devor, 1992). Consistent with this hypothesis has been the observation that interruption of fast axonal transport decreases ectopic impulse generation in injured peripheral nerves

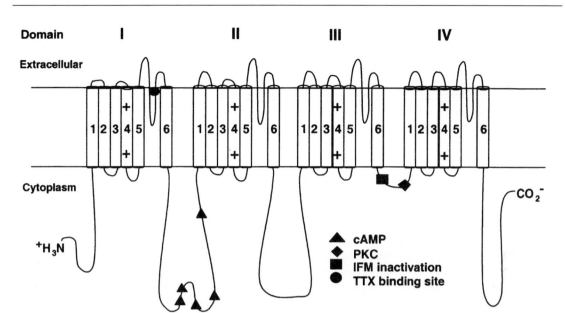

**Figure 7.3** This is a drawing of the subunit of the voltage gated sodium channel. The subunit is made up of 4 domains. The human gene loci for different sodium channels together with the corresponding rat orthologue is shown. Each channel has different sensitivity to tetradotoxin and has characteristic activation thresholds and inactivation rates.

| Gene Loci | Rat Orthologs | TTX sensitivity | Activation Threshold | Inactivation Rate |
|---|---|---|---|---|
| SCN1A | Brain I | - | Low | Fast |
| SCN2A | Brain IIA | 18 nM | Low | Fast |
| SCN3A | Brain III | 15 nM | Low | fast |
| SCN5A | Heart 1 | 1.8 μM | Low | Medium |
| SCN8A | SCP6, PN4 | 1.0 nM | Low | Fast |
| SCN9A | PN1 | 4.3 nM | Low | Fast |
| SCN10A | PN3 (A), SNS | 100 μM | High | Slow |
| SCN11A | NaN, SNS2 | 1.0 μM | Low | Medium |

without blocking nerve conduction (Devor and Govrin-Lippmann, 1983). Abnormal firing of DRG cells after injury may not be confined to local areas of damage alone. The axonal hillock near the DRG cell body also has a high concentration of sodium channels (Devor, 1999) and redistribution of VGSCs may also contribute to the rhythmic discharges seen in these axons.

Therefore, alterations in either the level of expression or distribution of sodium channels within the injured nerve have a major influence on the pathophysiology of pain associated with nerve damage. This concept is supported by numerous pharmacological studies involving the use of sodium channel modulating agents in animal models and in the clinic.

## Local anaesthetics

Local anaesthetics have traditionally been used to prevent acute pain by regional infiltration and local blocking of nerve conduction. However, the use of local anaesthetics both via systemic and topical administration for treating chronic pain is also gaining acceptance (Backonja, 1994; Tanelian and Victory, 1995; Rowbotham et al., 1995).

Bartlett and Hutaserani first reported the use of intravenous lignocaine for treating postoperative pain in 1961. The use of systemic local anaesthetics for acute pain was then abandoned because of safety concerns over potential CNS and cardiac toxicity (Cassuto et al., 1985; Birch et al., 1987). Large systemic doses of local anaesthetics, sufficient to achieve analgesia, have very narrow therapeutic margins. Therefore their use is restricted to local or regional blockade. Interest in the use of systemic local anaesthetics then reappeared 20 years later, this time for treating chronic pain. Boas et al. (1982) demonstrated a possible reduction in central and deafferented pain when patients were treated with intravenous lignocaine. More recently, there is an emerging appreciation for the ability of these agents to provide pre-emptive analgesia at low, non-toxic, systemic concentrations in order to limit any potential nociceptive sensitization to surgery in the nervous system (Woolf and Chong, 1993).

In animal models of neuropathic pain, the systemic administration of local anaesthetics appears to be effective for reducing pain. The most commonly tested animal models available are those in which neuroma are induced by nerve injury similar to the original model of Wall and Gutnick (1974), or else a painful neuropathy is induced either by chronic constriction injury to the sciatic nerve (the CCI animal model) (Bennett and Xie, 1988) or by ligation of the L5/L6 spinal nerve (the spinal nerve ligation or SNL animal model) (Kim and Chung, 1992). Neurophysiological recordings show that intravenous lignocaine can suppress the ectopic discharges in the neuroma (Chabal et al., 1989), CCI (Sotgiu et al., 1994) and SNL (Abdi et al., 1998) models of neuropathic pain. Behavioural observations show that systemic administration of local anaesthetics is effective against both mechanical and thermal hyperalgesia as well as tactile and cold allodynia, but with differential sensitivity and limited efficacy (Abram and Yaksh, 1994; Hedley et al., 1995). In most cases, a ceiling effect was observed with the appearance of side-effects such as sedation, loss of righting reflex and, at high doses, convulsions, that limited further escalation of the dose. In another model representative of facilitated processing of sensory information, the formalin test, lidocaine (lignocaine) (Abram and Yaksh, 1994) and mexiletine (Jett et al., 1997) attenuated both phases of the behavioural response. Interestingly, these changes were achieved at much higher doses than those observed to diminish the hyperaesthetic state following a peripheral nerve injury. Lignocaine and mexiletine are ineffective against an acute, high threshold thermal noxious stimulus in the rat tail flick test (Hedley et al., 1995). This may be consistent with the predicted use-dependent nature of the sodium channel blockage produced by these agents. One important aspect of this analgesic action is the ability of systemically administered local anaesthetics at these low subanaesthetic concentrations to block spontaneous and/or evoked afferent activity (impulse initiation) without affecting nerve conduction (impulse propagation) (Chabal et al., 1989; Devor et al., 1992; Matzner and Devor, 1994). Consequently, these agents have an advantage in being able to target injured nerves (neuropathic) on the basis of their high frequency, repetitive firing without affecting normal somatosensory (i.e. nociceptive) neuronal function.

In humans, local anaesthetics have been shown to be effective for treating many acute, subacute and chronic pain syndromes. Local anaesthetics administered subcutaneously (Brose and Cousins, 1991) as well as intravenously (Ellemann et al., 1989; Bruera et al., 1992) has been reported to be effective for relieving malignant neuropathic pain. As mentioned above, Boas et al. (1982) treated their patients with an intravenous bolus of lignocaine 3 mg/kg over 3 minutes followed by a continuous infusion of 4 mg/kg over 60 minutes. Relief from trigeminal neuralgia, phantom limb and central thalamic pain was reported by the authors. A much larger series of over 200 patients with a mixture of central and peripheral neuropathic pain was also reported to benefit from intravenous lignocaine infusion (Edwards et al., 1985).

Since then, numerous case series and small controlled studies have reported effective pain relief from painful diabetic polyneuropathy (Kastrup et al., 1987; Dejgard et al., 1988), neuralgic pain (Lindstrom and Lindblom, 1987; Rowbotham et al., 1991, 1995; Marchettini et al., 1992), lumbar radiculopathies (Nagaro et al., 1995; Ferrante et al., 1996), reflex sympathetic dystrophy (Edwards et al., 1985; Galer et al., 1993) and peripheral nerve injury (Tanelian and Brose, 1991; Chabal et al., 1992a, b; Galer et al., 1996). Very few controlled trials have been reported. Bach et al. (1990) performed a double-blinded placebo-controlled study in patients with painful diabetic neuropathy. They found intravenous lignocaine at 5 mg/kg but not saline to be effective for reducing pain and improve sleep in these patients. The effect of a single lignocaine infusion may last up to 21 days. Data from this study when used to calculate the accepted measure of treatment efficacy, the number needed to treat, (NNT) give a figure of 3 (Sindrup and Jensen, 1999). This means that for every three patients treated with intravenous lignocaine at the above stated dose, one will achieve over 50% reduction in pain. In another study, intravenous lignocaine and morphine was compared to saline for alleviating the pain of post-herpetic neuralgia (Rowbotham et al., 1991). Intravenous lignocaine was superior to placebo but 11 out of 19 patients expressed a preference for morphine as opposed to only four patients for lignocaine. As a general rule systemic local anaesthetics are more effective against neuropathic pain originating in the peripheral nervous system with known aetiology rather than in the CNS or where pathogenesis is unclear (Galer et al., 1993). Central pain following stroke, thalamic lesions and multiple sclerosis has been reported to respond to local anaesthetics but with a mixed degree of success when compared to the peripheral neuropathic pain syndromes (Awerbuch and Sandyk, 1990; Backonja and Gombar, 1992; Edmondson et al., 1993; Sakurai and Kanazawa 1999; Attal et al., 2000). Intravenous lignocaine even at plasma levels of 3 $\mu$g/ml appears to have little effect on the allodynia from complex regional pain syndromes 1 and 2 (causalgia and reflex sympathetic dystrophy) (Wallace et al., 2000).

Some important conclusions can be drawn from these clinical trials. If lignocaine is effective, the route of administration does not appear to greatly influence analgesic effect. Subcutaneous administration appears to be as effective as the intravenous infusions so long as adequate plasma levels are achieved (Devulder et al., 1993). Pain relief often outlasts drug elimination from the plasma (Petersen et al., 1986; Arner et al., 1990; Bach et al., 1990). The half-life of lignocaine is measured in hours, yet analgesic effect can last for days. The mechanisms to explain this phenomenon are presently unknown.

Parenteral administration of local anaesthetics is cumbersome and not feasible for most patients. Oral forms of local anaesthetic-like drugs are much easier to administer and have been used to treat neuropathic pain. Flecainide has been reported to be effective for treating cancer-related neuropathic pain (Sinnott et al., 1991). However, this drug is associated with causing life-threatening cardiac arrhythmias and its use is generally confined to patients with cancer. Another orally active local anaesthetic-like drug is tocainide. This has been reported to be effective for treating trigeminal neuralgia (Lindstrom and Lindblom, 1987). It has since been withdrawn from use because of its association with disastrous bone marrow suppression. The most common orally active local anaesthetic-like drug presently used is mexiletine, a type Ib antiarrhythmic agent. In their systemic analysis of drugs used for treating neuropathic pain, Sindrup and Jensen (1999) identified four placebo-controlled trials of mexiletine. Both Dejgard et al. (1988) and Oskarsson et al. (1997) reported mexiletine to be effective for treating painful diabetic neuropathy. However, two other studies reported that mexiletine is either no better than placebo (Wright et al., 1997) or an effect is identified only by using subgroup analysis with no difference from placebo found using the primary outcome measure (Stracke et al., 1992). At an average dose of 675 mg a day, mexiletine was calculated to have an NNT value of 10 (3.0 to $\infty$). Mexiletine had significant side-effects with nausea, dizziness, drowsiness and ataxia being common, particularly with rapid dose escalation. Rarely, mexiletine can be effective for treating neuropathic pain where other drugs have failed, but it is not a first line agent for treating chronic pain. Clinicians using mexiletine are also unclear as to whether it should be used only after a successful initial lignocaine infusion, which might predict a good mexilitine response. The case report by Tanelian and Brose (1991) and the small study reported by Galer *et al.* (1996) would support this.

One other method of using local anaesthetic type drugs that is gaining popularity is by topical administration. Studies have shown that neuropathic pain syndromes, where peripheral sensitization plays an important role, are eminently treatable with topical local anaesthetics. Good pain relief with the use of lignocaine gel patches is reported in patients with post-herpetic neuralgia, particularly the 'angry C-fibre subtype' (Rowbotham *et al.*, 1995; Rowbotham, 1999).

Despite producing varying degrees of relief in many different types of chronic pain conditions, the full analgesic potential of local anaesthetic-like drugs are limited by problems with optimal dosage, route and schedule of administration, and side-effects. They retain an important role for managing acute pain, particularly as pre-emptive analgesia. As for treating chronic pain, it can be argued that the presently available local anaesthetic-like drugs are best used topically for treating mainly peripheral forms of neuropathic pain where the principal mechanism of pain pathogenesis is the 'irritable' nociceptor.

## Anticonvulsants

In 1885, Trousseau noted that the paroxysmal component of trigeminal neuralgia was remarkably similar to epilepsy and termed it 'epileptiform neuralgia' (for review see Swerdlow, 1984). This early observation was then followed by successful trials of novel, anticonvulsant therapies as they became available, including diphenylhydantoin (or phenytoin; Swerdlow, 1984) and carbamazepine (Blom, 1962). Anticonvulsant drugs have subsequently remained among the more commonly used pharmacological interventions for the treatment of chronic pain (Swerdlow, 1984; McQuay *et al.*, 1995; Sindrup and Jensen, 1999). One of the largest placebo-controlled trials was carried out by Cambell *et al.* (1966). In their

crossover study nearly 80 patients were recruited and carbamazepine was shown to be clearly superior to placebo for treating trigeminal neuralgia.

It has been a common perception, possibly influenced by these early reports, that drugs of this class are more efficacious where there is a paroxysmal, lancinating component to the pain, e.g. trigeminal neuralgia (Campbell *et al.*, 1966; Killian and Fromm, 1968). Trial evidence to support this is sparse, possibly because this is not a parameter specifically reported in many studies.

Both carbamazepine and phenytoin have been reported to be effective for treating painful neuropathies. For painful diabetic neuropathy, the studies by Rull *et al.* (1969) using carbamazepine and Saudek *et al.* (1977) and Chadda and Mathur (1978) with phenytoin are often quoted. All three of these were small studies using crossover design with very narrow measures of efficacy. The study by Chadda and Mathur actually found phenytoin to be no better than placebo. Similarly, carbamazepine does not appear to be significantly better than placebo (Leijon and Boivie, 1989) when used to treat central post-stroke pain. However, carbamazepine can be effective for treating specific types of central pain. Chronic pain is common in patients with multiple sclerosis and from a case series report (Espir and Millac, 1970) as well as the personal experience of many clinicians, carbamazepine can be very effective in this situation. The reason for this may be the very specific nature of damage to central axons cause by demyelination and alterations in sodium channel function associated with it. Carbamazepine was also reported to be effective for treating the pain from Fabry's disease, possibly giving a clue to the pathogenesis of pain in this condition (Filling-Katz *et al.*, 1989).

Even though there is limited evidence from large placebo-controlled studies, carbamazepine is still the commonest antiepileptic drug prescribed by clinicians for neuropathic pain. Its efficacy is variable and when prescribed at anticonvulsant dosage, pain relief was almost always obtained concomitantly with numerous side-effects (Campbell *et al.*, 1966; Killian and Fromm, 1968; Rull *et al.*, 1969). The adverse reactions to these anticonvulsants include CNS effects such as dizziness, ataxia, light-headedness, somnolence and alterations in mood. Hepatic dysfunction, hyponatrae-mia and leucopenia have also been reported to occur with carbamazepine.

This questionable analgesic efficacy of pheny-toin and, to a lesser extent, carbamazepine, at doses not associated with side-effects, is also a consistent observation in most experimental ani-mal models of peripheral nerve injury (Koch et al., 1996) and inflammation (Nakamura-Craig and Follenfant, 1995). Since the use-dependent block of sodium channels produced by both carba-mazepine and phenytoin is analogous to that ob-tained with the local anaesthetics, it has been proposed that the reduced efficacy of carbamaze-pine and phenytoin may be related to the manner in which these drugs bind to the sodium channel (Kuo and Bean, 1994; Kuo et al., 1997). Relative to the local anaesthetics, both drugs, especially phenytoin, require a sustained membrane depolar-ization in order to bind with optimal affinity to the fast inactivated state of the sodium channel. Such a state of sustained depolarization may only be achieved during abnormal neuronal discharges of the intensity and duration often associated with certain types of epilepsy but probably not with peripheral nerve injury (Kuo and Bean, 1994; Kuo et al., 1997).

Recently, we have seen the emergence of sev-eral novel antiepileptic agents, exemplified by lamotrigine (Lamictal ®; Fitton and Goa, 1995), with a potential for treating chronic pain and possibly with an improved therapeutic window. Lamotrigine produces a voltage- and frequency-dependent block of sodium channels leading to stabilization of neuronal membrane excitability. Subsequent alterations in the presynaptic release of the excitatory amino acids glutamate and aspar-tate, may contribute to the anticonvulsant action. These postulated changes underlie lamotrigine's theoretical potential as an analgesic (Leach et al., 1986; Cheung et al., 1992).

In rodents, lamotrigine has been tested in mod-els of both neuropathic and inflammatory pain with variable results. In rat sciatic nerve injury models, lamotrigine produced a reversal of cold allodynia but was ineffective against tactile allo-dynia (Hunter et al., 1997). In two inflammatory pain models, lamotrigine reversed both prosta-glandin $E_2$ and streptozotocin-induced mechanical

hyperalgesia (Nakamura-Craig and Follenfant, 1995). Lamotrigine, however, appeared to have a negligible effect against acute, high threshold noxious stimuli, e.g. it was inactive in the rat tail immersion test at 52°C (Hunter et al., 1997). This would imply a selective interaction with pathways associated with pathophysiological events rather than with those associated with normal sensory nociceptive function, a difference that would be consistent with lamotrigine's use-dependent block of sodium channels.

Lamotrigine has been tested in only a limited number of clinical studies. One small controlled trial of trigeminal neuralgia patients showed lamo-trigine to be superior to carbamazepine and phe-nytoin (Zakrzewska et al., 1997). In open label case series of patients with diabetic neuropathy (Eisenberg et al., 1996) and either post-herpetic neuralgia, causalgia or phantom limb pain (Harbi-son et al., 1997), lamotrigine was reported to provide effective pain relief with minimal side-effects. One placebo-controlled study has reported that lamotrigine is effective, at least for non-evoked pain in diabetic neuropathy (Luria et al., 2000). Other studies, however, have cast doubt on the role of lamotrigine for treating neuropathic pain. The largest placebo-controlled randomized study in the literature involved 100 patients and reported that lamotrigine up to 200 mg a day was no better than placebo for treating neuropathic pain (McClean, 1999). Another study then re-ported that the addition of lamotrigine to gabapen-tin was no better than gabapentin alone for treating neuropathic pain (Polati et al., 1999). Therefore, there is much uncertainty over the role of lamotrigine for treating pain. One possible explanation is that it may be effective if admin-istered before or soon after injury, but become less effective once pain is established. The study re-ported by Bonicalzi et al. (1997) would tend to support this. Their patients who were given lamo-trigine, 200 mg preoperatively, required less post-operative analgesia than those given a placebo.

The overall profile of newer antiepileptic drugs such as lamotrigine indicate that they may be effective for treating neuropathic pain but the timing of administration may be crucial. This in turn suggests that different subtypes of VGSCs are important only at specific times in the temporal sequence of events occurring during the initiation and maintenance of chronic pain (see below).

## Peripheral neuron specific sodium channels

It is recognized that sodium channels located in the primary sensory neurons play an important role, not only in the initial injury discharge but also in spontaneous ongoing and stimulus-evoked pain, in many types of neuropathic pain syndromes. As mentioned above, lignocaine applied topically to the skin (Rowbotham et al., 1995), and also in regions of the nerve supplying the painful foci (Arner et al., 1990; Gracely et al., 1992; Koltzenburg et al., 1994) or neuroma (Chabal et al., 1992b), produces complete relief of spontaneous, ongoing and stimulus-evoked pain. Extensive data from animal experiments also testi-

fy to the importance of VGSCs. In animal models of inflammatory and neuropathic pain respectively, local application of bupivacaine produces a reversal of mechanical hyperalgesia (Fletcher et al., 1997) and allodynia (Yoon et al., 1996). Following sciatic nerve transection in anaesthetized rats, either systemic (Chabal et al., 1989; Devor et al., 1992) or perineuronal (Matzner and Devor, 1994) application of subanaesthetic doses of lignocaine silences the ectopic discharge recorded from the nerve-end neuroma. Similarly, systemic administration of QX-314, the quaternarized derivative of lignocaine, reduces ectopic neuronal activity originating from the neuroma and DRG at doses considerably below those required to affect spinal dorsal horn neuron hyperexcitability (Omana-Zapata et al., 1997a). In conscious animals, QX-314, at doses shown not to penetrate the CNS, produced an antiallodynic effect in the CCI model on days 3–5 of chronic twice a day

# PN3 Sodium Channel (Neuron-Specific)

◆ **In situ hybridization and immunohistochemical studies demonstrate specific localization of PN3 to sensory neurons**

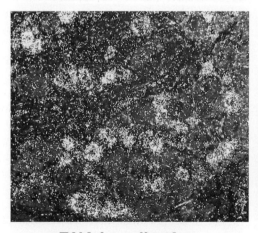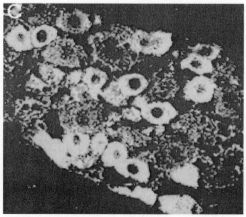

*mRNA Localization*                    *Protein Distribution*

**Figure 7.4** The PN3 sodium channels are only expressed in certain subgroups of primary afferent neurons in the dorsal root ganglion. Using co-localization techniques, the present evidence suggests that, in the physiological stage, these channels are only expressed in small diameter unmyelinated primary afferent neurons.

dosing that was comparable to the near-maximal effect of acutely administered lignocaine (Hunter *et al.*, 1995). These studies would suggest that, in chronic pain of inflammatory or neuropathic origin where there is nociceptor modulated central sensitization, sustained blockade of peripheral sodium channels may cause 'wind-down' of neuronal hyperexcitability and subsequent reversion to the physiological state.

A potential and logical exploitation of this hypothesis would be to target individual VGSC subtypes that may be either specific to sensory, nociceptive neurons (Akopian *et al.*, 1996; Sangameswaran *et al.*, 1996) or selectively regulated (Waxman *et al.*, 1994) in response to a peripheral nerve injury. DRG neurons are a heterogeneous population of cells expressing multiple sodium channel genes including those responsible for the rapidly inactivating, TTX-sensitive (TTX-S $I_{na}$) and the more slowly inactivating, TTX-resistant (TTX-R $I_{na}$) sodium currents (Roy and Narahashi, 1992; Elliott and Elliott, 1993; Ogata and Tatebayashi, 1993). TTX-S currents are the predominant $I_{Na}$ in all types of DRG cells at all stages of development. In adults, TTX-S VGSCs are the main, if not sole, $I_{Na}$ associated with the large diameter, fast conducting, myelinated A$\beta$ fibres (Roy and Narahashi, 1992; Elliott and Elliott, 1993; Rizzo *et al.*, 1994). By contrast, TTX-R $I_{Na}$ appears to have a more restricted distribution, appearing predominantly in a subpopulation of small diameter, unmyelinated, capsaicin-sensitive neurons (Roy and Narahashi, 1992; Elliott and Elliott, 1993; Arbuckle and Docherty, 1995). This different subdivision of VGSC expression is further supported by behavioural studies of SNS/PN3 knock-out mice. They do not appear to respond to noxious mechanical stimuli, have reduced response to noxious heat stimuli and take much longer to develop hyperalgesia in the model of inflammatory pain when caraggeenan was injected into their paw. Large myelinated primary afferent function however appears intact and they behave like wild type mice with Von Frey hair stimulation (Akopian *et al.*, 1999). In another set of experiments antisense oligodeoxynucleotides were used to reduce the expression of different VGSC subtypes. Selective reduction of SNS/PN3 expression in animals was associated with altera-

tion in behaviour in two models of chronic pain. Both mechanical allodynia and thermal hyperalgesia were reduced in the inflammatory Freund's adjuvant injection and neuropathic spinal nerve ligation (SNL) models of pain (Porecca *et al.*, 2000). In contrast, animals with knock-down of the SNS2/NaN TTX-S VGSCs behaved the same as wild type mice in these two models of pain. More recently, behavioural changes in other models of painful peripheral neuropathy, namely diabetic, vincristine and NGF induced in rats were reversed by treatment with SNS/PN3 oligodeoxynucleotides (Porreca *et al.*, 2000). A similar study also reported reduced reaction to prostaglandin-induced hyperalgesia when the rats were treated with antisense oligodeoxynucleotide to TTX-R VGSC (Khasar *et al.*, 1998).

Thus, all the evidence points to TTX-R VGSCs as the best target for developing drugs to alleviate inflammatory and neuropathic pain. The paradox, however, is that TTX-R channels are found to be down-regulated after nerve injury, while TTX-S receptors are up-regulated (Cummins and Waxman, 1997). Similar findings have been reported in an animal model of neuropathic pain (Dibb-Haj *et al.*, 1999). The increase in TTX-S current is due to the up-regulation of the $\alpha$-III channel that is normally absent in the adult DRG neurons (Waxman *et al.*, 1994). The greater role of TTX-S current after injury is demonstrated by the finding that following transection of the sciatic nerve, topical (Matzner and Devor, 1994) or systemically (Omana-Zapata *et al.*, 1997b) administered TTX eliminates ectopic nerve activity recorded from the neuroma or DRG.

This does not mean that TTX-R currents do not have a role in pathogenesis of neuropathic pain. In a rat model of neuropathic pain, a re-distribution of PN3/SNS protein has been shown to occur leading to intraneural channel accumulation just proximal to the site of injury (Novakovic *et al.*, 1998). The onset and subsequent reversal of PN3/SNS channel redistribution appeared to correlate closely with temporal changes in behavioural thermal hyperalgesia and, morphologically, with the damage and recovery of primary afferent fibres following this type of nerve ligation (Coggeshall *et al.*, 1993). Neurophysiological recordings of DRG neurons harvested from humans with neuropathic pain reported the presence of spontaneous firing in capsaicin sensitive cells (C-fibres) that appear to be mediated by TTX-R currents (Baumann and Martenson, 2000).

In summary, the available evidence suggests that there is an initial increase in TTX-S current after nerve injury mediated by the up regulation of $\alpha$-III channels. This appears to cause subthreshold oscillation of the membrane potential in the damaged primary afferents. The neurons that are affected are then more susceptible to depolarization by other stimuli like mechanical, efferent sympathetic or cross-depolarization from an adjacent axon (Amir et al., 2000). From the evidence described so far, it would appear that the maintenance of this hyperexcitable state is dependent on TTX-R currents. Very simplistically, one can speculate that there is a dynamic change in the role of different subtypes of VGSC in the pathogenesis of neuropathic pain: first TTX-S subtypes dominate followed by TTX-R subtypes.

It remains to be determined whether selective blockade of TTX-R VGSCs like PN3/SNS or, alternatively, any of the TTX-S channels in peripheral sensory neurons will produce an improvement in analgesic efficacy or a better therapeutic index compared to currently available non-selective agents. It is likely that a combined blockade of TTX-S and TTX-R currents is necessary to completely suppress chronic pain after nerve injury. The promising antihyperalgesic agent GW2040W92 not only causes a use-dependent block against TTX-R currents, but is also effective against TTX-S activity (Trezise et al., 1998). Thus it can be argued that looking for agents anatomically specific to DRG's VGSCs, whether TTX-R or TTX-S, may be more important than seeking agents with particular selectivity against either sodium channel subtype. The discrete anatomical localization of such VGSCs would produce an improvement in the safety profile of drugs targeted at these channels. The aim is to produce selective blockade of these channels to obtain pain relief without unwanted effects in other peripheral tissues or within the central nervous system.

# PN3 Sodium Channel (Neuron-Specific)

◆ **PN3 accumulation demonstrated at the site of a peripheral nerve injury in two rat models (CCI, SNL) and in humans**

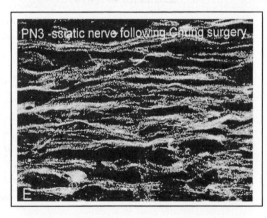

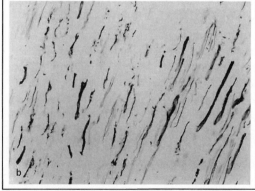

### Sciatic Nerve Injury In Rat After Spinal L5/L6 Nerve Ligation

### Human proximal nerve following avulsion injury

**Figure 7.5** After nerve injury in rats and humans, there is a translocation of PN3 VGSCs to sites of injury.

# Calcium channels

Voltage-gated calcium channels (VGCCs) are involved in many cellular and subcellular functions throughout the peripheral and central nervous systems. Calcium influx through neuronal VGCCs contributes to membrane depolarization in many excitable cells and plays a critical role in the presynaptic regulation of neurotransmitter release, second messenger signal transduction pathways and gene transcription (for reviews see Hofmann et al., 1994; Catterall, 1995; Miljanich and Ramachandran, 1995; Reuter, 1996). Multiple isoforms of neuronal VGCCs have been identified and differentiated on the basis of unique, primary structural features of each $\alpha_1$ subunit and distinct biophysical properties. Low voltage activated (LVA) channels, designated T-type, mediate transient calcium currents and high voltage activated (HVA) channels, designated L-, N-, P-, Q- and R-, mediate calcium currents with varying rates of inactivation depending on the composition of subunits. However, many of these VGCC subtypes are best distinguished pharmacologically, by agents that selectivity block channel function (Miljanich and Ramachandran, 1995; Reuter, 1996). For L-type channels these agents can be subdivided on the basis of chemical class into the dihydropyridines (e.g. nifedipine, nimodipine), phenylalkylamines (e.g. verapamil) and benzothiazepines (e.g. diltiazem). The N-type channel can be differentiated from other VGCCs by selective sensitivity to the $\omega$-conotoxins GVIA and MVIIA, members of a family of polypeptides isolated from the venom of several species of the marine snail, Conus. P- and Q-type channels are relatively insensitive to either the dihydropyridines or conotoxins, but can be distinguished on the basis of sensitivity to low (P-type) and high (Q-type) concentrations of the peptide $\omega$-agatoxin IVA, a toxin from the American funnel web spider, Agelenopsis aperta (Miljanich and Ramachandran, 1995; Reuter, 1996).

Several lines of evidence have implicated calcium channels in the processing of nociceptive information and in the pathogenesis of chronic pain. DRG cells differentially express various types of calcium current ($I_{Ca}$) including L-, N-, P/Q- and T-type $I_{Ca}$ (Scroggs and Fox, 1992;

Mintz et al., 1992; Cardenas et al., 1995). L- and N-type currents are expressed by all sizes of DRG cells, although their relative contribution to overall $I_{Ca}$ appears highest in small diameter, capsaicin-sensitive cells with the characteristics of nociceptors (Scroggs and Fox, 1992; Cardenas et al., 1995). In contrast, P- (Mintz et al., 1992) and T-type (Scroggs and Fox, 1992; Cardenas et al., 1995) currents, although present in some small diameter cells, appear to be preferentially expressed by medium and large diameter capsaicin-insensitive neurons. These neurons possess biophysical and morphological properties consistent with $A\beta$ fibres or non-nociceptors. In the spinal cord, L-type channels are present in the dorsal horn with a density comparable to many brain areas (Gandhi and Jones, 1988). N-type channels, however, appear to have a much more discrete localization with the highest densities found in the superficial laminae I and II (Kerr et al., 1988; Gohil et al., 1994) of the spinal dorsal horn. These are the areas where small diameter primary afferent neurons terminate. All VGCCs, however, have a widespread distribution throughout the peripheral and central nervous systems.

While more than one type of VGCC has been identified in the sensory pathways known to be important for nociceptive signalling, the N-type VGCC has emerged as the predominant calcium channel. They appear to be most important in the processing of nociceptive information at a spinal level. The N-type selective inhibitors, $\omega$-conopeptide GVIA and MVIIA, as well as numerous synthetic homologues, are antinociceptive in several animal models of acute and chronic pain (Malmberg and Yaksh, 1994, 1995). For example, $\omega$-conotoxin GVIA and SNX-111 or ziconotide (a synthetic homologue of $\omega$-conopeptide MVIIA) produce antinociceptive effect against acute, high threshold, thermal stimulus in the rat tail flick (Wei et al., 1996) and hot plate tests (Malmberg and Yaksh, 1994, 1995). In addition to this direct antinociceptive effect, $\omega$-conotoxin GVIA has been found to potentiate the antinociceptive response to both morphine and the $\alpha_2$-agonist clonidine in the tail flick test (Wei et al., 1996). SNX-111 and various N-type selective synthetic derivatives, when administered by either acute or continuous intrathecal infusion, inhibited both the early, acute and late, tonic phases of flinching behaviour following an intraplantar injection of formalin in the rat (Malmberg and Yaksh, 1994, 1995; Bowersox et al., 1996). In these studies, the conopeptides also produced a range of general behaviours and motor effects, but at doses usually in excess of those producing antinociception. These effects may be related to a non-specific, non-N-type blocking action. In an electrophysiological study of dorsal horn neuron activity *in situ*, $\omega$-conotoxin GVIA reduced both phases of the formalin response in a manner comparable to the behavioural studies (Diaz and Dickenson, 1997). $\omega$-conotoxin GVIA has also been shown to reduce the excitability of dorsal horn neurons receiving either nociceptive or innocuous mechanosensory input from the knee joint, both under normal conditions and in the presence of inflammation induced by either carrageenan or kaolin (Neugebauer et al., 1996). In the rat spinal nerve (L5/L6) ligation model of neuropathic pain, the administration of SNX-111 and a close analogue, $\omega$-conotoxin MVIIA (SNX-239) via continuous intrathecal administration over 7 days reversed tactile allodynia (Chaplan et al., 1994; Bowersox et al., 1996). However, when administered intravenously or by regional application to the nerve, neither agent was effective (Chaplan et al., 1994). In rats with a CCI sciatic nerve injury, bolus administration of SNX-111 and SNX-124 (a synthetic homologue of $\omega$-conopeptide GVIA) applied directly to the site of injury via chronically implanted perineural cannulae, reduced thermal hyperalgesia and mechano-allodynia but not mechanical hyperalgesia (Xiao and Bennett, 1995).

SNX-111 or ziconotide has undergone clinical trials for the treatment of chronic malignant and non-malignant pain. In an open label feasibility study of 31 patients, SNX-111, administered intrathecally, has been reported to produce partial to complete pain relief in a patient population previously found to be opioid-resistant (Brose et al., 1996). The pain syndromes included cancer and HIV-related neuropathic pain, phantom limb pain, post-herpetic neuralgia, spinal cord injury and thalamic pain. The most commonly reported side-effects were (in order of prevalence): nausea, dizziness and lightheadedness, headache, consti-

pation, confusion and nystagmus. Orthostatic hypotension without reflex tachycardia has also been noted within the analgesic dose-range (Bowersox and Luther, 1994). Controlled clinical trials are currently in progress. Preliminary evidence in over 150 patients treated with ziconitide reported a 30% reduction in pain measured by the VAS scale compared to placebo. Once again, a reduction in the reported level of pain was seen even in patients previously resistant to intrathecal opioids (Gouke et al., 2000).

Ziconitide is an important novel agent for treating intractable neuropathic pain. One important practical disadvantage is that it has to be administered intrathecally via an implantable pump with the potential risk that this entails. Other agents that may act on the N-type VGCC and that do not need to be administered intrathecally are being developed (Hu et al., 1999; Lotarski et al., 1999). The other problem with non-specific N-type VGCC antagonists is that they are likely to have a relatively narrow therapeutic window. As with some of the sodium channel blockers, many side-effects of ziconitide are CNS related and are likely to be due to the widespread localization of N-type calcium channels in the peripheral and central nervous systems. The existence of a peripheral VGCC N-type isoform with distinct structural and functional characteristics was recently reported in the superior cervical ganglion (Lin et al., 1997). If this discovery is indicative of the existence of additional N-channel subtypes that may be selectively expressed in the sensory system, then it may provide the opportunity for drug targeting in the search for analgesics with improved side-effect profile.

In comparison to the N-type VGCC, evidence in support of an antinociceptive effect mediated through a selective block of the L-type VGCC has been more limited and controversial. In the rodent hot plate or tail flick test of acute, thermal nociception, L-type VGCC antagonists, when administered alone, do not display any significant antinociceptive effect (Miranda et al., 1992; Omote et al., 1993; Hodoglugil et al., 1996). However, many of these agents potentiate the antinociception produced in these tests by either morphine or the $\alpha_2$-agonist clonidine (Omote et al., 1993; Hodoglugil et al., 1996; Wei et al.,

1996). In a postoperative pain study in patients, nifedipine, administered sublingually, potentiated the analgesic effect of epidural morphine (Pereira et al., 1993). Furthermore, nimodipine has enhanced opiate analgesia in cancer patients (Santillan et al., 1994, 1998), although this evidence has been challenged (Roca et al., 1996). More intriguing is the possibility that L-type VGCC blockers may prevent opioid tolerance. Chronic administration of opioids has been shown to increase dihydropyridine binding sites in the spinal dorsal horn, periaqueductal grey matter, thalamus and somatosensory cortex (Diaz et al., 1999). Co-administration of nimodipine and an opioid not only prevented tolerance but caused supersensitivity to the antinociceptive effect of the opioid (Diaz et al., 1995). If this is confirmed in humans, it could have important practical implications in the way opioids are prescribed for treating chronic pain. L-type antagonists also attenuate the acute antinociceptive response to a variety of cholinomimetic agents (nicotine, epibatidine, oxotremorine, physostigmine) acting through either nicotinic or muscarinic receptors (Damaj et al., 1993; Pavone et al., 1993; Bannon et al., 1995).

L-type VGCC antagonists have been found to be intrinsically antinociceptive when administered systemically under conditions of both acute inflammation in the acetic acid induced abdominal constriction test (Miranda et al., 1992) and in the formalin model of acute, persistent nociception (Coderre and Melzack, 1992; Miranda et al., 1992). However, the latter observations are more controversial as both behavioural (Malmberg and Yaksh, 1994) and electrophysiological (Diaz and Dickenson, 1997) studies have found that intraspinal administration of L-type antagonists are ineffective in the formalin test. Furthermore, in models of peripheral nerve injury, L-type antagonists appear universally ineffective at modulating either the spontaneous discharge recorded from a sciatic neuroma (Matzner and Devor, 1994) or the tactile allodynic behavioural response to tight ligation of spinal nerves L5 and L6 (Chaplan et al., 1994).

Very little information is available on the potential involvement of other VGCCs in the control of nociceptive transmission. The P/Q type channel blocker, $\omega$-agatoxin IVA, appears to have no effect in acute tests of nociception such as rat hot plate (Malmberg and Yaksh, 1994). However, behavioural and electrophysiological studies have demonstrated $\omega$-agatoxin IVA selective attenuation of the late, tonic phase in the formalin test of acute, persistent nociception. This would suggest a potential role for the P/Q channel in facilitated, rather than acute, processing of nociceptive information in the spinal cord (Malmberg and Yaksh, 1994; Diaz and Dickenson, 1997). $\omega$-Agatoxin IVA, however, had no effect on tactile allodynia in a peripheral neuropathy model (Chaplan et al., 1994). In humans, the P/Q VGCCs may play a role in certain forms of migraine. The discovery of specific mutations of the $\alpha$1A subunit of the P/Q VGCC linked to familial hemiplegic migraine (Ophoff et al., 1996) has led to intensive search for other mutations linked to this class of channel (see Chapter 19). It would be interesting to know if any link exists between mutations or altered function of P/Q VGCC and chronic pain.

One of the most widely used of the new drugs for treating neuropathic pain is gabapentin. Double-blind, placebo-controlled studies have reported the efficacy of gabapentin for alleviating postherpetic neuralgia (Rowbotham et al., 1998) and painful diabetic neuropathy (Backonja et al., 1998). The mechanism of action of gabapentin is unknown, but it binds avidly to the $\alpha$2$\delta$ site of voltage-sensitive calcium channels (for review see Taylor et al., 1998). A possible modulating role in VGCC current may explain the antihyperalgesic effect of gabapentin. This is also supported by studies of other gabapentinoids. The S-(+)-enantiomer of pre-gabalin that binds to this site is shown to have an antihyperalgesic effect in animals models of chronic pain while the R-(−)-enantiomer which is ten times weaker in binding does not have such an antihyperalgesic effect (Field et al., 1999). The actual effect of gabapentinoids binding to this site is unknown. It is possible that the antihyperalgesic effects of gabapentinoids have nothing to do with binding to calcium channels but are due to its numerous other actions (Taylor et al., 1998).

In conclusion, in animal models of neuropathic pain and inflammation, N-type channel blockers appear capable of producing effective analgesia at a spinal level, but may have to operate within a relatively narrow therapeutic window. It will therefore be of clinical interest to see whether direct, intrathecal application of a drug, like SNX-111, to the potential target site of action in the spinal cord, at doses sufficient to cause a sustained analgesic effect, will enable a suitable therapeutic window to be achieved. The therapeutic potential of L-type VGCC antagonists appears to be extremely limited but may find use as a combination therapy with morphine to enhance opioid efficacy and to prevent opioid tolerance. The P/Q-type VGCC may also have a role in the production of chronic pain and headaches. If so the development of orally active, selective antagonists could be beneficial.

## Potassium channels

Comparatively little is known about potassium channels as a potential target for the development of novel analgesics. This might be considered surprising since the role of potassium channels in the control of membrane excitability is as well established as that of the other types of voltage-gated channels (Pongs, 1992; Catterall, 1995; Kaczorowski et al., 1996; Isomoto et al., 1997). Potassium channel activation in the cell membrane allows potassium ions to move out of the cell causing membrane repolarization and after-hyperpolarization. Therefore, they play an integral role in setting the firing rhythm of the cell. Potassium currents ($I_K$) have a major impact on spike repolarization and interspike interval as well as burst adaptation. Several members of the potassium channel family have been identified and can be differentiated on the basis of voltage-dependency, kinetics, calcium-dependency and pharmacology (Rudy, 1988; Cook, 1988; Pongs, 1992; Catterall, 1995; Kaczorowski et al., 1996). The main types of voltage-sensitive potassium channels include those mediating a transient, rapidly inactivating A-type current $I_{K(A)}$ and a family of delayed rectifiers mediating currents characterized by delayed activation and slowed inactivation. Several variants of each have been identified (Pongs, 1992). The major $Ca^{2+}$-activated potassium channel is a voltage-dependent, large conductance channel termed maxi K or BK (Kaczorowski

et al., 1996). There is a super-family of voltage-insensitive, inwardly rectifying potassium channels mediating a series of inward currents activated either by hyperpolarization ($K_{IR}$) or regulated by a variety of G-protein coupled inhibitory neurotransmitter receptors ($K_G$), ATP ($K_{ATP}$) or sodium ($K_{Na}$) (Isomoto et al., 1997).

Cutaneous primary afferent neurons heterogeneously express both transient and sustained voltage-gated potassium currents, as well as the major $Ca^{2+}$-dependent BK current. Each subtype can be identified on the basis of distinct biophysical and pharmacological features. In adult DRG neurons, an A-type current ($I_A$) sensitive to 4-aminopyridine and TEA is preferentially expressed in the small diameter, capsaicin-sensitive cells (Akins and McCleskey, 1993; Pearce and Duchen, 1994; Gold et al., 1996b). However, additional A-type currents have also been reported from adult DRG neurons that display either slower inactivation kinetics or insensitivity to TEA when compared to the predominant $I_A$ (Gold et al., 1996b). Interestingly, the TEA insensitive $I_{K(Af)}$ was found to be exclusively expressed by large diameter DRG cells that would correspond to $A\beta$ fibres or non-nociceptors (Gold et al., 1996b). At least three types of sustained, delayed rectifier $I_{K(V)}$ and a $Ca^{2+}$-activated BK current have also been recorded from DRG cells. While each of these currents is found in all categories of DRG neurons, most have a higher frequency of expression in the small diameter, capsaicin-sensitive, nociceptors (Akins and McCleskey, 1993; Gold et al., 1996b). In addition to the voltage-sensitive currents, two types of voltage-insensitive, inwardly rectifying currents have been described in DRG neurons (Scroggs et al., 1994). $I_H$ and $I_{IR}$ appear to be preferentially expressed by large and medium diameter cells respectively, which were insensitive to capsaicin and thought to be non-nociceptors (Scroggs et al., 1994; Cardenas et al., 1995).

The preferential expression of specific categories of potassium currents in subpopulations of DRG neurons may be important from several perspectives. It suggests that certain types of voltage-sensitive potassium channels could play an important role in the functional diversity of primary afferent neurons with the ability to respond to nerve or tissue injury. This was illustrated by the increase in either the spontaneous firing of active fibres, or in the recruitment of quiescent fibres, when the voltage-sensitive potassium channel blocker TEA was applied to sciatic (Matzner and Devor, 1994) or saphenous (Burchiel and Russell, 1985) nerve neuromas. A similar response was seen with another potassium channel blocker, 4-AP. In a rat saphenous nerve–skin *in vitro* preparation, 4-AP and TEA also induced bursting discharges in all cutaneous primary afferent neurons by an action at or near the action potential generator region at the nerve terminal (Kirchhoff *et al.*, 1992). In conscious animals, however, evidence for the involvement of voltage-sensitive potassium channels in the transmission of nociceptive information has been limited to a few studies of acute nociception. TEA and 4-AP have been shown to block the antinociceptive effect of the $GABA_B$ agonist baclofen, but appear ineffective against either $\mu$-opioid or $\alpha_2$-agonist antinociception (Ocana and Baeyens, 1993; Ocana *et al.*, 1996). Different effects are seen with modulation of $K_{ATP}$, the voltage- and calcium-insensitive potassium channel regulated by ATP. Both $K_{ATP}$ channel activation and inhibition have been shown to be ineffective at modulating baclofen-mediated antinociception (Ocana *et al.*, 1996). In contrast, although not possessing antinociceptive action *per se*, chemicals that open $K_{ATP}$ channels potentiate the central antinociceptive effect of $\mu$- and $\delta$-opioid agonists (Wild *et al.*, 1991; Ocana and Baeyens, 1993; Ocana *et al.*, 1995, 1996) and the $\alpha_2$-adrenoceptor agonist clonidine (Ocana *et al.*, 1996). Conversely, chemicals that close the $K_{ATP}$ channels inhibit the antinociceptive effects of opioids and $\alpha_2$-adrenoceptor agonist. However, although potentiation of morphine is consistently observed, not all $\mu$-opioid agonists are similarly affected (Ocana *et al.*, 1995; Raffa and Martinez, 1995). The $K_{ATP}$ channel opener, cromakalim, failed to potentiate the antinociceptive properties of the $\kappa$-opioid agonist, U-50,488. In the mouse tail flick test, the antinociceptive response to the tricyclic antidepressants, clomipramine and amitriptyline, was blocked by an antisense oligodeoxynucleotide to the mouse $K_v1.1$ delayed rectifier (Galeotti *et al.*, 1997).

Therefore, the function of voltage-gated potassium channels appears to be to limit neuronal excitability by regulating action potential thresholds and accommodation. Consequently, modulation of these channels by agents that selectively increase potassium conductance could play an important role in the control of baseline rhythmogenesis (impulse initiation) and burst firing in a chronically injured axon. However, the relative importance of the voltage-gated potassium channel family to primary afferent neuronal function and by extension, to acute and facilitated processing of nociceptive information at a peripheral and spinal level, still remains a largely unexplored area. This is due to the lack of potent and/or selective channel activators. There are mixed results with antisense oligodeoxynucleotide against voltage gated potassium channel Kv1.1 (Galeotti *et al.*, 1997; 1999). On the other hand, it is reported that ATP gated potassium channel openers have been reported to possess anti-nociceptive effect (Welch and Dunlow, 1993) and calcium gated potassium channel may be responsible for the peripheral analgesic effect of opioids (Rodriques and Duarante, 2000). At present, potassium channels remain an unknown quantity for the treatment of pain and we need to accumulate more data on human studies with all potassium channel openers (Jang *et al.*, 2000).

## Future perspective

Modulation of voltage-gated ion channels or at least blockade of sodium channels has been an area where there has been moderate success at producing effective relief in a number of chronic pain conditions. Clinically, the full analgesic potential of these drugs is rarely realized due to side-effects. Therefore, future drug development must address not solely analgesic efficacy but the therapeutic window of newer agents. There is no shortage of potential targets among the sodium, calcium and potassium channels to achieve this goal. The major limitation, however, is the ubiquitous distribution of these channels throughout the peripheral and central nervous systems. It is likely that side-effects would continue to limit therapeutic potential. One possible solution is to develop agents that target channels specific to the peripheral nociceptive pathways, e.g. the TTX-resistant sodium channel PN3/SNS. This may allow the development of antinociceptive agents relatively free of autonomic and motor side-effects. An alternative strategy would be to select biophysical and temporal specific channels to target. For example, the repetitive firing behaviour of peripheral and central neurons following injury may be modulated by specific channels that differentiate them from other voltage-gated channels. The biophysical properties that modulate the abnormal activation pattern of injured neurons may also be time dependent. Thus, even a less specific channel blocker may be clinically acceptable when it is used for a limited period to act on a subtype of channels with temporally restricted biophysical properties contributing to the pathogenesis of chronic pain.

The future for developing new analgesic agents looks very bright. Animal experimentation has greatly advanced the understanding of voltage-gated channels and their importance in nociception and pain pathogenesis. This, in turn, has opened up many avenues in the search for medications to relieve pain. However, it should be borne in mind that some of the most effective medications found for treating neuropathic pain (e.g. tricyclics, gabapentin) have arisen by serendipity. Such serendipitous drugs have tended to have multiple sites of action suggesting that it would be unwise for all efforts in the search for new analgesic drugs to be confined to narrow molecular targets.

# References

Abdi, S., Lee, D. H. and Chung, J. M. (1998). The anti-allodynic effects of amitriptyline, gabapentin and lidocaine in a rat model of neuropathic pain. *Anesth Analg.*, **87**, 1360–6.

Abram, S. E. and Yaksh, T. L. (1994). Systemic lidocaine blocks nerve injury-induced hyperalgesia and nociceptor-driven spinal sensitization in the rat. *Anesthesiology*, **80**, 383–91.

Ackerman, M. J. and Clapham, D. E. (1997). Ion channels – basic science and clinical disease. *New Eng J Med.*, **336**, 1575–86.

Akins, P. T. and McCleskey, E. W. (1993). Characterization of potassium currents in adult rat sensory neurons and modulation by opioids and cyclic AMP. *Neuroscience*, **56**, 759–69.

Akopian, A. N., Sivilotti, L. and Wood, J. N. (1996). A tetrodotoxin-resistant voltage-gated sodium channel expressed by sensory neurons. *Nature*, **379**, 257–62.

Akopian, A. N., Souslova, V., England, S., Okuse, K., Ogata, N. *et al.* (1999). The tetrodotoxin-resistant sodium channel SNS has a specialized function in pain pathways. *Nat. Neurosci.*, **2**, 541–8.

Amir, R., Michaelis, M. and Devor, M. (2000). Ectopic discharge in primary sensory neurons depends on intrinsic membrane potential oscillations. In *Proceedings of the 9th World Congress on Pain, Prog. In Pain Research and Management*, Vol.16 (eds Devor, M., Rowbotham, M. C. and Wiesenfeld-Hallin, Z.), pp. 93–100, Seattle: IASP Press.

Arbuckle, J. B. and Docherty, R. J. (1995). Expression of tetrodotoxin-resistant sodium channels in capsaicin-sensitive dorsal root ganglion neurons of adult rats. *Neurosci Letts.*, **185**, 70–3.

Arner, S., Lindblom, U., Meyerson, B. A. and Molander, C. (1990). Prolonged relief of neuralgia after regional anesthetic blocks. A call for further experimental and systematic clinical studies. *Pain*, **43**, 287–97.

Attal, N., Gaude, V., Brasseur, L. *et al.* (2000). Intravenous lidocaine in central pain: a double-blind, placebo-controlled, psychophysical study. *Neurology*, **54**, 564–74.

Awerbuch, G. I. and Sandyk, R. (1990). Mexiletine for thalamic pain syndrome. *Int J Neurosci.*, **55**, 129–33.

Bach, F. W., Jensen, T. S., Kastrup, J., Stigsby, B. and Dejgard, A. (1990). The effect of intravenous lidocaine on nociceptive processing in diabetic neuropathy. *Pain*, **40**, 29–34.

Backonja, M. and Gombar, K. A. (1992). Response of central pain syndromes to intravenous lidocaine. *J Pain Symp Manag.*, **7**, 172–8.

Backonja, M. M. (1994). Local anesthetics as adjuvant analgesics. *J Pain Symp Manag.*, **9**, 491–9.

Backonja, M., Beydoun, A., Edwards, K. R. *et al.* (1998). Gabapentin for the symptomatic treatment of painful neuropathy in patients with diabetes mellitus. A randomised controlled trial. *J Am Med Assoc.*, **280**, 1831–6.

Bannon, A. W., Gunther, K. L., Decker, M. W. and Arneric, S. P. (1995). The influence of Bay K 8644 treatment on (+/−):-epibatidine-induced analgesia. *Brain Res.*, **678**, 44–250.

Bartlett, E. E. and Hutanserani, O. (1961). Xylocaine for the relief of postoperative pain. *Anest Analg.*, **40**, 296–304.

Baumann, T. K., Martenson, M. E. (2000). Spontaneous action potential discharge in cultured dorsal root ganglion neurons from patients with neuropathic pain. In: *Proceedings of the 9th World Congress on Pain, Prog. In Pain Research and Management*, Vol. 16 (eds Devor, M., Rowbotham, M. C. and Wiesenfeld-Hallin, Z.), pp. 101–8. Seattle: IASP Press.

Bennett, G. J. and Xie, Y. K. (1988). A peripheral

mononeuropathy in rat that produces disorders of pain sensation like those seen in man. *Pain*, **33**, 87–107.

Birch, K., Jorgensen, J., Chraemmer-Jorgensen, B. and Kehlet, H. (1987). Effect of i.v. lignocaine on pain and the endocrine metabolic responses after surgery. *Br J Anaesth.*, **59**, 721–4.

Blom, S. (1962). Trigeminal neuralgia: its treatment with a new anticonvulsant drug (G-32883). *Lancet,* **1**, 839–40.

Boas, R. A., Covino, B. G. and Shahnarian, A. (1982). Analgesic response to IV lidocaine. *Br J Anest.*, **54**, 501–5.

Bonicalzi, V., Canavero, S., Cerutti, F., Piazza, M., Clemente, M. and Chio, A. (1997). Lamotrigine reduces total postoperative analgesic requirement: a randomised double-blind, placebo-controlled pilot study. *Surgery*, **122**, 567–70.

Bowersox, S. S., Gadbois, T., Singh, T., Pettus, M., Wang, Y. X. and Luther, R. R. (1996). Selective N-type neuronal voltage-sensitive calcium channel blocker, SNX-111, produces spinal antinociception in rat models of acute, persistent and neuropathic pain. *J Pharmacol Exp Ther.*, **279**, 1243–9.

Bowersox, S. S. and, Luther, R. R. (1994). SNX-111. N-Type voltage-sensitive calcium channel antagonist. *Drugs of the Future*, **19**, 128–30.

Brose, W. G., Pfeiffer, B. L., Hassenbusch, S. J. *et al.* (1996). Analgesia produced by SNX-111 in patients with morphine-resistant pain. *Am Pain Soc Abstr.,* A-122.

Brose, W. G. and Cousins, M. J. (1991). Subcutaneous lidocaine for treatment of neuropathic cancer pain. *Pain,* **45**, 145–8.

Bruera, E., Ripamonti, C., Brenneis, C., Macmillan, K. and Hanson, J. (1992). A randomized double-blind crossover trial of intravenous lidocaine in the treatment of neuropathic cancer pain. *J Pain Symp Manag.,* **7**, 138–40.

Burchiel, K. J. and Russell, L. C. (1985). Effects of potassium channel-blocking agents on spontaneous discharges from neuromas in rats. *J Neurosurg.*, **63**, 246–9.

Campbell, F. G., Graham, J. G. and Zilkha, K. J. (1966). Clinical trial of carbamazepine (Tegretol) in trigeminal neuralgia. *J Neurol Neurosurg Psychiatr.*, **29**, 265–7.

Cardenas, C. G., Del Mar, L. P. and Scroggs, R. S. (1995). Variation in serotonergic inhibition of calcium channel currents in four types of rat sensory neurons differentiated by membrane properties. *J Neurophysiol.*, **74**, 1870–9.

Cassuto, J., Wallin, G., Hogstrom, S., Faxen, A. and Rimback, G. (1985). Inhibition of postoperative pain by continuous low-dose intravenous infusion of lidocaine. *Anesth Analg.*, **64**, 971–4.

Catterall, W. A. (1987). Common modes of drug action on $Na^+$ channels: Local anesthetics, antiarrhythmics and anticonvulsants. *Trends Pharmacol Sci.*, **8**, 57–65.

Catterall, W. A. (1992). Cellular and molecular biology of voltage-gated sodium channels. *Physiol Rev.* **72**, S15–48.

Catterall, W. A. (1995). Structure and function of voltage-gated ion channels. *Ann Rev Biochem.*, **64**, 493–531.

Chabal, C., Russell, L. C. and Burchiel, K. J. (1989). The effect of intravenous lidocaine, tocainide, and mexiletine on spontaneously active fibers originating in rat sciatic neuromas. *Pain*, **38**, 333–8.

Chabal, C., Jacobson, L., Mariano, A., Chaney, E. and Britell, C. W. (1992a). The use of oral mexiletine for the treatment of pain after peripheral nerve injury. *Anesthesiology*, **76**, 513–7.

Chabal, C., Jacobson, L., Russell, L. C. and Burchiel, K. J. (1992b). Pain response to perineuromal injection of normal saline, epinephrine, and lidocaine in humans. *Pain*, **49**, 9–12.

Chadda, V. S. and Mathur, M. S. (1978). Double blind study of the effects of diphenylhydantoin sodium on diabetic neuropathy. *J Assoc Phys India*, **26**, 403–6.

Chaplan, S. R., Pogrel, J. W. and Yaksh, T. L. (1994). Role of voltage-dependent calcium channel subtypes in experimental tactile allodynia. *J Pharmacol Exp Ther.*, **269**, 1117–23.

Cheung, H., Kamp, D. and Harris, E. (1992). An in vitro investigation of the action of lamotrigine on neuronal voltage-activated sodium channels. *Epilepsy Res.*, **13**, 107–12.

Coderre, T. J. and Melzack, R. (1992). The role of NMDA receptor-operated calcium channels in persistent nociception after formalin-induced tissue injury. *J Neurosci.*, **12**, 3671–5.

Coggeshall, R. E., Dougherty, P. M., Pover, C. M. and Carlton, S. M. (1993). Is large myelinated fiber loss associated with hyperalgesia in a model of experimental peripheral neuropathy in the rat? *Pain*, **52**, 233–42.

Cook, N. S. (1988). The pharmacology of potassium channels and their therapeutic potential. *Trends Pharmacol Sci.*, **9**, 21–8.

Cummins, T. R. and Waxman, S. G. (1997) Downregulation of tetradotoxin resistant sodium currents and upregulation of a rapidly repriming tetradotoxin sensitive current in small spinal neurons after nerve injury. *J. Neurosci.*, **17**, 3503–14.

Damaj, M. I., Welch, S. P. and Martin, B. R. (1993). Involvement of calcium and L-type channels in nicotine-induced antinociception. *J Pharmacol Exp Ther.*, **266**, 1330–8.

Dejgard, A., Petersen, P. and Kastrup, J. (1988). Mexiletine for treatment of chronic painful diabetic neuropathy. *Lancet*, **1**, 9–11.

Devor, M. (1999). Unexplained peculiarities of the dorsal root ganglion. *Pain*, **Suppl. 6**, S27–S35.

Devor, M., Wall, P. D. and Catalan, N. (1992). Systemic

lidocaine silences ectopic neuroma and DRG discharge without blocking nerve conduction. *Pain*, **48**, 261–8.

Devor, M., Govrin-Lippmann, R. and Angelides, K. (1993). Na$^+$ channel immunolocalization in peripheral mammalian axons and changes following nerve injury and neuroma formation. *J Neurosci.*, **13**, 1976–92.

Devor, M. (1994). The pathophysiology of damaged peripheral nerves. In *Textbook of Pain*, 3rd edn (eds Wall, P. D. and Melzack, R.), pp. 79–100. Edinburgh: Churchill Livingstone.

Devor, M. and Govrin-Lippmann, R. (1983). Axoplasmic transport block reduces ectopic impulse generation in injured peripheral nerves. *Pain*, **16**, 73–85.

Devulder, J. E., Ghys, L., Dhondt, W. and Rolly, G. (1993). Neuropathic pain in a cancer patient responding to subcutaneously administered lignocaine. *Clin J Pain*, **9**, 220–3.

Diaz, A. and Dickenson, A. H. (1997). Blockade of spinal N- and P-type, but not L-type, calcium channels inhibits the excitability of rat dorsal horn neurones produced by subcutaneous formalin inflammation. *Pain*, **69**, 93–100.

Diaz, A., Florez, J., Pazos, A. and Hurle, M. A. (1999). Opioid tolerance and supersensitivity induces regional changes in the autoradiographic density of dihydropyridine-sensitive calcium channels in the rat central nervous system. *Pain*, **86**, 227–35.

Diaz, A., Florez, J., Pazos, A. and Hurle, M. A. (1995). Regulation of dihydropyridine sensitive calcium channels during opioid tolerance and supersensitivity in rats. *J Pharmacol Exp Ther.*, **274**, 1538–44.

Dib-Hajj, S. D., Fjell, J., Cummins, T. R. *et al.* (1999). Plasticity of sodium channel expression in DRG neurons in the chronic constriction injury model of neuropathic pain. *Pain*, **83**, 591–600.

Dietrich, P. S., McGivern, J. G., Delgado, S. G. *et al.* (1998). Functional analysis of a voltage-gated sodium channel and its splice variant from rat dorsal root ganglia. *J Neurochem.*, **70**, 2262–72.

Eccles, J. C., Libet, B. and Young, R. R. (1958). The behavior of chromatolysed motorneurons studied by intracellular recordings. *J Physiol (Lond).*, **143**, 11–40.

Edmondson, E. A., Simpson, R. K. Jr, Stubler, D. K. and Beric, A. (1993). Systemic lidocaine therapy for poststroke pain. *Southern Med J.*, **86**, 1093–6.

Edwards, W. T., Habib, F., Burney, R. G. and Begin, G. (1985). Intravenous lidocaine in the management of various chronic pain states. A review of 211 cases. *Reg Anesth.*, **10**, 1–6.

Eisenberg, E., Alon, N., Yarnitsky, D., Ishay, A. and Daoud, D. (1996). Lamotrigine for the treatment of painful diabetic neuropathy. *8th World Congress on Pain Abstr.*, p. 372. Vancouver, Canada.

Ellemann, K., Sjogren, P., Banning, A. M., Jensen, T. S., Smith, T. and Geertsen, P. (1989). Trial of intravenous lidocaine on painful neuropathy in cancer patients. *Clin J Pain*, **5**, 291–4.

Elliott, A. A. and Elliott, J. R. (1993). Characterization of TTX-sensitive and TTX-resistant sodium currents in small cells from adult rat dorsal root ganglia. *J Physiol.*, **463**, 39–56.

England, J. D., Happel, L. T., Kline, D. G. *et al.* (1996). Sodium channel accumulation in humans with painful neuromas. *Neurology*, **47**, 272–6.

Espir, M. L. E. and Millac, P. (1970). Treatment of paroxysmal disorders in multiple sclerosis with carbamezepine (Tetretol). *JNNP*, **33**, 528–31.

Ferrante, F. M., Paggioli, J., Cherukuri, S. and Arthur, G. R. (1996). The analgesic response to intravenous lidocaine in the treatment of neuropathic pain. *Anesth Analg.*, **82**, 91–7.

Field, M. J., McCleary, S., Hughes, J. and Singh, L. (1999). Gabapentin and pregabalin, but not morphine and amitriptyline block both static and dynamic components of mechanical allodynia induced by streptozocin in the rat. *Pain*, **80**, 391–8.

Filling-Katz, M. R., Merrick, H. F., Fink, J. K., Miles, R. B., Sokol, J. and Barton, N. W. (1989). Carbamezepine in Fabry's disease: effective analgesia with dose dependent exacerbation of autonomic dysfunction. *Neurology*, **39**, 598–600.

Fitton, A. and Goa, K. L. (1995). Lamotrigine. An update of its pharmacology and therapeutic use in epilepsy. *Drugs,* **50**, 691–713.

Fletcher, D., Le Corre, P., Guilbaud, G. and Le Verge, R. (1997). Antinociceptive effect of bupivacaine encapsulated in poly(D,L):-lactide-co-glycolide microspheres in the acute inflammatory pain model of carrageenin-injected rats. *Anesth Analg.,* **84**, 90–4.

Galeotti, N., Ghelardini, C., Papucci, L., Capaccioli, S., Quattrone, A. and Bartolini, A. (1997). An antisense oligonucleotide on the mouse Shaker-like potassium channel Kv1.1 gene prevents antinociception induced by morphine and baclofen. *J Pharmacol Exp Ther.*, **281**, 941–9.

Galeotti, N., Ghelardini, C. and Bartolini, A. (1999). The role of potassium channels in antihistamine analgesia. *Neuropharmacology*, **38**, 1893–901.

Galer, B. S., Miller, K. V. and Rowbotham, M. C. (1993). Response to intravenous lidocaine infusion differs based on clinical diagnosis and site of nervous system injury. *Neurology*, **43**, 1233–5.

Galer, B. S., Harle, J. and Rowbotham, M. C. (1996). Response to intravenous lidocaine infusion predicts subsequent response to oral mexiletine: a prospective study. *J Pain Symp Manag.*, **12**, 161–7.

Gandhi, V. C. and Jones, D. J. (1988). Identification and characterization of [$^3$H]nitrendipine binding sites in rat spinal cord. *J Pharmacol Exp Ther.*, **247**, 473–80.

Gohil, K., Bell, J. R., Ramachandran, J. and Miljanich, G. P. (1994). Neuroanatomical distribution of receptors for a novel voltage-sensitive calcium-channel antagonist, SNX-230 ($\omega$-conopeptide MVIIC). *Brain Res.*, **653**, 258–66.

Gold, M. S., Shuster, M. J. and Levine, J. D. (1996b). Characterization of six voltage-gated K$^+$ currents in adult rat sensory neurons. *J Neurophysiol.*, **75**, 2629–46.

Goucke, C. R., Mathur, V. and Luther, R. (1999). The complex patient with opioid resistant chronic pain: the analgesic effect of intrathecal ziconitide. *IASP 9th World Congress on Pain.* Vienna, 1999, pp. 446: 236.

Gracely, R. H., Lynch, S. A. and Bennett, G. J. (1992). Painful neuropathy: altered central processing maintained dynamically by peripheral input. *Pain*, **51**, 175–94.

Harbison, J., Dennehy, F. and Keating, D. (1997). Lamotrigine for pain with hyperalgesia. *Irish Med J.,* **90**, 56.

Hedley, L. R., Martin, B., Waterbury, L. D., Clarke, D. E. and Hunter, J. C. (1995). A comparison of the action of mexiletine and morphine in rodent models of acute and chronic pain. *Proc West Pharmacol Soc.,* **38**, 103–4.

Hodoglugil, U., Guney, H. Z., Savran, B., Guzey, C., Gorgun, C. Z. and Zengil, H. (1996). Temporal variation in the interaction between calcium channel blockers and morphine-induced analgesia. *Chronobiol Intl.,* **13**, 227–34.

Hofmann, F., Biel, M. and Flockerzi, V. (1994). Molecular basis for Ca2$^+$ channel diversity. *Ann Rev Neurosci.*, **17**, 399–418.

Hu, L. Y., Ryder, T. R., Rafferty, M. F. *et al.* (1999). Structure–activity relationship of N~methyl-N-aralkyl-peptidylamines as novel N-type calcium channel blockers. *Bioorg Med Chem Lett.*, **9**, 2151–6.

Hunter, J. C., Martin, B., Lewis, R., Smith, L., Fontana, D. J. and Lee, C.-H. (1995). The contribution of peripheral sensory neuronal input towards the maintenance of neuropathic pain. *Soc Neurosci Abstr.*, **21**, 1411.

Hunter, J. C., Gogas, K. R., Hedley, L. R. *et al.* (1997). The effect of novel anti-epileptic drugs in rat experimental models of acute and chronic pain. *Eur J Pharmacol.,* **324**, 153–60.

Isomoto, S., Kondo, C. and Kurachi, Y. (1997). Inwardly rectifying potassium channels: their molecular heterogeneity and function. *Jap J Physiol.*, **47**, 11–39.

Jett, M. F., McGuirk, J., Waligora, D. and Hunter, J. C. (1997). The effects of mexiletine, desipramine and fluoxetine in rat models involving central sensitization. *Pain*, **69**, 161–9.

Kaczorowski, G. J., Knaus, H. G., Leonard, R. J., McManus, O. B. and Garcia, M. L. (1996). High-conductance calcium-activated potassium channels: structure, pharmacology, and function. *J Bioenerg Biomembr.,* **28**, 255–67.

Kallen, R. G., Cohen, S. A. and Barchi, R. L. (1993). Structure, function and expression of voltage-dependent sodium channels. *Mol Neurobiol.*, **7**, 383–428.

Kastrup, J., Petersen, P., Dejgard, A., Angelo, H. R. and Hilsted, J. (1987). Intravenous lidocaine infusion – a new treatment of chronic painful diabetic neuropathy? *Pain*, **28**, 69–75.

Kerr, L. M., Filloux, F., Olivera, B. M., Jackson, H. and Wamsley, J. K. (1988). Autoradiographic localization of calcium channels with [125]w-conotoxin in rat brain. *Eur J Pharmacol.*, **146**, 181–3.

Killian, J. M. and Fromm, G. H. (1968). Carbamazepine in the treatment of neuralgia. Use of side-effects. *Arch Neurol.*, **19**, 129–36.

Khasar, S. G., Gold, M. S. and Levine, J. D. (1998). A tetrodotoxin-resistant sodium current mediates inflammatory pain in the rat. *Neurosci Lett.*, **256**, 17–20.

Kim, S. H. and Chung, J. M. (1992). An experimental model for peripheral neuropathy produced by segmental spinal nerve ligation in the rat. *Pain,* **50**, 355–63.

Kirchhoff, C., Leah, J. D., Jung, S. and Reeh, P. W. (1992). Excitation of cutaneous sensory nerve endings in the rat by 4-aminopyridine and tetraethylammonium. *J Neurophysiol.*, **67**, 125–31.

Kirk, E. J. (1994). Impulses in dorsal spinal rootlets in cats and rabbits arising from dorsal root ganglia isolated from the periphery. *J Comp Neurol.*, **155**, 165–75.

Koch, B. D., Faurot, G. F., McGuirk, J. R., Clarke, D. E. and Hunter, J. C. (1996). Modulation of mechanohyperalgesia by clinically effective analgesics in rats with a peripheral mononeuropathy. *Analgesia*, **2**, 157–64.

Koltzenburg, M., Torebjork, H. E. and Wahren, L. K. (1994). Nociceptor modulated central sensitization causes mechanical hyperalgesia in acute chemogenic and chronic neuropathic pain. *Brain*, **117**, 579–91.

Kuo, C.-C. and Bean, B. P. (1994). Slow binding of phenytoin to inactivated sodium channels in rat hippocampal neurons. *Mol Pharmacol.*, **46**, 716–25.

Kuo, C. C., Chen, R. S., Lu, L. and Chen, R. C. (1997). Carbamazepine inhibition of neuronal Na$^+$ currents: quantitative distinction from phenytoin and possible therapeutic implications. *Mol Pharmacol*, **51**, 1077–83.

Leach, M. J., Marden, C. M. and Miller, A. A. (1986). Pharmacological studies on lamotrigine, a novel potential antiepileptic drug. Part II: Neurochemical studies on the mechanism of action. *Epilepsia*, **27**, 490–7.

Leijon, G. and Boivie, J. (1989). Central post-stroke pain – a controlled trial of amitriptyline and carbamazepine. *Pain*, **36**, 27–36.

Lin, Z., Haus, S., Edgerton, J. and Lipscombe, D. (1997). Identification of functionally distinct isoforms of the N-type Ca2$^+$ channel in rat sympathetic ganglia and brain. *Neuron*, **18**, 153–66.

Lindstrom, P. and Lindblom, U. (1987). The analgesic effect of tocainide in trigeminal neuralgia. *Pain,* **28**, 45–50.

Lotarski, S. M., Taylor, C. P., Wang, Y.-X., Bowersox, S. and Song, Y. (1999). PD 0176078, a potent blocker of voltage-gated calcium channels, prevents pain related behavior in mice and rats. *18th Annual Scientific Meeting American Pain Society.* Fort Lauderdale, 1999, pp. 167; 870.

Luria, Y., Brecker, C., Daoud, D., Ishay, A. and Eisenberg, E. (2000). Lamotrigine in the treatment of painful diabetic neuropathy: a randomised placebo-controlled study. In *Proceedings of the 9th World Congress on Pain, Prog. In Pain Research and Management*, Vol.16 (eds Devor, M., Rowbotham, M. C. and Wiesenfeld-Hallin, Z.), pp. 857–862. Seattle: IASP Press.

McClean, G. (1999). Two-hundred milligrams a day of lamotrigine has no effect in neuropathic pain: a randomiZed, double-blind placebo-controlled trial. *Pain*, **83**, 105–7.

Maizels, M., Scott, B., Cohen, W. and Chen, W. (1996). Intranasal lidocaine for treatment of migraine: a randomized, double-blind, controlled trial. *JAMA*, **276**, 319–21.

Malmberg, A. B. and Yaksh, T. L. (1994). Voltage-sensitive calcium channels in spinal nociceptive processing: blockade of N- and P-type channels inhibits formalin-induced nociception. *J Neurosci.*, **14**, 4882–90.

Malmberg, A. B. and Yaksh, T. L. (1995). Effect of continuous intrathecal infusion of $\omega$-conopeptides, N-type calcium-channel blockers, on behavior and antinociception in the formalin and hot-plate tests in rats. *Pain*, **60**, 83–90.

Marchettini, P., Lacerenza, M., Marangoni, C., Pellegata, G., Sotgiu, M. L. and Smirne, S. (1992). Lidocaine test in neuralgia. *Pain*, **48**, 377–82.

Matzner, O. and Devor, M. (1992). Na$^+$ conductance and the threshold for repetitive neuronal firing. *Brain Res.*, **597**, 92–8.

Matzner, O. and Devor, M. (1994). Hyperexcitability at sites of nerve injury depends on voltage-sensitive Na$^+$ channels. *J Neurophysiol.*, **72**, 349–59.

McQuay, H., Carroll, D., Jadad, A. R., Wiffen, P. and Moore, A. (1995). Anticonvulsant drugs for the management of pain: a systematic review. *Br Med J.*, **311**, 1047–52.

Miljanich, G. P. and Ramachandran, J. (1995). Antagonists of neuronal calcium channels: structure, function, and therapeutic implications. *Ann Rev Pharmacol Toxicol.*, **35**, 707–34.

Mintz, I. M., Adams, M. E. and Bean, B. P. (1992). P-type calcium channels in rat central and peripheral neurons. *Neuron*, **9**, 85–95.

Miranda, H. F., Bustamante, D., Kramer, V. *et al.* (1992). Antinociceptive effects of Ca2$^+$ channel blockers. *Eur J Pharmacol.*, **217**, 137–141.

Nagaro, T., Shimizu, C., Inoue, H. *et al.* (1995). The efficacy of intravenous lidocaine on various types of neuropathic pain. *Jap J Anesth.*, **44**, 862–7.

Nakamura-Craig, M. and Follenfant, R. L. (1995). Effect of lamotrigine in the acute and chronic hyperalgesia induced by PGE$_2$ and in the chronic hyperalgesia in rats with streptozotocin-induced diabetes. *Pain*, **63**, 33–7.

Neugebauer, V., Vanegas, H., Nebe, J., Rumenapp, P. and Schaible, H. G. (1996). Effects of N- and L-type calcium channel antagonists on the responses of nociceptive spinal cord neurons to mechanical stimulation of the normal and the inflamed knee joint. *J Neurophysiol.*, **76**, 3740–9.

Novakovic, S. D., Tzoumaka, E., McGivern, J. G. *et al.* (1998). Distribution of the tetrodotoxin-resistant sodium channel, PN3, in rat sensory neurons in normal and neuropathic conditions. *J Neurosci.*, **18**, 2174–87.

Ocana, M,. Del Pozo, E., Barrios, M. and Baeyens, J. M. (1995). Subgroups among $\mu$-opioid receptor agonists distinguished by ATP-sensitive K$^+$ channel-acting drugs. *Br J Pharmacol.*, **114**, 1296–1302.

Ocana, M., Barrios, M. and Baeyens, J. M. (1996). Cromakalim differentially enhances antinociception induced by agonists of $\alpha$(2): adrenoceptors, gamma-aminobutyric acid(B):, mu and kappa opioid receptors. *J Pharmacol Exp Ther.*, **276**, 1136–42.

Ocana, M. and Baeyens, J. M. (1993). Differential effects of K$^+$ channel blockers on antinociception induced by $\alpha$ 2-adrenoceptor, GABA$_B$ and kappa-opioid receptor agonists. *Br J Pharmacol.*, **110**, 1049–54.

Ogata, N. and Tatebayashi, H. (1993). Kinetic analysis of two types of Na$^+$ channels in rat dorsal root ganglia. *J Physiol.*, **466**, 9–37.

Omana-Zapata, I., Khabbaz, M. A., Hunter, J. C. and Bley, K. R. (1997a). QX-314 inhibits ectopic nerve activity associated with neuropathic pain. *Brain Res.*, **771**, 228–37.

Omana-Zapata, I., Khabbaz, M. A., Hunter, J. C., Clarke, D. E. and Bley, K. R. (1997b). Tetrodotoxin inhibits neuropathic ectopic activity in neuromas, dorsal root ganglia and dorsal horn neurons. *Pain*, **72**, 41–9.

Omote, K., Sonoda, H., Kawamata, M., Iwasaki, H. and Namiki, A. (1993). Potentiation of antinociceptive effects of morphine by calcium-channel blockers at the level of the spinal cord. *Anesthesiology*, **79**, 746–52.

Ophoff, R. A., Terwindt, G. M., Vergouwe, M. N., van Eijk, R., Oefner, P. J. *et al.* (1996). Familial hemiplegic migraine and episodic ataxia type-2 are caused by mutations in the Ca2$^+$ channel gene CACNL1A4. *Cell*, **87**, 543–52.

Oskarsson, P., Lins, P. E. and Lunggren, J. G. (1997). Mexilitene Study Group. Efficacy and safety of mexilitene in the treatment of painful diabetic neuropathy. *Diabetes Care* **20**, 1594–7.

Pavone, F., Battaglia, M. and Sansone, M. (1993). Attenuation of cholinergic analgesia by nifedipine. *Brain Res.*, **623**, 308–10.

Pearce, R. J. and Duchen, M. R. (1994). Differential expression of membrane currents in dissociated mouse primary sensory neurons. *Neuroscience*, **63**, 1041–56.

Pereira, I. T., Prado, W. A. and Dos Reis, M. P. (1993). Enhancement of the epidural morphine-induced analgesia by systemic nifedipine. *Pain*, **53**, 341–5.

Petersen, P., Kastrup, J., Zeeberg, I. and Boysen, G. (1986). Chronic pain treatment with intravenous lidocaine. *Neurol Res.*, **8**, 189–90.

Polati, E., Benedini, B., Finco, G., Gottin, L., Orlandi, L. and Schweiger, V. (1999). Gabapentin and Gabapentin+lamotrigine in the treatment of neuropathic pain. 18th Annual Scientific Meeting APS Fort Lauderdale, Oct 21–24, 713, p. 114.

Pongs, O. (1992). Molecular biology of voltage-dependent potassium channels. *Physiol Rev.*, **72**, S69–88.

Porreca, F., Ossipov, M., Lai, J. *et al.* (2000). Blockade of diabetic, chemotherapeutic and NGF-induced pain by antisense knockdown of PN3/SNS, a TTX-resistant sodium channel. In *Proceedings of the 9th World Congress on Pain, Prog. In Pain Research and Management* Vol.16 (eds Devor, M., Rowbotham, M. C. and Wiesenfeld-Hallin, Z.), pp. 273–80. Seattle: IASP Press.

Raffa, R. B. and Martinez, R. P. (1995). The 'glibenclamide-shift' of centrally-acting antinociceptive agents in mice. *Brain Res.*, **677**, 277–82.

Reuter, H. (1996). Diversity and function of presynaptic calcium channels in the brain. *Curr Opin Neurobiol.*, **6**, 331–7.

Rizzo, M. A., Kocsis, J. D. and Waxman, S. G. (1994). Slow sodium conductances of dorsal root ganglion neurons: intraneuronal homogeneity and interneuronal heterogeneity. *J Neurophysiol.*, **72**, 2796–815.

Rizzo, M. A., Kocsis, J. D. and Waxman, S. G. (1995). Selective loss of slow and enhancement of fast Na$^+$ currents in cutaneous afferent dorsal root ganglion neurones following axotomy. *Neurobiol Dis.*, **2**, 87–96.

Roca, G., Aguilar, J. L., Gomar, C., Mazo, V., Costa, J. and Vidal, F. (1996). Nimodipine fails to enhance the analgesic effect of slow release morphine in the early phases of cancer pain treatment. *Pain*, **68**, 239–43.

Rowbotham, M. C., Petersen, K. L. and Fields, H. L. (1999). Is postherapeutic neuralgia more than one disorder? IASP Newsletter, Fall, pp. 3–7.

Rowbotham, M. C., Reisner-Keller, L. A. and Fields, H. L. (1991). Both intravenous lidocaine and morphine reduce the pain of postherpetic neuralgia. *Neurology*, **41**, 1024–8.

Rowbotham, M. C., Davies, P. S. and Fields, H. L. (1995). Topical lidocaine gel relieves postherpetic neuralgia. *Ann Neurol.*, **37**, 246–53.

Rowbotham, M., Harden, N., Stacey, B., Berstein, P. and Magnus-Miller, L. (1998). Gabapentin for the treatment of postherpetic neuralgia: a randomized controlled trial. *JAMA*, **280**, 1837–42.

Roy, M. L. and Narahashi, T. (1992). Differential properties of tetrodotoxin-sensitive and tetrodotoxin-resistant sodium channels in rat dorsal root ganglion neurons. *J Neurosci.*, **12**, 2104–11.

Rudy, B. (1988). Diversity and ubiquity of K-channels. *Neuroscience*, **25**, 729–49.

Rull, J., Quibrera, R., Gonzalez-Millan, H. and Lozano Castenada, O. (1969). Symptomatic treatment of peripheral diabetic neuropathy with carbamazepine: double-blind crossover study. *Diabetologia*, **5**, 215–20.

Sakurai, M. and Kanazawa, I. (1999). Positive symptoms in multiple sclerosis; their treatment with sodium channel blockers lidocaine and mexiletine. *J Neurol Sci.*, **162**, 162–8.

Sangameswaran, L., Delgado, S. G., Fish, L. M. *et al.* (1996). Structure and function of a novel voltage-gated, tetrodotoxin-resistant sodium channel specific to sensory neurons. *J Biol Chem.*, **271**, 5953–6.

Sangameswaran, L., Fish, L. M., Koch, B. D. *et al.* (1997). A novel tetrodotoxin-sensitive, voltage-gated sodium channel expressed in rat and human dorsal root ganglia. *J Biol Chem.*, **272**, 14805–9.

Santillan, R., Maestre, J. M., Hurle, M. A. and Florez, J. (1994). Enhancement of opiate analgesia by nimodipine in cancer patients chronically treated with morphine: a preliminary report. *Pain*, **58**, 129–32.

Santillan, R., Maestre, J. M., Hurle, M. A. and Florez, J. (1998). Nimodipine-enhanced opiate analgesia in cancer patients requiring morphine dose escalation: a double blind placebo controlled study. *Pain*, **76**, 17–26.

Saudek, C. D., Werns, S. and Reidenberg, M. M. (1977). Phenytoin in the treatment of diabetic symmetrical polyneuropathy. *Clin Pharmacol Ther.*, **22**, 196–9.

Schaller, K. L., Krzemien, D. M., Yarowsky, P. J., Krueger, B. K. and Caldwell, J. H. (1995). A novel, abundant sodium channel expressed in neurons and glia. *J Neurosci.*, **15**, 3231–42.

Scroggs, R. S., Todorovic, S. M., Anderson, E. G. and Fox, A. P. (1994). Variation in IH, IIR, and ILEAK between acutely isolated adult rat dorsal root ganglion neurons of different size. *J Neurophysiol.*, **71**, 271–9.

Scroggs, R. S. and Fox, A. P. (1992). Calcium current variation between acutely isolated adult rat dorsal root ganglion neurons of different size. *J Physiol.*, **445**, 639–58.

Sindrup, S. H. and Jensen, T. S. (1999). Efficacy of pharmacological treatments of neuropathic pain: an update and effect related to mechanism of drug action. *Pain* **83**, 389–400.

Sinnott, C., Edmonds, P., Cropley, I. *et al.* (1991). Flecainide in cancer nerve pain. *Lancet*, **337**, 1347.

Sotgiu, M. E., Biella, G., Castagna, A., Lacerenza, M., Marchettini, P. (1994). Different time-courses of IV lidocaine effect on ganglionic and spinal units in neuropathic rats. *NeuroReport*, **5**, 873–6.

Stracke, H., Meyer, U. F., Schumacher, H. F. and Federlin, K. (1992). Mexiletene in the treatment of diabetic neuropathy. *Diabetes Care*, **15**, 1550–5.

Swerdlow, M. (1984). Anticonvulsant drugs and chronic pain. *Clin Neuropharmacol.*, **7**, 51–82.

Tanelian, D. L. and Victory, R. A. (1995). Sodium channel-blocking agents: their use in neuropathic pain conditions. *Pain Forum*, **4**, 75–80.

Tanelian, D. L. and Brose, W. G. (1991). Neuropathic pain can be relieved by drugs that are use-dependent sodium channel blockers: lidocaine, carbamazepine, and mexiletine. *Anesthesiology*, **74**, 949–51.

Taylor, C. P., Gee, N. S., Su, T. Z. *et al.* (1998). A summary of mechanistic hypotheses of gabapentin pharmacology. *Epilepsy Res.*, **29**, 233–49.

Toledo-Aral, J. J., Moss, B. L., He, Z. J. *et al.* (1997). Identification of PN1, a predominant voltage-dependent sodium channel expressed principally in peripheral neurons. *Proc Natl Acad Sci (USA)*, **94**, 1527–32.

Trezise, D. J., John, V. H. and Xie, X. M. (1998). Voltage and use-dependent inhibition of sodium channels in rat sensory neurons by 430W92, a new antihyperalgesic agent. *Br J Pharmacol.*, **124**, 953–63.

Wall, P. D. and Devor, M. (1983). Sensory afferent impulses originate from dorsal root ganglia as well as from the periphery in normal and nerve injured rats. *Pain*, **17**, 321–39.

Wall, P. D. and Gutnick, M. (1974). Ongoing activity in peripheral nerves: the physiology and pharmacology of impulses originating from a neuroma. *Exp Neurol.* **43**, 580–93.

Wallace, M. S., Ridgway, B., Leung, A. and Yaksh, A. (2000). Concentration-effect relationship of intravenous lidocaine on the allodynia of complex regional pain syndromes 1 and 2. *Anesthesiology*, **92**, 75–83.

Waxman, S. G., Kocsis, J. D. and Black, J. A. (1994). Type III sodium channel mRNA is expressed in embryonic but not adult spinal sensory neurons, and is re-expressed following axotomy. *J Neurophysiol.*, **72**, 466–70.

Wei, Z. Y., Karim, F. and Roerig, S. C. (1996). Spinal morphine/clonidine antinociceptive synergism: involvement of G proteins and N-type voltage-dependent calcium channels. *J Pharmacol Exp Ther.*, **278**, 1392–1407.

Wild, K. D., Vanderah, T., Mosberg, H. I. and Porreca, F. (1991). Opioid delta receptor subtypes are associated with different potassium channels. *Eur J Pharmacol.*, **193**, 135–6.

Woolf, C. J. and Chong, M. S. (1993). Preemptive analgesia – treating postoperative pain by preventing the establishment of central sensitization. *Anesth Analg.*, **77**, 362–79.

Woolf, C. J. and Doubell, T. P. (1994). The pathophysiology of chronic pain – increased sensitivity to low threshold Aβ-fibre inputs. *Curr Opin Neurobiol.*, **4**, 525–34.

Wright, J. M., Oki, J. C. and Graves, L. (1997). Mexiletine in the symptomatic treatment of diabetic peripheral neuropathy. *Ann Pharmacother.*, **31**, 29–34.

Xiao, W. H. and Bennett, G. J. (1995). Synthetic ω-conopeptides applied to the site of nerve injury suppress neuropathic pains in rats. *J Pharmacol Exp Ther.*, **274**, 666–72.

Yoon, Y. W., Na, H. S. and Chung, J. M. (1996). Contributions of injured and intact afferents to neuropathic pain in an experimental rat model. *Pain*, **64**, 27–36.

Zakrzewska, J. M., Chaudhry, Z., Nurmikko, T. J., Patton, D. W. and Mullens, E. L. (1997). Lamotrigine (Lamictal) in refractory trigeminal neuralgia: results from a double-blind placebo controlled crossover trial. *Pain*, **73**, 223–30.

# The role of ion channel distribution, dysfunction and gene expression in demyelinating disease

*Paul A. Felts*

## Introduction

Primary demyelination, the loss of the myelin sheath with axonal sparing, is a prominent feature in a number of disorders of both the central and peripheral nervous systems (CNS, PNS). Several of the most commonly studied demyelinating disorders, such as multiple sclerosis (MS), Guillain-Barré syndrome (GBS) and chronic inflammatory demyelinating polyradiculoneuropathy (CIDP) have an inflammatory aetiology (see Smith and McDonald, 1999; Hughes *et al.*, 1999; Pouly and Antel, 1999; Van der Meche and Van Dorn, 1999). However, demyelinating disorders with toxic (e.g. diphtheritic neuropathy, buckthorn neuropathy) or genetic (e.g. metachromatic or globoid-cell leukodystrophies) causes are also known. Although each of these disorders has unique, defining features, they probably have a shared sequela which results directly from the loss of myelin. Demyelinating diseases are not known to be associated with defects in individual ion channels, however, there is no doubt that ion channels play a major role in the often devastating effects of these disorders. In particular, the heterogeneous distribution of channels along the myelinated axon, although integral to normal action potential transmission, contributes to dysfunction following demyelination. In addition, blocking factors that interfere with ion channel function, and alterations in the expression and localization of ion channel subtypes, may also contribute to the effects of demyelinating disease. Study of the latter mechanism is in its infancy. This chapter will examine the role of ion channels in the flawed impulse transmission that is at the heart of symptom production in demyelinating disease.

## Ion channel distribution in demyelinating disease

### Distribution of ion channels in normal myelinated axons

Myelinated axons effect the rapid, faithful transmission of impulses within the nervous system. Chief among the adaptations which permit this efficient form of transmission are the myelin sheath itself, which reduces the loss of action potential current along the internode, and a heterogeneous distribution of ion channels. The rapid depolarizing current at the rising phase of the axonal action potential is conducted through voltage-gated sodium channels. In normal mammalian myelinated axons, sodium channels are present at a very high density at the node of Ranvier ($1000-2000/\mu m^2$ (Chiu, 1980)). These channels are found in the internodal axolemma at only $2-6$ % of the nodal density (Shrager 1989). In addition to the voltage-gated sodium channel, several types of potassium channel have been identified in the mammalian myelinated axon. These include rapidly-gated and slowly-gated voltage-sensitive potassium channels (Chiu and Ritchie, 1980; Smith and Schauf, 1981) and ligand- and ion-gated (Safronov *et al.*, 1993) forms. Unlike myelinated axons in amphibians (Frankenhaeuser, 1963), voltage-gated potassium currents are largely absent during action potential conduction in mammals (Chiu and Ritchie, 1980; Kocsis and Waxman, 1980; Smith and Schauf, 1981) because the channels responsible for these currents are sequestered beneath the myelin sheath. The role of potassium channels in normal adult axons is not known, however, recent evidence suggests that they serve to prevent repetitive firing in nerves (Vabnick et al., 1999) and motor nerve terminals (Zhou et al., 1998) in very young animals. In adult rodent CNS (Wang et al., 1993, 1994; Rasband et al., 1999a) and PNS (Mi et al., 1995; Vabnick et al., 1999) voltage-gated Kv1.1 and Kv1.2 potassium channels are found at a high density in the juxtaparanodes, the internodal axolemma immediately adjacent to the paranode.

Finally, although most studies of ion channels in mammalian axons have been performed on rats and mice, those studies which have examined human axons have found that the types and distributions of currents are broadly similar to those found in rodents (Scholz et al., 1993; Schwarz et al., 1995; Reid et al., 1999).

## Conduction in demyelinated and remyelinated axons

### Demyelination results initially in conduction block

The loss of entire internodes of myelin, or segmental demyelination, uncovers the internodal axolemma, unmasking voltage-gated potassium channels (Chiu and Ritchie, 1980, 1981; Smith and Schauf, 1981; Schwarz et al., 1991) and exposing an axon membrane with a relatively low density of sodium channels (Chiu and Schwarz, 1987; Shrager, 1989). Although such a low density of sodium channels will allow conduction to occur in very small calibre axons (Waxman et al., 1989; Waxman and Ritchie, 1993), the likely immediate consequence of segmental demyelination in most axons is conduction block. A number of experimental studies have demonstrated conduction block following demyelination (e.g. McDonald and Sears, 1970; Shrager and Rubinstein, 1990; Felts and Smith, 1992). In disorders such as MS, conduction block undoubtedly contributes to the production of 'negative' symptoms, that is symptoms arising from a failure of conduction, such as blindness, numbness or paralysis. In the past, these symptoms have often been wholly attributed to demyelination, however, it is now clear that other mechanisms are also involved, and these will be discussed later in this chapter.

Although the conduction block that immedi-

ately follows myelin loss is inevitable in most axons, conduction can be restored prior to remyelination of the demyelinated internode in both the PNS (Bostock and Sears, 1978; Smith et al., 1982; Shrager and Rubinstein, 1990) and the CNS (Felts et al., 1997a). Conduction in demyelinated axons is characterized by decreased conduction velocity, increased refractory period of transmission (the maximum interval at which the second of two impulses just fails to be transmitted) and an inability faithfully to transmit trains of impulses. This conduction, albeit imperfect, almost certainly provides relief from symptoms. Many MS patients exhibit delayed evoked responses in the absence of clinically demonstrable visual loss (Celesia and Daly, 1977), and it has been suggested that the delay in these responses results from the slowing of conduction in demyelinated axons (Bostock, 1994). However, it is clear that conduction along these pathways provides useful visual information to the patients (Wisniewski et al., 1976).

### Ectopic activity in demyelinated axons

In addition to negative symptoms resulting from conduction block, demyelinating diseases are also characterized by the presence of symptoms such as paresthesiae and phosphenes (see Smith et al., 1997). In a 1999 survey of 224 MS patients, 12 % reported that the worst symptom that they experienced was pain, which the authors describe as neuropathic pain (Rae-Grant et al., 1999). These 'positive' symptoms are believed to arise from the ectopic initiation of action potentials in hyperexcitable axons along regions of demyelination. These ectopic action potentials may be triggered by conducted impulses (Ostermann and Westerberg, 1975), and there is evidence that ephaptic spread of excitation occurs (Rasminsky, 1978). Such ephaptic spread could account for the paroxysmal nature of some symptoms. Ectopic action potentials can also be initiated by mechanical deformation, for example Lhermitte's sign, in which neck flexion in patients with demyelinating lesions of the cervical dorsal columns results in radiating electric shock-like sensations (Nordin et al., 1984). Similar mechanosensitive and spontaneously active axons have been demonstrated in demyelinated lesions in experimental animals (e.g. Smith and McDonald, 1982). These ectopic impulses are generated by inappropriate membrane excitability which almost certainly involves ion channels. The exact mechanisms of impulse initiation are not known, however, experimental evidence suggests several potential causes. Baker and Bostock (1992) found that ectopic firing in demyelinated rat spinal roots was related to a pacemaker potential mediated by a slow potassium conductance. Potassium loading of the internodal, periaxonal space in normal axons produces ectopic action potentials (David et al., 1993; Kapoor et al., 1993), and these are associated with a periodic, prolonged conductance across the internodal axolemma resulting in a local depolarizing potential shift in the axon. This prolonged current can be eliminated by the potassium channel blockers tetraethylammonium (TEA) or 4-aminopyridine (4-AP), and is probably the result of potassium entering the axon following local reversal of its electrochemical gradient. Ectopic spikes were recorded in demyelinated axons associated with similar potential shifts (Felts et al., 1995a), suggesting that localized potassium accumulation in a compartment adjacent to demyelinated axons could account for some spontaneous activity. Potassium channel blockers have also been shown to increase, rather than decrease, spontaneous activity in demyelinated axons, particularly in sensory fibres (Bowe et al., 1987; Baker and Bostock, 1992; Kapoor et al., 1997). These ectopic impulses can also occur in the absence of potassium channel block, and are associated with an oscillating generator potential which is eliminated by the sodium channel blocker tetrodotoxin (TTX) (Kapoor et al., 1997). The time course of these potential changes suggests that a slowly inactivating sodium channel is responsible, and indeed, such channels have been described in sensory axons (Honmou et al., 1994).

Symptoms caused by spontaneous activity in demyelinating disorders like MS and GBS are typically treated with drugs such as phenytoin and carbamazepine, which produce a potential- and frequency-dependent block of sodium currents in axons (David et al., 1986; Schwarz and Grigat, 1989). Other sodium channel blockers, such as lidocaine and mexiletine, have recently been used in MS, and were found to be particularly effective on paroxysmal symptoms (Sakurai and Kanazawa, 1999). However, these drugs are not ideal therapeutic agents because demyelinating lesions often contain axons with a safety factor for conduction which is just above unity, that is they produce just enough current for conduction to proceed. Any decrease in depolarizing current resulting from therapeutic sodium channel block is likely to decrease the number of conducting axons and worsen negative symptoms, or unmask latent lesions (Sakurai et al., 1992). A greater understanding of the mechanisms involved in generation of these impulses will hopefully allow the development of compounds which can prevent the ectopic activity without blocking the insecure conduction along demyelinated axons.

## Distribution of ion channels in demyelinated and remyelinated axons

In most demyelinated axons, restoration of conduction is likely to require changes in ion channel distribution. This redistribution is strongly suggested by the electrophysiological demonstration of conduction in demyelinated and remyelinated axons (Smith et al., 1979; Smith and Hall, 1980; Felts and Smith, 1992; Felts et al., 1997a). Rapid and secure conduction in remyelinated axons indicates ion channel redistribution because new internodes are shorter than the original internodes, therefore new nodes of Ranvier are located at sites which previously had a low density of sodium channels. Axolemmal remodelling of sodium channel distribution is clearly demonstrated in an electrophysiological study which revealed new regions of focal, high density, inward current (termed 'phi' nodes) on rat ventral root axons several days after demyelination by lysolecithin and prior to remyelination (Smith et al., 1982).

### Morphological studies

Considerable insights into membrane reorganization following demyelination came from freeze-fracture and histochemical studies (Foster et al.,

1980; Rosenbluth and Blakemore, 1984; Black et al., 1987), however, these techniques are not specific for ion channels. In the past decade, antibodies against sodium channels and potassium channels have been developed which can be used for immunohistochemical labelling of mammalian tissues. These antibodies have substantially increased our knowledge of ion channel distributions both during development and following pathological changes.

## Changes in sodium channel distribution following demyelination and remyelination: immunohistochemical studies

Sodium channel distribution has been examined in animal models of both focal demyelination and genetic myelin disruption. In the rat sciatic nerve, demyelinated by lysolecithin, sodium channel distribution was examined using a channel-specific antibody (Dugandzija-Novakovic et al., 1995; Novakovic et al., 1996). Sodium channel labelling is evident at heminodes at the edges of the lesion and at occasional sites scattered along the demyelinated axons. When Schwann cells begin to ensheath the demyelinated axons, sodium channel immunoreactivity appears at the edges of these regions of contact. As the Schwann cell processes extend along the axon, these regions of high sodium channel density appear to be swept ahead until neighbouring Schwann cell processes are in close proximity to one another and the new node of Ranvier is formed. This new node exhibits highly focal sodium channel labelling, similar to that in normal fibres. Inhibition of Schwann cell proliferation demonstrates that these cells are necessary for the maintenance of sodium channel clustering. In the absence of Schwann cell association, even the labelling at the original heminodes at the edge of the demyelinating lesion is eventually lost (Dugandzija-Novakovic et al., 1995).

The lysolecithin model of demyelination provides a relatively synchronized, focal lesion for study, however, its similarity to clinical disorders is limited. Experimental allergic neuritis (EAN) is a model of GBS which mimics some of the important features of the disorder, such as nerve oedema and perivenular lymphocyte infiltration

(see Hughes et al., 1999). Approximately 10 days after injection with peripheral myelin and adjuvant, experimental animals exhibit a progressive neurological deficit that gradually resolves between days 20 and 40. In these animals, the pattern of sodium channel labelling in regions of segmental demyelination is similar to that seen in the lysolecithin lesion (Novakovic et al., 1998). However, before the onset of clinical signs or segmental demyelination, sodium channel labelling of nodes is disordered, and electrophysiological recordings from spinal roots exhibit evidence of conduction block. These findings indicate that demyelination is not the only process contributing to the deficits observed in these animals. Conduction block correlates with a paucity of sodium channel labelling at the nodes, and as clinical signs appear and progress, labelling disperses to include the paranodes, and finally, at most nodes, disappears (Novakovic et al., 1998). In MS and GBS, the rapid onset of dysfunction which is sometimes observed has cast doubt on the idea that demyelination alone can account for the symptoms (see Rose, 1963; Smith, 1994). Blocking factors have been cited to explain this observation (see below), however, the relatively rapid loss of sodium channels from nodes, in the absence of segmental demyelination, may provide another mechanism.

In the optic nerves of *Shiverer* mice, which have a gene defect resulting in severe CNS hypomyelination, most, but not all of the axonal sodium channel labelling is located adjacent to cell processes with paranodal characteristics (Rasband et al., 1999b). The dystrophic mouse, which has a genetic defect resulting in regions of packed amyelinated axons in the spinal roots, was used in an elegant electron microscopy study which showed patches of axolemmal sodium channel labelling in the absence of adjacent glial cell contact (Deerinck et al., 1997). It should be noted that axons in these models are either hypomyelinated or amyelinated, rather than demyelinated, and it is possible that the sodium channel distributions will vary between these different forms of myelin pathology.

Myelination of axons during development also offers an opportunity to examine the process of nodal development and comparison with repair following demyelination may demonstrate important differences. In the rat PNS, aggregates of sodium channels initially appear in the axolemma adjacent to ensheathing Schwann cell processes. As the processes approach close to one another, sodium channel immunoreactivity either fills the space as a broad, uniform band, or exhibits two intensely labelled rings at either end of the gap (Vabnick et al., 1996). In the CNS, aggregates of axolemmal sodium channels are found adjacent to developing oligodendrocyte structures which are indicative of paranodes. Aggregates in the CNS appear about one week later than in the PNS (Rasband et al., 1999b; see Rasband and Shrager, 2000). These studies, and particularly the finding that sodium channel aggregates only appear after glial contact, suggest that glial cells may play the lead role in nodal development. However, there is some evidence that aggregates can form in the absence of glial contact. Such aggregates have been described in mouse peripheral nerve during early development (Vabnick et al., 1997), in the axolemma of amyelinated dystrophic mouse spinal roots (Deerinck et al., 1997), and in the axolemma of retinal ganglion cells in vitro following exposure to oligodendrocyte-conditioned medium (Kaplan et al., 1997). Taken together, the above studies suggest that axons and glial cells act in concert to produce the nodal sodium channel aggregations. The relative contributions of the axon and the glial cell are still the subject of considerable debate.

## Changes in potassium channel distribution following demyelination and remyelination: immunohistochemical studies

Changes in the distribution of Shaker-type potassium channels following demyelination have been examined in lysolecithin lesions and in animals with mutations in myelin-associated genes. Rat sciatic nerves normally exhibit juxtaparanodal Kv1.1 and Kv1.2 labelling. Rasband et al. (1998) found that one week after the injection of lysolecithin, when the nerves exhibit prominent demyelination, 79% of the original nodes of Ranvier do not label with a potassium channel antibody. The sites of the original nodes are still obvious due to

the retention of focal sodium channel labelling, indicating that the potassium channels are more labile than the nearby nodal sodium channels. The authors suggest that the more ephemeral nature of potassium channel aggregation is due to a greater dependence on signals from the Schwann cells overlying the juxtaparanodes (Rasband et al., 1998). During early remyelination, when Schwann cells are extending processes along the demyelinated axons, and sodium channel labelling is present, Kv1.1 labelling is not seen. As remyelination progresses, an increasing number of fibres show intense Kv1.1 labelling, and perhaps surprisingly, the label is located not at the juxtaparanode, but at the new node. With time, the label extends into the paranodes and juxtaparanodes, and is finally lost from the nodal gap. However, even after 10 weeks the original distribution is not regained, and potassium channel label is present at the paranode, in addition to the normal juxtaparanodal location. The period of nodal potassium channel labelling correlates with an increase in the effect of the potassium channel blocker 4-AP on conduction. Application of 4-AP at this time enhances the compound action potential, suggesting that these channels impede conduction (Rasband et al., 1998). However, these channels may have other important actions, such as the prevention of ectopic firing (see above). The ability of potassium channel blockers to enhance conduction through demyelinated lesions has been recognized for two decades. In 1980, Sherratt et al. showed that the direct application of 4-AP to a demyelinated dorsal root causes an increase in the size of the compound action potential conducted along the root. This report spawned a number of clinical trials in MS patients which demonstrated that, despite the relatively narrow therapeutic window of this pro-convulsive drug, it does provide at least partial alleviation of negative symptoms in many patients (e.g. Stefoski et al., 1987). However, the interpretation that the clinical improvement results from increased conduction in demyelinated axons has recently been disputed. Smith et al. (2000) found no evidence of an increase in conduction through demyelinating lesions in the rat spinal cord following systemic administration of clinically relevant doses of 4-AP. They note that the maximal concentration of the drug which can be attained in patients is 250–1000 times lower than that which Sherratt et al. (1980) applied directly to the demyelinated axons. Physiological changes which are known to occur at concentrations which can be attained in patients include synaptic potentiation and enhanced muscle contraction, and the authors suggest that these probably account for much of the observed symptomatic improvement.

Potassium channel distribution has been examined in a number of mutant animals: Jimpy mouse, which has an X-linked mutation in the proteolipid protein (PLP) gene, PLP transgenic mouse, which has extra copies of the PLP gene (Baba et al., 1999), connexin32 deficient mouse (Neuberg et al., 1999), Shiverer mouse, which has a defect in the myelin basic protein gene (Wang et al., 1995; Rasband et al., 1999a), and Trembler mouse, which has a point mutation in the peripheral myelin protein 22 gene (Wang et al., 1995). These studies demonstrate that, unlike clusters of sodium channels in the nodal gap, potassium channel aggregation requires mature paranodal axo-glial interactions typical of myelinated fibres for their initiation and maintenance. This conclusion is supported by the observation that mice with disrupted paranodal axo-glial interactions, in the absence of segmental demyelination, lack high density juxtaparanodal potassium channel labelling, but retain nodal sodium channel aggregation (Dupree et al., 1999). Several studies show more diffuse potassium channel labelling along axons with disrupted myelin (Wang et al., 1995; Rasband et al., 1999a), and Baba et al. (1999) have shown that PLP transgenic mouse CNS and normal mouse CNS have similar amounts of total potassium channel Kv1.1 protein, suggesting that the channels are simply redistributed. However, Wang et al. (1995) found increased mRNA for Kv1.1 and Kv1.2 in both white matter glia and neurons from Shiverer mice. These different results may reflect the dissimilarities between a demyelinating mutant (PLP transgenic mouse) and a hypomyelinating mutant (Shiverer).

In the developing rat PNS, at the end of the first postnatal week, Kv1.1 and Kv1.2 potassium channels first appear in the axolemma at the paranodes and at nodal gaps between adjacent Schwann cells (Vabnick et al., 1999). However, during the third and fourth postnatal weeks these channels become sequestered in the juxtaparanode (Vabnick et al., 1999). Therefore potassium channel segregation in the PNS is similar during developmental myelination and during remyelination in the adult (Rasband et al., 1998). In CNS development, potassium channel clustering appears later, beginning at about P14 (rat) or P16 (mouse), it is associated with myelination, and it is initially observed in the juxtaparanode (Baba et al., 1999; Rasband et al., 1999a; see Rasband and Shrager, 2000), rather than in the node and/or paranode as in the PNS. It is not known whether this developmental pattern, in which potassium channel labelling appears initially at the juxtaparanodes, is repeated during CNS remyelination.

The above animal-based studies on sodium and potassium channel distributions provide important clues to probable changes in human axons during demyelination and remyelination. Studies of ion channels in pathological human tissue would certainly be preferable, unfortunately such studies have not been reported. Tritiated saxitoxin, a sodium channel ligand, has been used to demonstrate that sodium channel density in demyelinated white matter from MS patient is two to four times higher than normal (Moll et al., 1991). The technique did not allow the determination of the distribution of these channels along the axon, however, this finding suggests that human axons respond to demyelination by increasing their complement of sodium channels.

## Channel-blocking factors

In addition to the role played by ion channels in demyelinating diseases due to their distribution within the axolemma, there is also evidence that they may contribute to symptom production as a result of compromised function. As mentioned previously, the rapid onset and remission of symptoms in MS has suggested to many that factors other than demyelination and remyelination are also likely to be involved in symptom production. This is supported by reports that the extent of demyelination in animals with experimental allergic encephalomyelitis (EAE) often appears to be insufficient to explain the observed deficits (e.g. Panitch and Ciccone, 1981), although later evidence contradicts this suggestion (Pender, 1987). Several studies have shown that sera from MS patients or animals with EAE are capable of inhibiting evoked reflex activity in the CNS (e.g. Bornstein and Crain, 1965), and the unknown factor responsible for this was termed the 'neuro-electric blocking factor'. The exact nature and site of action of this factor is still unknown, although action on an ion channel is a distinct possibility. Interest in this factor waned, however, following reports that sera from healthy volunteers and control animals also inhibit activity in this system (e.g. Seil et al., 1976). For an excellent review of this literature see Smith (1994).

From the literature which is briefly summarized above, it is often difficult to draw conclusions regarding the specific effects of factors on ion channels because of the complexity of the poly-synaptic assay that was frequently used. A number of studies within the past decade have examined more directly the effects on ion channel function of blocking factors found in the serum or cerebrospinal fluid (CSF) of patients with demyelinating disease. In one series of experiments lasting nearly a decade, a group at the University of Ulm in Germany (Brinkmeier et al., 1992) examined a factor in the CSF of patients with demyelinating disorders which inhibits sodium conductance. This factor is present in patients with non-inflammatory disorders, however, it is elevated in patients with GBS and MS (Brinkmeier et al., 1992; 1993; Weber et al., 1999). The inhibitory effect on sodium channel conductance is associated with a negative shift in the steady state inactivation curve (Wurz et al., 1995), resulting in a decrease in the number of channels available for activation at the resting potential. CSF samples from GBS patients inhibit transient sodium currents by 10–40% (Brinkmeier et al., 1992) and cause a negative shift of approximately 10 mV in the steady state inactivation curve (Weber et al., 1999). This latter finding has also been reported by another group examining CSF from MS patients (Koller et al., 1996). The factor has been identified as a penta-peptide (Gln-Tyr-Asn-Ala-Asp) which mimics lidocaine in terms of its electrophysiological actions on the sodium channel. At equimolar concentrations it is a more potent sodium channel blocker than lidocaine and a similar block is ob-

served with the synthetic pentapeptide. The term 'endocaine', indicating an endogenous lidocaine, has been coined by the authors (Brinkmeier et al., 2000). If this peptide proves to be important in the production of conduction block in patients, it presents a significant opportunity for therapeutic intervention in demyelinating disorders.

A number of cytokines and inflammatory mediators have been found which directly alter ion conductances in neurons. Tumour necrosis factor-$\alpha$ (TNF-$\alpha$) decreases sodium conductance, interleukin-2 (IL-2) increases gamma-aminobutyric acid-induced chloride current, and nitric oxide donors increase a sodium conductance in identified Aplysia neurons (Sawada et al., 1991, 1992, 1995). Nitric oxide has the opposite effect on sodium conductance in mammalian dorsal root ganglion neurons, since block of its endogenous production increases sodium conductance (Renganathan et al., 2000). In cell line NH15-CA2, a neuroblastoma-glioma hybrid, both IL-1$\beta$ and IL-2 produce an inhibition of sodium current, however, their effects on channel kinetics differ (Hamm et al., 1996). In guinea-pig hippocampal CA1 neurons, both IL-1$\beta$ and IL-2 depress voltage-gated calcium currents (Plata-Salaman and ffrench-Mullen, 1992, 1993). Most symptoms in demyelinating diseases are thought to arise from conduction deficits in white matter tracts or nerves. Although changes in neuronal conductances will probably be reflected in disturbances of axonal conduction, this cannot be assumed. Examination of axonal conduction following TNF-$\alpha$ exposure in vitro did not provide evidence of conduction changes (Dugandzija-Novakovic and Shrager, 1995). Nitric oxide, however, has been shown to produce a reversible conduction block in axons, and interestingly, demyelinated axons were more susceptible than normal axons (Redford et al., 1997; Shrager et al., 1998; Kapoor et al., 1999). It is not known whether this effect of nitric oxide results from an action on ion channels.

Disorders such as MS and GBS are generally considered to be autoimmune, and so it is perhaps not surprising that it has been suggested that antibodies might have a direct effect on ion channel function. Animal sera containing antibodies against the $GM_1$ ganglioside (a glycosphingolipid found in axons and myelin) increases potassium current and reduces sodium current in rat myelinated sciatic nerve axons (Takigawa *et al.*, 1995). Sera which are positive for antibodies against $GM_1$ ganglioside from patients with GBS or CIDP also reduce sodium current (Takigawa *et al.*, 2000). Hirota *et al.* (1997) investigated the effects of similar sera using a high resolution recording technique that allows tracking of transmembrane currents. These recordings do not show sodium channel block. The authors suggest that the increase in potassium current and the decrease in sodium current observed by Takigawa *et al.* (1995) are probably due to exposure of potassium channels following paranodal retraction, and a reduction in the sodium concentration gradient, respectively. The absence of any effect on sodium channels was confirmed by Benatar *et al.* (1999). Using a motor neuron cell line, they found that following the application of plasma from GBS patients, there was no change in the flux of radioactive sodium across the cell membranes. The mechanism of the effect of antiganglioside antibodies on axonal conduction is still open to question. However, on balance, current evidence suggests that they do not act directly on ion channels.

## Sodium channel gene expression in demyelinating disease

We now have substantial insights into the altered ion channel distributions which accompany demyelination, however, we know little about the changes in channel gene expression which may also occur. Voltage-gated sodium channels are typically composed of a large $\alpha$-subunit and two smaller subunits, $\beta1$ and $\beta2$. The $\alpha$-subunit is the product of a multigene family and at least eight different types have been cloned and expressed (for reviews see Catterall, 2000; Waxman, Chapter 6). During development, $\alpha$-subunit mRNA expression is both temporally and spatially regulated in the nervous system (Bech *et al.*, 1989; Brysch *et al.*, 1991; Waxman *et al.*, 1994; Felts *et al.*, 1997b). However, this expression pattern can be altered by pathological processes. Nerve injury

has been shown to alter the subunit expression pattern in the affected neurons. Expression of mRNA for the SNS/PN3 $\alpha$-subunit is down-regulated in DRG neurons after nerve injury (Dib-Hajj *et al.*, 1996, 1999; Okuse *et al.*, 1997), and there is evidence that this down-regulation results from the interruption of the flow of trophic factors from the periphery to the neurons (Dib-Hajj *et al.*, 1998). In contrast to the SNS/PN3 $\alpha$-subunit, the type III $\alpha$-subunit is up-regulated in dorsal root ganglion neurons following axonal injury (Waxman *et al.*, 1994). When expressed in oocytes, the SNS/PN3 gene encodes a channel which is TTX-resistant, and slowly inactivating (Akopian *et al.*, 1996; Sangameswaran *et al.*, 1996), whereas the type III gene encodes a channel which is TTX-sensitive, and fast inactivating. The switch in sodium channel subtype expression may explain changes observed in DRG neurons following axotomy, including alterations in excitability (Amir *et al.*, 1999), current kinetics (Cummins and Waxman, 1997; Kral *et al.*, 1999) and the shape of somatic action potentials (Stebbing *et al.*, 1999). Similar changes in excitability along the axon following demyelination might be adaptive for conduction, and so changes in neuronal ion channel gene expression in response to demyelination might also be expected.

The study of changes in ion channel gene expression following demyelination is still in its infancy, few studies having been performed. Black *et al.* (1999) showed that demyelination in the *taiep* myelin mutant rat is accompanied by an up-regulation of mRNA for the SNS/PN3 $\alpha$-subunit in cerebellar Purkinje cells. Immunolabelling with a subtype-specific antibody did reveal increased channel protein in the somata and apical dendrites of these cells, but not in the axon. This group also compared the cerebella obtained at post-mortem from MS patients with those from controls who had no neurological disorders (Black *et al.*, 2000). Tissue from two out of three MS patients exhibited clear up-regulation of SNS/PN3 mRNA expression in Purkinje cells. Using subtype-specific antibody they showed that SNS/PN3 protein was similarly increased. Comparable changes in SNS/PN3 expression also occurred in animals with a relapsing/remitting form of EAE. The cause of this change in expression remains unknown.

Although these findings suggest that the extent of myelination of the axon may play a role in determining the channel expression pattern of the neuron, other factors, such as inflammatory mediators or axonal degeneration, may be involved. Felts *et al.* (1995b) compared the developmental progression from an embryonic to an adult sodium channel subunit pattern in *myelin-deficient* (*md*) and normal rats. Despite the almost complete lack of myelin in the CNS of the *md* rat, similar patterns were observed in both. This study suggests that, at least in development, the extent of myelination does not affect channel expression patterns. However, it should be noted that the study by Felts *et al.* was published prior to the cloning of the SNS/PN3 channel, and the effect of the *md* mutation on the distribution of this channel is not known. Whether demyelination *per se* is capable of altering channel expression in the adult remains to be seen.

## Summary

Production of many of the symptoms in disorders such as MS and GBS is closely related to the distribution and functional state of voltage-gated ion channels. The heterogeneous distribution of ion channels, coupled with the electrical properties of myelin, allow for rapid conduction in normal fibres. However, immediately following the loss of the myelin sheath, this channel distribution contributes to conduction block in most axons and symptoms resulting from a lack of conduction, such as blindness and paralysis, will ensue. At least some demyelinated axons regain the ability to transmit impulses as sodium channel distributions are altered. This conduction will be comparatively slow, but it will very likely provide substantial relief from symptoms. Conduction at this time is not secure, and is liable to block. There is evidence that a peptide present within the CSF and some inflammatory mediators are capable of decreasing sodium conductances. If the connection between these electrophysiological findings and symptom production can be made, it will open a promising new avenue for the treatment of symptoms. As well as leading to conduction block, demyelination of axons can also lead to the gen-

eration of ectopic impulses, which results in symptoms, such as paresthesiae. The treatment of these symptoms is complicated by the fact that reducing axonal excitability may also decrease the current available for conduction to occur in the demyelinated axons. In most demyelinating disorders repair by remyelination occurs, and rapid, secure conduction is restored to the remyelinated axons. Voltage-gated sodium channels and voltage-gated potassium channels at mature nodes of Ranvier in remyelinated axons have distributions which are similar to those at normal nodes. However, in diseases such as MS, repair by remyelination is often impermanent, resulting in regions of persistent demyelination.

## References

Akopian, A. N., Sivilotti, L. and Wood, J .N. (1996). A tetrodotoxin-resistant voltage-gated sodium channel expressed by sensory neurons. *Nature*, **379**, 257–62.

Amir, R., Michaelis, M. and Devor, M. (1999). Membrane potential oscillations in dorsal root ganglion neurons: role in normal electrogenesis and neuropathic pain. *J Neurosci.*, **19**, 8589–96.

Baba, H., Akita, H., Ishibashi, T. *et al.* (1999). Completion of myelin compaction, but not the attachment of oligodendroglial processes triggers $K^+$ channel clustering. *J Neurosci Res.*, **58**, 752–64.

Baker, M. and Bostock, H. (1992). Ectopic activity in demyelinated spinal root axons of the rat. *J Physiol (Lond.)*, **451**, 539–52.

Beckh, S., Noda, M., Lubbert, H., and Numa, S. (1989). Differential regulation of three sodium channel messenger RNAs in the rat central nervous system during development. *EMBO J.*, **8**, 3611–6.

Benatar, M., Willison, H. J. and Vincent, A. (1999). Immune-mediated peripheral neuropathies and voltage-gated sodium channels. *Muscle Nerve*, **22**, 108–10.

Black, J. A., Waxman, S. G. and Smith, M. E. (1987). Macromolecular structure of axonal membrane during acute experimental allergic encephalomyelitis in rat and guinea pig spinal cord. *J Neuropathol Exp Neurol.*, **46**, 167–84.

Black, J. A., Fjell, J., Dib-Hajj, S. *et al.* (1999). Abnormal expression of SNS/PN3 sodium channel in cerebellar Purkinje cells following loss of myelin in the taiep rat. *Neuroreport*, **10**, 913–8.

Black, J. A., Dib-Hajj, S., Baker, D. *et al.* (2000). Sensory Neuron Specific sodium channel SNS is abnormally expressed in the brains of mice with experimental allergic encephalomyelitis and humans with multiple sclerosis. *Proc Natl Acad Sci USA*, **97**, 11598–602.

Bornstein, M. B. and Crain, S.M. (1965). Functional studies of cultured brain tissues as related to 'demyelinative disorders'. *Science*, **148**, 1242–4.

Bostock, H. (1994). The pathophysiology of demyelination. In *Multiple Sclerosis: Current Status of Research and Treatment*. (eds Herndon, R. M and Seil, F. J.,) pp. 89–112, Demos Publications, Inc., London.

Bostock, H. and Sears, T. A. (1978). The internodal axon membrane: electrical excitability and continuous conduction in segmental demyelination. *J Physiol (Lond.)*, **280**, 273–301.

Bowe, C. M., Kocsis, J. D., Targ, E. F. and Waxman, S. G. (1987). Physiological effects of 4-aminopyridine on demyelinated mammalian motor and sensory fibers. *Ann Neurol.*, **22**, 264–8.

Brinkmeier, H., Wollinsky, K. H., Hulser, P. J. *et al.* (1992). The acute paralysis in Guillain-Barré Syndrome is related to a Na+ channel blocking factor in the cerebrospinal fluid. *Pflugers Arch.*, **421**, 552–7.

Brinkmeier, H., Wollinsky, K. H., Seewald, M. J. *et al.* (1993). Factors in the cerebrospinal fluid of multiple sclerosis patients interfering with voltage-dependent sodium channels. *Neurosci Lett.*, **156**, 172–5.

Brinkmeier, H., Aulkemeyer, P., Wollinsky, K. H. and Rudel, R. (2000). An endogenous pentapeptide acting as a sodium channel blocker in inflammatory autoimmune disorders of the central nervous system. *Nature Med.*, **6**, 808–11.

Brysch, W., Creutzfeldt, O. W., Luno, K. *et al.* (1991). Regional and temporal expression of sodium channel messenger RNAs in the rat brain during development. *Exp Brain Res.*, **86**, 562–7.

Catterall, W. A. (2000). From ionic currents to molecular mechanisms: The structure and function of voltage-gated sodium channels. *Neuron*, **26**, 13–25.

Celesia, G. G. and Daly, R. F. (1977). Visual electroencephalographic computer analysis (VECA). A new electrophysiologic test for the diagnosis of optic nerve lesions. *Neurology*, **27**, 637–41.

Ching, W., Zanazzi, G., Levinson, S. R. and Salzer, J. L. (1999). Sodium channel clustering at the node of Ranvier requires contact with myelinating Schwann cells. *Soc Neurosci Abstr.*, **25**, 999.

Chiu, S. Y. (1980). Asymmetry currents in the mammalian myelinated nerve. *J Physiol (Lond.)*, **309**, 499–519.

Chiu, S. Y. and Ritchie, J. M. (1980). Potassium channels in nodal and internodal axonal membrane of mammalian myelinated fibres. *Nature*, **284**, 170–1.

Chiu, S. Y. and Ritchie, J. M. (1981). Evidence for the presence of potassium channels in the paranodal region of acutely demyelinated mammalian single nerve fibres. *J Physiol (Lond.)*, **313**, 415–37.

Chiu, S. Y. and Schwarz, W. (1987). Sodium and potassium currents in acutely demyelinated internodes

of rabbit sciatic nerves. *J Physiol (Lond.)*, **391**, 631–49.

Cummins, T. R. and Waxman, S. G. (1997). Down-regulation of tetrodotoxin-resistant sodium currents and upregulation of a rapidly repriming tetrodotoxin-sensitive sodium current in small spinal sensory neurons after nerve injury. *J Neurosci.*, **17**, 3503–14.

David, G., Selzer, M. E. and Yaari, Y. (1986). Activity-dependent depression of nerve action potential by phenytoin. *Neurosci Lett.*, **66**, 163–8.

David, G., Barrett, J. N. and Barrett, E. F. (1993). Activation of internodal potassium conductance in rat myelinated axons. *J Physiol (Lond.)*, **472**, 177–202.

Deerinck, T. J., Levinson, S. R., Bennett, G. V. and Ellisman, M. H. (1997). Clustering of voltage-sensitive sodium channels on axons is independent of direct Schwann cell contact in the dystrophic mouse. *J Neurosci.*, **17**, 5080–8.

Dib-Hajj, S., Black, J. A., Felts, P. and Waxman, S. G. (1996). Down-regulation of transcripts for Na channel alpha-SNS in spinal sensory neurons following axotomy. *Proc Natl Acad Sc. USA*, **93**, 14950–4.

Dib-Hajj, S. D., Black, J. A., Cummins, T. R. *et al.* (1998). Rescue of alpha-SNS sodium channel expression in small dorsal root ganglion neurons after axotomy by nerve growth factor in vivo. *J Neurophysiol.*, **79**, 2668–76.

Dib-Hajj, S. D., Fjell, J., Cummins, T.R. *et al.* (1999). Plasticity of sodium channel expression in DRG neurons in the chronic constriction injury model of neuropathic pain. *Pain*, **83**, 591–600.

Dugandzija-Novakovic, S. and Shrager, P. (1995). Survival, development, and electrical activity of central nervous system myelinated axons exposed to tumor necrosis factor in vitro. *J Neurosci Res.*, **40**, 117–26.

Dugandzija-Novakovic, S., Koszowski, A. G., Levinson, S. R. and Shrager, P. (1995). Clustering of Na+ channels and node of Ranvier formation in remyelinating axons. *J Neurosci.*, **15**, 492–503.

Dupree, J. L., Girault, J.-A. and Popko, B. (1999). Axoglial interactions regulate the localization of axonal paranodal proteins. *J Cell Biol.*, **147**, 1145–51.

Felts, P. A. and Smith, K. J. (1992). Conduction properties of central nerve fibers remyelinated by Schwann cells. *Brain Res.*, **574**, 178–92.

Felts, P. A., Kapoor, R. and Smith, K. J. (1995a). A mechanism for ectopic firing in central demyelinated axons. *Brain*, **118**, 1225–31.

Felts, P. A., Black, J. A. and Waxman, S. G. (1995b). Expression of sodium channel alpha- and beta-subunits in the nervous system of the myelin-deficient rat. *J Neurocytol.*, **24**, 654–66.

Felts, P. A., Baker, T. A. and Smith, K. J. (1997a). Conduction in segmentally demyelinated mammalian central axons. *J Neurosci.*, **17**, 7267–77.

Felts, P. A., Yokoyama, S., Dib-Hajj, S. *et al.* (1997b). Sodium channel alpha-subunit mRNAs I, II, III, NaG, Na6 and hNE (PN1): Different expression patterns in developing rat nervous system. *Mol Brain Res.*, **45**, 71–82.

Foster, R. E., Whalen, C. C. and Waxman, S. G. (1980). Reorganization of the axon membrane in demyelinated peripheral nerve fibers: morphological evidence. *Science*, **210**, 661–3.

Frankenhaeuser, B. A. (1963). A quantitative description of potassium currents in myelinated nerve fibers of Xenopus laevis. *J Physiol (Lond.)*, **169**, 424–30.

Hamm, S., Rudel, R. and Brinkmeier, H. (1996). Excitatory sodium currents of NH15-CA2 neuroblastoma × glioma hybrid cells are differently affected by interleukin-2 and interleukin-1beta. *Pflugers Arch – Europ J Physiol.*, **433**, 160–5.

Hirota, N., Kaji, R., Bostock, H. *et al.* (1997). The physiological effect of anti-GM1 antibodies on saltatory conduction and transmembrane currents in single motor axons. *Brain*, **120**, 2159–69.

Honmou, O., Utzschneider, D. A., Rizzo, M. A. *et al.* (1994). Delayed depolarization and slow sodium currents in cutaneous afferents. *J Neurophysiol.*, **71**, 1627–37.

Hughes, R. A. C., Hadden, R. D. M., Gregson, N. A. and Smith, K. J. (1999). Pathogenesis of Guillain-Barré syndrome. *J Neuroimmunol.*, **100**, 74–97.

Kaplan, M. R., Meyer-Franke, A., Lambert, S. *et al.* (1997). Induction of sodium channel clustering by oligodendrocytes. *Nature*, **386**, 724–8.

Kapoor, R., Smith, K. J., Felts, P. A. and Davies, M. (1993). Internodal potassium currents can generate ectopic impulses in mammalian myelinated axons. *Brain Res.*, **611**, 165–9.

Kapoor, R., Li, Y. G. and Smith, K. J. (1997). Slow sodium-dependent potential oscillations contribute to ectopic firing in mammalian demyelinated axons. *Brain*, **120**, 647–52.

Kapoor, R., Davies, M. and Smith, K. J. (1999). Temporary axonal conduction block and axonal loss in inflammatory neurological disease: a potential role for nitric oxide? *Ann NY Acad Sci.*, **893**, 304–8.

Kocsis, J. D. and Waxman, S. G. (1980). Absence of potassium conductance in central myelinated axons. *Nature*, **287**, 348–9.

Koller, H., Buchholz, J. and Siebler, M. (1996). Cerebrospinal fluid from multiple sclerosis patients inactivates neuronal $Na^+$ current. *Brain*, **119**, 457–63.

Kral, M. G., Xiong, Z. and Study, R. E. (1999). Alteration of $Na^+$ currents in dorsal root ganglion neurons from rats with a painful neuropathy. *Pain*, **81**, 15–24.

McDonald, W. I. and Sears, T. A. (1970). The effects of experimental demyelination on conduction in the central nervous system. *Brain*, **93**, 583–98.

Mi, H., Deerinck, T. J., Ellisman, M. H. and Schwarz, T. L. (1995). Differential distribution of closely related potassium channels in rat Schwann cells. *J Neurosci.*, **15**, 3761–74.

Moll, C., Mourre, C., Lazdunski, M. and Ulrich, J.

(1991). Increase of sodium channels in demyelinated lesions of multiple sclerosis. *Brain Res.*, **556**, 311–6.

Neuberg, H. -R., Sancho, S. and Suter, U. (1999). Altered molecular architecture of peripheral nerves in mice lacking the Peripheral Myelin Protein 22 or Connexin 32. *J Neurosci Res.*, **58**, 612–23.

Nordin, M., Nystrom, B., Wallin, U. and Hagbarth, K. E. (1984). Ectopic sensory discharges and paresthesiae in patients with disorders of peripheral nerves, dorsal roots and dorsal columns. *Pain*, **20**, 231–45.

Novakovic, S. D., Deerinck, T. J., Levinson, S. R. *et al.* (1996). Clusters of axonal $Na^+$ channels adjacent to remyelinating Schwann cells. *J Neurocytol.*, **25**, 403–12.

Novakovic, S. D., Levinson, S. R., Schachner, M. and Shrager, P. (1998). Disruption and reorganization of sodium channels in experimental allergic neuritis. *Muscle Nerve*, **21**, 1019–32.

Okuse, K., Chaplan, S. R., McMahon, S. B. *et al.* (1997). Regulation of expression of the sensory neuron-specific sodium channel SNS in inflammatory and neuropathic pain. *Mol Cell Neurosci.*, **10**, 196–207.

Osterman, P. O. and Westerberg, C. E. (1975). Paroxysmal attacks in multiple sclerosis. *Brain*, **98**, 189–202.

Panitch, H. and Ciccone, C. (1981). Induction of recurrent experimental allergic encephalomyelitis with myelin basic protein. *Ann Neurol.*, **9**, 433–8.

Pender, M. P. (1987). Demyelination and neurological signs in experimental allergic encephalomyelitis. *J Neuroimmunol.*, **15**, 11–24.

Plata-Salaman, C. R. and ffrench-Mullen, J. M. (1992). Interleukin-1 beta depresses calcium currents in CA1 hippocampal neurons at pathophysiological concentrations. *Brain Res Bull.*, **29**, 221–3.

Plata-Salaman, C. R. and ffrench-Mullen, J. M. (1993). Interleukin-2 modulates calcium currents in dissociated hippocampal CA1 neurons. *Neuroreport*, **4**, 579–81.

Pouly, S. and Antel, J. P. (1999). Multiple sclerosis and central nervous system demyelination. *J Autoimmun.*, **13**, 297–306.

Rae-Grant, A. D., Eckert, N. J., Bartz, S. and Reed, J. F. (1999). Sensory symptoms of multiple sclerosis: A hidden reservoir of morbidity. *Multiple Sclerosis*, **5**, 179–83.

Rasband, M. N. and Shrager P. (2000). Ion channel sequestration in central nervous system axons. *J Physiol (Lond.)*, **525**, 63–73.

Rasband, M. N., Trimmer, J. S., Schwarz, T. L. *et al.* (1998). Potassium channel distribution, clustering, and function in remyelinating rat axons. *J Neurosci.*, **18**, 36–47.

Rasband, M. N., Trimmer, J. S., Peles, E. *et al.* (1999a). $K^+$ channel distribution and clustering in developing and hypomyelinated axons of the optic nerve. *J Neurocytol.*, **28**, 319–31.

Rasband, M. N., Peles, E., Trimmer, J. S. *et al.* (1999b). Dependence of nodal sodium channel clustering on paranodal axoglial contact in the developing CNS. *J Neurosci.*, **19**, 7516–28.

Rasminsky, M. (1978) Ectopic generation of impulses and cross-talk in the spinal nerve roots of 'dystrophic' mice. *Ann Neurol.*, **3**, 351–7.

Redford, E. J., Kapoor, R. and Smith, K. J. (1997). Nitric oxide donors reversibly block axonal conduction: demyelinated axons are especially susceptible. *Brain*, **120**, 2149–57.

Reid, G., Scholz, A., Bostock, H. and Vogel, W. (1999). Human axons contain at least five types of voltage-dependent potassium channel. *J Physiol (Lond.)*, **518**, 681–6.

Renganathan, M., Cummins, T. R., Hormuzdiar, W. N. *et al.* (2000). Nitric oxide is an autocrine regulator of $Na^+$ currents in axotomized C- type DRG neurons. *J Neurophysiol.*, **83**, 2431–42.

Rose, A. S. (1963). Demyelinating disease: clinical features. In *Mechanisms of Demyelination* (eds Rose, A. S. and Pearson, C. M.,) pp. 199–217, McGraw-Hill, New York.

Rosenbluth, J. and Blakemore, W. F. (1984). Structural specializations in cat of chronically demyelinated spinal cord axons as seen in freeze-fracture replicas. *Neurosci Lett.*, **48**, 171–7.

Safronov, B. V., Kampe, K. and Vogel, W. (1993). Single voltage-dependent potassium channels in rat peripheral nerve membrane. *J Physiol (Lond.)*, **460**, 675–91.

Sakurai, M. and Kanazawa, I. (1999). Positive symptoms in multiple sclerosis: Their treatment with sodium channel blockers, lidocaine and mexiletine. *J Neurol Sci.*, **162**, 162–8.

Sakurai, M., Mannen, T., Kanazawa, I. and Tanabe, H. (1992). Lidocaine unmasks silent demyelinative lesions in multiple sclerosis. *Neurology*, **42**, 2088–93.

Sangameswaran, L., Delgado, S. G., Fish, L .M. *et al.* (1996). Structure and function of a novel voltage-gated, tetrodotoxin-resistant sodium channel specfic to sensory neurons. *J Biol Chem.*, **271**, 5953–6.

Sawada, M., Hara, N. and Maeno, T. (1991). Analysis of a decreased $Na^+$ conductance by tumor necrosis factor in identified neurons of Aplysia kurodai. *J Neurosci Res.*, **28**, 466–73.

Sawada, M., Hara, N. and Ichinose, M. (1992). Interleukin-2 inhibits the GABA-induced $Cl^-$ current in identified Aplysia neurons. *J Neurosci Res.*, **33**, 461–5.

Sawada, M., Ichinose, M. and Hara, N. (1995). Nitric oxide induces an increased $Na^+$ conductance in identified neurons of Aplysia. *Brain Res.*, **670**, 248–56.

Scholz, A., Reid, G., Vogel, W. and Bostock, H. (1993). Ion channels in human axons. *J Neurophysiol.*, **70**, 1274–9.

Schwarz, J. R. and Grigat, G. (1989). Phenytoin and carbamazepine: potential- and frequency-dependent block of Na currents in mammalian myelinated nerve fibers. *Epilepsia*, **30**, 286–94.

Schwarz, J. R., Corrette, B. J., Mann, K. and Wietholter, H. (1991). Changes of ionic channel distribution in myelinated nerve fibres from rats with experimental allergic neuritis. *Neurosci Lett.*, **122**, 205–9.

Schwarz, J. R., Reid, G. and Bostock, H. (1995). Action potentials and membrane currents in the human node of Ranvier. *Pflugers Arch.*, **430**, 283–92.

Seil, F. J., Leiman, A. L. and Kelly, J. M. (1976). Neuroelectric blocking factors in multiple sclerosis and normal human sera. *Arch Neurol.*, **33**, 418–22.

Sherratt, R. M., Bostock, H. and Sears, T. A. (1980). Effects of 4-aminopyridine on normal and demyelinated mammalian nerve fibres. *Nature*, **283**, 570–2.

Shrager, P. (1989). Sodium channels in single demyelinated mammalian axons. *Brain Res.*, **483**, 149–154.

Shrager, P., Custer, A. W., Kazarinova, K. *et al.* (1998). Nerve conduction block by nitric oxide that is mediated by the axonal environment. *J Neurophysiol.*, **79**, 529–36.

Shrager, P. and Rubinstein, C. T. (1990). Optical measurement of conduction in single demyelinated axons. *J Gen Physiol.*, **95**, 867–90.

Smith, K. J. (1994). Conduction properties of central demyelinated and remyelinated axons, and their relation to symptom production in demyelinating disorders. *Eye*, **8**, 224–37.

Smith, K. J. and Hall, S. M. (1980). Nerve conduction during peripheral demyelination and remyelination. *J Neurol Sci.*, **48**, 201–19.

Smith, K. J. and Schauf, C. L. (1981). Gallamine triethiodide (flaxedil): tetraethylammonium- and pancuronium-like effects in myelinated nerve fibers. *Science*, **212**, 1170–2.

Smith, K. J. and McDonald, W. I. (1982). Spontaneous and evoked electrical discharges from a central demyelinating lesion. *J Neurol Sci.*, **55**, 39–47.

Smith, K. J. and McDonald, W. I. (1999). The pathophysiology of multiple sclerosis: the mechanisms underlying the production of symptoms and the natural history of the disease. *Phil Trans R Soc Lond B*, **354**, 1649–73.

Smith, K. J., Blakemore, W. F. and McDonald, W. I. (1979). Central remyelination restores secure conduction. *Nature*, **280**, 395–6.

Smith, K. J., Bostock, H. and Hall, S. M. (1982). Saltatory conduction precedes remyelination in axons demyelinated with lysophosphatidyl choline. *J Neurol Sci.*, **54**, 13–31.

Smith, K. J., Felts, P. A. and Kapoor, R. (1997). Axonal hyperexcitability: mechanisms and role in symptom production in demyelinating diseases. *Neuroscientist*, **3**, 237–46.

Smith, K. J., Felts, P. A. and John, G. R. (2000). Effects of 4-aminopyridine on demyelinated axons, synapses and muscle tension. *Brain*, **123**, 171–84.

Stebbing, M. J., Eschenfelder, S., Habler, H. J. *et al.* (1999). Changes in the action potential in sensory neurones after peripheral axotomy in vivo. *Neuroreport*, **10**, 201–6.

Stefoski, D., Davis, F. A., Faut, M. and Schauf, C. L. (1987). 4-Aminopyridine improves clinical signs in multiple sclerosis. *Ann Neurol.*, **21**, 71–7.

Strichartz, G., Hahin, R. and Cahalan, M. (1982). Pharmacological models for sodium channels producing abnormal impulse activity. In *Abnormal Nerves and Muscles as Impulse Generators.* (eds Culp, W. J. and Ochoa, J.) pp. 98–129, Oxford University Press, Oxford.

Takigawa, T., Yasuda, H., Kikkawa, R. *et al.* (1995). Antibodies against GM1 ganglioside affect $K^+$ and $Na^+$ currents in isolated rat myelinated nerve fibers. *Ann Neurol.*, **37**, 436–442.

Takigawa, T., Yasuda, H., Terada, M. *et al.* (2000). The sera from GM1 ganglioside antibody positive patients with Guillain-Barré syndrome or chronic inflammatory demyelinating polyneuropathy blocks $Na^+$ currents in rat single myelinated nerve fibres. *Internal Med.*, **39**, 123–7.

Vabnick, I., Novakovic, S. D., Levinson, S. R. *et al.* (1996). The clustering of axonal sodium channels during development of the peripheral nervous system. *J Neurosci.*, **16**, 4914–22.

Vabnick, I., Messing, A., Chiu, S. Y. *et al.* (1997). Sodium channel distribution in axons of hypomyelinated and MAG null mutant mice. *J Neurosci Res.*, **50**, 321–36.

Vabnick, I., Trimmer, J. S., Schwarz, T. L. *et al.* (1999). Dynamic potassium channel distributions during axonal development prevent aberrant firing patterns. *J Neurosci.*, **19**, 747–58.

Van der Meche, F. G. and Van Doorn, P. A. (1999). Chronic inflammatory demyelinating polyneuropathy (CIDP). *Electroencephal Clin Neurophys Suppl.*, **50**, 493–8.

Wang, H., Kunkel, D. D., Martin, T. M. *et al.* (1993). Heteromultimeric $K^+$ channels in terminal and juxtaparanodal regions of neurons. *Nature*, **365**, 75–9.

Wang, H., Kunkel, D. D., Schwartzkroin, P. A. and Tempel, B. L. (1994). Localization of Kv1.1 and Kv1.2, two K channel proteins, to synaptic terminals, somata, and dendrites in the mouse brain. *J Neurosci.*, **14**, 4588–99.

Wang, H., Allen, M. L., Grigg, J. J. *et al.* (1995). Hypomyelination alters $K^+$ channel expression in mouse mutants shiverer and Trembler. *Neuron*, **15**, 1337–47.

Waxman, S. G. and Ritchie, J. M. (1993). Molecular dissection of the myelinated axon. *Ann Neurol.*, **33**, 121–36.

Waxman, S. G., Black, J. A., Kocsis, J. D. and Ritchie, J. M. (1989). Low density of sodium channels supports action potential conduction in axons of neonatal rat optic nerve. *Proc Natl Acad Sci USA*, **86**, 1406–10.

Waxman, S. G., Kocsis, J. D. and Black, J. A. (1994). Type III sodium channel mRNA is expressed in embryonic but not adult spinal sensory neurons, and is reexpressed following axotomy. *J Neurophysiol.*, **72**, 466–70.

Weber, F., Brinkmeier, H., Aulkemeyer, P. *et al.* (1999). A small sodium channel blocking factor in the cerebrospinal fluid is preferentially found in Guillain-Barré syndrome: a combined cell physiological and HPLC study. *J Neurol.*, **246**, 955–60.

Wisniewski, H. M., Oppenheimer, D. and McDonald, W. I. (1976). Relation between myelination and function in MS and EAE. *J Neuropathol Exp Neurol.*, **35**, 327.

Wurz, A., Brinkmeier, H., Wollinsky, K. H. *et al.* (1995). Cerebrospinal fluid and serum from patients with inflammatory polyradiculoneuropathy have opposite effects on sodium channels. *Muscle Nerve*, **18**, 772–81.

Zhou, L., Zhang, C. -L., Messing, A. and Shing, Y. C. (1998). Temperature-sensitive neuromuscular transmission in Kv1.1 null mice: Role of potassium channels under the myelin sheath in young nerves. *J Neurosci.*, **18**, 7200–15.

# Neuromuscular channel gene disorders (genetic)

# Chloride and sodium channel myotonias

## Karin Jurkat-Rott, Frank Lehmann-Horn and Reinhardt Rüdel

## Introduction

The first diseases for which an ion channel defect was functionally identified as pathogenetically decisive were skeletal muscle disorders associated with myotonia, i.e. muscle stiffness (Bryant, 1969; Lehmann-Horn *et al.*, 1987a, b). Identification of the causative genes (Fontaine *et al.*, 1990; Rojas *et al.*, 1991; Koch *et al.*, 1992) led to the coining of the term channelopathies for these hereditary ion channel diseases (Lehmann-Horn *et al.*, 1993).

Myotonic disorders can be divided into two major subgroups according to differences in clinical features and pathogenetic mechanisms: the dystrophic myotonias (myotonic dystrophies DM-1 and DM-2) and the here-described non-dystrophic myotonias or ion channel myotonias (chloride and sodium channel diseases). There are two forms of chloride channel myotonia: autosomal dominant Thomsen and autosomal recessive Becker. Both types are caused by mutations in the *CLCN-1* gene encoding the skeletal muscle chloride channel ClC-1. Sodium channel myotonias are caused by mutations in the *SCN4A* gene encoding the adult skeletal muscle sodium channel $\alpha$-subunit hSkm. These diseases are called hyperkalaemic periodic paralysis, paramyotonia congenita and potassium-aggravated myotonia. Hyperkalaemic periodic paralysis is dealt with in more detail in Chapter 10 on dyskalaemic periodic paralyses, not all of which are associated with myotonia. For more information on the clinical features of the diseases, detailed overviews on the subject are available (Rüdel *et al.*, 1994; Lehmann-Horn *et al.*, 1994; Lehmann-Horn and Jurkat-Rott, 1999).

## Clinical myotonia

The word 'myotonia' was coined by Strümpell (1891) as a composition of the Greek words for muscle and tension. Myotonia is characterized by an uncontrolled temporary muscle stiffness caused by a transient hyperexcitability of the muscle fibre membrane. In myotonia congenita, both Thomsen and Becker, the myotonia decreases with continued muscle activity, a phenomenon termed warm-up. In contrast, myotonia that increases with muscle activity is termed paradoxical myotonia or paramyotonia. Clinical examination reveals percussion myotonia, i.e. muscles react to a blow with the percussion hammer by becoming indented for a few seconds. Erb, who first described percussion myotonia, also observed that myotonic muscles have a lowered electrical threshold and an increased tendency to react to direct current with a prolonged contraction. The combination of these mechanical and electrical abnormalities is called the myotonic reaction. Its presence was used to diagnose a myotonic disease in the early days of electrophysiology, but has now been replaced by the electromyogram (EMG), which shows that the muscles exhibit myotonic runs, i.e. repetitive activity. In very mild cases, myotonic stiffness might not be clinically present, yet the EMG might reveal myotonic runs, so called latent myotonia.

## Chloride channel myotonia congenita

Myotonia congenita comprises two forms: Thomsen's disease, or dominant myotonia congenita,

(Thomsen, 1876), and Becker's disease or recessive myotonia congenita (Becker, 1977). Thomsen's disease was the first myotonic disease to be described, but Becker's disease is more frequent. Both are non-progressive and non-dystrophic muscle diseases. They have been shown to be due to allelic mutations in the gene coding for the chloride channel of the skeletal muscle fibre membrane located on chromosome 7q35. Hence, they were classified by an International Consortium as 'muscle chloride channel diseases' (Lehmann-Horn et al., 1993).

In Thomsen's disease, the myotonia is usually recognized in early childhood. It is generalized with the legs being most affected causing the children to fall frequently. Upper limb and cranial musculature can be severely affected; even chewing is sometimes impaired. The myotonic stiffness is most pronounced when a forceful movement is abruptly initiated after the patient has rested for a few minutes. For instance, after making a hard fist, the patient may not be able to extend the fingers fully for several seconds. The myotonia decreases or vanishes completely when the same movement is repeated several times ('warm-up phenomenon'), but recurs after a few minutes of rest. The patient may experience much difficulty while getting up from a chair or stepping into a bus in a hurry. Occasionally, a sudden noise may cause instantaneous generalized stiffness. The patient may then fall to the ground and remain rigid and helpless for some seconds or even minutes. Some patients have hypertrophied muscles and an athletic appearance. Their muscle strength is normal or even greater than normal and they can be quite successful in athletic disciplines in which strength is more important than speed. Lid lag is usually present, and in some patients myotonia of the lid muscles causes blepharospasm after forceful eye closure. The tendon reflexes are normal. In some families, the degree of myotonia fluctuates at a very slow and irregular periodicity of up to several months; the afflicted members may sometimes suffer from muscle pain due to muscle spasms.

In Becker-type myotonia, the clinical picture is similar, however, more severe than that of the dominant form. In some patients, the myotonia does not manifest until the age of 10 years or even later, although, in a few it is present by the age of 2–3 years. The severity of the myotonia may slowly increase for a number of years, but usually not after the age of 25–30 years. Patients with Becker myotonia are quite handicapped in daily life. The disability arises mainly from myotonic stiffness affecting the lower limbs. In severely affected young patients the contracted calf muscles may lead to toe-walking and lumbal lordosis. Muscular contractures can also be seen in other joints, e.g. the elbow. Even more disabling in Becker patients is a peculiar transient weakness best demonstrated when the patient makes a tight fist after a period of rest: the force exerted by the finger flexors vanishes almost completely within a few seconds. With repeated muscle contractions, the force returns within 20–60 s. This transient weakness is often generalized and troublesome, typically occurring when a patient attempts to rise from a recumbent position after rest or sleep (Deymeer et al., 1998). The leg and gluteal muscles are often markedly hypertrophied. In contrast, the neck, shoulder and arm muscles appear poorly developed resulting in a characteristic disproportionate figure (Becker, 1977). Patients with severe recessive myotonia congenita are limited in their choice of occupation and they are unsuited for military service. They may develop continuous muscle weakness in the forearm and lower extremity muscles. In a few families, the heterozygotes can be identified by showing repetitive action potentials on EMG. Typical for Thomsen and Becker myotonias are short bursts of action potentials with amplitude and frequency modulation, so called dive-bombers, on the acoustic EMG.

The intensive search for mutations that followed the discovery of the CLCN1 gene showed that the dominant form is very rare, as less than 10 different families were identified at the molecular level. The recessive form is much more frequent, and the estimation by Becker (1977) of a frequency between 1:2300 and 1:5000 might still hold. Males seem to be affected more often than females with a ratio of 3:1 when only the typical clinical features are taken into account. However, family studies disclosed that women are affected at the same frequency though to a much lesser degree (Becker, 1977; Deymeer et al., 1999).

## Molecular pathology

The muscle stiffness is caused by the fact that, following voluntary excitation, the membranes of individual muscle fibres may continue to generate runs of action potentials for several seconds that prevent immediate muscle relaxation. Experiments with muscles of an animal model, the myotonic goat, showed that the over-excitability is caused by a permanent reduction of the resting chloride conductance of the muscle fibre membranes (Bryant, 1969). A normal chloride conductance is necessary for a fast repolarization of the transverse tubular membranes, otherwise these tend to stay depolarized due to potassium accumulated in the tubules during tetanic muscle excitation. Both human dominant and recessive myotonia congenita are caused by this common mechanism of pathogenesis (Lipicky 1979; Rüdel *et al.*, 1988; Franke *et al.*, 1991).

The starting point for an understanding of myotonia congenita on the molecular level was the cloning of the chloride channel, *Clc-0*, from the electric organ of the fish *Torpedo marmorata* (Jentsch *et al.*, 1990). Rat skeletal muscle chloride channel cDNA, was then cloned by homology screening (Steinmeyer *et al.*, 1991). This was followed by the demonstration of linkage of both dominant and recessive myotonia congenita to chromosome 7q35 (Koch *et al.*, 1992) and to *CLCN1*, the gene encoding the chloride channel. *CLCN1* spans at least 40 kb and contains 23 exons whose boundaries have been defined (Lorenz *et al.*, 1994).

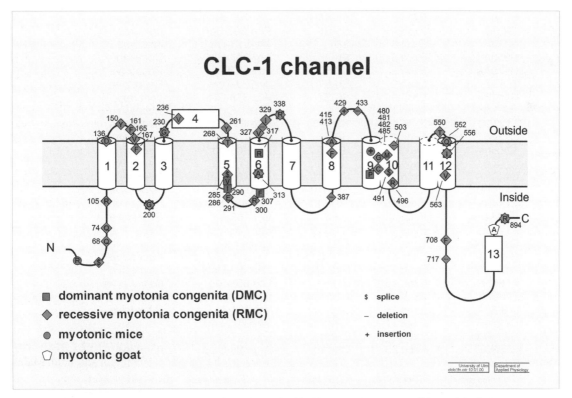

**Figure 9.1** Membrane topology model of the skeletal muscle chloride channel monomer, ClC-1, originally based on hydropathy analysis (Jentsch *et al.*, 1990). The functional channel is a homodimer. The different symbols used for the known mutations leading to dominant Thomsen-type myotonia and recessive Becker-type myotonia are explained on the left-hand bottom. Conventional 1-letter abbreviations were used for replaced amino acids (modified after Pusch and Jentsch, 1994).

**Table 9.1** *CLCN1* mutations causing myotonia congenita. The gene encodes the major chloride channel of skeletal muscle.

| Genotype | Segment | Region | Mutation | Trait |
|---|---|---|---|---|
| +3/A→T | Intron 1 | N-term | splice site | Recessive |
| C202T | Exon 2 | N-term | Gln-68-Stop | Recessive |
| C220T | Exon 2 | N-term | Gln-74-Stop | Recessive |
| C313T | Exon 3 | N-term | Arg-105-Cys | Recessive |
| A407G | Exon 3 | S1 | Asp-136-Gly | Recessive |
| A449G | Exon 4 | S1-S2 | Tyr-150-Cys | Recessive |
| T481G | Exon 4 | S1-S2 | Phe-161-Val | Recessive |
| T494G | Exon 4 | S2 | Val-165-Gly | Recessive |
| C501G | Exon 4 | S2 | Phe-167-Leu | Recessive |
| G598A | Exon 5 | S3-S4 | Gly-200-Arg | Dominant |
| G689A | Exon 5 | S3-S4 | Gly-230-Glu | dom./rec. |
| G706C | Exon 6 | S4 | Val-236-Leu | Recessive |
| A782G | Exon 7 | S4-S5 | Tyr-261-Cys | Recessive |
| G854A* | Exon 8 | S5 | splice site | Recessive |
| G854A* | Exon 8 | S5 | Gly-285-Glu | Recessive |
| T857C | Exon 8 | S5 | Val-286-Ala | Dominant |
| C870G | Exon 8 | S5-S6 | Ile-290-Met | Dominant |
| G871A | Exon 8 | S5-S6 | Glu-291-Lys | Recessive |
| C898T | Exon 8 | S5-S6 | Arg-300-Stop | Recessive |
| T920C | Exon 8 | S5-S6 | Phe-307-Ser | dom./rec. |
| G937A | Exon 8 | S6 | Ala-313-Thr | dom./rec. |
| G950A | Exon 8 | S6 | Arg-317-Gln | Dominant |
| G979A | Exon 8 | S6-S7 | splice site | Recessive |
| T986C | Exon 9 | S6-S7 | Ile-329-Thr | Recessive |
| G1013A | Exon 9 | S6-S7 | Arg-338-Gln | dom./rec. |
| 1095-96Δ | Exon 10 | S7 | fs 387-Stop | Recessive |
| T1238G | Exon 11 | S8 | Phe-413-Cys | Recessive |
| C1244T | Exon 11 | S8 | Ala-415-Val | Recessive |
| 1262insC | Exon 12 | S8-S9 | fs 429-Stop | Recessive |
| 1278-81Δ | Exon 12 | S8-S9 | fs 433-Stop | Recessive |
| C1439T | Exon 13 | S9-S10 | Pro-480-Leu | Dominant |
| 1437-50Δ | Exon 13 | S9-S10 | fs 503-Stop | Recessive |
| C1443A | Exon 13 | S9-S10 | Cys-481-Stop | Recessive |
| G1444A | Exon 13 | S9-S10 | Gly-482-Arg | Recessive |
| A1453G | Exon 13 | S9-S10 | Met-485-Val | Recessive |
| G1471A | Exon 13 | S10 | splice site | Recessive |
| G1488T | Exon 14 | S10-S11 | Arg-496-Ser | Recessive |
| C1649T | Exon 15 | S11-S12 | Thr-550-Met | Recessive |
| A1655G | Exon 15 | S12 | Gln-552-Arg | dom. Levior |
| T1667A | Exon 15 | S12 | Ile-556-Asn | dom./rec. |
| G1687A | Exon 15 | S12 | Val-563-Ile | Recessive |
| C2124G | Exon 17 | C-term | Phe-708-Leu | Recessive |
| G2149Δ | Exon 17 | C-term | Glu-717-Stop | Recessive |
| C2680T | Exon 23 | C-term | Arg-894-Stop | dom./rec. |

fs = frame shift due to an insertion (ins) and/or deletion (Δ); sp = splice site mutation; * both events cause altered amino acid sequence usually followed by premature termination, sometimes indicated by the given stop codon number.

## Functional expression

Functional expression of *CLCN1* has been accomplished in *Xenopus* oocytes (Steinmeyer *et al.*, 1991; Pusch *et al.*, 1994; Pusch and Jentsch, 1994; Jentsch *et al.*, 1995), human embryonic kidney (HEK-293) cells (Fahlke *et al.*, 1995) and the insect cell line Sf-9 (Rychkov *et al.*, 1997). The resulting currents were similar to those found in native muscle fibres (Fahlke and Rüdel, 1995). Electrophysiological studies of wildtype and mutant channel proteins have provided first insight into the pharmacology and structure-function relationships of ClC-1, and led to the identification of regions involved in gating and permeation (Steinmeyer *et al.*, 1991; Fahlke *et al.*, 1995, 1996, 1997a; Pusch *et al.*, 1995; Kürz *et al.*, 1997). Inferences from experiments with the chloride channel ClC-0 (Ludewig *et al.*, 1996; Middleton *et al.*, 1996) and studies of ClC-1 constructs (Fahlke *et al.*, 1997b) strongly suggest that functional channels are formed as homodimers.

More than 40 mutations have been found in the channel gene, and they cause either dominant or recessive myotonia congenita (Figure 9.1, Table 9.1) by producing change or loss of function of the gene product. Experiments with myotonia-generating drugs showed that blockade of 50 % of the physiological chloride current is not sufficient to produce myotonic activity. This could be the reason why heterozygous carriers of recessive mutations that completely destroy the channel function and therefore have 50% chloride current do not present with clinical myotonia. Dominant inheritance is explained by the dominant negative effect of a mutant monomer on ClC-1 heteromultimers, i.e. capability to produce loss of function when coassembling with wildtype. The most common feature of the thereby resulting chloride currents is a shift of the activation curve towards more positive membrane potentials reducing the total chloride conductance at the resting potential (Figure 9.2). Surprisingly, the degree of the shift and clinical severity do not always correlate, e.g. Gln-552-Arg causes an unusually large potential shift but a very mild clinical phenotype, so called myotonia levior (Pusch *et al.*, 1995; Lehmann-Horn *et al.*, 1995).

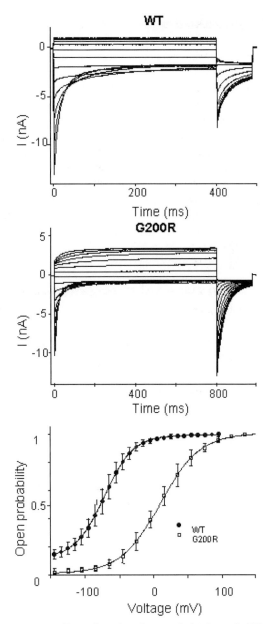

**Figure 9.2** Recordings from human skeletal muscle ClC-1 channels expressed in a mammalian cell line. Compared are currents from normal (WT) and dominant myotonia-causing mutant (Gly-200-Arg) channels. Upper and middle panels: macroscopic currents, recorded in the whole-cell mode, were activated from a holding potential of 0 mV by voltage steps to potentials of −145 to +95 mV, and deactivated after 400 ms by polarization to −105 mV. Lower panel: voltage dependence of the relative open probability that is much reduced for the mutant channel in the physiological potential range. All mutations that cause such a voltage shift have dominant effects (modified after Wagner *et al.*, 1998).

## Therapeutic drugs

Many myotonia congenita patients can manage their disease without medication. Should treatment be necessary, myotonic stiffness responds well to drugs that reduce the increased excitability of the cell membrane by interfering with the sodium channels, i.e. local anaesthetics, antifibrillar and antiarrhythmic substances, and related agents. These treatments suppress myotonic runs by decreasing the number of available sodium channels and have no known effect on chloride channels. Of the many drugs tested that can be administered orally, mexiletine is the drug of choice (Rüdel et al., 1994).

# Sodium channel myotonias and paralyses

## Hyperkalaemic periodic paralysis (HyperPP)

This disease is transmitted as an autosomal dominant trait. Patients experience generalized attacks of flaccid weakness that usually begin in the first decade of life. Symptoms commonly start in the morning before breakfast, last from minutes to hours, and then spontaneously disappear. Between attacks affected individuals have normal strength. Rest often provokes the attack, and prior strenuous work usually aggravates it. Potassium loading, cold environment, emotional stress, glucocorticoids, and pregnancy provoke or worsen the attacks. After strenuous exercise, weakness can follow within a few minutes of rest. Sustained mild exercise after a period of strenuous exercise may postpone or prevent the weakness in the exercising muscle groups while the resting muscles become weak. The generalized weakness is usually accompanied by significant increase in the serum potassium concentration.

## Paramyotonia congenita (PC)

The hallmarks of this condition as first described by Eulenburg (1886) and later confirmed in many families by Becker (Becker, 1970) are: (i) para-doxical myotonia; (ii) severe worsening of the myotonia by cold; and (iii) weakness after longer exposure to cold in most cases. In some families, patients have spontaneous attacks of weakness similar to those occurring in HyperPP. The condition is transmitted as a dominant trait with complete penetrance. Paramyotonic symptoms are present at birth and remain often unchanged for the entire lifetime. In the cold, the face may appear mask-like, and for a few seconds the eyes cannot be opened normally. Working in the cold makes the fingers so stiff that the patient becomes unable to move them within minutes of exposure. After a short time, the stiffness gives way to weakness. Upon rewarming, hands may not regain strength for several hours. Under warm conditions many patients have no complaints. Muscle pain or muscle atrophy are not features of this disease.

The diagnosis of PC is usually made clinically and supported by a positive family history. Serum CK may be elevated up to 10 times above normal. EMG shows generalized spontaneous activity in the form of fibrillation-like potentials and myotonic discharges which are usually present at room temperature but, if not, can be provoked by cooling of hand and forearm in a water bath at about 15°C for 15–30 minutes. Cooling induces muscle stiffness and later weakness corresponding to a reduction of the amplitude of the evoked compound muscle action potential (Subramony et al., 1983; Gutmann et al., 1986; Jackson et al., 1994). A more precise measurement of myotonia and weakness can be obtained by determining the isometric force and relaxation time of the long finger flexor muscles before and after cooling (Ricker et al., 1986). Relaxation time can be prolonged from 0.5 s up to 50 s and contraction force reduced by more than 50%. A muscle biopsy is not necessary to diagnose PC. The diagnosis may be confirmed genetically by identifying a mutation within the SCN4A gene.

## Potassium-aggravated myotonia (PAM)

This disease was newly defined by updating long-known clinical knowledge with recent genetic and molecular biological information (Ptacek et al.,

1992b, 1994; Lerche *et al.*, 1993, Heine *et al.*, 1993). Becker (1977) had investigated more than 100 families with non-dystrophic dominant myotonia and proposed several subtypes of what he thought was myotonia congenita. Molecular biology revealed that many of these conditions were in fact caused by mutations in the gene encoding a muscle sodium channel subunit. A few forms could be classified as special types of paramyotonia, because they showed cold- and exercise-induced stiffness, albeit no cold-induced weakness. Other conditions, however, were too inconsistent to fit the definition of PC.

PAM can be distinguished by the fact that patients never experience muscle weakness and are not substantially sensitive to cold. Four clinical phenotypes can be delineated based upon the severity of the myotonia and the response to therapy. One group of affected persons experiences muscle stiffness that tends to fluctuate from day to day, hence the name 'myotonia fluctuans' (Ricker *et al.*, 1990, 1994, Lennox *et al.*, 1992). Their muscle stiffness is provoked by exercise, and often it occurs with some delay during rest after heavy exercise. The stiffness may then last for 0.5 to 2 h. On many days or even for weeks, afflicted persons experience no symptoms at all. A second group is more severely affected with generalized moderate myotonia which may show a kind of delayed warm-up phenomenon. A third group has the most severe form of PAM and of myotonia in general called 'myotonia permanens' (Lerche *et al.*, 1993). It is characterized by very severe and persistent myotonia. When the myotonia is aggravated, e.g. by intake of potassium-rich food, ventilation might be impaired by stiffness of the thoracic muscles. In particular, children can suffer from acute hypoventilation which may lead to cyanosis and unconsciousness, so that such episodes are occasionally mistaken for epileptic seizures. In spite of such misdiagnosis, antiepileptic medication, e.g. administration of carbamazepine, can be useful in these cases because of its antimyotonic effects. Such patients would probably not survive without continuous treatment. A fourth subtype of PAM presents with acetazolamide-responsiveness of myotonia (Trudell *et al.*, 1987), also described as atypical myotonia congenita (Ptacek *et al.*, 1992b, 1994). In addition to stiffness, patients also complain of muscle pain. Both the stiffness and pain are relieved by acetazolamide.

In PAM, depolarizing agents such as potassium or suxamethonium may aggravate the myotonia, but do not induce weakness. It is well known for myotonic disorders that the risk of depolarizing relaxants to induce anaesthesia-related events is increased. The incidence of such events seems to be highest in myotonia fluctuans families (Ricker *et al.*, 1994, Vita *et al.*, 1995). There seems to be no other biological reason for this than the frequent absence of clinical myotonia in these patients making the anaesthesiologists unaware of the condition.

The diagnosis of PAM is suggested by a generalized myotonia with dominant inheritance, by the absence of weakness and cold sensitivity. The clinical severity varies considerably from very slight myotonia with fluctuating degrees of stiffness to permanent severe myotonia with changes in facial morphology. In intermediate cases PAM cannot be clinically differentiated from myotonia congenita (MC) Thomsen. In this situation oral potassium loading, which induces a myotonic attack in PAM but not in MC Thomsen, might differentiate these two diseases. This test is contraindicated in patients with myotonia permanens since it may provoke severe attacks. Another important differentiating feature is that PAM patients show paramyotonia of the orbicularis oculi muscles.

## Common features

Before *SCN4A*, the gene encoding the $\alpha$-subunit of the human adult skeletal muscle sodium channel was cloned, an extensive electrophysiological investigation, carried out with excised muscle specimens from all kinds of myotonia patients, had yielded evidence that in two of these rare hereditary conditions the inactivation of the muscular sodium channels was defective (Lehmann-Horn *et al.*, 1987a, 1987b). Genetic studies of large families performed with an intragenic marker quickly revealed that they are indeed linked to *SCN4A* (Fontaine *et al.*, 1990; Koch *et al.*, 1991; Ptacek *et al.*, 1992b). Intron-exon boundaries of the gene are known; primer sets consisting of intron sequences for amplification of all 24 exons by use of PCR are available (George *et al.*, 1993). To date, 21 missense mutations have been discovered leading to the different symptoms described above (Figure 9.3; Table 9.2).

The three allelic diseases do not always appear in their pure forms, e.g. PC patients often suffer from spontaneous episodes of weakness which may go along with an elevated serum potassium level. However, HyperPP patients never show substantial stiffness when cooled, and muscle weakness never occurs in PAM. Although intermediate forms are frequent, it seems reasonable to maintain the classification of three separate nosological entities because, in the pure forms, not only the symptoms but also the recommended treatments differ (Ricker *et al.*, 1983).

As in most other channelopathies, the clinical symptoms of the three diseases, muscle stiffness and, in HyperPP and PC, muscle weakness, are not present all the time. Rather, they are elicited by various stimuli. A typical trigger for an episode of weakness in HyperPP would be rest after a heavy work load; stiffness and weakness in paramyotonia congenita are triggered by muscle exercise and/or exposure of the muscles to cold; ingestion of potassium-rich food may induce muscle stiffness in PAM patients. In each case, the symptoms taper off spontaneously within a few hours. The episodes aggravate the patient's life considerably, although they may be prevented to a certain extent by appropriate lifestyle changes and symptomatic drug treatment (for review see Lehmann-Horn *et al.*, 1994).

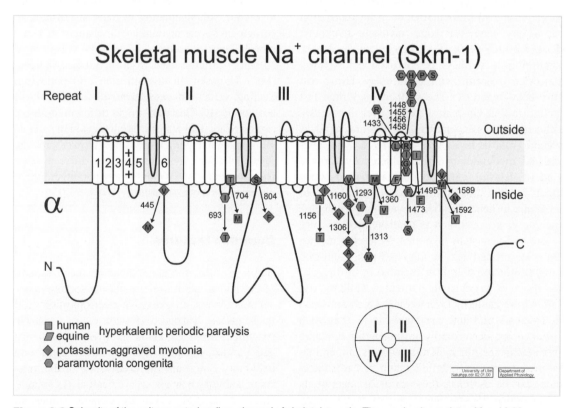

**Figure 9.3** Subunits of the voltage-gated sodium channel of skeletal muscle. The $\alpha$-subunit consists of four highly homologous domains (repeats I–IV) containing six transmembrane segments each (S1–S6). The S5–S6 loops form the ion selective pore, and the S4 segments contain positively charged residues conferring voltage dependence to the protein. The repeats are connected by intracellular loops; one of them, the III–IV linker, contains the supposed inactivation particle of the channel. When inserted in the membrane, the four repeats of the protein fold to generate a central pore as schematically indicated on the right-hand bottom of the figure.

**Table 9.2 Mutations in *SCN4A*, the gene encoding the α-subunit of the human skeletal muscle sodium channel.**

| Genotype | Channel region | Mutation | Exon | Phenotype |
|---|---|---|---|---|
| *Hyperkalaemic periodic paralysis* | | | | |
| C2188T | IIS5$_i$ | Thr-704-Met | 13 | Permanent weakness (non)-myotonic most frequent |
| G3466A | IIIS4-S5 | Ala-1156-Thr | 19 | Reduced penetrance |
| A4078G | IVS1 | Met-1360-Val | 23 | Reduced penetrance |
| T4484C | IVS5 | Ile-1495-Phe | 24 | Potential atrophy |
| A4774G | IVS6$_i$ | Met-1592-Val | 24 | Myotonic, frequent |
| *Paramyotonia congenita* | | | | |
| T2078C | IIS4-S5 | Ile-693-Thr | 13 | No paralysis |
| G3877A | IIIS6$_i$ | Val-1293-Ile | 21 | No paralysis |
| C3938T | III/IV | Thr-1313-Met | 22 | Frequent |
| T4298G | IVS3 | Leu-1433-Arg | 24 | |
| C4342T | IVS4 | Arg-1448-Cys | 24 | Potential atrophy |
| C4342A | IVS4 | Arg-1448-Ser | 24 | |
| G4343A | IVS4 | Arg-1448-His | 24 | |
| G4343C | IVS4 | Arg-1448-Pro | 24 | Potential atrophy |
| T4364C | IVS4 | Ile-1455-Thr | 24 | |
| G4372T | IVS4 | Val-1458-Phe | 24 | |
| T4418C | IVS4-S5 | Phe-1473-Ser | 24 | |
| *Potassium-aggravated myotonias* | | | | |
| G1333A | IS6$_i$ | Val-445-Met | 9 | Painful myotonia |
| C2411T | IIS6$_i$ | Ser-804-Phe | 14 | Paramyotonic features myotonia fluctuans |
| A3478G | III-IV | Ile-1160-Val | 19 | Acetazolamide-responsive |
| G3917A | III-IV | Gly-1306-Glu | 22 | Myotonia permanens |
| G3917C | III-IV | Gly-1306-Ala | 22 | Myotonia fluctuans |
| G3917T | III-IV | Gly-1306-Val | 22 | Paramyotonic features, myotonia |
| G4765A | IVS6$_i$ | Val-1589-Met | 24 | Myotonia |

i = internal end of a transmembrane segment (S) situated in one of the 4 repeats (I–IV).

## Electrophysiological basis

The key symptoms of stiffness and weakness are caused by the same pathogenetic mechanism, namely a long-lasting depolarization of the muscle fibre membranes (Lehmann-Horn *et al.*, 1987a, b). For the explanation of the pathogenesis of the diseases it is important to remember that such patients possess two populations of sodium channels, i.e. mutant and wild-type.

When, after an action potential, the membrane does not repolarize completely, but remains slightly depolarized by 5–10 mV because of the inactivation defects of the mutant channels, the wild-type sodium channels that physiologically recover from inactivation can be reactivated. Consequently, one or more successive action potentials are initiated, and this repetitive firing is the basis for the involuntary muscle activity that the patients experience as muscle stiffness. Such a hyperexcitable state can be computer-simulated and mimicked with anemone toxin (Cannon *et al.*, 1993; Cannon and Corey, 1993).

When the depolarization brought about by the mutant channels is stronger, say 20–30 mV, the majority of the wild-type sodium channels remain in the state of inactivation and this gradually renders the muscle fibres inexcitable leading to muscle weakness or even paralysis. This state is also temporary, as excitability of the muscle fibres returns when, by action of the sodium-potassium pumps, the membrane resting potential slowly assumes the physiological value of about −80 mV (Lehmann-Horn *et al*., 1987a, b).

## Functional expression

A more detailed specification of the altered channel properties produced by the various disease-causing mutations was possible by heterologous expression of the respective mutant cDNA in cultured cells and subsequent studies of the sodium currents conducted by the membranes of such cells upon depolarizing steps. Both whole-cell and patch-clamp recordings showed that all mutations affected the channel inactivation in one or the other way (Figures 9.3 and 9.4). The alterations that were observed with such mutant channels were a reduced speed of current decay following a depolarization step, a more or less incomplete decay of the current, an increased

## Hinged-lid model for Na channel inactivation

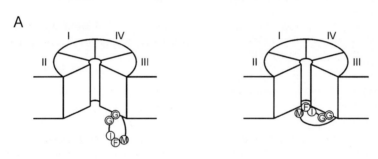

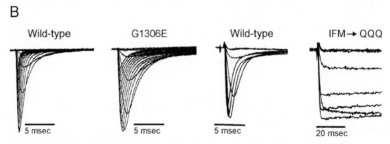

**Figure 9.4** Hinged-lid model of fast inactivation of sodium channels and the effects of mutations at various locations on the current decay. (A) Bird's eye view on the channel consisting of four similar repeats (I to IV). The channel is cut and spread open between repeats II and III to allow the view on the intracellular loop between repeats III and IV (after West *et al*., 1992). The loop acts as the inactivation gate whose 'hinge' GG (= a pair of glycines) allows it to 'swing' between two positions, i.e. the non-inactivated channel state, (pore open, left panel) and the inactivated state (pore blocked by the 'plug' IMF = amino acid sequence isoleucine, phenylalanine, methionine, right panel). (B) The substitution of E (Glu) for Gly-1306 slows channel inactivation (left two panels, c.f. fast current decay in wild-type channel on far left) and leads to a life-threatening form of potassium-aggravated myotonia. The designed substitution of QQQ for IFM completely abolishes channel inactivation (two right hand panels) proving that the loop between repeats III and IV is indeed the inactivation gate (adapted from Mitrovic *et al*., 1995).

speed of the recovery from inactivation, a shifted position of the steady-state inactivation curve (Hodgkin and Huxley's $h_\infty$ curve) and an altered degree of uncoupling of inactivation from activation (Chahine et al., 1994, Mitrovic et al., 1994).

The various mutations produce either one or several of these changes (Table 9.3). For example, slowing of the current decay is most pronounced with substitutions for Arg-1448 causing paramyotonia (Chahine et al., 1994, Lerche et al., 1996), whereas a large persistent sodium current is found with the HyperPP mutation Met-1592-Val (Cannon and Strittmatter, 1993) and the PAM mutation Val-1589-Met (Mitrovic et al., 1994). Persistent current should be decreased by slow channel inactivation (Ruff, 1994), however, this type of inactivation seems to be disturbed by some HyperPP mutants situated at the cytoplasmic ends of segments S5 and S6 (Cummins and Sigworth, 1996). In contrast, mutations within the III/IV linker abolish fast inactivation and have no effect on slow inactivation (Cummins and Sigworth, 1996; Hayward et al., 1997).

The alterations found with the different disease-causing mutants are summarized in Table 9.1. They can be generalized as follows: i) sodium currents conducted by *HyperPP mutants* show a large fraction of persistent current and an incomplete slow inactivation; these changes may cause strong and long-lasting membrane depolarization which is the basis of weakness in HyperPP; ii) sodium currents conducted by *PC mutants* are characterized by a slowing of fast inactivation; this change explains paradoxical myotonia; another typical change is acceleration of recovery from inactivation and a left-shift of the steady-state inactivation curve; in combination with an increased persistent current, it could explain the cold-induced weakness; iii) sodium currents conducted by *PAM mutants* are characterized by an increased persistent fraction and/or slowing of fast inactivation; these alterations explain the slight depolarization which causes the myotonia. The right-shift of the steady-state inactivation curve also found might be the reason why PAM patients do not experience weakness.

## Phenotype–genotype correlations

Looking at the positions of amino acid substitutions caused by disease-causing mutations along the sequence of the *SCN4A* product, it is remarkable that most of them are in the 'inactivating' linker between repeats III and IV or adjacent in the 'voltage-sensing' segment S4 of repeat IV. Almost all remaining mutations are situated at the inner side of the membrane where they could impair the docking site for the inactivation particle.

Three of the mutations in the III/IV linker

**Table 9.3 Summary of main locations and electrophysiological effects of the disease-causing sodium channel mutations. For details see text.**

|  | Paramyotonia congenita | Potassium-aggravated myotonia | Hyperkalaemic periodic paralysis | Hypokalaemic periodic paralysis |
|---|---|---|---|---|
| Mutation region | IV/S4 | III/IV loop | Intracellular side of segments | II/S4 |
| Fast inactivation | Slowed | Normal to slowed | Normal | Normal |
| Persistent current | Small | Zero | Large | Zero |
| Steady-state fast inactivation | Left-shift | Right-shift | normal | Large left-shift |
| Recovery from fast inactivation | Accelerated | Not or slightly accelerated | Normal |  |
| Slow inactivation | Normal | Normal | Reduced | Increased |

(Gly-1306-Ala/Val/Glu) produce different amino acid substitutions for one of a pair of glycines proposed to act as the 'hinge' for the inactivation gate. They all cause PAM and, interestingly, the more the structure of the substituting amino acid differs from the physiological Gly-1306 (longer side chains and/or greater charge) the more intensive is the hyperexcitability of the muscles and the more severe the myotonia:

- Alanine, with a short side-chain, results in a benign, often 'subclinical' form of myotonia
- Valine (Figure 9.5), having a side-chain of intermediate size, causes moderate exercise-induced myotonia
- Glutamic acid, an amino acid with a long side-chain, causes permanent myotonia, the most severe form of the disease.

Thus the natural mutations affecting Gly-1306 provided evidence for an increased rigidity of the amino acid chain at the position of the highly conserved pair of glycines increasingly hampering channel inactivation (Mitrovic *et al.*, 1995). Mutations at this hinge site also altered channel activation and deactivation.

A similar correlation between the structural differences between wild-type and mutant amino acids on one side, and the severity of clinical symptoms on the other, was found for four PC-causing mutants at another identical site (Arg-1448-Cys/His/Pro/Ser) (Ptacek *et al.*, 1992a) near the extracellular face of IVS4. This finding led to a systematic application of site-directed mutagenesis in this supposed channel activation domain. All tested mutants primarily affected channel inactivation (Chahine *et al.*, 1994). There-

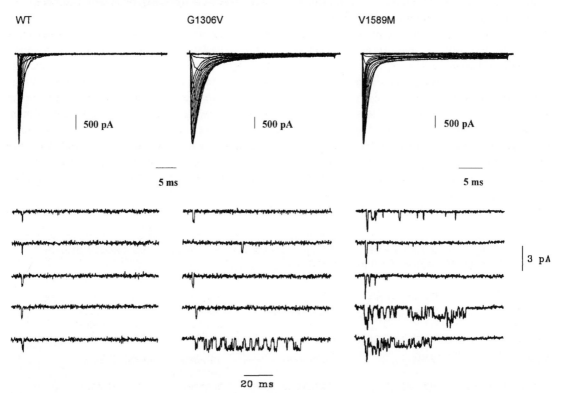

**Figure 9.5** Two examples of faulty mutant sodium channel inactivation. Patch-clamp recordings from normal (WT), Gly-1306-Val and Val-1589-Met channels expressed in HEK-293 cells. Upper panels: families of sodium currents recorded at various test potentials in the whole-cell mode show slowed decay and failure to return completely to baseline. Slowed inactivation is more pronounced with Gly-1306-Val, persistent inward sodium current is larger for Val-1589-Met. Lower panels: traces of 5 single-channel recordings each obtained by clamping the membrane potential to −20 mV. Mutant channels show re-openings which are the reason for the 'macroscopic' current alterations shown in the upper panels (modified after Mitrovic *et al.*, 1995, 1996).

fore, it was hypothesized that depolarization-induced movements in IVS4 concern both the inactivation gate and the docking site for the inactivation particle (Yang et al., 1996).

## Pathogenesis

Although the symptoms in PC are very much aggravated in the cold, the sodium currents conducted by PC-causing mutants expressed in heterologous cells did not show a corresponding dependence on temperature. The mechanism by which cold enhances muscle stiffness in PC patients is not completely clear. Both the time constant of fast inactivation and the persistent current increase with cooling, and mutant and normal channels show the same temperature dependence; however, the absolute figures are larger for mutant channels at all temperatures. Therefore, it was proposed that a certain threshold has to be exceeded in the cold environment to induce myotonic and/or paralytic symptoms (Fleischhauer et al., 1998). In contrast to the cold-induced symptoms, the pathogenesis of the potassium-induced stiffness and paralysis is well understood. The physiological depolarization which, according to Nernst, follows an elevation of serum potassium, increases the open probability of the sodium channels and unmasks their inactivation defect. Thus, potassium exerts its effect via depolarization.

## Therapy

Local anaesthetics and antiarrhythmic drugs of class IB, such as mexiletine and other lidocaine analogues, very effectively prevent muscle stiffness and weakness in PC (Ricker et al., 1980; Streib, 1987). They also relieve stiffness in PAM. In addition, these drugs prevent or reduce muscle stiffness in the chloride channel myotonias and in myotonic dystrophy, both of them having a different pathogenesis (Rüdel et al., 1980). This beneficial effect is due to their well-known use-dependent block of sodium channels (Hille, 1992). The block prevents the membranes from repetitive firing, the common path in the generation of

myotonia. This 'non-specific' antimyotonic action seems to be most effective in PC and PAM, probably because it does actually directly influence the function at fault, namely sodium channel inactivation. Mexiletine stabilizes the inactivated channel by a left-shift of the steady-state inactivation curve and a slowing of the recovery from inactivation (Fan et al., 1996; Fleischhauer et al., 1998).

The effects of mexiletine have been studied in cell lines expressing sodium channel mutants affecting regions known to be essential for channel inactivation. Compared to wild-type, the use-dependent block was increased for R1448C, located in the IVS4 voltage sensor, and decreased for F1473S (IVS4-S5), G1306E and T1313M, both within the III/IV loop (Fan et al., 1996; Fleischhauer et al., 1998). For the latter mutant only, reduced affinity of the drug to the inactivated state has been reported, suggesting both less beneficial drug effects for this mutation and a binding site for local anaesthetics and antiarrhythmics in this loop. Data on minor therapeutic effects are not available for this mutation, and studies on drug binding mainly focus on the cytoplasmic end of segment IVS6 (Ragsdale et al., 1994; Qu et al., 1995).

In contrast to the stiffness and the cold-induced weakness, spontaneous as well as potassium-induced attacks of weakness, typical for HyperPP and also often in PC, are not influenced by mexiletine. Diuretics such as hydrochlorothiazide and acetazolamide can decrease frequency and severity of paralytic episodes by lowering serum potassium (Lehmann-Horn et al., 1994) and perhaps by shifting the pH to lower values (Lehmann-Horn et al., 1987a).

## Conclusions and open questions

Many basic questions on myotonia congenita are now understood. We know the mutated gene and its product, and understand the physiological mechanisms underlying the pathology of muscle stiffness fairly well. No studies have yet been able to explain the warm-up phenomenon, which remains an unanswered question from pre-molecular biology days (Birnberger and Klepzig, 1979). Several mutations have been found in families with myotonia congenita which, under certain circumstances, can be either dominantly or recessively transmitted, but what the decisive circumstances are remains to be elucidated. Even though all dominant mutations have been found to shift the activation curve of ClC-1 towards more positive membrane potentials, there is no simple relation between the amount of shift that was measured with the various mutant ClC-1 channels and the severity of symptoms usually seen with patients carrying the respective mutation. Presumably other not yet recognized factors influence disease expression. Such factors may also play a role in cases of recessive myotonia where the symptoms fluctuate (Wagner et al., 1998).

Even more enigmatic is the finding that some 'recessive' mutations do not lead to the loss of a gene product but rather to channels that, when expressed in one of the usual expression systems, conduct chloride currents with normal amplitude and normal gating behaviour. Relatively little – in comparison to our knowledge on cation channels – is known about the structure/function relation of ClC-1. This is of course due to the fact that the ClC family of chloride channels was detected only recently and that the structure of its members is totally different from that of the well understood cation channel families. Several groups of investigators are involved in finding the pore region of the channel and the mechanism of gating (Fahlke et al., 1998; Rychkov et al., 1998; Kürz et al., 1999). Hopefully molecular biological methods, such as site-directed mutagenesis and the use of channel chimeras, will fill this current unsatisfactory gap in our knowledge.

The pathology of the sodium channelopathies has been well elucidated by detailed in-vitro studies of the alterations of the sodium currents conducted by the various mutant channels. Parallels with sodium channel disorders of heart and brain highlight recurring common underlying disease patterns. It is not entirely clear why patients with PC are temperature-sensitive and those with PAM and HyperPP are not, since a specific temperature dependence could not be found with any of the PC-causing mutants in vitro. On the other hand, the cold-induced weakness is clearly linked to

membrane depolarization due to increased sodium inward current, and so a mechanism other than that related to the sodium channel seems unlikely. The aggravation of the clinical symptoms upon potassium intake seen with PAM and HyperPP patients is consistent with studies on PAM- or PC-causing mutants showing sensitivity to extracellular potassium (Chahine et al., 1994; Mitrovic et al., 1994; 1995). The effect of potassium is most likely explained by a membrane depolarization. This may not be the only mechanism involved because, in hypokalaemic periodic paralysis, attacks of generalized flaccid weakness are associated with membrane depolarization upon hypokalaemia. The recent discovery of sodium channel mutations in hypokalaemic periodic paralysis (Bulman et al., 1999; Jurkat-Rott et al., 2000) may give interesting insights into additional channel dysfunction mechanisms involved in generating muscle weakness.

# References

Becker, P. E. (1970). *Paramyotonia congenita (Eulenburg). Fortschritte der allgemeinen und klinischen Humangenetik*. Georg Thieme, Stuttgart.

Becker, P. E. (1977). *Myotonia Congenita and Syndromes Associated with Myotonia*. Georg Thieme, Stuttgart.

Birnberger, K. L. and Klepzig, M. (1979). Influence of extracellular potassium and intracellular pH on myotonia. *J Neurol.*, **222**, 23–35.

Bryant, S. H. (1969). Cable properties of external intercostal muscle fibres from myotonic and nonmyotonic goats. *J Physiol. (Lond.)*, **204**, 539–50.

Bulman, D. E., Scoggan, K. A., van Oene, M. D. *et al.* (1999). A novel sodium channel mutation in a family with hypokalemic periodic paralysis. *Neurology*, **53**, 1932–6.

Cannon, S. C., Brown, R.H. Jr and Corey, D. P. (1993). Theoretical reconstruction of myotonia and paralysis caused by incomplete inactivation of sodium channels. *Biophys J.*, **65**, 270–88.

Cannon, S. C. and Corey, D. P. (1993). Loss of $Na^+$ channel inactivation by anemone toxin (ATX II) mimics the myotonic state in hyperkalaemic periodic paralysis. *J Physiol (Lond.)*, **466**, 501–20.

Cannon, S. C. and Strittmatter, S. M. (1993). Functional expression of sodium channel mutations identified in families with periodic paralysis. *Neuron*, **10**, 317–26.

Chahine, M., George, A. L. Jr, Zhou, M. *et al.* (1994). Sodium channel mutations in paramyotonia congenita uncouple inactivation from activation. *Neuron*, **12**, 281–94.

Cummins, T. R. and Sigworth, F. J. (1996). Impaired slow inactivation in mutant sodium channels. *Biophys J.*, **71**, 227–36.

Deymeer, F., Cakirkaya, S., Serdaroglu, P. *et al.* (1998). Transient weakness and compound muscle action potential decrement in myotonia congenita. *Muscle Nerve*, **21**, 1334–7.

Deymeer, F., Lehmann-Horn, F., Serdaroglu, P. *et al.* (1999). Electrical myotonia in heterozygous carriers of recessive myotonia congenita. *Muscle Nerve*, **22**, 123–5.

Eulenberg (1886) Ueber eine familiaere durch 6 Generationen verfolgbare Form congenitaler Paramyotonie. *Neurologisches Zentralblatt*, **5**, 265–72.

Fahlke, C., Beck, C. L. and George, A. L. Jr (1997a). A mutation in autosomal dominant myotonia congenita affects pore properties of the muscle chloride channel. *Proc Natl Acad Sci USA*, **94**, 2729–34.

Fahlke, C., Knittle, T., Gurnett, C. A., Campbell, K. P. and George, A. L. Jr (1997b). Subunit stoichiometry of human muscle chloride channels. *J Gen Physiol.*, **109**, 93–104.

Fahlke, C., Rhodes, T. H., Desai, R. R. and George, A. L. Jr (1998). Pore stoichiometry of a voltage-gated chloride channel. *Nature*, **394**, 687–90.

Fahlke, C. Rosenbohm, A., Mitrovic, N., George, A. L. Jr and Rüdel, R. (1996). Mechanism of voltage-dependent gating in skeletal muscle chloride channels. *Biophys J.*, **71**, 695–706.

Fahlke, C., Rüdel, R., Mitrovic, N., Zhou, M. and George, A. L. Jr (1995). An aspartic acid residue important for voltage-dependent gating of human muscle chloride channels. *Neuron*, **15**, 463–72.

Fahlke, C. and Rüdel, R. (1995). Chloride currents across the membrane of mammalian skeletal muscle fibres. *J Physiol (Lond.)*, **484**, 355–68.

Fan, Z., George, A. L. Jr, Kyle, J. W. and Makielski, J. C. (1996). Two human paramyotonia congenita mutations have opposite effects on lidocaine block of Na$^+$ channels expressed in a mammalian cell line. *J Physiol (Lond.)*, **496**, 275–86.

Fleischhauer, R., Mitrovic, N., Deymeer, F., Lehmann-Horn, F. and Lerche, H. (1998). Effects of temperature and mexiletine on the F1473S Na$^+$ channel mutation causing paramyotonia congenita. *Pflügers Arch.*, **436**, 757–65.

Fontaine, B., Khurana, T. S., Hoffman, E. P. *et al.* (1990). Hyperkalemic periodic paralysis and the adult muscle sodium channel $\alpha$-subunit gene. *Science*, **250**, 1000–2.

Franke, C., Iaizzo, P. A., Hatt, H., Spittelmeister, W., Ricker, K. and Lehmann-Horn, F. (1991). Altered Na$^+$ channel activity and reduced Cl$^-$ conductance cause hyperexcitability in recessive generalized myotonia (Becker). *Muscle Nerve*, **14**, 762–70.

George, A. L. Jr, Iyer, G. S., Kleinfeld, R., Kallen, R. G.

and Barchi, R. L. (1993). Genomic organization of the human skeletal muscle sodium channel gene. *Genomics*, **15**, 598–606.

Gutmann, L., Riggs, J. and Brick, J. (1986). Exercise-induced membrane failure in paramyotonia congenita. *Neurology*, **36**, 130–2.

Hayward, L. J., Brown, R. H. Jr and Cannon, S. C. (1997). Slow inactivation differs among mutant Na channels associated with myotonia and periodic paralysis. *Biophys J.*, **72**, 1204–19.

Heine, R., Pika, U. and Lehmann-Horn, F. (1993). A novel SCN4A mutation causing myotonia aggravated by cold and potassium. *Hum Mol Genet.*, **2**, 1349–53.

Hille, B. (1992). *Ionic Channels of Excitable Membranes*. Sunderland, Massachusetts.

Jackson, C. E., Barohn, R. J.and Ptacek, L. J. (1994). Paramyotonia congenita: abnormal short exercise test, and improvement after mexiletine therapy. *Muscle Nerve*, **17**, 763–8.

Jentsch, T. J., Günther, W., Pusch, M. and Schwappach, B. (1995). Properties of voltage-gated chloride channels of the ClC gene family. *J Physiol (Lond.)*, **482**, 19S–25S.

Jentsch, T. J., Steinmeyer, K. and Schwarz, G. (1990). Primary structure of *Torpedo marmorata* chloride channel isolated by expression cloning in *Xenopus* oocytes. *Nature*, **348**, 510–4.

Jurkat-Rott, K., Mitrovic, N., Hang, C., Iaizzo, P., Herzog, J., Lerche, H. *et al.* (2000). Novel voltage sensor sodium channel mutations cause hypokalemic periodic paralysis type 2 by enhanced inactivation and reduced current. *Proc Natl Acad Sci USA*, **97**, 549–54.

Koch, M. C., Ricker, K., Otto, M. *et al.* (1991). Linkage data suggesting allelic heterogeneity for paramyotonia congenita and hyperkalemic periodic paralysis on chromosome 17. *Hum Gen.*, **88**, 71–4.

Koch, M. C., Steinmeyer, K., Lorenz, C. *et al.* (1992). The skeletal muscle chloride channel in dominant and recessive human myotonia. *Science*, **257**, 797–800.

Kürz, L. L., Klink, H., Jakob, I. *et al.* (1999). Identification of three cysteines as targets for the Zn$^{2+}$ blockade of the human skeletal muscle chloride channel. *J Biol Chem.*, **274**, 11687–92.

Kürz, L. L., Wagner, S., George, A. L. Jr and Rüdel, R. (1997). Probing the major skeletal muscle chloride channel with Zn$^{2+}$ and other sulfhydryl-reactive compounds. *Pflügers Arch.*, **433**, 357–63.

Lehmann-Horn, F., Engel, A. G., Ricker, K. and Rüdel, R. (1994). The periodic paralyses and paramyotonia congenita. In *Myology* (eds Engel, A.G. and Franzini-Armstrong, C.) pp. 1303–1334. McGraw-Hill, New York.

Lehmann-Horn, F. and Jurkat-Rott, K. (1999). Voltage-gated ion channels and hereditary disease. *Physiol Rev.*, **79**, 1317–71.

Lehmann-Horn, F., Küther, G., Ricker, K., Grafe, P., Ballanyi, K. and Rüdel, R. (1987a). Adynamia episodica hereditaria with myotonia: a non-inactivating sodium current and the effect of extracellular pH. *Muscle Nerve*, **10**, 363–74.

Lehmann-Horn, F., Mailänder, V., Heine, R. and George, A. L. Jr (1995). Myotonia levior is a chloride channel disorder. *Hum Mol Genet.*, **4**, 1397–1402.

Lehmann-Horn, F., Rüdel, R. and Ricker, K. (1993). Non-dystrophic myotonias and periodic paralyses. A European Neuromuscular Center Workshop held 4-6 October 1992, Ulm, Germany. *Neuromuscul Disord.*, **3**, 161–8.

Lehmann-Horn, F., Rüdel, R. and Ricker, K. (1987b). Membrane defects in paramyotonia congenita (Eulenburg). *Muscle Nerve*, **10**, 633–41.

Lennox, G., Purves, A. and Marsden, D. (1992). Myotonia fluctuans. *Arch Neurol.*, **49**, 1010–1.

Lerche, H., Heine, R., Pika, U. *et al.* (1993). Human sodium channel myotonia: slowed channel inactivation due to substitutions for glycine within the III/IV linker. *J Physiol (Lond.)*, **470**, 13–22.

Lerche, H., Mitrovic, N., Dubowitz, V. and Lehmann-Horn, F. (1996). Paramyotonia congenita: the R1448P Na$^+$ channel mutation in adult human skeletal muscle. *Ann Neurol.*, **39**, 599–608.

Lipicky, R. J. (1979). Myotonic syndromes other than myotonic dystrophy. In *Handbook of Clinical Neurology* (eds Vinken, P. J. and Bruyn, G. W.) pp. 533–571, Elsevier, Amsterdam.

Lorenz, C., Meyer-Kleine, C., Steinmeyer, K., Koch, M. C. and Jentsch, T. J. (1994). Genomic organization of the human muscle chloride channel ClC-1 and analysis of novel mutations leading to Becker-type myotonia. *Hum Mol Genet.*, **3**, 941–6.

Ludewig, U., Pusch, M. and Jentsch, T. J. (1996). Two physically distinct pores in the dimeric ClC-0 chloride channel. *Nature*, **383**, 340–3.

Middleton, R. E., Pheasant, D. J. and Miller, C. (1996). Homodimeric architecture of a ClC-type chloride ion channel. *Nature*, **383**, 337–40.

Mitrovic, N., George, A. L. Jr, Heine, R. *et al.* (1994). K$^+$-aggravated myotonia: destabilization of the inactivated state of the human muscle Na$^+$ channel by the V1589M mutation. *J Physiol (Lond.)*, **478**, 395–402.

Mitrovic, N., George, A. L. Jr, Lerche, H., Wagner, S., Fahlke, C. and Lehmann-Horn, F. (1995). Different effects on gating of three myotonia-causing mutations in the inactivation gate of the human muscle sodium channel. *J Physiol (Lond.)*, **487**, 107–14.

Mitrovic, N., Lerche, H., Heine, R. *et al.* (1996). Role in fast inactivation of conserved amino acids in the IV/S4-S5 loop of the human muscle Na$^+$ channel. *Neurosci Lett.*, **214**, 9–12.

Ptacek, L. J., George, A. L. Jr, Barchi, R. L. *et al.* (1992a). Mutations in an S4 segment of the adult skeletal muscle sodium channel cause paramyotonia congenita. *Neuron*, **8**, 891–7.

Ptacek, L. J., Tawil, R., Griggs, R. C. *et al.* (1994). Sodium channel mutations in acetazolamide-responsive myotonia congenita, paramyotonia congenita and hyperkalemic periodic paralysis. *Neurology*, **44**, 1500–3.

Ptacek, L. J., Tawil , R., Griggs, R. C., Storvick, D. and Leppert, M. (1992b). Linkage of atypical myotonia congenita to a sodium channel locus. *Neurology*, **42**, 431–3.

Pusch, M. and Jentsch, T. J. (1994). Molecular physiology of voltage-gated chloride channels. *Physiol Rev.*, **74**, 813–27.

Pusch, M., Steinmeyer, K. and Jentsch, T. J. (1994). Low single channel conductance of the major skeletal muscle chloride channel, ClC-1. *Biophys J.*, **66**, 149–52.

Pusch, M., Steinmeyer, K., Koch, M. C. and Jentsch, T. J. (1995). Mutations in dominant human myotonia congenita drastically alter the voltage dependence of the ClC-1 chloride channel. *Neuron*, **15**, 1455–63.

Qu, Y. S., Rogers, J., Tanada, T., Scheuer, T. and Catterall, W. A. (1995). Molecular determinants of drug access to the receptor site for antiarrhythmic drugs in the cardiac Na$^+$ channel. *Proc Natl Acad Sci USA*, **92**, 11839–43.

Ragsdale, D. S., McPhee, J. C., Scheuer, T. and Catterall, W. A. (1994). Molecular determinants of state-dependent block of Na$^+$ channels by local anesthetics. *Science*, **265**, 1724–28.

Ricker, K., Böhlen, R. and Rohkamm, R. (1983). Different effectiveness of tocainide and hydrochlorothiazide in paramyotonia congenita with hyperkalemic episodic paralysis. *Neurology*, **33**, 1615–8.

Ricker, K., Haass, A., Rüdel, R., Böhlen, R. and Mertens, H. G. (1980). Successful treatment of paramyotonia congenita (Eulenburg): muscle stiffness and weakness prevented by tocainide. *J Neurol Neurosurg Psychiatr.*, **43**, 268–71.

Ricker, K., Lehmann-Horn, F. and Moxley, R. T. (1990). Myotonia fluctuans. *Arch Neurol.*, **47**, 268–72.

Ricker, K., Moxley, R. T., Heine, R. and Lehmann-Horn, F. (1994). Myotonia fluctuans, a third type of muscle sodium channel disease. *Arch Neurol.*, **51**, 1095–102.

Ricker, K., Rohkamm, R. and Böhlen, R. (1986). Adynamia episodica and paralysis periodica paramyotonica. *Neurology*, **36**, 682–6.

Rojas, C. V., Wang, J., Schwartz, L., Hoffman, E. P., Powell, B. R. and Brown, R. H. Jr (1991). A Met-to-Val mutation in the skeletal muscle sodium channel α-subunit in hyperkalemic periodic paralysis. *Nature*, **354**, 387–9.

Rüdel, R., Dengler, R., Ricker, K., Haass, A., and Emser, W. (1980). Improved therapy of myotonia with the lidocaine derivative tocainide. *J Neurol.*, **222**, 275–8.

Rüdel, R., Lehmann-Horn, F. and Ricker, K. (1994). Altered excitability of the muscle cell membrane. In *Myology* (eds Engel, A. G. and Franzini-Armstrong, C.) pp. 1291–302, McGraw-Hill, New York.

Rüdel, R., Ricker, K. and Lehmann-Horn, F. (1988). Transient weakness and altered membrane characteristic in recessive generalized myotonia (Becker). *Muscle Nerve*, **11**, 202–11.

Ruff, R. L. (1994). Slow $Na^+$ channel inactivation must be disrupted to evoke prolonged depolarization-induced paralysis. *Biophys J.*, **66**, 542–5.

Rychkov, G. Y., Astill, D. S., Bennetts, B., Hughes, B. P., Bretag, A. H., and Roberts, M. L. (1997). pH-dependent interactions of $Cd^{2+}$ and a carboxylate blocker with the rat ClC-1 chloride channel and its R304E mutant in the Sf-9 insect cell line. *J Physiol (Lond.)*, **501**, 355–62.

Rychkov, G. Y., Pusch, M., Roberts, M. L., Jentsch, T. J. and Bretag, A. H. (1998). Permeation and block of the skeletal muscle chloride channel, ClC-1, by foreign anions. *J Gen Physiol.*, **111**, 653–5.

Steinmeyer, K., Ortland, C. and Jentsch, T. J. (1991). Primary structure and functional expression of a developmentally regulated skeletal muscle chloride channel. *Nature*, **354**, 301–4.

Streib, E. W. (1987). Paramyotonia congenita: successful treatment with tocainide. Clinical and electrophysiologic findings in seven patients. *Muscle Nerve*, **10**, 155–62.

Subramony, S. H., Malhotra, C. P. and Mishra, S. K. (1983). Distinguishing paramyotonia congenita and myotonia congenita by electromyography. *Muscle Nerve*, **6**, 374–9.

Thomsen, J. (1876). Tonische Krämpfe in willkürlich beweglichen Muskeln in Folge von ererbter psychischer Disposition. *Arch Psychiatr Nervenkrankh.*, **6**, 702–18.

Trudell, R. G., Kaiser, K. K. and Griggs, R. C. (1987). Acetazolamide responsive myotonia congenita. *Neurology*, **37**, 488–91.

Vita, G. M., Olckers, A., Jedlicka, A. E. *et al.* (1995). Masseter muscle rigidity associated with glycine[1306]-to-alanine mutation in adult muscle sodium channel $\alpha$-subunit gene. *Anesthesiology*, **82**, 1097–103.

Wagner, S., Deymeer, F., Kürz, L. L. *et al.* (1998). The dominant chloride channel mutant G200R causing fluctuating myotonia: clinical findings, electrophysiology, and channel pathology. *Muscle Nerve*, **21**, 1122–8.

West, J. W., Patton, D. E., Scheuer, T., Wang, Y., Goldin, A. L. and Catterall, W. A. (1992). A cluster of hydrophobic amino acid residues required for fast $Na^+$-channel inactivation. *Proc Natl Acad Sci USA.*, **89**, 10910–4.

Yang, N., George, A. L. Jr and Horn, R. (1996). Molecular basis of charge movement in voltage-gated sodium channels. *Neuron*, **16**, 113–22.

# The periodic paralyses: hyperkalaemic and hypokalaemic paralysis

*Rabi Tawil*

## Introduction

The primary periodic paralyses are inherited disorders of skeletal muscle specific, sarcolemmal ion channels. Although clinically and pathophysiologically heterogeneous, the episodic muscle weakness, a hallmark of these conditions, is always the result of transient inexcitability of the sarcolemmal membrane. For years, the classification of the periodic paralyses was based on the determination of serum potassium levels, during a spontaneous attack or in response to hypokalaemic or hyperkalaemic challenges. Thus, the periodic paralyses were divided into hyperkalaemic (HyperKPP) and hypokalaemic (HypoKPP) groups in addition to a poorly defined normokalaemic group, in which consistent abnormalities in serum potassium levels cannot be documented. Recent studies showing that the periodic paralyses are the result of mutations in muscle-specific membrane ion channel genes have confirmed the general outline of the clinically-based classification system, and provided new insights into the pathophysiology of these conditions.

## Clinical presentation

Both HypoKPP and HyperKPP are inherited in an autosomal dominant fashion although sporadic cases have been reported (Tawil *et al.*, 1999). Penetrance is variable, and women are less severely affected. The common clinical feature in both HypoKPP and HyperKPP is the occurrence of transient muscle weakness, lasting minutes to hours triggered by rest following physical exertion or following prolonged rest. Thus, rest following

exercise, prolonged car rides and sleep are common precipitants. Attacks are almost always confined to the limbs sparing bulbar and respiratory muscles. Abnormalities of cardiac rhythm, although rare, can occur with extreme fluctuations in serum potassium levels. The onset of muscle weakness typically does not occur as a sudden cataclysmic event but, rather, progresses over minutes, and is often heralded by vague discomfort in the muscles. During an attack, muscle stretch reflexes are hypoactive to absent in weakened muscles. Although the frequency of paralytic attacks lessens with age, it is frequently replaced by persistent and progressive interattack weakness.

In addition to these common clinical features, HypoKPP and HyperKPP have several distinguishing features (Table 10.1).

### HypoKPP

Age of symptom onset is usually in adolescence with a range of 6 to 25 years. The most characteristic precipitating factor is the ingestion of large, carbohydrate rich meals. Attacks can also occur with alcohol ingestion, exposure to cold or emotional stress. Medications, such as corticosteroids and diuretics that lower serum potassium levels, can also potentially induce attacks of weakness.

### HyperKPP

Paralytic attacks typically start early in childhood. In contrast to hypokalaemic periodic paralysis, fasting can induce attacks of weakness in HyperKPP. Cold is a more consistent precipitant of

**Table 10.1 Distinguishing clinical features of the periodic paralyses**

|  | HypoKPP | Hyper KPP |
| --- | --- | --- |
| Age at onset | 6–25 years | < 10 years |
| Attack duration (typical) | 1–6 h | < 2 h |
| Precipitating factors | Rest post-exercise | Rest post-exercise |
|  | Carbohydrates | Fasting |
|  | Cold | Cold |
| Myotonia | Absent | Often present |
| Progressive weakness | Frequent | Frequent |
| Chromosome/gene | 1q/calcium channel | 17q/sodium channel |

weakness in hyperkalaemic periodic paralysis. Stiffness due to myotonia, absent in HypoKPP, is a variable symptom in HyperKPP. Myotonia may be asymptomatic and detectable only by EMG in HyperKPP. Lid lag myotonia and paradoxical eye closure myotonia are often present on examination. Well-developed musculature is common in HyperKPP.

## Diagnosis

Since, between attacks, patients often have a normal exam, obtaining an accurate and detailed medical history is critical. The clinician has to decide first if the episodes of weakness are consistent with periodic paralysis, and if so, are they due to a primary inherited or secondary form of peri-odic paralysis. Patients should be asked details of their dietary habits, and a careful inventory of their prescription and over-the-counter medications should be taken. Clues suggesting the presence of a systemic illness (i.e. hyperthyroidism) should be sought in the review of systems.

The differential diagnosis of periodic paralysis includes a long list of conditions associated with changes in serum potassium levels that can result in transient muscle paralysis (Table 10.2). Thus, renal, adrenal and gastrointestinal conditions that significantly alter potassium homeostasis should be considered. Of the conditions listed in Table 10.2, hypokalaemic paralysis secondary to hyperthyroidism is the most common single cause.

The simplest and most direct way to confirm the diagnosis of periodic paralysis is to examine a patient during an attack and determine their serum

**Table 10.2 Secondary causes of periodic paralysis**

|  | Hypokalaemic | Hyperkalaemic |
| --- | --- | --- |
| Endocrine | Hyperthyroidism | Hypoaldosteronism |
|  | Primary hypoaldosteronism |  |
| Gastrointestinal | Gastroenteritis |  |
|  | Villous adenoma |  |
| Renal | Renal tubular acidosis, type 1, 2 | Renal failure |
| Drugs/toxins | Glycirrhizin (present in liquorice, snuff) | Diuretics: K sparing |
|  | Diuretics | ACE inhibitors |
|  | Laxatives | Cyclosporin |
|  | Alcohol |  |
|  | Barium |  |

potassium levels. Yet, patients are rarely seen during an acute episode. Moreover, serum potassium levels, even when obtained in a timely fashion may not be clearly abnormal. Whereas in HypoKPP, serum potassium levels are consistently and profoundly low during an acute attack, serum potassium levels may be normal in the recovery phase of an acute attack. In HyperKPP, on the other hand, serum potassium levels are less consistently abnormal. To rule out secondary forms of periodic paralysis, screening blood tests should also include thyroid function tests, serum electrolytes and renal function. Thyroid functions should include a measurement of T3 since isolated T3 thyrotoxicosis has been associated with periodic paralysis (Griggs *et al.*, 1996). If adrenal or renal tubular disease is suspected, assessment of urinary electrolytes or screening for adrenal dysfunction should be performed. If the history, supported by the blood tests, suggests a specific primary periodic paralysis, the diagnosis can then be confirmed by DNA molecular diagnostic techniques where available.

If the initial workup is not diagnostic and molecular diagnosis is not available, additional diagnostic tests may be helpful. Nerve conduction studies and EMG are helpful in establishing the presence of periodic paralysis. The exercise nerve conduction test demonstrates the presence of an exercise-induced decrement in compound muscle action amplitudes (Figure 10.1) (McManis *et al.*, 1986). This test has a sensitivity of 71% and is essentially 100% specific. A positive test establishes the diagnosis of periodic paralysis but does not distinguish between the various forms of primary or secondary periodic paralyses. It is thus helpful in establishing a diagnosis of periodic paralysis when the history is vague and the episodic weakness has not been witnessed. On the other hand, if the exercise test is positive and EMG documents the presence of myotonic discharges, then the diagnosis of HyperKPP is essentially confirmed. Engel *et al.* (1965) describe a variation of the exercise test which is combined with local intra-arterial injection of epinephrine and is reported to be highly specific for hypokalaemic periodic paralysis.

When it is not possible to measure serum

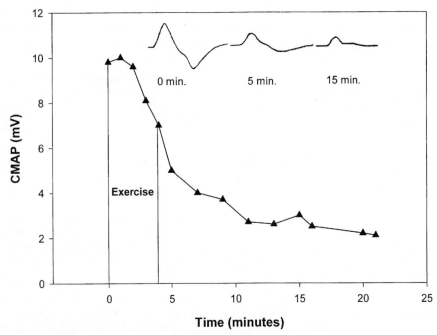

**Figure 10.1** Exercise nerve conduction test in a patient with HypoKPP. The ulnar nerve at the wrist is stimulated and the compound muscle action potential recorded at the abductor digiti minimi. The muscle is contracted isometrically for 20 second intervals followed by 5 seconds for a total of 4 minutes.

potassium levels during an acute attack, the use of hypo- and hyperkalaemic challenges to induce an attack remains a useful diagnostic test (Griggs *et al.*, 1995). These challenges should always be performed in an inpatient setting with appropriate cardiac monitoring. A baseline ECG is always obtained with particular attention to the QTc interval. Patients with periodic paralysis and prolonged QTc interval likely have Andersen's syndrome, a rare periodic paralysis variant (see Chapter 22) (Sansone *et al.*, 1997). Inducing hypokalaemia in such a situation may worsen the QT prolongation and potentially induce a fatal ventricular arrhythmia. Another diagnostic test involving rest followed by vigorous exercise has been described and avoids the potential morbidity associated with pharmacological induction of hypo- or hyperkalaemia (Kantola and Tarssanan, 1992).

Muscle biopsy often demonstrates specific pathological changes that can help confirm the clinical suspicion of periodic paralysis. However, as with other diagnostic tests, the usefulness of the biopsy has been superceded by the availability of molecular diagnostic testing. The biopsy remains a useful diagnostic test only when other diagnostic modalities have been uninformative and when molecular confirmation is not possible. Early in the disease, a muscle biopsy may show no pathological changes. With recurrent attacks, the muscle shows variable non-specific myopathic changes. Vacuoles, most often central and of considerable size, are the characteristic histopathological feature, seen in both forms of primary periodic paralysis. In a detailed study of hypokalaemic periodic paralysis biopsies, the evolution of these vacuoles from dilated sarcoplasmic reticulum filled with cellular debris is described (Lehmann-Horn *et al.*, 1994).

## Pathophysiology

### HypoKPP

Early investigations of the cause of HypoKPP naturally focused on metabolic disturbances that can potentially cause hypokalaemia. Thus it was established early on that total body potassium was not depleted in these patients but that the hypoka-

laemia is due to an exaggerated intracellular shift (Grob *et al.*, 1957; Zierler and Andres, 1957). Hoffman *et al.* (1983) found increased insulin binding to monocytes of patients with hypokalaemic periodic paralysis concluding that they may have a supraphysiological response to insulin. Another study suggested that hypokalaemic periodic paralysis patients are disproportionately sensitive to the action of insulin on potassium independent of its action on glucose (Rudel *et al.*, 1984). *In vitro* electrophysiological experiments demonstrated lower than normal resting potential in muscle membranes from patients with hypokalaemic periodic paralysis (Hoffman *et al.*, 1983; Grafe *et al.*, 1990). Moreover, hypokalaemic periodic paralysis muscle instead of becoming hyperpolarized, becomes depolarized and inexcitable in response to insulin or reduction in extracellular potassium concentrations, an effect not blocked by the sodium channel blocker tetrodotoxin (Grafe *et al.*, 1990). A pathogenic role for potassium channels was suggested several years ago by the demonstration of improved contraction force in HypoKPP muscle exposed to potassium channel openers (Grafe *et al.*, 1990).

Based on these physiological studies, one would not have anticipated that HypoKPP would be linked to the dihydropyridine (DHP) receptor gene, CACNL1A3, on chromosome 1q (Jurkatt-Rott *et al.*, 1994). Two point mutations have been identified in two adjacent positions in the S4 segment of domain 4 of the gene (Jurkatt-Rott *et al.*, 1994; Fouad *et al.*, 1997). Subsequently a third mutation was identified in the S4 segment of domain 2 (Figure 10.2) (Ptacek *et al.*, 1994a). Together, these mutations are present in about two-thirds of HypoKPP families screened.

The DHP receptor is a calcium channel that has important functions in EC-coupling and calcium conductance (Ptacek, 1998). Functional studies of the mutated channel have been mixed, with most not showing significant abnormalities in L-type $Ca^{2+}$ currents and one study noting slowed channel activation but normal inactivation (Cannon, 1996; Lapie *et al.*, 1996; Jurkatt-Rott *et al.*, 1998; Morrill *et al.*, 1998). How mutations of the dihydropyridine receptors explain the abnormal depolarization of the affected muscle fibres, the unusual response to insulin and the associated

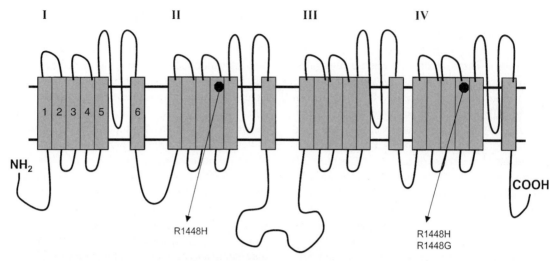

**Figure 10.2** A model of the calcium channel with the three defined HypoKPP mutations. This calcium channel is known to interact with the ryanodine receptor at the sarcoplasmic reticulum membrane.

hypokalaemia remains largely unknown. A recent study demonstrated reduced sarcolemmal ATP-sensitive $K(K_{ATP})$ channel currents in affected HypoKPP muscle which is partially restored by cromakalim, a potassium channel opener (Tricarico *et al.*, 1999). Moreover, it appears that abnormal $Ca^{2+}$ homeostasis influences the $K_{ATP}$ channel currents. Thus, this mechanism provides one possible explanation as to how mutations within the DHP receptor gene could influence $K_{ATP}$ currents leading to hypokalaemia, muscle fibre depolarization and ultimately the episodic weakness observed in HypoKPP (Tricarico *et al.*, 1999).

Although DHP mutations account for most cases of HypoKPP, the demonstration of a typical HypoKPP family not linked to the DHP gene locus suggests the presence of genetic heterogeneity in HypoKPP (Plassart *et al.*, 1994). One such small HypoKPP pedigree was reported to have an arginine to histidine substitution in a highly conserved area of the skeletal muscle sodium channel on chromosome 17q also implicated in HyperKPP (see below) (Bulman *et al.*, 1999). Confirmation of this surprising finding will be accomplished by demonstrating that this mutation, rather than representing a rare polymorphism, results in abnormal channel function (Bulman *et al.*, 1999). On a practical level, the above finding means that typical HypoKPP patients without identifiable DHP

mutations should be screened for the presence of skeletal muscle sodium channel mutations.

## HyperKPP

A number of *in vitro* physiological studies had implicated the sodium channel as an important factor in the pathophysiology of HyperKPP (Rudel and Ricker, 1985). It was therefore not surprising that HyperKPP was linked to a gene coding the alpha-subunit of the skeletal muscle sodium channel (SCN4A) on 17q (Figure 10.3) (Fontaine *et al.*, 1990). It soon became apparent that related clinical entities such as paramyotonia congenita with and without periodic paralysis and even some purely myotonic disorders are all allelic disorders resulting from mutations at the same skeletal muscle sodium channel (Ptacek *et al.*, 1991a, 1992). Four mutations account for the majority of patients with pure HyperKPP with another eight mutations described in patients who also have cold induced myotonia and weakness (Ptacek *et al.*, 1991b, 1994b; Rojas *et al.*, 1991). Although some correlation exists between the site of specific mutations (genotype) and the resultant clinical phenotype, it is rough at best. This is illustrated by a kindred with a demonstrated sodium channel mutation whose members exhibited either paramyotonia without periodic paralysis or pure HyperKPP (DeSilva *et*

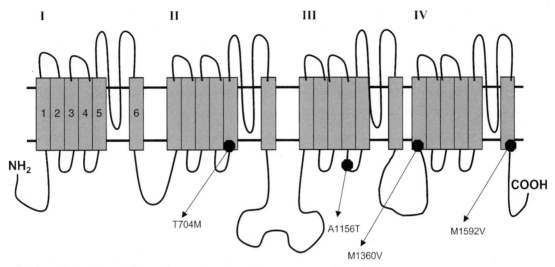

**Figure 10.3** A model of the sodium channel with the four common HyperKPP mutations. More than 20 mutations in the sodium channel have been defined that encompass HyperKPP, paramyotonia congenita and of allelic purely myotonic disorders. As with the calcium channel, the sodium channel is composed of four domains (I–IV) each with six putative membrane spanning segments ($S_1$–$S_6$).

*al.*, 1990). Thus, the genetic background and perhaps other epigenetic factors may influence the clinical expression of a particular mutation.

## Treatment

The optimal treatment of the periodic paralyses requires a two-pronged approach: prophylactic interventions to prevent or reduce the frequency and severity of the episodic weakness; and abortive interventions for the treatment of acute attacks. Prophylactic treatment regimens include a combination of dietary and lifestyle changes as well as pharmacological interventions. Abortive treatment of an acute attack is usually aimed at rapid correction of serum potassium abnormalities as well as the management of associated complications. Most attacks are self-limited and uncomplicated, requiring little intervention. However, attacks can be prolonged, have associated severe bulbar involvement and, when serum potassium changes are profound, are associated with disturbance of cardiac rhythm. Whether effective prevention of attacks lessens the chances of developing the persistent, often progressive, myopathy seen in many patients with periodic paralysis is not known. However, since structural changes observed in periodic paralysis muscle biopsies appear later in the course of the illness, it seems a reasonable assumption that reducing the number of hypokalaemic or hyperkalaemic insults to the muscle may be protective.

### HypoKPP

#### Prophylactic treatment

Institution of a low-salt, low-carbohydrate diet is recommended, although studies of their efficacy are limited and the results mixed. The first line of pharmacological treatment is the use of carbonic anhydrase inhibitors. Non-randomized, single-blind studies have demonstrated that acetazolamide can reduce attack frequency and improve interattack weakness (Resnick *et al.*, 1968; Griggs *et al.*, 1970). Dichlorphenamide, a more potent carbonic anhydrase inhibitor, in a small series of cases, was shown to be effective when the beneficial effects of acetazolamide appeared to be waning (Dalakas and Engel, 1983; Sander 1988). Definitive proof of the effectiveness of the carbonic anhydrase inhibitors comes from a recent randomized trial of dichlorphenamide in hypokalaemic periodic paralysis, which demonstrated its efficacy in the prevention of episodic weakness (Tawil *et al.*, 2000). The average dose of dichlorphenamide used in that study was 100 mg/day (Tawil *et al.*, 2000). Carbonic anhydrase inhibitors are associated with an increased incidence of nephrolithiasis necessitating a baseline KUB or renal ultrasound followed by yearly studies while patients are being treated.

Alternatives to the carbonic anhydrase inhibitors are potassium sparing diuretics and oral potassium supplementation (De Graeff and Lameijer, 1965). Many patients with HypoKPP take large daily doses of supplemental potassium, especially at night, to try to prevent early morning attacks. The usefulness of this strategy has not been well studied.

## Treatment of acute attacks

Patients often learn that, at the first sign of an impending attack, continued physical activity can blunt the severity of an attack. Intake of oral potassium at the start of an attack can also effectively shorten or lessen its severity. The total dose should not exceed 200 mEq of KCl in a 12-hour period. Intravenous potassium replacement is necessary only if severe dysphagia or vomiting is present and oral replacement is not possible. This should always be done with cardiac monitoring. Intravenous potassium given in saline or glucose solutions should be avoided as they may cause an initial acute fall in serum levels (Kunin *et al.*, 1962; Griggs *et al.*, 1983). Mannitol is the preferred diluent for intravenous KCl with 0.05–0.1 mEq/kg body weight of KCl given in bolus form (Moreno *et al.*, 1969). Serial potassium levels should be checked, as life-threatening rebound hyperkalaemia can occur with either oral or intravenous replacement (Sestoft, 1967).

### HyperKPP

## Prophylactic treatment

Dietary recommendations include having frequent meals rich in carbohydrates and the avoidance of fasting and of potassium rich foods. Pharmacological treatments include the use of thiazide diuretics to keep serum potassium in the low normal range (3.7 mmol/l). The use of carbonic anhydrase inhibitors, such as acetazolamide (125–1000 mg/day) has been recommended but not proven to be effective until recently. As with HypoKPP, dichlorphenamide (100 mg/day) also effectively reduces attack frequency in HyperKPP (Tawil *et al.*, 2000).

## Treatment of acute attacks

Mild attacks, as in HypoKPP, can often be 'walked off'. Intake of oral glucose (2 g/kg) and, if necessary, combined with subcutaneous insulin (15–20 u) can be helpful in aborting an attack. Other strategies have included the use of calcium gluconate and inhaled beta agonists (Hanna *et al.*, 1998).

## Summary

Significant advances in our understanding of the periodic paralyses have occurred over the last ten years. Yet, despite clear definition of the molecular lesions in these disorders, much remains to be learned. As with many genetic disorders, the relationship between the molecular defect and the clinical phenotype is proving to be complex. Although much is known about the abnormal sodium channel physiology in HyperKPP, it is not clear how adjacent mutations in the sodium channel gene produce such vastly differing clinical phenotypes. In HypoKPP, the relationship of the mutated calcium channel to the pathophysiology of HypoKPP remains poorly understood. In both periodic paralyses, the intrafamilial and gender-related variability in clinical phenotype suggest the presence of epigenetic factors. Nevertheless, our increasing understanding of these channelopathies will eventually translate into more rational therapeutic options for these disorders.

## References

Bulman, D. E., Scoggan, K. A., van Oene, M. D. *et al.* (1999). A novel sodium channel mutation in a family with hypokalemic periodic paralysis. *Neurology*, **53**, 1932–6.

Cannon, S. C. (1996). Ion-channel defects and aberrant excitability in myotonia and periodic paralysis. *Trends Neurosci.*, **19**, 3–10.

Dalakas, M. C. and Engel, W. K. (1983) Treatment of 'permanent' weakness in familial hyopkalemic periodic paralysis. *Muscle Nerve*, **6**, 182–6.

De Graeff, J. and Lameijer, L. D. F. (1965). Periodic paralysis. *Am J Med.*, **39**, 70–80.

DeSilva, S. M., Kunel, R. W., Griggin, J. W. *et al.* (1990). Paramyotonia congenita or hyperkalemic periodic paralysis? Clinical and electrophysiologic features of each entity in one family. *Muscle Nerve*, **13**, 21–6.

Engel, A. G., Lambert, E. H., Resevear, J. W. *et al.* (1965). Clinical and electrophysiologic studies in a patient with primary hypokalemic periodic paralysis. *Am J Med.*, **38**, 626–40.

Fontaine, B., Khurana, T. S., Hoffmann, E. P. *et al.* (1990). Hyperkalemic periodic paralysis and the adult muscle sodium channel alpha-subunit gene. *Science*, **250**, 1000–2.

Fouad, G., Dalakas, M., Servedei, S. *et al.* (1997). Genotype-phenotype correlations of the DHP receptor alpha-1 gene mutations causing hypokalemic periodic paralysis. *Neuromusc disord.*, **7**, 33–8.

Grafe, P., Quasthoff, S., Strupp, M. *et al.* (1990). Enhancement of $K^+$ conductance improves in vitro the contraction force of skeletal muscle in hypokalemic periodic paralysis. *Muscle Nerve*, **13**, 451–7.

Griggs, R. C., Engel, W. K. and Resnick, J. S. (1970). Acetazolamide treatment of hypokalemic periodic paralysis: prevention of attack and improvement of persistent weakness. *Ann Int Med.*, **73**, 39–48.

Griggs, R. C., Resnick, J. and Engel, W. K. (1983). Intravenous treatment of hypokalemic periodic paralysis. *Arch Neurol.*, **40**, 539–40.

Griggs, R. C., Mendell, J. R. and Miller, R. G. (1995). Periodic paralysis and myotonia. In *Evaluation and Treatment of Myopathies*, pp 318–354. Philadelphia: F. A. Davis Company.

Griggs, R. C., Bender, A. N. and Tawil, R. (1996). A puzzling case of periodic paralysis. *Muscle Nerve*, **19**, 362–4.

Grob, D., Johns, R. J. and Liljestrand, A. (1957). Potassium movement in patients with familial periodic paralysis. *Am J Med.*, **23**, 356–75.

Hanna, M. G., Stewart, J., Schapira, A. H. *et al.* (1998). Salbutamol treatment in a patient with hyperkalemic periodic paralysis due to a mutation in the skeletal muscle sodium channel (SCN4A). *J Neurol Neurosurg Psychiatr.*, **65**, 248–50.

Hoffman, W. W., Adornato, B. T. and Reich, H. (1983). The relationship of insulin receptors to hypokalemic periodic paralysis. *Muscle Nerve*, **6**, 48–51.

Jurkatt-Rott, K., Lehmann-Horn, F., Elbaz, A. *et al.* (1994). A calcium channel mutation causing hypoka-

lemic periodic paralysis. *Hum Mol Genet.*, **3**, 1415–9.

Jurkatt-Rott, K., Uetz, U., Pika-Hartlaub, U. *et al.* (1998). Calcium currents and transients of native and heterologous expressed mutant skeletal muscle DHP receptor alpha 1 subunits. *FEBS Lett.*, **423**, 198–204.

Kantola, I. M. and Tarssanan, L. T. (1992). Diagnosis of familial hypokalemic periodic paralysis: role of potassium exercise test. *Neurology*, **42**, 2158–61.

Kunin, A. S., Surawicz, B. and Sims, E. A. H. (1962). Decrease in serum potassium concentrations and appearance of cardiac arrhythmias during infusion of potassium with glucose in potassium depleted patients. *N Engl J Med.*, **266**, 228–33.

Lapie, P., Goudet, C., Nargeot, J. *et al.* (1996). Electrophysiological properties of the hypokalaemic periodic paralysis mutation (R528) of the skeletal muscle $a_{1s}$ subunit as expressed in mouse L cell. *FEBS Lett.*, **382**, 244–8.

Lehmann-Horn, F., Engel, A. G., Ricker, K. *et al.* (1994). The periodic paralyses and paramyotonia congenita. In *Myology*, (eds Engel, A.G., Franzini-Armstrong, C.) pp. 1303–1334. New York: McGraw Hill.

McManis, P. G., Lambert, E. H. and Daube, J. R. (1986). The exercise test in periodic paralysis. *Muscle Nerve*, **9**, 704–10.

Moreno, M., Murphy, C. and Goldsmith, C. (1969). Increase in serum potassium resulting from the administration of hypertonic mannitol and other solutions. *J Lab Clin Med.*, **73**, 291–8.

Morrill, J. A., Brown, R. H. Jr. and Cannon, S. C. (1998). Gating of the L-type Ca channel in human skeletal myotubes: an activation defect caused by the hypokalemic periodic paralysis mutation R528H. *J Neurosci.*, **18**, 10320–34.

Plassart, E., Elbaz, A., Santos, J. V. *et al.* (1994). Genetic heterogeneity in hypokalemic periodic paralysis (hypoPP). *Hum Genet.*, **94**, 551–6.

Ptacek, L. J., Trimmer, J. S., Agnew, W. S. *et al.* (1991a) Paramyotonia congenita and hyperkalemic periodic paralysis map to the same sodium channel gene locus. *Am J Hum Genet.*, **49**, 851–4.

Ptacek, L. J., George, A. L. Jr., Griggs, R. C. *et al.* (1991b). Identification of a mutation in the gene causing hyperkalemic periodic paralysis. *Cell*, **67**, 1021–7.

Ptacek, L. J., Tawil, R., Griggs, R. C. *et al.* (1992). Linkage of atypical myotonia congenita to a sodium channel locus. *Neurology*, **42**, 431–3.

Ptacek, L. J., Tawil, R., Griggs, R. C. *et al.* (1994a). Dihydropyridine receptor mutations cause hypokalemic periodic paralysis. *Cell*, **77**, 863–8.

Ptacek, L. J., Tawil, R., Griggs, R. C. *et al.* (1994b). Sodium channel mutations in acetazolamide-responsive myotonia congenita, paramyotonia congenita, and hypekalemic periodic paralysis. *Neurology*, **44**, 1500–3.

Ptacek, L. (1998). The familial periodic paralyses and nondystrophic myotonias. *Am J Med.*, **105**, 58–70.

Resnick, J. S., Engel, W. K., Griggs, R. C. *et al.* (1968). Acetazolamide prophylaxis in hypokalemic periodic paralysis. *N Engl J Med.*, **278**, 582–6.

Rojas, C. V., Wang, J. Z., Schwartz, L. S. *et al.* (1991). A Met-to-Val mutation in the skeletal muscle $Na^+$ channel alpha subunit in hypekalemic periodic paralysis. *Nature*, **354**, 387–9.

Rudel, R., Lehman-Horn, F., Ricker, K. *et al.* (1984). Hypokalemic periodic paralysis: in vitro investigation of muscle fiber membrane parameters. *Muscle Nerve*, **7**, 110–20.

Rudel, R. and Ricker, K. (1985). The periodic paralyses. *Trends Neurosci.*, **8**, 467–70.

Sander, C. (1988). Treatment of hypokalemic periodic paralysis with diclofenamid. *Monatsschr Kinderheilkd.*, **136**, 149–50.

Sansone, V., Griggs, R. C., Meola, G. *et al.* (1997). Andersen's syndrome: a distinct periodic paralysis. *Ann Neurol.*, **42**, 305–12.

Sestoft, L. (1967). Direct transition from hypo- to hyperkalemic paralysis during potassium treatment of familial periodic paralysis. *Dan Med Bull.*, **14**, 157–60.

Tawil, R., Griggs, R. C. and Rose, M. (1999). Channelopathies. In *Neurogenetics,* (ed. Pulst, S.M.) pp 45–47. New York: Oxford University Press.

Tawil, R., McDermott, M. P., Brown, R. Jr. *et al.* (2000) Randomized clinical trials of dichlorphenamide in the periodic paralyses. *Ann Neurol.*, **47**, 46–53.

Tricarico, D., Servidei, S., Tonali, P. *et al.* (1999). Impairment of skeletal muscle adenosine triphosphate-sensitive $K^+$ channels in patients with hypokalemic periodic paralysis. *J Clin Invest.*, **103**, 675–82.

Zierler, K. L. and Andres, R. (1957). Movement of potassium into skeletal muscle during spontaneous attack in familial periodic paralysis. *J Clin Invest.*, **36**, 730–7.

# 11

# Malignant hyperthermia

*Terry D. Heiman-Patterson*

## Introduction and historical perspective

Malignant hyperthermia (MH) is an anaesthetic-induced syndrome that results in a hypermetabolic state. The pharmacological triggers are the volatile halogenated inhalation anaesthetics and depolarizing neuromuscular junction blockade (suxamethonium). The term MH was coined since there was a 70% mortality in untreated patients and initial case reports underscored the rapid rise in temperature occurring during anaesthesia. While the earliest descriptions of MH probably date back to 1900, when postoperative heat stroke was described (Tuttle, 1900); the first clear description of MH is credited to Denborough and Lovell (1960) who described a young man surviving an episode of hypotension, cyanosis, tachycardia, hyperthermia, and weakness following inhalation anaesthesia. He had told the physicians that 10 of 24 relatives who had previously undergone general anaesthesia had died. This history suggested an inherited disorder. Subsequently, additional cases described were found to have rhabdomyolysis with elevated creatine kinase (CK) (Denborough *et al.*, 1970). Further reports of an MH kindred with an autosomal dominant pattern of CK elevation suggested an association of MH with a myopathy and autosomal dominant inheritance (Isaacs and Barlow, 1970a, b). Thus, a connection between MH and underlying muscle disease was first suggested. Subsequent reports have documented several specific muscle disorders that are associated with MH and MH-like symptoms. The clinical picture is further complicated by the association of clinical events similar to MH with non-anaesthetic triggers, including neuroleptic malignant syndrome

triggered by neuroleptics. Thus MH may be considered a syndrome with several underlying causes, one of which is a genetic disease. It is likely that the underlying causes of the syndrome share some underlying pathophysiological mechanisms resulting in the clinical picture of MH. The most likely commonality relates to the regulation of $Ca^{2+}$ in muscle and elevated sarcoplasmic $Ca^{2+}$.

At the same time that clinical reports were appearing, diagnostic testing for MH susceptibility was described by Kalow and colleagues (1970). These investigators observed an increased contracture in muscle exposed to halothane and caffeine. This test could be applied to family members who had not undergone anaesthesia and a spectrum of susceptibility was defined (Britt, 1989). In some patients, family history and diagnostic testing indicated an inherited disorder with an autosomal dominant inheritance. While most families demonstrated an autosomal dominant inheritance of anaesthetic susceptibility, there were some families in which contracture testing suggested two different non-allelic genes were present and other families in which inheritance was multifactorial (McPherson and Taylor, 1981; Britt, 1989). Thus, the genetics of MH are complex (see below). Linkage studies assuming an autosomal dominant pattern of inheritance have identified at least four loci, with 20% of susceptible families linked to the Ryanodine receptor (RYR1) on chromosome 19q12-13.2 (McCarthy *et al.*, 1990).

The mainstay of treatment for an MH event is dantrolene; first described in MH swine (Harrison, 1975) and subsequently in humans (Austin and Denborough, 1977). Dantrolene, which decreases the release of $Ca^{2+}$ from the sarcoplasmic reticulum, has dramatically reduced the mortality of MH from 65% to under 10% (Britt and Kalow, 1970).

## Clinical presentation

### Epidemiology

MH is estimated to occur in 1 in 15 000 paediatric and 1 in 50 000–100 000 adult anaesthetic procedures (Britt, 1989). It is more common in males (3:1). Non-depolarizing muscle relaxants, including succinylcholine, as well as potent inhalation agents, including halothane, isoflurane, trichloroethylene, diethyl ether, enflurane, methoxyflurane, chloroform, cyclopropane, and ketamine, have all been identified as potential triggers. In addition, non-anaesthetic triggers have also been reported (see below). There may be a history of a previously uneventful anaesthetic in up to half the patients (Britt, 1989). This is likely related to variability in factors that influence whether an anaesthetic event will occur. These factors include the concentration of the anaesthetic agent, the use of succinylcholine with a potent inhalation agent, the duration of anaesthesia, the type of premedication, the state of the sympathetic nervous system, and the degree of susceptibility of the patient (Britt, 1989).

### Clinical evolution

Malignant hyperthermia is a hypermetabolic reaction. The initial sign of an episode is the rise in end-tidal $CO_2$ caused by an increased production of $CO_2$ as a byproduct of the hypermetabolic state (Gronert, 1981, 1983; Rosenberg, 1989). There is central venous desaturation along with the elevated end-tidal $CO_2$ in the context of a combined respiratory and metabolic acidosis. The initial clinical sign may be a failure to relax with succinylcholine. This is followed by tachycardia and tachypnoea with subsequent cyanosis in the face of a high inspired oxygen level and adequate ventilation. Acidosis develops along with rhabdomyolysis, and muscle rigidity. In one-third of patients there will be temperature elevations of 2–4°C/h with temperatures of 42.2°C(108°F) re-

ported. However, the hyperthermia can be delayed. Arrhythmias and hypertension are frequent and death often results from ventricular arrhythmia. Increases in serum CK, along with myoglobinuria, occur during the event. Hyperkalaemia, hyperphosphataemia, and hypercalcaemia can be found associated with rhabdomyolysis and muscle breakdown. Late complications include seizures, disseminated intravascular coagulopathy, acute renal failure, and acute pulmonary and cerebral oedema. With early recognition and aggressive treatment with datrolene sodium, the mortality has been reduced from 65% to 7% (see Treatment). The name 'malignant hyperthermia' was coined because of the high mortality and the marked rise in temperature. However, fever occurs late in the evolution of the MH episode, and often MH is recognized and treated before the temperature elevation occurs. Thus the term malignant hyperthermia may be a misnomer.

### Atypical presentations

#### Anaesthetic-induced atypical clinical presentations

There is large variability in the clinical picture and some, but not all, of the clinical features of an MH episode may be present. The first indication of an MH episode may be cardiac arrest or arrhythmia. The onset may be prolonged and symptoms mild, or there may be a fulminant evolution with rapid death. Of special interest is the group of children who exhibit masseter muscle rigidity when they receive succinylcholine with halogenated volatile anaesthetic. Approximately 50% of these patients will have a positive contracture test, indicating susceptibility for MH (Rosenberg and Fletcher, 1986; O'Flynn et al., 1994; see below: Diagnosis). It is important to recognize the presence of atypical masseter spasm so that the MH syndrome can be diagnosed early and therapy initiated.

#### Non-anaesthetic related clinical presentations

MH can present without an anaesthetic trigger (Denborough, 1996, 1998). Patients have been reported who present as heat stroke, rhabdomyolysis, chronically raised CK, myalgias, neuroleptic malignant syndrome, and sudden infant death syndrome. These patients had abnormal CK and positive contracture testing for MH susceptibility (see below: Diagnosis). Thus, while their clinical presentation was not associated with anaesthestic administration, the positive contracture test indicated MH susceptibility. Furthermore, in some of the cases, family members were also MH susceptible.

## Heat stroke

There have been at least five patients described who presented with heat stroke after vigorous exercise in hot weather (Denborough, 1982, 1996, 1998). These MH patients had rhabdomyolysis during exercise and subsequent contracture testing in the probands and other family members was positive. Furthermore, in a series of 55 patients with heat stroke, six patients were found to be MH susceptible on contracture testing along with some of their relatives (Kozak-Ribbens et al., 1994). These data suggest MH susceptible patients can trigger without anaesthetic exposure and present as heat stroke.

## Rhabdomyolysis

There have also been patients reported who developed rhabdomyolysis with elevated CK after a variety of triggers and were found to have positive contracture tests. In some of these cases, other family members also demonstrated MH susceptibility by contracture testing. Among the triggers reported were viral infections, exertion, and exposure to bromochlorodifluoromethane (a halothane-like gas) (Denborough, 1996, 1998). Myalgias with exercise but without rhabdomyolysis have also been described (Denborough, 1996).

## Neuroleptic malignant syndrome (NMS)

Neuroleptic malignant syndrome is an idiosyncratic disorder whose primary features include the development of rigidity and hyperthermia during the administration of neuroleptics or the withdrawal of dopaminergic agents. More than 25 pharmacological agents have been implicated, including most commonly the butyrophenones, phenothiazines, and thioxanthines. Treatment includes cessation of the pharmacological agent and administration of dantrolene along with dopaminergic agents.

Since NMS and MH share several common features, including muscle rigidity with elevated CK, hyperthermia, and a clinical response to dantrolene, there is concern that MH susceptible patients can present with NMS events. Both syndromes are induced by pharmacological agents. While MH is inherited, there is no genetic basis for NMS. There has been ongoing controversy over the relationship of NMS to MH. While some patients who have presented with NMS have demonstrated positive contracture testing, indicating MH susceptibility (Caroff et al., 1983; Downey et al., 1984), others report negative contracture tests in NMS patients (Tolefson 1982; Adnet et al., 1989). Studies have demonstrated that neuroleptic drugs also raise the sarcoplasmic $Ca^{2+}$ levels but by a different mechanism than halothane. While halothane increases sarcoplasmic reticulum release of $Ca^{2+}$, neuroleptics not only increase the efflux of $Ca^{2+}$ from the sarcoplasmic reticulum, they also inhibit $Ca^{2+}$-dependent ATPase and ATP-dependent $Ca^{2+}$ uptake by the sarcoplasmic reticulum (Collins et al., 1987). These findings may explain why neuroleptics can trigger MH-like events in MH susceptible patients. However, it is likely that not all patients with NMS events are MH susceptible.

## Sudden infant death syndrome (SIDS)

MH has also been associated with SIDS. An early report reviewed a case in which a man's son died of SIDS and who himself had had three cardiac arrests following an appendectomy. The patients contracture test was positive (Denborough, 1981). Subsequently, biopsies were performed on 15 parents who had babies with SIDS. Five of these parents had positive tests (Denborough et al., 1982). Epidemiological studies have demonstrated an excess number of anaesthetic deaths in SIDS families (Peterson and Davis, 1986). Finally, MH susceptible swine exposed to a heat challenge as newborns developed MH and a significant proportion died (Denborough et al., 1996). This further supports the view that the MH myopathy predisposes to both MH and SIDS.

## Diagnosis

The diagnosis of MH involves not only the intra-operative assessment of patients with suggestive symptoms but also the evaluation of patients potentially at risk for MH. The 'at risk' group includes patients who have had an event during anaesthesia and relatives of MH patients. Additional indications for MH testing are controversial but include patients with neuromuscular diseases, osteogenesis imperfecta, or those who have conditions that can be associated with MH.

The intraoperative diagnosis of MH relies on the recognition of the clinical picture by the anaesthesiologist. In some patients, the earliest sign is the failure of the masseter to relax with succinylcholine, while in others it is a rise in end-tidal $CO_2$. The diagnosis is supported by the presence of a mixed respiratory and metabolic acidosis in conjunction with elevated end-tidal $CO_2$ and tachycardia. Other signs include tachypnoea, hypertension, and muscle rigidity. Patients may demonstrate lactic acidosis along with hyperkalaemia, elevated phosphate, elevated CK, and myoglobinuria. There can be a delay in the onset of symptoms with patients presenting as postoperative fevers. Once the syndrome is suspected, treatment should be initiated immediately (see Treatment below).

The differential diagnosis includes disorders with symptoms similar to MH such as phaeochromocytoma and thyrotoxicosis. However, acute treatment of symptoms suggestive of MH should begin immediately and should not be delayed by tests to investigate these alternative diagnoses. In addition, hyperthermia can occur in the context of non-anaesthetic drugs including neuroleptics, anticholinergic poisoning, and serotonin syndrome (Chan et al., 1997), thereby mimicking one aspect of MH.

While many non-invasive tests for MH susceptibility have been suggested, invasive testing with muscle biopsy and contracture testing remains the most reliable method to determine MH status. CK testing was frequently used to screen at risk patients in a family since CK increases were demonstrated in 50% of subjects in a large MH kindred (Isaacs and Barlow, 1970b). This suggested an autosomal dominant inheritance and the possibi-

lity that CK might provide a non-invasive screen for at risk patients for MH susceptibility. However, in a large study that examined the relationship of elevated CK to contracture tests results, there was no predictive value for CK levels (Paasuke and Brownell, 1986). Furthermore, while histological changes are common in MH susceptible patients, the changes are non-specific (Harriman et al., 1977; Isaacs, 1977; Harriman, 1988). Similarly, other non-invasive blood tests that have been suggested, including halothane-induced calcium uptake into lymphocytes, platelet aggregation with nucleotide depletion in the presence of halothane, and red cell fragility; have all proved unreliable (Rosenberg, 1989b). Future tests based on genetic analysis of DNA isolated from the leukocytes of patients and relatives may prove useful in selected cases; however, owing to the heterogeneity of MH, a single genetic test is not a reasonable expectation (Hogan, 1997). Furthermore, there are reports of families in which mutations have been identified but in which there is not strict genotype and phenotype (positive contracture test) correlation (Deufel et al., 1995; O'Brien et al., 1995; Serfas et al., 1996). Finally, nuclear MRI techniques show an increased ratio of inorganic phosphate to phosphocreatine at rest, as well as abnormalities of the high energy phosphate recovery curve following exercise (Olgin et al., 1988). Although no false negative results were identified when spectroscopy results were compared to contracture testing response, there was overlap between some normal patients and MH-susceptible patients. Furthermore, similar results have been seen in patients with other neuromuscular diseases.

Invasive procedures using skeletal muscle obtained during muscle biopsy for in vitro contracture testing remain the most reliable method for predicting MH susceptibility (Gronert, 1981, 1983; Rosenberg and Reed, 1983; Rosenberg, 1989b). The halothane-caffeine contracture test first suggested by Kalow et al. (1970) consists of exposing thin strips (1 cm × 1 mm) of muscle to Krebs-Ringer solution at 37°C, bubbled with 95% oxygen and 5% carbon dioxide. The strips are stimulated electrically to achieve a supramaximal response. Once equilibration is obtained, strips are exposed to 3% halothane and/or caffeine and the amount of contracture (increase in resting tension) that develops is recorded. The strength of the muscle contracture is related to the free $Ca^{2+}$ within the myoplasm. In MH there is an elevated myoplasmic $Ca^{2+}$ at baseline. Halothane causes release of calcium from the sarcoplasmic reticulum thereby further elevating the myoplasmic calcium. Therefore the increased contracture that develops upon exposure to halothane and/or caffeine supports the notion that raised $Ca^{2+}$ plays a primary role in the genesis of the syndrome (see below: Pathogenesis). Halothane, in causing the increased sarcoplasmic $Ca^{2+}$, results in the *in-vitro* contracture and the '*in vivo*' MH syndrome.

The contracture test requires that muscle be viable and therefore the biopsy must be done on site and cannot be shipped. There are two basic protocols for the tissue: the North American Group protocol and the European Malignant Hyperthermia Group protocol. Both protocols utilize halothane or caffeine addition to the tissue baths containing the muscle and measure the tension that develops in the strips of muscle. In the European protocol, incremental doses of halothane up to 2% are used as well as incremental doses of caffeine. The North American protocol uses a single dose of halothane (3%) and incremental doses of caffeine. Patients with MH susceptibility have increased contracture '*in vitro*' upon exposure to halothane and caffeine. Standards for increased contracture of the muscle on exposure to halothane, caffeine, or halothane plus caffeine have been defined to identify MH susceptibility. A patient is considered positive if their skeletal muscle develops a contracture of 0.5 g or more to 3% halothane or a contracture of 0.2 g or more to 2 mmol/l caffeine (Moulds and Denborough, 1974). The contracture test performed using the North American protocol demonstrates 92% sensitivity and 74% specificity. Up to 5–15% of patients may have ambiguous results and are considered positive in the North American protocol. The ambiguity may relate to variability of the biological test, the variability in pathophysiology of the MH syndrome, or the non-specificity of the test. Unfortunately, since all patients who have undergone biopsy cannot be exposed to anaesthetic challenge to verify results, the true predictive value, sensitivity, and specificity of the test cannot be ascertained.

# Treatment and prognosis

Once an episode of MH is suspected, the triggering anaesthetic must be immediately stopped. The patient should be hyperventilated with 100% oxygen. Dantrolene sodium is the mainstay of pharmacological treatment for both an MH event as well as being preventative treatment in a susceptible individual. Its efficacy was described in susceptible swine in 1975 (Harrison, 1975) and its use in humans reported first in 1977 (Austin and Denborough, 1977). Dantrolene sodium likely acts at the level of the sarcoplasmic reticulum to inhibit the release of $Ca^{2+}$ stimulated by halothane. The usual starting dose for an event is 2.5 mg/kg intravenously. Doses as high as 10 mg/kg may be required for control. Repeat doses of dantrolene sodium are administered every 6 h until the event resolves, with close monitoring of blood gases, electrolytes, glucose, CK, and urine myoglobin. In addition to the administration of dantrolene, the acidosis is treated with bicarbonate at doses of 2–4 mEq/kg (Gronert, 1981, 1983). The patient should also be iced as necessary to reduce temperature. If hyperkalaemia occurs, it should be treated with glucose, insulin, calcium, and bicarbonate. Care needs to be taken to avoid hypokalaemia since potassium replacement can retrigger the syndrome. The patient requires an intensive care unit, continued dantrolene, and treatment of rhabdomyolysis if it occurs. Finally, there should be close monitoring of coagulation studies to monitor for the presence of disseminated intravascular coagulopathy. Prior to the availability of dantrolene as the treatment of choice for malignant hyperthermia, the mortality rate from an MH event was as high as 60–70%. Presently, the mortality has been reduced to under 10% (Britt and Kalow, 1970).

Patients who are at risk for an MH event should have anaesthesia with non-triggering agents. This includes patients with a previous history of an event, patients with positive contracture tests, patients with a family history of MH, and patients with an associated disorder including the myopathies (See below: Associated disorders). Safe agents include antibiotics, antihistamines, antipyretics, atracurium, barbiturates, benzodiazepines, droperidol, ketamine, local anaesthetics, mivacurium, opioids, nitrous oxide, pancuronium, propofol, propranolol, vasoactive drugs, and vecuronium. Phenothiazines should be avoided. Careful monitoring of exhaled $CO_2$, heart rate, muscle tone, and temperature and an available supply of dantrolene should be sufficient precaution. The anaesthesia machine should be prepared by draining or removing the vaporizers used for triggering volatile anaesthetics. Also, the tubing and $CO_2$ absorbant should be changed and the oxygen flow maintained at 10 l/minute for 10 to 20 minutes prior to use.

Regional, local, or major conduction anaesthetics with either amide or ester local anaesthetic are advised when appropriate. In other cases, barbiturate or narcotic induction followed by nitrous oxide/oxygen and non-depolarizing neuromuscular blockade (not curare) and opioid supplementation may be appropriate. Induction can also be safely produced with diazepam, droperidol, midazolam, and propofol. Anticholinesterase and anticholinergics are safe for use.

# Associated disorders

## Musculoskeletal abnormalities

Musculoskeletal abnormalities are common both in patients and first degree relatives (Britt, 1989). The most common abnormalities include kyphosis, scoliosis, pectus deformities, strabismus, ptosis, dislocated patella, poor dentition with crowded teeth, cryptorchidism, hernias, and cramps.

## King-Denborough syndrome

The King-Denborough syndrome is characterized by MH, myopathy, and skeletal dysmorphisms. It occurs predominantly in young boys and dysmorphic features have included short stature, cryptorchidism, webbed neck, lordosis, kyphosis, low set ears, winged scapula, pectus excavatum, and an antimongoloid slant of the palpebral fissures (King and Denborough, 1973; Heiman-Patterson et al., 1986). Muscle biopsies in these children have shown non-specific changes suggestive of a myopathy including variation in fibre size, increased central nuclei, regeneration and degeneration, poor fibre type differentiation, and type I hypertrophy. We performed halothane contracture testing for MH susceptibility in a young boy with King-Denborough syndrome and also in other family members (Heiman-Patterson et al., 1986). A positive contracture test was found in the boy as well as his mother who had only scoliosis and a history of three previous anaesthetics all of which were uneventful. These results have several explanations. First, King-Denborough syndrome may be part of an autosomal dominantly inherited MH syndrome with the disparate number of dysmorphisms between the boy and his mother emphasizing the phenotypic heterogeneity of the MH syndrome. A second possibility is that MH and King-Denborough syndrome may be closely linked and inherited together. Finally, the association of MH and King-Denborough could be coincidental.

## Myopathies and neuromuscular diseases

MH was first associated with neuromuscular disease in 1970. At that time Isaacs and Barlow (1970a) described an MH kindred with elevated CK in an autosomal dominant pattern. They suggested that there was a subclinical myopathy in patients with MH. Additionally, in a follow-up study of the first reported MH patient, the young man and his family were evaluated for the presence of elevated CK and myopathy. In fact, it was found that the boy's father, paternal aunt and sister all had elevated CK and his father and aunt had a myopathy (Denborough et al., 1970). Furthermore, many non-specific abnormalities have been described on histopathological examination of biopsied muscle from patients with MH (Harriman et al., 1977; Harriman, 1988). The most frequently described changes include variation in fibre size, increased internal nuclei, and architectural changes on reduced nicotinamide-adenine dinucleotide staining. There may also be small angulated fibres and type II atrophy. Other changes including regeneration and necrosis have also been reported. We studied histopathological findings in 102 patients with positive contracture tests for

MH susceptibility and 104 patients who tested negatively for MH susceptibility. Almost 50% of the positively testing patients had no pathological changes, while 88% of the patients testing negatively were normal (Heiman-Patterson, 1991). The most frequent abnormalities in our patients were variation in fibre size, angulated fibres, type II atrophy, and architectural changes. Three of our patients had central core disease. These findings were similar to those reported in the literature, further validating the presence of muscle abnormalities in MH. However, negatively testing patients had similar findings albeit less frequent.

The *Evans myopathy*, named for the family in which MH was first described, is usually applied to the mild subclinical myopathy seen in association with MH to distinguish this mild myopathy from the specific diseases that have been associated with MH events (Denborough *et al.*, 1970; Harriman *et al.*, 1977). Patients with Evans myopathy often have no weakness, although there can be wasting of the lower thighs. The CK can be elevated but is frequently normal. Muscle biopsy findings are non-specific.

Several specific neuromuscular disorders have also been identified in patients who have experienced anaesthetic events that were similar, if not identical to MH (Heiman-Patterson, 1991; Heiman-Patterson *et al.*, 1988). In 1973, an aunt of the original proband reported by Denborough and Lovell was found to have *central core disease* (Denborough *et al.*, 1973; Isaacs and Barlow, 1974). Several additional reports documenting this association have appeared in the literature (Eng *et al.*, 1978). Anaesthetic events have also been reported with *myotonia congenita* (Heiman-Patterson *et al.*, 1988), *myotonic dystrophy* (Saidman *et al.*, 1964), *Duchenne and Beckers muscular dystrophy* (Brownell *et al.*, 1983; Heiman-Patterson *et al.*, 1986), and *congenital muscular dystrophy* (Fletcher *et al.*, 1982).

In order to determine if the neuromuscular population is at a higher risk of MH, we performed contracture tests in 25 patients undergoing diagnostic biopsies (Heiman-Patterson *et al.*, 1988). Positive contracture tests were observed in seven out of 18 patients with myopathic disorders and three of seven patients with neurogenic disorders. Similar results were reported with caffeine contracture tests in 21 patients with myopathic and four patients with neurogenic disorders (Takagi *et al.*, 1983). These authors reported positive tests in a variety of disorders including Duchenne muscular dystrophy, adult onset muscular dystrophy, infantile hypotonia, congenital muscular dystrophy, central core disease, and polyradiculitis. We found positive halothane contracture tests in similar groups of patients as well as in spinal muscle atrophy, fascioscapulohumeral dystrophy, limb girdle dystrophy, and Beckers muscular dystrophy. Thus, both the standard halothane testing of muscle fibres and the caffeine skinned fibre contracture testing have shown an abnormal response in various neuromuscular diseases.

The positive contracture tests in patients with neuromuscular diseases suggests that these disorders may share pathogenetic mechanisms with MH resulting in the development of muscle contracture on exposure of skeletal muscle to halothane. One possible shared abnormality is elevated calcium concentration in the muscle cell, since elevated myoplasmic calcium has been reported in MH as well as several neuromuscular disorders including Duchenne and Beckers muscular dystrophy (Bodensteiner and Engel, 1978; Lopez *et al.*, 1985). It has been suggested that when the myoplasmic calcium levels in MH muscle surpass a critical threshold, a chain of biochemical events is triggered that leads to the development of the MH syndrome (Eng *et al.*, 1978; see below: Pathogenesis). Halothane exposure induces an efflux of calcium from the sarcoplasmic reticulum in skeletal muscle. Thus, if the intracellular calcium is already elevated at baseline, a critical threshold may be reached on exposure to halothane, leading to the initiation of a cascade of biochemical events that results in a positive contracture test *in vitro* or an anaesthetic event *in vivo*.

Although the presence of an abnormal contracture test in the neuromuscular population might simply suggest that the test is non-specific and the abnormal response due to diseased tissue, suspicious anaesthetic events have been reported in patients with a variety of neuromuscular diseases (Waters *et al.*, 1977; Brownell *et al.*, 1983; Rosenberg and Heiman-Patterson, 1983; Heiman-Patterson *et al.*, 1988) and the contracture test is still the most specific test of MH susceptibility. Thus, patients with neuromuscular disorders may be at higher risk than the general population for the development of MH-like episodes.

## Other disorders

In addition to the association of MH with various neuromuscular disorders, there have been reports of MH-like anaesthetic events and positive contracture testing with non-neuromuscular disorders such as osteogenesis imperfecta and myelomeningocele (Nelson and Flewellen, 1983; Rampton et al., 1984).

## Genetics

While autosomal dominant inheritance is most common, studies indicate in some families there may be two different non-allelic genes present and in other families inheritance is multifactorial (McPherson and Taylor, 1981; Britt, 1989). The gene for MH is estimated to occur in from one in 10 000 to 1 in 250 000 people based on the clinical presentation (Britt and Kalow, 1970; Ording, 1985). Since many people with MH do not develop MH on some or all exposures the true incidence of the gene is unknown.

Linkage studies in autosomal dominant kindreds have suggested that one gene causing MH in humans resides close to or at the gene locus of the skeletal muscle ryanodine receptor RYR1; the calcium release channel of the sarcoplasmic reticulum, on chromosome 19q13.1 (McCarthy et al., 1990). There are at least 18 different mutations identified in this locus including a small number of unrelated kindreds with the C1840T mutation, which results in a change in arginine to cystine at the 614 position. This is the same mutation identified in the recessive porcine malignant hyperthermia with a lod score of 101.75 at a recombination fraction of theta = 0.00 (Otsu et al., 1991).

Mutations in the RYR1 receptor are linked to 50% of kindreds. However, there has been discordance reported between contracture test results and the presence of the Arg614Cys mutation of the RYR1 gene in some kindreds (Serfas et al.,

1996; Fortunato et al., 1999) and, in two of the families, recombination events between the MH susceptibility and the C1840T mutation have been reported (Fagerlund et al., 1997). Thus, it is necessary to reconsider both the specificity of contracture testing and the role of the C1840T mutation as a cause for MH susceptibility. However, strong evidence exists for the C1840T mutation as causal in MH in both swine and humans. Both the high lod score in the swine linkage studies, combined with the association of the mutation with MH across species provides strong genetic evidence. Further, purified ryanodine receptors from MH swine that were reconstituted into lipid bilayers, demonstrated prolonged open times and shortened closed times compared with normal calcium release channels (Shomer et al., 1993). Finally, expression of RYR1 cDNA containing the Arg614Cys mutation in muscle cells and COS-7 cells leads to hypersensitive gating of $Ca^{2+}$ release in the transfected cells (Otsu et al., 1994; Treves et al., 1994).

Other loci identified include the regions at or close to the alpha-subunit of the adult sodium channel on chromosome 17q (Olckers et al., 1992), the alpha2/delta-subunits of the dihydropyridine receptor on chromosome 7q (Iles et al., 1994), the region near the alpha subunit of the dihydropyridine receptor on chromosome 1q (Robinson et al., 1977), a region on chromosome 5p (Robinson et al., 1977), and a region on chromosome 3q13.1 (Sudbrak et al., 1995). In addition to the primary gene defect, there appears to be a modulator that is crucial in precipitating the syndrome (Fletcher et al., 1993).

## Pathogenesis

Studies of MH pathogenesis have focused on swine models, which closely resemble the human disorder clinically and biochemically. These inbred strains of swine were first reported to develop convulsions and death with succinylcholine in 1966 (Hall et al., 1966). Subsequently, there were additional reports of pigs that developed hyperthermia and seizures with halothane (Harrison et al., 1968). Exposure of these pigs to halothane provided a window into the earliest biochemical changes that occur during an MH event. In these pigs, the first change to occur was lactic acidosis with a drop in blood pH. This rise in lactic acid was accompanied by a rise in $CO_2$ and drop in bicarbonate levels (Denborough *et al.*, 1973). Temperature elevation follows the lactic acidosis. The most suggestive abnormalities are related to the control of $Ca^{2+}$.

Elevated levels of calcium in the sarcoplasm have been reported and are likely caused by an abnormality of the sarcoplasmic reticulum $Ca^{2+}$ release mechanisms (Endo *et al.*, 1983; Mickelson *et al.*, 1986). The major calcium release channel of the sarcoplasmic reticulum is the ryanodine channel (RYR1), a homotetrameric complex constructed from a 565-kilodalton subunit (Mac-Lennan and Phillips, 1992). It is named for the plant alkaloid, ryanodine, which binds the receptor releasing $Ca^{2+}$ from the sarcoplasmic reticulum (Sutko *et al.*, 1985; Zorzato *et al.*, 1990; McPherson and Campbell, 1993). Abnormalities in ryanodine channel function have been reported in both the swine and humans with MH (Mickelson *et al.*, 1986, 1988). Furthermore, as described above, mutations in the ryanodine receptor gene have been found in 50% of MH kindreds and a specific point mutation at C1840T has been found in MH susceptible swine in some human families.

Elevated myoplasmic calcium that results from the abnormal function of the RYR1 receptor has been postulated to set off a cascade of biochemical events resulting in lactic acidosis, muscle rigidity, and heat production along with an energy crisis (Eng *et al.*, 1978; Gronert, 1981; MacLennan and Phillips, 1992). Elevated myoplasmic $Ca^{2+}$ stimulates phosphorylase kinase leading to increased glycolysis that results in the formation of lactic acid and initiates muscle contraction by binding to troponin. It also increases the use of adenosine triphosphate (ATP) through the stimulation of myosin ATPase and leads to the sequestering of $Ca^{2+}$ within mitochondria in an energy (ATP) requiring process despite the already depleted ATP stores. This results in further ATP loss, increased carbon dioxide production, and worsening acidosis. Finally, uncoupling of oxidative phosphorylation and uncontrolled heat production occur. In the swine model, $^{31}P$ nuclear magnetic resonance studies have shown that the elevated temperature is due to the continued $Ca^{2+}$-induced synthesis and hydrolysis of ATP (Foster *et al.*, 1989). Soon ATP depletion surpasses ATP production, and energy necessary for critical cell functions is not available. The integrity of the sarcolemma can no longer be maintained and additional $Ca^{2+}$ leaks into muscle while CK, potassium, and myoglobin leak out. In addition, there are data suggesting that an increase in phospholipase A2 activity occurs and leads to increased mitochondrial free fatty acids (FFA) as well as increased calcium release (Cheah and Cheah, 1981).

Thus, whatever mechanism leads to elevated myoplasmic $Ca^{2+}$, once present, it can cause biochemical changes that lead to the MH syndrome. The elevated $Ca^{2+}$ may be the shared mechanism between MH and the disorders associated with MH-like symptoms. For instance, in Duchenne muscular dystrophy, there is an elevated myoplasmic $Ca^{2+}$ which may underlie the MH-like events that have been reported.

While some families with MH have been shown to have a mutation in the skeletal muscle RYR1 calcium receptor of the sarcoplasmic reticulum and abnormal RYR1 receptor function could lead to elevated myoplasmic $Ca^{2+}$ and disturbed $Ca^{2+}$ regulation occurring with anaesthesia, other kindreds have been identified in which MH susceptibility does not link to the ryanodine receptor (Olckers *et al.*, 1992; Iles *et al.*, 1994; Sudbrak *et al.*, 1995, see above). In these families, different genetic defects could lead to elevated myoplasmic $Ca^{2+}$ through different mechanisms resulting in the MH syndrome under anaesthesia.

# References

Adnet, P. J., Krivosic-Horber, R. M., Adamantidis, M. M. *et al.* (1989). The association between neuroleptic malignant syndrome and malignant hyperthermia. *Acta Anaesthesiol Scand.*, **33**, 676–80.

Austin, K. L. and Denborough, M. A. (1977). Drug treatment of malignant hyperpyrexia. *Anaesth Intens Care*, **5**, 207–13.

Bodensteiner, J. B. and Engel, A. G. (1978). Intracellular calcium accumulation in Duchenne dystrophy and other myopathies: A study of 567,000 muscle fibers in 114 biopsies. *Neurology*, **28**, 439–46.

Britt, B. A. (1989). Hereditary and epidemiologic

aspects of malignant hyperthermia. In *Malignant Hyperthermia: Current Concepts* (eds Naida Felipe, M. A., Gottman, S. and Khambata, H. J.). pp 19–44. Bad Hamburg: Normed Verlag.

Britt, B. A. and Kalow, W. (1970). Malignant hyperthermia: A statistical review. *Can Anaesth Soc J.*, **17**, 293–315.

Brownell, A. K. W., Paasuke, R. T, Elash, A. *et al.* (1983). Malignant hyperthermia in Duchenne muscular dystrophy. *Anesthesiology*, **58**, 182–4.

Caroff, S., Rosenberg, H. and Gerber, J. C. (1983). Neuroleptic malignant syndrome and malignant hyperthermia. *Lancet*, i, 244.

Chan, T. C., Evans, S. D. and Clark, R. F. (1997). Drug-induced hyperthermia. *Crit Care Clin.*, **13**, 785–808.

Cheah, K. S. and Cheah, A. M. (1981). Skeletal muscle mitochondrial phospholipase A2 and the interaction of mitochondria and sarcoplasmic reticulum in porcine malignant hyperthermia. *Biochim Biophys Acta.* **12**, 638(1), 40–9.

Collins, S. P., White, M. D. and Denborough, M. A. (1987). The effects of calmodulin antagonist drugs on isolated sarcoplasmic reticulum from malignant hyperpyrexia susceptible swine. *Int J Biochem.*, **19**, 819–26.

Denborough, M. A. (1981). Sudden infant death syndrome and malignant hyperthermia. *Med J Aust.*, i, 649–50.

Denborough, M. A. (1982). Heat stroke and malignant hyperpyrexia. *Med J Aust.*, i, 204–5.

Denborough, M. A. (1996). Clinical classification and incidence of malignant hyperthermia in Australia. In *Proceedings of the 3rd International Symposium on Malignant Hyperthermia* (eds Morio, M., Kikuchi, H. and Yuge, O). pp 43–47. Tokyo: Springer Verlag.

Denborough, M. A. (1998). Malignant hyperthermia (seminar). *Lancet*, **352**, 1131–6.

Denborough, M. A., Dennet, X. and Anderson, R. M. (1973). Central core disease and malignant hyperthermia. *Br Med J.*, **1**, 272–3.

Denborough, M. A., Ebeling, P. , King, J. O. and Zapf, P. (1970). Myopathy and malignant hyperpyrexia. *Lancet*, i, 1138–40.

Denborough, M. A., Forster, J. F. A., Hudson, M. C. *et al.* (1970). Biochemical changes in malignant hyperpyrexia. *Lancet*, i, 1137–8.

Denborough, M. A., Galloway, G. J. and Hopkinson, K. C. (1982). Malignant hyperpyrexia and sudden infant death. *Lancet*, ii, 1068–9.

Denborough, M. A., Hird, F. J. R., King, J. O. *et al.* (1973). Mitochondrial and other studies in Australian Landrace pigs affected with malignant hyperpyrexia. In *International Symposium on Malignant Hyperthermia* (eds Gordon, R. A., Britt, B. A. and Kalow, W.) pp 229–237. Charles C. Thomas.

Denborough, M. A., Hopkinson, K. C., O'Brien, R. O. and Foster, P. S. (1996). Overheating alone can trigger malignant hyperthermia in piglets. *Anaesth Intens Care*, **24**, 348–54.

Denborough, M. A. and Lovell, R. R. H. (1960). Anaesthetic deaths in a family. *Lancet*, ii, 45.

Deufel, T., Sudbrak, R., Feist, Y. *et al.* (1995). Discordance in a malignant hyperthermia pedigree between in vitro contracture test phenotypes and haplotypes for the MHS1 region on chromosome 19q12-q13.2, comprising the C1840T transition in the RYR1 gene. *Am J Hum Genet.*, **56**, 1334–6.

Downey, G. P., Rosenberg, H., Caroff, S. *et al.* (1984). Neuroleptic malignant syndrome: patient with unique clinical and physiological features. *Am J Med.*, **77**, 338–40.

Endo, M., Yagi, S., Ishizuka, T. M. *et al.* (1983). Changes in the Ca-induced Ca release mechanisms in the sarcoplasmic reticulum of the muscle from a patient with malignant hyperthermia. *Biomed Res.*, **4**, 83–92.

Eng, G. D., Epstein, B. S., Engel, K. *et al.* (1978). Malignant hyperthermia and central core disease in a child with congenital dislocating hips. *Arch Neurol.*, **35**, 189–92.

Fagerlund, T. H., Ording, H., Bendixen, D. *et al.* (1997). Discordance between malignant hyperthermia susceptibility and RYR1 mutation C1840T in two Scandinavian MH families exhibiting this mutation. *Clin Genet.*, **52**, 416–21.

Fletcher, J. E., Calvo, P. A. and Rosenberg, H. (1993). Phenotypes associated with malignant hyperthermia susceptibility in swine genotyped as homozygous or heterozygous for the ryanodine receptor mutation. *Br J Anaesth.*, **71**, 410–7.

Fletcher, R., Blennow, G., Olsson, A. K. *et al.* (1982). Malignant hyperthermia in a myopathic child: Prolonged post-operative course requiring dantolene. *Acta Anaesthiol Scand.*, **26**, 435–8.

Fortunato, G., Carsana, A., Tinto, N. *et al.* (1999). A case of discordance between genotype and phenotype in a malignant hyperthermia family. *Eur J Hum. Genet.*, 7, 415–20.

Foster, P. S., Hopkinson, K. and Denborough, M. A. (1989). 31P-NMR spectroscopy: the metabolic profile of malignant hyperpyrexia porcine skeletal muscle. *Muscle Nerve*, **12**, 390–6.

Gronert, G. (1981). Puzzles in malignant hyperthermia. *Anesthesiology*, **54**, 1–2.

Gronert, G. (1983). Malignant hyperthermia. *Semin Anaesthesia*, **2**, 97–204.

Hall, L. W., Woolf, N., Bradley, J. W. P. and Jolly, D. W. (1966). Unusual reaction to suxamethonium chloride. *Br Med J*, **2**, 1305.

Harriman, D. G. F. (1988). Malignant hyperthermia myopathy – a critical review. *Br J Anaesth.*, **60**, 309–16.

Harriman, D. G. F., Ellis, F. R., Franka, A. J. *et al.* (1977). Malignant hyperthermia myopathy in man: An investigation of 75 families. In *Second International Symposium on Malignant Hyperthermia* (eds

Aldrette, J. A. and Britt, B. A.) pp 67-87. New York: Grune and Stratton.

Harrison, G. G. (1975). Control of the malignant hyperpyrexic syndrome in MHS swine by dantrolene sodium. *Br J Anaesth.*, **47**, 62–5.

Harrison, G. G., Biebuyck, J F., Terblanche, J. *et al.* (1968). Hyperpyrexia during anesthesia. *Br Med J.*, **3**, 594–5.

Heiman-Patterson, T. D. (1991). Malignant hyperthermia. *Sem Neurol.*, **11**, 220–7.

Heiman-Patterson, T. D., Binning, C. P. S. and Tahmoush, A.J. (1986). King Denborough Syndrome: Contracture Testing and Review of the Literature. *Pediatr Neurol.*, **2**, 175–8.

Heiman-Patterson, T. D., Martino, C., Rosenberg, H., Fletcher, J. and Tahmoush, A. J. (1988). Malignant Hyperthermia in Myotonia Congenita. *Neurology*, **38**, 810–2.

Heiman-Patterson, T. D., Natter, H. M., Rosenberg, H., Fletcher, J. E. and Tahmoush, A. J. (1986). Malignant Hyperthermia Susceptibility in X-Linked Muscle Dystrophies. *Pediatr Neurol.*, **2**, 356–8.

Heiman-Patterson, T. D., Rosenberg, H., Fletcher, J. E. and Tahmoush, A. J. (1988). Contracture Testing for Malignant Hyperthermia in Neuromuscular Diseases. *Muscle Nerve*, **38**, 810–2.

Hogan, K. (1997). Molecular medicine and malignant hyperthermia: A step ahead. *Anesthesiology*, **86**, 511–3.

Iles, D. E., Lehmann-Horn, F., Scherer, S. W. *et al.* (1994). Localization of the gene encoding the alpha2/delta-subunits of the L-type voltage-dependent calcium channel to chromosome 7q and analysis of the segregation of flanking markers in malignant hyperthermia susceptible families. *Hum Mol Genet.*, **3**, 969–75.

Isaacs, H. (1977). Myopathy and malignant hyperthermia. In *Second International Symposium on Malignant Hyperthermia* (eds Aldrette, J. A. and Britt, B. A.) pp 89–101. New York: Grune and Stratton.

Isaacs, H. and Barlow, M. B. (1970a). Malignant hyperpyrexia during anesthesia: Possible association with subclinical myopathy. *Br Med J.*, **2**, 275–7.

Isaacs, H. and Barlow, M. B. (1970b). The genetic background to malignant hyperpyrexia revealed by serum creatine phosphokinase estimation in asymptomatic relatives. *Br J Anaesth.*, **42**, 1077.

Isaacs, H. and Barlow, M. B. (1974). Central core disease associated with elevated creatine kinases: Two members of a family known to be susceptible to malignant hyperpyrexia. *South Afr Med J.*, **46**, 640–2.

Kalow, W., Britt, B. A., Terreau, M. E. *et al.* (1970). Metabolic error of muscle metabolism after recovery from MH. *Lancet*, ii, 895–8.

King, J. O. and Denborough, M. A. (1973). Anesthetic induced malignant hyperpyrexia in children. *J Pediatr.*, **83**, 37–40.

Kozak-Ribbens, G., Rodet, L., Petrognani, R. *et al.*

(1994). Hyperthermie d'effort (HE): resultats des explorations de 55 patients. In *Workshop in Anaesthesia and Pharmacogenetic Diseases: malignant hyperthermia* (eds Novelli, G. P. and Tegazzini, V.) *Minerva Anestesiol.*, **60** (suppl. 3), 177–81.

Lopez, J. R., Alamo, L., Caputo, C. *et al.* (1985). Intracellular ionized calcium concentration in muscle from humans with malignant hyperthermia. *Muscle Nerve*, **8**, 355–8.

MacLennan, D. H. and Phillips, M. S. (1992). Malignant hyperthermia. *Science*, **256**, 789–93.

McCarthy, T. V., Healy, J. M. S., Heffron, J. J. A. *et al.* (1990). Localization of the malignant hyperthermia susceptibility locus to human chromosome 19q12-13.2. *Nature*, **343**, 562–4.

McPherson, P. S. and Campbell, D. P. (1993). The ryanodine receptor/$Ca^{2+}$ release channel. *J Biol Chem.*, **268**, 13765–68.

McPherson, E. W. and Taylor, C. A. Jr (1981). The genetics of malignant hyperthermia: Evidence for heterogeneity. *Am J Med Genet.*, **8**, 159–65.

Mickelson, J. R., Gallant, E. M., Litterer, L. A. *et al.* (1988). Abnormal sarcoplasmin reticulum ryanodine receptor in malignant hyperthermia. *J Biol Chem.*, **263**, 9310–5.

Mickelson, J. R., Ross, J. A., Reed, B. K. *et al.* (1986). Enhanced $Ca^{2+}$-induced calcium release by isolated sarcoplasmic reticulum vesicles from malignant hyperthermia susceptible pig muscle. *Biochem Biophys Acta*, **862**, 318–328.

Moulds, R. F. W. and Denborough, M. A. (1974). Identification of susceptibility to malignant hyperthermia. *Br Med J.*, **2**, 245–7.

Nelson, T. E. and Flewellen, E. H. (1983). The malignant hyperthermia syndrome. *N Eng J Med.*, **309**, 416–8.

O'Brien, R. O., Taske, N. L., Hansboro, P. M. *et al.* (1995). Exclusion of defects in the skeletal muscle specific regions of the DHPRa1 subunit as frequent causes of malignant hyperthermia. *J Med Genet.*, **32**, 913–4.

O'Flynn, R. P., Shutack, J. G., Rosenberg, H. *et al.* (1994). Masseter muscle rigidity and malignant hyperthermia susceptibility in pediatric patients. An update on management and diagnosis. *Anesthesiology*, **80**, 1228–33.

Olckers, A., Meyers, D. A., Meyers, S. *et al.* (1992) Adult muscle sodium channel alpha-subunit is a gene candidate for malignant hyperthermia susceptibility. *Genomics*, **14**, 829–31.

Olgin, J., Argov, Z., Rosenberg, H. *et al.* (1988). Non-invasive testing of malignant hyperthermia susceptibility with phosphorus nuclear magnetic resonance spectroscopy. *Anesthesiology*, **68**, 507–13.

Ording, H. (1985). Incidence of malignant hyperthermia in Denmark. *Anesth Analg.*, **64**, 700–4.

Otsu, K., Nishida, K., Kimura, Y. *et al.* (1994). The point mutation Arg615Cys in the 4Calcium $2^+$ release channel of skeletal sarcoplasmic reticulum is responsible for hypersensitivity to caffeine and halothane in malignant hyperthermia. *J Biol Chem.*, **269**, 9413–5.

Otsu, K., Khanna, V. K., Archibald, A. L. and MacLennan, D. H. (1991). Cosegregation of porcine malignant hyperthermia and a probable causal mutation in the skeletal muscle ryanodine receptor gene in backcross families. *Genomics*, **11**, 744–50.

Paasuke, R. T. and Brownell, A. K. (1986). Serum creatine kinase level as a screening for susceptibility to malignant hyperthermia. *JAMA*, **255**, 769–74.

Peterson, D. R. and Davis, N. (1986). Sudden infant death syndrome and maligant hyperthermia diathesis. *Aust J Paediatr.*, **22** (suppl), 33–5.

Rampton, A. J., Kelly, D. A., Shanahan, E. C. *et al.* (1984). Occurence of malignant hyperthermia in a patient with osteogenesis imperfecta. *Br J Anaesth.*, **56**, 1443–4.

Robinson, R. L., Monnier, N., Wolz, W. *et al.* (1997). A genome wide search for susceptibility loci in three European malignant hyperthermia pedigrees. *Hum Mol Genet.*, **6**, 953–61.

Rosenberg, H. (1989). Clinical presentation of malignant hyperthermia. In *Malignant Hyperthermia: Current Concepts* (eds Naida Felipe, M. A., Gottman, S. and Khambata, H. J.) pp. 40–46. Bad Hamburg: Normed Verlag.

Rosenberg, H. (1989b). Testing for malignant hyperthermia. In *Malignant Hyperthermia: Current Concepts* (eds Naida Felipe, M. A., Gottman, S. and Khambata, H. J.) pp 47–52. Bad Hamburg: Normed Verlag.

Rosenberg, H. and Fletcher, J. E. (1986). Masseter muscle rigidity and malignant hyperthermia susceptibility. *Anesth Analg.*, **65**, 161–4.

Rosenberg, H. and Heiman-Patterson, T. D. (1983). Duchenne's Muscular Dystrophy in Malignant Hyperthermia. Another Warning. *Correspondence Anesthesiology*, **59**, 362.

Rosenberg, H. and Reed, S. (1983). In vitro contracture tests for susceptibility to malignant hyperthermia. *Anesth Analg.*, **62**, 415–20.

Saidman, L. J., Harvard, E. S. and Eger, E. L. (1964).

Hyperthermia during anesthesia. *JAMA.*, **190**, 1029–32.

Serfas, K. D., Deepak, M. D., Patel, L. *et al.* (1996). Comparison of the segregation of the RYR1 C1840t Mutation with segregation of the Caffeine/Halothane Contracture Test results for Malignant Hyperthermia Susceptibility in a Large Manitoba Mennonite Family. *Anesthesiology*, **84**, 322–9.

Shomer, N. H., Louis, C. F., Fill, M. *et al.* (1993). Reconstitution of abnormalities in the malignant hyperthermia-susceptible pig ryanodine receptor. *Am J Physiol.*, **264**, C125–35.

Sudbrak, R., Procaccio, V., Klausnitzer, M., Curran, J. L. *et al.* (1995). Mapping of a further malignant hyperthermia susceptibility locus to chromosome 3q13.1. *Am J Hum Genet.*, **56(3)**, 684–91.

Sutko, J. L., Ito, K. and Kenyon, J. L. (1985). Ryanodine: a modifier of sarcoplasmic calcium release in striated muscle. *Fed Proc.*, **44**, 2984–8.

Takagi, A., Sunohara, N., Ishiahara, T. *et al.* (1983). Malignant hyperthermia and related neuromuscular disease: caffeine contracture of the skinned muscle fibers. *Muscle Nerve*, **6**, 510–4.

Tolefson, G. (1982). A case of neuroleptic malignant syndrome: In vitro muscle comparison with malignant hyperthermia. *J Clin Psychpharmacol.*, **2**, 266–70.

Treves, S., Larini, F., Menigazzi, P. *et al.* (1994). Alteration of intracellular Calcium $2^+$ transients in COS-7 cells transfected with cDNA encoding skeletal muscle ryanodine receptor carrying a mutation associated with malignant hyperthermia. *Biochem J.*, **301**, 661–5.

Tuttle, J. P. (1900). Heat-stroke as a postoperative complication. *JAMA.*, **35**, 1685.

Waters, G., Karpati, G. and Kaplan, B. (1977). Post anesthetic augmentation of muscle damage as a presenting sign in three patients with Duchenne muscular dystrophy. *Can J Neurol Sci.*, **9**, 228.

Zorzato, F., Fujii, J, Otsu, K. *et al.* (1990). Molecular cloning of DNA encoding human and rabbit forms of the $CA2^+$ release channel (Ryanodine receptor) of skeletal muscle sarcoplasmic reticulum. *J Biol Chem.*, **265**, 2244–56.

# CHAPTER 12

# Acetylcholine receptor channelopathies and other congenital myasthenic syndromes

*Andrew G. Engel, Kinji Ohno and Steven M. Sine*

## Introduction: Overview of the congenital myasthenic syndromes

Congenital myasthenic syndromes (CMS) are inherited disorders in which the safety margin of neuromuscular transmission is compromized by one or more specific mechanisms. The slow-channel CMS is transmitted by dominant inheritance; all other CMS recognized to date are transmitted by autosomal recessive inheritance (Engel *et al.*, 1999). In 125 CMS kinships investigated at the Mayo Clinic, the defect was presynaptic in nine, synaptic in 17, post-synaptic in 95, and unclassified in four. Except for the CMS associated with plectin deficiency (Banwell *et al.*, 1999), which will not be considered here, all post-synaptic CMS stem from a defect in the nicotinic muscle acetylcholine receptor (AChR) (Table 12.1). There-fore, on the average, three out of four CMS patients suffer from an AChR channelopathy.

## Diagnosis

CMS are not uncommon, but are commonly undiagnosed or diagnosed incorrectly. A *generic diagnosis* of a CMS can be made on clinical grounds from a history of fatiguable weakness involving ocular, bulbar and limb muscles since infancy or early childhood, a history of similarly affected relatives, a decremental EMG response, and negative tests for acetylcholine receptor (AChR) antibodies. In some CMS, however, the onset is delayed, the EMG abnormalities are not present in all muscles, or are present only intermittently, and the weakness has a restricted distribution. Sometimes clinical or EMG clues can point to the correct diagnosis:

| Table 12.1 Classification of CMS and index patients investigated at the Mayo Clinic | |
|---|---|
| *Presynaptic defects* | |
| Defect in ACh resynthesis/packaging (CMS with episodic apnoea) | 7 |
| Paucity of synaptic vesicles | 1 |
| Lambert Eaton syndrome-like CMS | 1 |
| *Synaptic defect* | |
| Endplate AChE deficiency | 17 |
| *Post-synaptic defects* | |
| Primary kinetic abnormality with/without AChR deficiency | 30 |
| Primary AChR deficiency with/without minor kinetic abnormality | 64 |
| Myasthenic syndrome with plectin deficiency | 1 |
| No identified defect | 4 |
| *Total* | 125 |

1. A repetitive compound muscle action potential (CMAP) in response to a single stimulus occurs in endplate (EP) acetylcholinesterase (AChE) deficiency (Engel *et al.*, 1977) and in the slow-channel CMS (Engel *et al.*, 1982).
2. Refractoriness to cholinesterase inhibitors and delayed pupillary light reflexes suggest EP AChE deficiency (Engel *et al.*, 1977; Hutchinson *et al.*, 1993).
3. Selectively severe weakness of cervical and wrist and finger extensor muscles is found in the slow-channel CMS (Engel *et al.*, 1982) and in older patients with EP AChE deficiency (Hutchinson *et al.*, 1993).
4. A history of recurrent apnoeic episodes provoked by stress suggests a defect in the resynthesis or vesicular packaging of acetylcholine (ACh). Here a decremental EMG is not found in rested muscle but appears after a few minutes of stimulation at 10 Hz (Mora *et al.*, 1987).

## Differential diagnosis

In the neonatal period, infancy and childhood, the differential diagnosis includes spinal muscular atrophy, morphologically distinct congenital myopathies, congenital muscular dystrophies, infantile myotonic dystrophy, mitochondrial myopathy, brainstem anomaly, Möbius syndrome, congenital fibrosis of the extraocular muscles, infantile botulism, and seropositive and seronegative autoimmune myasthenia gravis (MG). In older patients, the differential diagnosis includes motor neuron disease, limb girdle or facioscapulohumeral dystrophy, mitochondrial myopathy, chronic fatigue syndrome, and seropositive and seronegative MG. Radial nerve palsy, peripheral neuropathy, and syringomyelia have been incorrectly diagnosed in some cases of the slow-channel CMS.

## Investigation of the CMS

A deeper understanding of disease mechanisms and a precise classification of the CMS requires estimation of the number of AChRs per EP, light and electron microscopic analysis of EP morphology, and electrophysiologic assessment of EP function *in vitro*. Conventional microelectrode studies of EP potentials and currents readily reveal presynaptic defects in quantal release and altered post-synaptic responses to the released quanta, while patch-clamp recordings of currents flowing through single AChR channels provide precise information on the conductance and kinetic properties of the channels. If the foregoing studies point to a defect in a candidate gene or protein, then molecular genetic analysis becomes feasible. If a mutation is discovered in the candidate gene, then expression studies with the genetically engineered mutant molecule can be used to confirm pathogenicity and to analyse the properties of the mutant molecule. To date, the candidate gene approach has resulted in discovery of more than 70 mutations in different subunits of the AChR and of 18 mutations in the collagenic tail subunit of the EP species of AChE.

## Acetylcholine receptor channelopathies

### The nicotinic acetylcholine receptor

The muscle nicotinic AChR is a pentameric transmembrane macromolecule with a subunit composition of $\alpha_2\beta\delta\varepsilon$ at adult endplates, and $\alpha_2\beta\delta\gamma$ at fetal endplates and extrajunctional sites (Figure 12.1). In humans, the genes encoding the $\alpha$-, $\delta$-, and $\gamma$-subunits are at different loci on chromosome 2q; the genes encoding the $\beta$- and $\varepsilon$-subunits are at different loci on chromosome 17p. Neuronal AChRs are also pentameric, composed of moieties of two $\alpha$- ($\alpha_2-\alpha_7$) and three $\beta$- ($\beta_2-\beta_4$) subunits, or exist as $\alpha$-homopentamers. Both muscle and neuronal AChRs are members of a superfamily of ligand-gated ion channels that also includes receptors for 5-hydroxytryptamine, $\gamma$-aminobutyric acid, and glycine. Subunits of these receptors have similar sequences; hence they fold similarly and assemble into receptors that have similar secondary, tertiary, and quaternary structures. A characteristic feature of subunits in this superfamily is two cysteine (Cys) residues separated by 13 other residues in the N-terminal extracellular domain.

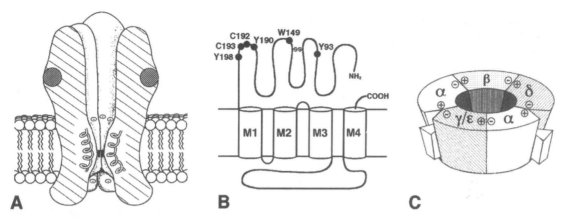

**Figure 12.1** Schematic diagrams: (A) AChR in lipid bilayer showing putative ACh binding pockets (shaded circles) and the central pore of the channel. (B) Folding pattern of the $\alpha$-subunit; residues indicated on 3 peptide loops are implicated in governing affinity for ACh. (C) Cross-section of AChR at the level of the ACh binding pocket. Note circular arrangement of AChR subunits and that the ACh binding pockets appear at the interfaces between $\alpha$- and $\varepsilon/\gamma$-subunits, and between the $\alpha$- and $\delta$-subunits.

The two Cys residues are disulphide-linked in the mature receptor to form a 15-residue loop. For this reason, members of the superfamily are also known as Cys-loop receptors (Karlin and Akabas, 1994). We here discuss channelopathies arising from mutations in muscle AChR. Chapter 16 deals with the channelopathies arising from mutations in neuronal AChRs.

The five subunits of AChR are organized like barrel staves around a central cation-permeable channel. Each subunit has an N-terminal extracellular domain that comprises ~50% of the primary sequence, four putative transmembrane domains (M1–M4), and a small C-terminal extracellular domain. M2, which lines the ion channel, forms an $\alpha$-helix interrupted by a short stretch of $\beta$-sheet (see Figure 12.1). C-terminal residues of the M1 domain may also contribute to the channel lumen in the resting state (Akabas and Karlin, 1995). The transmembrane domains are connected by an extracellular M2/M3 linker and by intracellular M1/M2 and M3/M4 linkers (Figure 12.1B). The M3/M4 linker forms a long cytoplasmic loop that likely serves as an attachment site for cytoskeletal elements and bears phosphorylatable residues that may be important for desensitization. Each AChR has two ACh binding pockets positioned at the $\alpha/\varepsilon$- (or $\alpha/\gamma$) and $\alpha/\delta$-interfaces. Residues con-

tributing to the binding pocket appear on three peptide loops on $\alpha$, and on four peptide loops on $\varepsilon$, $\delta$, and $\gamma$ (Prince and Sine, 1998). An essential framework for activation of the AChR channel can be shown in a linear scheme

$$\begin{array}{ccc} k_{+1} & k_{+2} & \beta \\ A + R \rightleftarrows AR \rightleftarrows A_2R \rightleftarrows A_2R^* \\ k_{-1} & k_{-2} & \alpha \end{array}$$

where two ACh molecules (A) bind to the receptor R with association rates $k_{+1}$ and $k_{+2}$ and dissociate from it with rates $k_{-2}$ and $k_{-1}$. The double-liganded receptor ($A_2R$) opens with rate $\beta$, and the open receptor ($A_2R^*$) closes with rate $\alpha$. The scheme predicts that the mean duration of channel opening episodes is approximately $(1 + \beta/k_{-2})/\alpha$. This value also corresponds to the decay time constant of the miniature EP current (MEPC) in response to the instantaneous release of a quantum of ACh at EPs where AChE activity is intact.

The scheme represented above is simplified by not showing the following:

1. Reversible transitions of AR into the open state $AR^*$; such transitions are likely to occur at low concentrations of ACh and decrease in frequency with increasing concentration of ACh.
2. Reversible transitions of the receptor into a

non-conducting desensitized state on prolonged exposure to high concentrations of the agonist.

3. Very fast blockages of the open channel by ACh when the ACh concentration exceeds 30 $\mu M$.

4. The allosteric model of AChR predicts that even the unliganded receptor R can enter the open state $R^*$, and that transitions can occur between $R^*$ and $AR^*$ as well as between $AR^*$ and $A_2R^*$, the different states thus forming a closed two-dimensional network (Edelstein and Changeux, 1998).

The linear model of receptor activation, which is a subset of the general allosteric model of activation, neglects the additional transitions because they occur at a very low probability. The additional transitions, however, become important with some mutations that perturb the balance between allosteric states. For example, replacement of a proline by a leucine residue at position 121 in the $\varepsilon$-subunit ($\varepsilon$ P121L) increases the equilibrium dissociation constant for ACh binding to $AR^*$ to form $A_2R^*$; this destabilizes the diliganded open state relative to the diliganded closed state, thereby reducing the probability and duration of channel opening events (Ohno et al., 1996a); and slow-channel mutations destabilize closed states, whether liganded or not, thereby increasing the probability and duration of all open states (Ohno et al., 1995a; Milone et al., 1997).

## Classification of the AChR channelopathies

All AChR channelopathies arise from mutations in AChR subunits that increase or decrease the response to ACh. An increased response to ACh is observed with gain-of-function mutations that slow the decay of the EP currents and prolong the duration of channel opening episodes. These disorders are referred to as slow-channel syndromes. A decreased response to ACh is caused by two types of loss-of-function mutations:

1. Mutations that act primarily by reducing the expression of EP AChR.

2. Mutations that speed the decay of EP currents

and decrease the duration of channel opening episodes; these syndromes are collectively referred to as fast-channel-syndromes.

The terms 'slow' and 'fast' are accurate in the strict sense of the term when they refer to the decay of EP currents. The duration of channel activation episodes, however, is determined by microscopic rate constants for agonist association ($k_{+1}$ and $k_{+2}$), and dissociation ($k_{-2}$ or $k_{-1}$), and by rates of channel opening ($\beta$) and closure ($\alpha$), and these may become faster or slower in either syndrome. For example, prolonged activation episodes could result from a faster than normal $\beta$, a slower than normal $\alpha$, a decrease in $k_{-2}$, or a combination of these changes; conversely, brief activation episodes could stem from reciprocal alteration of the same rate constants. Other names for the slow- and fast-channel syndromes would be slow- and fast-EP-current syndromes, or long- and short-channel-activation syndromes. Because these terms are awkward, the slow-channel syndromes are defined as CMS associated with prolonged EP currents and channel activation episodes; and the fast-channel syndromes are defined as CMS associated with abnormally brief EP currents and channel activation episodes (Figure 12.2B, C). In some fast-channel syndromes, however, miniature EP currents may be difficult to record or analyse owing to their low amplitude, very fast decay, or low probability of opening.

## Increased response to ACh: the slow-channel syndromes

The clinical phenotypes vary. Some slow-channel CMS present in early life and cause severe disability by the end of the first decade (Milone et al., 1997); others present later in life and progress slowly, resulting in little disability even in the sixth or seventh decade (Engel et al., 1982, 1999; Sine et al., 1995). Most patients show selectively severe involvement of cervical, wrist and finger extensor muscles.

The phenotypic consequences stem from prolonged opening episodes of the AChR channel in the presence of ACh (Figure 12.2B). Additionally, increased opening of unliganded receptors, plus

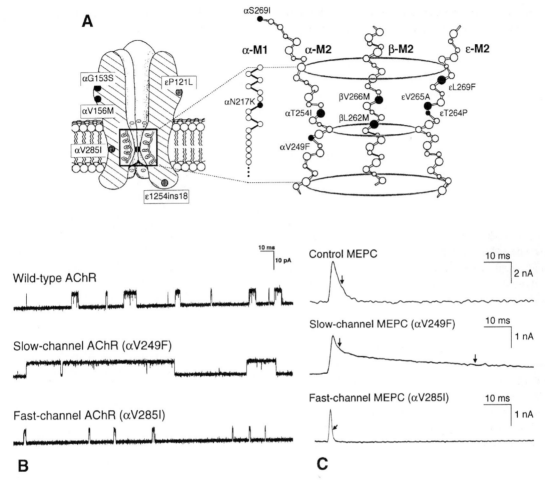

**Figure 12.2** (A) Schematic diagram of slow-channel (solid circles) and fast-channel (shaded circles) mutations reported to date. The drawing on the left shows a section through the acetylcholine receptor with two slow-channel mutations, αG153S and αV156M, in the extracellular domain near the ACh binding site of the α-subunit, and 3 fast channel mutations: εP121L near the ACh binding site of the ε-subunit, αV156M in the M3 domain of the α-subunit, and ε1254ins18 in the long-cytoplasmic loop of the ε-subunit. In the drawing on the right, dotted lines delimit transmembrane domains. Slow-channel mutations appear in the M2 domains of the α-, β-, and ε-subunits, and in the M1 domain of the α-subunit. The αS269I slow-channel mutation above the dotted line is in the extracellular M2–M3 linker. (B) Examples of single channel currents from wild-type, slow-channel (αV249F), and fast-channel (αV285I) AChRs expressed in HEK cells. (C) Miniature endplate currents (MEPC) recorded from endplates of a control subject, a patient harbouring the αV249F slow-channel mutation, and a patient harbouring the αV285I fast-channel mutation. Arrows indicate decay time constants. The slow-channel MEPC decays biexponentially due to expression of both wild-type and mutant AChRs at the EP, with one decay time constant that is normal and one that is markedly prolonged. (Reproduced from Engel, A. G. *et al.* Congenital Myasthenic Syndromes, in *Myasthenia Gravis and Myasthenic Disorders* (eg. Engel, A. G.), pp. 251–297. New York: Oxford University Press, 1999.)

activation by choline, normally present in serum at 10 $\mu$M, contribute to cationic overloading of the junctional sarcoplasm and an EP myopathy (Zhou *et al.*, 1999). The EP myopathy comprises degeneration of the junctional folds with loss of AChR, widening of the synaptic space, and subsynaptic alterations consisting of degeneration of organelles, apoptosis of nuclei, and vacuolar change (Engel *et al.*, 1982, 1996a, 1999; Milone *et al.*, 1997). The prolonged channel activation episodes prolong the EP potential beyond the refractory period of the muscle fibre, so that a single nerve stimulus elicits one or more repetitive CMAPs. During physiological activity, the prolonged EP potentials undergo staircase summation producing a depolarization block (Sine *et al.*, 1995; Ohno *et al.*, 1995a; Engel *et al.*, 1996a).

Eleven slow-channel mutations have been reported to date (Sine *et al.*, 1995; Ohno *et al.*, 1995a, 1998a, 2000; Engel *et al.*, 1996a; Gomez *et al.*, 1996; Croxen *et al.*, 1997; Milone *et al.*, 1997; Wang *et al.*, 1997) (Figure 12.2A, solid circles). The different mutations occur in different AChR subunits and in different functional domains of the subunits. Patch-clamp studies at the EP, mutation analysis, and expression studies in human embryonic kidney (HEK) cells indicate that the αG153S mutation near extracellular ACh binding site (Sine *et al.*, 1995) and the αN217K mutation in the N-terminal part of M1 (Wang *et al.*, 1997) act mainly by enhancing affinity for ACh. This slows dissociation of ACh from the binding site and results in repeated channel reopenings during the prolonged receptor occupancy. Another slow-channel mutation near the binding site region, αV156M, probably has the same effects, although its mechanistic consequences have not been investigated (Croxen *et al.*, 1997). Mutations in the M2 domain that lines the channel pore, such as βV266M, εL269F, εT264P and αV249F, promote the open state by affecting channel opening and closing steps (Ohno *et al.*, 1995a; Engel *et al.*, 1996a; Milone *et al.*, 1997). Increases in steady-state affinity for ACh are also observed, which are largely accounted for by an increased extent of desensitization; increased affinity is most marked in the case of αV249F (Milone *et al.*, 1997), pronounced with εL269F [17], εT264P (Ohno *et al.*, 1995a; Milone *et al.*, 1997) and not apparent with βV266M (Engel *et al.*, 1996a).

Following the lead that quinidine is a long-lived open-channel blocker of AChR (Sieb *et al.*, 1996), Fukudome and coworkers (1998) showed that clinically attainable levels of quinidine normalize the prolonged opening episodes of mutant slow-channels expressed in HEK cells. On the basis of these findings, Harper and Engel (1998) treated slow-channel patients with quinidine sulphate, 200 mg three to four times daily, producing serum levels of 0.7–2.5 $\mu$g/ml (2.1–7.7 $\mu$M/L), and

found that the patients were improved by clinical as well as by EMG criteria.

## Decreased response to ACh: the fast channel syndromes

These CMS are caused by recessive, loss-of-function mutations of AChR that reduce the affinity for ACh, primarily affect channel gating, or cause mode-switching kinetics. The common features of the syndromes are rapidly decaying EP currents, brief channel activation episodes (see Figure 12.2B and C), and a reduced probability of channel opening in the presence of ACh. Three fast-channel mutations have been reported to date (Figure 12.2A, shaded circles). In each disorder, the mutated allele causing the kinetic abnormality is accompanied by a null mutation in the second allele; therefore the kinetic mutation dominates the clinical phenotype. The fast-channel syndromes, and especially the low-affinity fast-channel syndrome, respond well to combined therapy with 3,4-diaminopyridine (1 mg per kg per day given in three to five divided doses) which increases the number of quanta released by nerve impulse, and cholinesterase inhibitors, which increase the number of AChRs activated by each quantum.

## Low-affinity fast channel syndrome

This is a severely disabling CMS whose clinical features closely resemble severe autoimmune myasthenia gravis. The MEPCs are very small but, unlike in autoimmune myasthenia gravis, EP ultrastructure and AChR counts per EP are normal. The phenotype is determined by a mutation in the extracellular domain of the ε-subunit, εP121L. Patch-clamp studies of genetically engineered εP121L-AChR expressed in human embryonic kidney (HEK) fibroblasts reveal a marked *decrease* of the channel opening rate, $\beta$, few if any channel reopenings, a reduced affinity for ACh in the open channel and desensitized states, resistance to desensitization on exposure to high concentrations of ACh, and a markedly reduced probability of channel opening (Ohno *et al.*, 1996a).

## Fast-channel syndrome due to a gating abnormality

Patients with this CMS have only mild myasthenic symptoms. The phenotype is determined by a mutation in the M3 domain of the AChR $\alpha$-subunit, $\alpha$V285I, which causes a kinetic abnormality (see Figure 12.2B, C) and also reduces the expression of AChR at the EP. Studies of the mutant receptor at the endplate and HEK cells reveal that the channel opening rate, $\beta$, is decreased, the channel closing rate, $\alpha$, is enhanced, and the probability of channel opening is reduced (Wang et al., 1998).

## Fast-channel syndrome due to mode-switching kinetics

This CMS causes moderately severe symptoms. The kinetically significant mutation is an in-frame duplication of six residues in the long cytoplasmic loop of $\varepsilon$, $\varepsilon$1254ins18, which also reduces AChR expression at the EP (Milone et al., 1998). At the EP, the $\varepsilon$1254ins18 mutant shows abnormally brief activation episodes during steady-state agonist application and is electrically silent or undetectable during the synaptic response to ACh. When expressed in HEK cells, the mutant AChR exhibits mode switching in the kinetics of activation in which the normal high efficiency of gating is accompanied by two new modes that gate inefficiently, opening more slowly and closing more rapidly than normal. In this disorder, the EP AChR deficiency and the reduced efficiency of synaptic transmission are partially compensated for by the expression of fetal AChR harbouring the $\gamma$-instead of the $\varepsilon$-subunit ($\gamma$-AChR); this restores electrical activity at EP and rescues the phenotype (Milone et al., 1998).

## Decreased response to ACh: mutations causing AChR deficiency with or without minor kinetic abnormalities

CMS with severe EP AChR deficiency result from different homozygous or, more frequently, heterozygous recessive mutations in AChR subunit genes. The mutations are concentrated in the $\varepsilon$-subunit (Figure 12.3, Table 12.2). There are two possible reasons for this:

1. Expression of the fetal type $\gamma$-subunit, although at a low level, may compensate for absence of the $\varepsilon$-subunit (Engel et al., 1996b; Ohno et al., 1997; Milone et al., 1998), whereas patients harbouring null mutations in subunits other than $\varepsilon$ might not survive for lack of a substituting subunit.
2. The gene encoding the $\varepsilon$-subunit, and especially the exons coding for the long cytoplasmic loop, have a high GC content that likely predisposes to DNA rearrangements (Krawczak and Cooper, 1991).

Morphological studies show an increased number of EP regions distributed over an increased span of the muscle fibre. The integrity of the junctional folds is preserved, but AChR expression on the folds is patchy and faint. Some EP regions are simplified and small, and there is a non-specific decrease in the number of openings between the primary and secondary synaptic clefts. The amplitude of miniature EP potentials (MEPPs) and currents is reduced, but quantal release by nerve impulse is often higher than

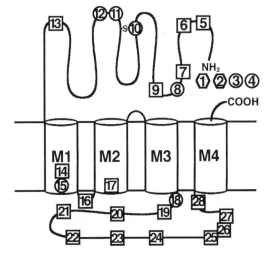

**Figure 12.3** Schematic diagram of AChR $\varepsilon$-subunit showing location of 28 recessive mutations that reduce AChR expression. □, null mutations; ○, missense mutations; hexagons, mutations in promoter region. Table 12.2 identifies the 28 mutations.

**Table 12.2 Identified mutations in the $\varepsilon$-subunit of AchR**

| | Mutations | Domains | Reference |
|---|---|---|---|
| 1 | $\varepsilon$-156C$\rightarrow$T | Ets binding site | Nichols *et al.* (1999) |
| 2 | $\varepsilon$-155G$\rightarrow$A | Ets binding site | Ohno *et al.* (1999) |
| 3 | $\varepsilon$V-13D | Signal peptide | Middleton *et al.* (1999) |
| 4 | $\varepsilon$G-8R | Signal peptide | Ohno *et al.* (1996a) |
| 5 | $\varepsilon$59ins5 | Extracellular domain | Ohno *et al.* (1998b) |
| 6 | $\varepsilon$70insG | Extracellular domain | Ohno *et al.* (1998b) |
| 7 | $\varepsilon$127ins5 | Extracellular domain | Ohno *et al.* (1997) |
| 8 | $\varepsilon$T51P | Extracellular domain | Middleton *et al.* (1999) |
| 9 | $\varepsilon$R64X | Extracellular domain | Ohno *et al.* (1997) |
| 10 | $\varepsilon$C128S | Disulphide loop | Milone *et al.* (1998) |
| 11 | $\varepsilon$S143L | N-glycosylation site | Ohno *et al.* (1996a) |
| 12 | $\varepsilon$R147L | Extracellular domain | Ohno *et al.* (1997) |
| 13 | $\varepsilon$553del7 | Extracellular domain | Ohno *et al.* (1995b, 1997); Milone *et al.* (1996) |
| 14 | $\varepsilon$723delC | M1 domain | Middleton *et al.* (1999) |
| 15* | $\varepsilon$P245L | M1 domain | Ohno *et al.* (1997) |
| 16 | $\varepsilon$IVS7+2T$\rightarrow$C | Link between M1 and M2 | Ohno *et al.* (1998b) |
| 17 | $\varepsilon$760ins8 | M2 domain | Middleton *et al.* (1999) |
| 18* | $\varepsilon$R311W | Long cytoplasmic loop | Ohno *et al.* (1997) |
| 19 | $\varepsilon$IVS9-1G$\rightarrow$C | Long cytoplasmic loop | Ohno *et al.* (1995b) |
| 20 | $\varepsilon$1012del20 | Long cytoplasmic loop | Ohno *et al.* (1996b) |
| 21 | $\varepsilon$1033delG | Long cytoplasmic loop | Brengman *et al.* (1998) |
| 22 | $\varepsilon$1101insT | Long cytoplasmic loop | Engel *et al.* (1996b) |
| 23 | $\varepsilon$IVS10+2T$\rightarrow$G | Long cytoplasmic loop | Middleton *et al.* (1999) |
| 24 | $\varepsilon$1206ins19 | Long cytoplasmic loop | Ohno *et al.* (1998b) |
| 25 | $\varepsilon$1259del23 | Long cytoplasmic loop | Brengman *et al.* (1998) |
| 26 | $\varepsilon$1267delG | Long cytoplasmic loop | Ohno *et al.* (1998b); Abicht *et al.* (1999); Croxen *et al.* (1999) |
| 27 | $\varepsilon$1276delG | Long cytoplasmic loop | Ohno *et al.* (1998b) |
| 28 | $\varepsilon$1293insG | Long cytoplasmic loop | Engel *et al.* (1996b) |

*Mutation also has significant kinetic effects.

normal. With null or low-expressor mutations in the $\varepsilon$-subunit, both single channel recordings (Milone *et al.*, 1996; Ohno *et al.*, 1997) and immunocytochemical studies (Engel *et al.*, 1996b) reveal $\gamma$-AchR at the EP, and the expression of $\gamma$-AchR at the EP likely rescues the phenotype. Most patients respond to anticholinesterase drugs, and some derive additional benefit from 3,4-diaminopyridine.

Different recessive mutations causing severe EP AchR deficiency have been identified:

1. Mutations causing premature termination of the translational chain – these mutations are frameshifting (Ohno *et al.*, 1995b, 1996b, 1997, 1998b; Engel *et al.*, 1996b; Croxen *et al.*, 1996

1999; Abicht *et al.*, 1999; Middleton *et al.*, 1999), occur at a splice site (Ohno *et al.*, 1995b, 1998b; Middleton *et al.*, 1999), or produce a stop codon directly (Ohno *et al.*, 1997).

2. Point mutations in the promoter region of a subunit gene $\varepsilon$-155G $\rightarrow$ A (Ohno *et al.*, 1999) and $\varepsilon$-156C $\rightarrow$ T (Nichols *et al.*, 1999).

3. Missense mutations in a signal peptide region, ($\varepsilon$G-8R) (Ohno *et al.*, 1996a) and $\varepsilon$V-13D (Middleton *et al.*, 1999).

4. Mutations involving residues essential for assembly of the pentameric receptor. Mutations of this type were observed in the $\varepsilon$-subunit at an N-glycosylation site ($\varepsilon$S143L) (Ohno *et al.*, 1996a), in cysteine 128 ($\varepsilon$C128S), a residue that is an essential part of the C128-C142

disulphide loop in the extracellular domain (Milone *et al.*, 1998), in arginine 147 ($\varepsilon$R147L) in the extracellular domain, which lies between isoleucine 145 and threonine 150, residues that contribute to subunit assembly (Ohno *et al.*, 1997), and in threonine 51 ($\varepsilon$T51P) (Middleton *et al.*, 1999); and with a 3 codon deletion in the long cytoplasmic loop of the $\beta$-subunit (Quiram *et al.*, 1999).

5. Missense mutations affecting both AChR expression and kinetics. For example, $\varepsilon$R311W in the long cytoplasmic loop between M3 and M4 decreases (Ohno *et al.*, 1997), whereas $\varepsilon$P245L in the M1 domain increases (Ohno *et al.*, 1997) the open duration of channel events. In the case of $\varepsilon$R311W and $\varepsilon$P245L, the kinetic consequences are modest and are likely overshadowed by the reduced expression of the mutant gene.

# Congenital myasthenic syndromes not due to AChR channelopathies

## Defect in ACh resynthesis or vesicular packaging (CMS with episodic apnoea)

The clinical features of this disorder were recognized more than three decades ago under the rubric of 'familial infantile myasthenia' (Greer and Schotland, 1960; Robertson *et al.*, 1980), but it was not differentiated from MG until the autoimmune origin of MG was established, and until electrophysiological and morphological differences were demonstrated between MG and the congenital syndrome (Hart *et al.*, 1979; Engel and Lambert, 1987; Mora *et al.*, 1987). Because all CMS can be familial and because most CMS present in infancy, the term 'familial infantile myasthenia' has become a source of confusion (Christodoulou *et al.*, 1997; Middleton *et al.*, 1999).

The distinguishing feature of this CMS is sudden episodes of apnoea precipitated by infections, fever, or excitement. In some patients the disease presents at birth with hypotonia, and severe bulbar and respiratory weakness requiring ventilatory support that gradually improves, but is followed by apnoeic attacks associated with bulbar paralysis in later life. Other patients are normal at birth and first experience the typical attacks during infancy or early childhood. Variable ptosis and fatiguable weakness may persist between the attacks. The ocular muscles are usually spared.

Endplate studies reveal no AChR deficiency and the post-synaptic region of the EP shows no abnormality. The MEPP is normal in rested muscle but decreases abnormally during 10 Hz stimulation for 5 minutes (Mora *et al.*, 1987). The number of quanta released by nerve impulse is not affected by 10 Hz stimulation (Tsujino *et al.*, 2000). The stimulation-dependent decrease of the MEPP amplitude points to a defect in choline reuptake by the nerve terminal, in choline acetyltransferase, or in vesicular filling with ACh. This hypothesis was recently confirmed by tracing the cause of the disease in five patients to different recessive mutations in choline acetyltransferase that either decrease the expression or reduce the catalytic efficiency, or both, of the enzyme (Ohno *et al.*, 2001).

## Paucity of synaptic vesicles and reduced quantal release

The clinical features of this syndrome closely mimic those of autoimmune MG, but EP studies reveal no AChR deficiency. A presynaptic defect is indicated by a severe decrease (to $\sim$20% of normal) in the number of ACh quanta ($m$) released by nerve impulse. The decrease in $m$ is due to a decrease in the number of readily releasable quanta ($n$), and this decrease is associated with a comparable decrease (to $\sim$20% of normal) in the numerical density of synaptic vesicles. The putative defect resides in the synthesis or axonal transport of vesicle precursors from the anterior horn cell to the nerve terminal or, less likely, is related to impaired recycling of the synaptic vesicles (Walls *et al.*, 1993).

## CMS resembling the Lambert Eaton myasthenic syndrome

In one patient reported with this syndrome, the amplitude of the CMAP was reduced but facilitated severalfold on tetanic stimulation and the symptoms were improved by guanidine (Bady et al., 1987). In a second patient, observed at the Mayo Clinic, quantal release by nerve impulse was very low at 1 Hz stimulation but increased markedly with stimulation rates >10 Hz. The pre- and post-synaptic regions were structurally intact by electron microscopy and the nerve terminals harboured abundant synaptic vesicles. The defect likely resides in a subunit of the presynaptic voltage-gated calcium channel or in a component of the synaptic vesicle release complex.

## Synaptic acetylcholinesterase deficiency

A highly disabling CMS is caused by the absence of AChE from the synaptic space (Hutchinson et al., 1993; Engel et al., 1997, 1999). Neuromuscular transmission is compromised by smallness of the nerve terminals and their encasement by Schwann cells, which reduces the number of releasable quanta, an EP myopathy from cholinergic

overactivity, and desensitization and depolarization block of AChR at physiological rates of stimulation. In the absence of AChE, the synaptic potentials are prolonged and evoke repetitive compound muscle fibre action potentials (CMAP). AChR kinetics and the dwell times of channel activation episodes are normal.

The EP species of AChE is a heteromeric asymmetric enzyme composed of 1, 2, or 3 homotetramers of globular catalytic subunits ($AChE_T$) attached to a triple-stranded collagenic tail (ColQ) (Rotundo and Fanbrough, 1994) (Figure 12.4B). $AChE_T$ and ColQ are encoded by $ACHE_T$ and $COLQ$, respectively. ColQ has an N-terminal proline-rich region attachment domain (PRAD), a collagenic central domain, and a C-terminal region enriched in charged residues and cysteines (Figure 12.4A). Each ColQ strand binds an $AChE_T$ tetramer to its PRAD (Bon et al., 1997). Two groups of charged residues in the collagen domain (heparan sulphate proteoglycan binding domains or HSPBD) (Deprez and Inestrosa, 1995; Krejci et al., 1997) plus other residues in the C-terminal region (Donger et al., 1998; Engel et al., 1999;

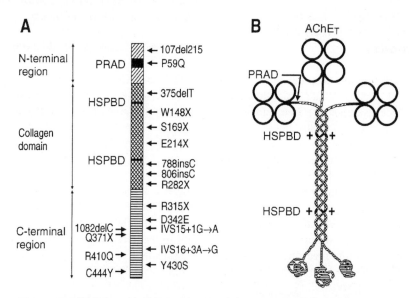

**Figure 12.4** (A) Schematic diagram showing domains of a ColQ strand with 18 identified ColQ mutations and (B) components of the $A_{12}$ species of asymmetric AChE. AChE = acetylcholinesterase; HSPD = heparan sulphate proteoglycan binding domain; PRAD = proline-rich attachment domain. (Reproduced from Engel, A. G. et al. Congenital Myasthenic Syndromes, in *Myasthenia Gravis and Myasthenic Disorders* (eg. Engel, A. G.), pp. 251–297. New York: Oxford University Press, 1999.)

Ohno *et al.*, 2000) assure that the asymmetric enzyme is inserted into the synaptic basal lamina. The C-terminal region is also required for initiating the triple helical assembly of the ColQ which proceeds from a C- to an N-terminal direction in a zipper-like manner (Prockop and Kivirikko, 1995).

In 1998, human *COLQ* cDNA was cloned (Donger *et al.*, 1998; Ohno *et al.*, 1998), the genomic structure of *COLQ* determined (Ohno *et al.*, 1998), and the molecular basis of EP AChE deficiency traced to recessive mutations in *COLQ*. Eighteen *COLQ* mutations in 15 kinships have been identified to date (Donger *et al.*, 1998; Ohno *et al.*, 1998, 1999, 2000) (see Figure 12.4A). The mutations are of three types (Ohno *et al.*, 1998, 2000):

1. PRAD mutations that prevent attachment of $AChE_T$ to ColQ;
2. Collagen domain mutations that produce a short, single-stranded ColQ that binds a single $AChE_T$ tetramer and is insertion incompetent.
3. C-terminal mutations that hinder the triple helical assembly of the collagen domain, or produce an insertion-incompetent asymmetric species of AChE, or both.

# References

Abicht, A., Stucka, R., Karcagi, V. *et al.* (1999). A common mutation (e1267delG) in congenital myasthenic patients of Gipsy ethnic origin. *Neurology*, **53**, 1564–9.

Akabas, M. H. and Karlin, A. (1995). Identification of acetylcholine receptor channel-lining residues in the M1 segment of the $\alpha$-subunit. *Biochemistry*, **34**, 12496–500.

Bady, B., Chauplannaz, G. and Carrier, H. (1987). Congenital Lambert-Eaton myasthenic syndrome. *J Neurol Neurosurg Psychiatr.*, **50**, 476–8.

Banwell, B. L., Russel, J., Fukudome, T., Shen, X.-M., Stilling, G. and Engel, A.G. (1999). Myopathy, myasthenic syndrome, and epidermolysis bullosa simplex due to plectin deficiency. *J Neuropathol Exp Neurol.*, **58**, 832–46.

Bon, S., Coussen, F. and Massoulié, J. (1997). Quaternary associations of acetylcholinesterase. II. The polyproline attachment domain of the collage tail. *J Biol Chem.*, **272**, 3016–21.

Brengman, J. M., Ohno, K., Shen, X.-M. and Engel,

A. G. (1998). Congenital myasthenic syndrome due to two novel mutations in the acetylcholine receptor $\varepsilon$ subunit gene. *Muscle Nerve*, **21** (Suppl. 7), S120 (Abstr).

Christodoulou, K., Tsingis, M., Deymeer F. *et al.* (1997). Mapping of the familial infantile myasthenia (congenital myasthenic syndrome type Ia) to chromosome 17p with evidence of genetic homogeneity. *Hum Mol Genet.*, **6**, 635–40.

Croxen, R., Beeson, D., Vincent, A. and Newsom-Davis, J. (1996). Congenital myasthenic syndrome with a single nucleotide deletion at the intron/exon boundary in exon 12 of the gene encoding the acetylcholine receptor $\varepsilon$ subunit. *Ann Neurol.*, **40**, 513 (Abstr).

Croxen, R., Newland, C., Beeson, D. *et al.* (1997). Mutations in different functional domains of the human muscle acetylcholine receptor $\alpha$ subunit in patients with the slow-channel congenital myasthenic syndrome. *Hum Mol Genet.*, **6**, 767–73.

Croxen, R., Newland, C., Betty, M., Vincent, A., Newsom-Davis, J. and Beeson, D. (1999). Novel functional $\varepsilon$-subunit polypeptide generated by a single nucleotide deletion in acetylcholine receptor deficiency congenital myasthenic syndrome. *Ann Neurol.*, **46**, 639–47.

Deprez, P. N. and Inestrosa, N. C. (1995). Two heparin-binding domains are present on the collagenic tail of asymmetric acetylcholinesterase. *J Biol Chem.*, **270**, 11043–6.

Donger, C., Krejci, E., Serradell, P. *et al.* (1998). Mutation in the human acetylcholinesterase-associated gene, *COLQ*, is responsible for congenital myasthenic syndrome with end-plate acetylcholinesterase deficiency. *Am J Hum Genet.*, **63**, 967–75.

Edelstein, S. J. and Changeux, J.-P. (1998). Allosteric transitions of the acetylcholine receptor. *Adv Protein Chem.*, **51**, 121–84.

Engel, A. G., Lambert, E. H. and Gomez, M. R. (1977). A new myasthenic syndrome with end-plate acetylcholinesterase deficiency, small nerve terminals, and reduced acetylcholine release. *Ann Neurol.*, **1**, 315–30.

Engel, A. G., Lambert, E. H., Mulder, D. M. *et al.* (1982). A newly recognized congenital myasthenic syndrome attributed to a prolonged open time of the acetylcholine-induced ion channel. *Ann Neurol.*, **11**, 553–69.

Engel, A. G. and Lambert, E. H. (1987). Congenital myasthenic syndromes. *Electroencephalogr Clin Neurophysiol.*, **39** (Suppl.), 91–102.

Engel, A. G., Ohno, K., Milone, M. *et al.* (1996a). New mutations in acetylcholine receptor subunit genes reveal heterogeneity in the slow-channel congenital myasthenic syndrome. *Hum Mol Genet.*, **5**, 1217–27.

Engel, A. G., Ohno, K., Bouzat, C., Sine, S. M. and Griggs, R. G. (1996b). End-plate acetylcholine receptor deficiency due to nonsense mutations in the $\varepsilon$ subunit. *Ann Neurol.*, **40**, 810–7.

Engel, A. G., Ohno, K. and Sine, S. M. (1999). Congenital myasthenic syndromes. In *Myasthenia Gravis and Myasthenic Disorders* (ed. Engel, A. G.). pp. 251–297. New York: Oxford University Press.

Fukudome, T., Ohno, K., Brengman, J. M. and Engel, A. G. Quinidine normalizes the open duration of slow-channel mutants of the acetylcholine receptor. *Neuroreport*, **9**, 1907–11.

Gomez, C. M., Maselli, R., Gammack, J. *et al.* (1996). A beta-subunit mutation in the acetylcholine receptor gate causes severe slow-channel syndrome. *Ann Neurol.*, **39**, 712–23.

Greer, M. and Schotland, M. (1960). Myasthenia gravis in the newborn. *Pediatrics*, **26**, 101–8.

Harper, C. M. and Engel, A. G. (1998). Quinidine sulfate therapy for the slow-channel congenital myasthenic syndrome. *Ann Neurol.*, **43**, 480–4.

Hart, Z., Sahashi, K., Lambert, E. H., Engel, A. G. and Lindstrom, J. (1979). A congenital, familial, myasthenic syndrome caused by a presynaptic defect of transmitter resynthesis of mobilization. *Neurology*, **29**, 559 (Abstr).

Hutchinson, D. O., Walls, T. J., Nakano, S. *et al.* (1993). Congenital endplate acetylcholinesterase deficiency. *Brain*, **116**, 633–53.

Karlin, A. and Akabas, M. H. (1994). Toward a structural basis for the function of nicotinic acetylcholine receptors and their cousins. *Neuron*, **15**, 1231–44.

Krawczak, M. and Cooper, D. N. (1991). Gene deletions causing human genetic disease: mechanisms of mutagenesis and the role of the local DNA sequence environment. *Hum Genet.*, **86**, 425–41.

Krejci, E., Thomine, S., Boschetti, N., Legay, C., Sketelj, J. and Massoulié, J. (1997). The mammalian gene of acetylcholinesterase-associated collagen. *J Biol Chem.*, **272**, 22840–7.

Middleton, L., Ohno, K., Christodoulou, K. *et al.* (1999). Congenital myasthenic syndromes linked to chromosome 17p are caused by defects in acetylcholine receptor ε subunit gene. *Neurology*, **53**, 1076–82.

Milone, M., Ohno, K., Pruitt, J. N., Brengman, J. M., Sine, S. M. and Engel, A. G. (1996). Congenital myasthenic syndrome due to frameshifting acetylcholine receptor epsilon subunit mutation. *Soc Neurosci Abstr.*, **22**, 1942.

Milone, M., Wang, H.-L., Ohno, K. *et al.* (1997). Slow-channel syndrome caused by enhanced activation, desensitization, and agonist binding affinity due to mutation in the M2 domain of the acetylcholine receptor alpha subunit. *J Neurosci.*, **17**, 5651–65.

Milone, M., Wang, H.-L., Ohno, K. *et al.* (1998). Mode switching kinetics produced by a naturally occurring mutation in the cytoplasmic loop of the human acetylcholine receptor ε subunit. *Neuron*, **20**, 575–88.

Mora, M., Lambert, E. H. and Engel, A. G. (1987). Synaptic vesicle abnormality in familial infantile myasthenia. *Neurology*, **37**, 206–14.

Nichols, P., Croxen, R., Vincent, A. *et al.* (1999).

Mutation of the acetylcholine receptor ε-subunit promoter in congenital myasthenic syndrome. *Ann Neurol.*, **45**, 439–43.

Ohno, K., Hutchinson, D. O., Milone, M. *et al.* (1995a). Congenital myasthenic syndrome caused by prolonged acetylcholine receptor channel openings due to a mutation in the M2 domain of the ε subunit. *Proc Natl Acad Sci USA*, **92**, 758–62.

Ohno, K., Engel, A. G., Milone, M., Brengman, J. M., Sieb, J. P. and Iannaccone, S. (1995b). A congenital myasthenic syndrome with severe acetylcholine receptor deficiency caused by heteroallelic frameshifting mutations in the epsilon subunit. *Neurology*, **45** (Suppl. 4), A283 (Abstr).

Ohno, K., Wang, H.-L., Milone, M. *et al.* (1996a). Congenital myasthenic syndrome caused by decreased agonist binding affinity due to a mutation in the acetylcholine receptor ε subunit. *Neuron*, **17**, 157–70.

Ohno, K., Fukudome, T., Nakano, S. *et al.* (1996b). Mutational analysis in a congenital myasthenic syndrome reveals a novel acetylcholine receptor epsilon subunit mutation. *Soc Neurosci Abstr.*, **22**, 234.

Ohno, K., Quiram, P., Milone, M. *et al.* (1997). Congenital myasthenic syndromes due to heteroallelic nonsense/missense mutations in the acetylcholine receptor ε subunit gene: identification and functional characterization of six new mutations. *Hum Mol Genet.*, **6**, 753–66.

Ohno, K., Brengman, J. M., Tsujino, A. and Engel, A. G. (1998). Human endplate acetylcholinesterase deficiency caused by mutations in the collagen-like tail subunit (ColQ) of the asymmetric enzyme. *Proc Natl Acad Sci USA*, **95**, 9654–9.

Ohno, K., Milone, M., Brengman, J. M. *et al.* (1998a). Slow-channel congenital myasthenic syndrome caused by a novel mutation in the acetylcholine receptor ε subunit. *Neurology*, **50**, A432 (Abstr).

Ohno, K., Anlar, B., Özdirim, E., Brengman, J. M., De Bleecker, J. and Engel, A. G. (1998b). Myasthenic syndromes in Turkish kinships due to mutations in the acetylcholine receptor. *Ann Neurol.*, **44**, 234–41.

Ohno, K., Brengman, J. M., Felice, K. J., Cornblath, D. R. and Engel, A. G. (1999). Congenital endplate acetylcholinesterase deficiency caused by a nonsense mutation and an A-to-G splice site mutation at position +3 of the collagen-like tail subunit gene (*COLQ*): How does G at position +3 result in aberrant splicing? *Am J Hum Genet.*, **65**, 635–44.

Ohno, K., Anlar, B. and Engel, A. G. (1999). Congenital myasthenic syndrome caused by a mutation in the Ets-binding site of the promoter region of the acetylcholine receptor ε subunit gene. *Neuromuscul Disord.*, **9**, 131–5.

Ohno, K., Wang, H.-L., Shen, X.-M. *et al.* (2000). Slow-channel mutations in the center of the M1 transmembrane domain of the acetylcholine receptor α subunit. *Neurology*, **54** (suppl. 3) A183.

Ohno, K., Engel, A. G., Brengman, J. M. *et al.* (2000).

The spectrum of mutations causing endplate acetylcholinesterase deficiency. *Ann Neurol.*, **47**, 162–70.

Ohno, K., Tsujino, A., Brengman, J. M., Harper, C. M., Bajzer, Z., Udd, B., Beyring, R., Robb, S., Kirkhan, F. J. and Engel, A. G. (2001). Choline acetyltransferase mutations cause myasthenic syndrome associated with episodic apnea in humans. *Proc Natl Acad Sci USA.* **98**, 2017–22.

Prince, R. J. and Sine, S. M. (1998). The ligand binding domains of the nicotinic acetylcholine receptor. In *The Nicotinic Acetylcholine Receptor: Current Views and Future Trends* (ed. Barrantes, F. J.) pp 31–59. Austin, TX: Landes Bioscience.

Prockop, D. J. and Kivirikko, K.I. (1995). Collagens: Molecular biology, diseases, and potentials for therapy. *Ann Rev Biochem.*, **64**, 403–34.

Quiram, P., Ohno, K., Milone, M. *et al.* (1999). Acetylcholine receptor β-subunit mutations causing endplate AChR deficiency and reduced assembly with the δ subunit. *Neurology*, **52** (Suppl. 2), A185 (Abstr).

Robertson, W. C., Chun, R. W. M. and Kornguth, S. E. (1980). Familial infantile myasthenia. *Arch Neurol.*, **37**, 117–9.

Rotundo, R. L. and Fambrough, D. M. (1994). Function and molecular structure of acetylcholinesterase. In *Myology*, 2nd edn. (eds Engel, A. G. and Franzini-Armstrong, C.) pp 607–623. New York: McGraw-Hill.

Sieb, J. P., Milone, M. and Engel, A. G. (1996). Effects of the quinoline derivatives quinine, quinidine, and chloroquine on neuromuscular transmission. *Brain Res.*, **712**, 179–89.

Sine, S. M., Ohno, K., Bouzat, C. *et al.* (1995). Mutation of the acetylcholine receptor α subunit causes a slow-channel myasthenic syndrome by enhancing agonist binding affinity. *Neuron*, **15**, 229–39.

Tsujino, A., Shen, X.-M., Milone, M., Harper, C. M., Ohno, K. and Engel, A. G. (2000). Abnormal decrease in quantal size, not in quantal content, accounts for congenital myasthenic syndrome with episodic apnea. *Neurology*, **54** (Suppl. 3), A139.

Walls, T. J., Engel, A. G., Nagel, A. S., Harper, C. M. and Trastek, V. F. (1993). Congenital myasthenic syndrome associated with paucity of synaptic vesicles and reduced quantal release. *Ann NY Acad Sci.*, **681**, 461–8.

Wang, H.-L., Auerbach, A., Bren, N., Ohno, K., Engel, A. G. and Sine, S. M. (1997). Mutation in the M1 domain of the acetylcholine receptor alpha subunit decreases the rate of agonist dissociation. *J Gen Physiol.*, **109**, 757–66.

Wang, H.-L., Milone, M., Ohno, K. *et al.* (1998). Acetylcholine receptor M3 domain: Stereochemical and volume contributions to channel gating. *Nature Neurosci.*, **2**, 226–33.

Zhou, M., Engel, A. G. and Auerbach, A. (1999). Serum choline activates mutant acetylcholine receptors that cause slow channel congenital myasthenic syndrome. *Proc Natl Acad Sci USA*, **96**, 10466–71.

# Neuromuscular channel disorders (acquired)

# 13 Myasthenia gravis and the Lambert Eaton syndrome

*Angela Vincent*

## Introduction

Over the last twenty years it has become increasingly clear that neurological disorders can be caused by autoantibodies, and that a frequent and functionally very important target of these antibodies are neuronal ion channels. There are now two well-defined conditions that are known to be caused by autoantibodies directed at neuronal ion channels that are essential for the function of the neuromuscular junction (NMJ). Myasthenia gravis (MG) and the Lambert Eaton myasthenic syndrome (LEMS) are due to antibodies to the muscle acetylcholine-gated ion channel (acetylcholine receptor, AChR) and the voltage-gated calcium channel (VGCC) respectively. A third condition, acquired neuromyotonia, that is associated with antibodies to voltage-gated potassium channels (VGKC), is considered in Chapter 14. In order to appreciate the importance of these ion channels in neuromuscular transmission, one first needs to consider the function of the NMJ, and the way in which it is formed during development. Many reviews describing the formation and function of the NMJ are available (e.g. Vincent and Wray, 1992; Hall and Sanes, 1993; Aidley 1999; Sanes and Lichtman, 1999).

## The neuromuscular junction and neuromuscular transmission

The neuromuscular junction is a synapse between the motor nerve terminal and the post-synaptic surface at the motor endplate. The myelinated motor nerve axon, which has its cell body in the spinal cord, can be over a metre in length and divides on the surface of the muscle into many motor nerve endings. Each of these loses its myelin sheath and synapse on the surface of a single muscle fibre at the motor endplate, which is the only point of contact between the motor nerve and the muscle that it innervates. The longest diameter of the motor endplate is around 30 $\mu$m, whereas the length of the motor nerve and of the muscle fibres can be up to many centimetres. Thus the successful transmission of impulses from the motor nerve to the muscle must depend on a highly efficient, fast and reliable process occurring at this tiny and remote point of contact (Figure 13.1A).

At the motor endplate, the muscle surface is slightly raised and the sarcoplasmic membrane is thrown into a series of deep folds (the post-synaptic folds). In between the nerve and the muscle, a basal lamina can be seen that extends into the folds. The surface of the muscle at the tops of the folds is noticeably denser in electron micrographs than that elsewhere, mainly due to the very high density of acetycholine receptors that are clustered there (Figure 13.1B).

Neuromuscular transmission is similar to that at most chemical synapses, and has long been considered to be a good model for synaptic transmission in general (Aidley, 1999). The nerve action potential, that is dependent on voltage-gated sodium channels, invades the motor nerve terminal bouton leading to opening of voltage-gated calcium channels that are present on the presynaptic membrane (Figure 13.1C). These channels are thought to be the active zone particles that can be seen in highly structured parallel arrays when the

A

B

0.5 μm

C

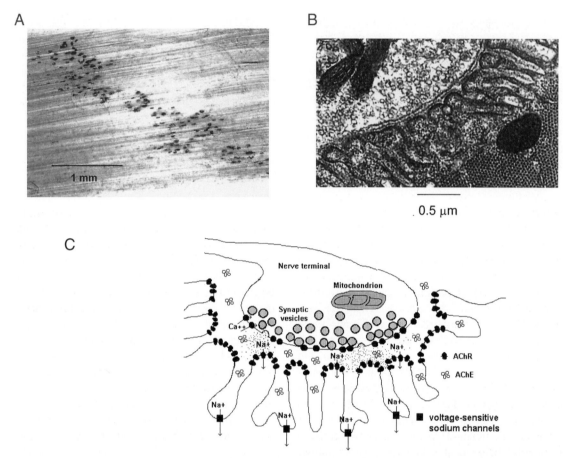

**Figure 13.1** The neuromuscular junction. (A) Neuromuscular junctions demonstrated on the surface of an intact muscle by staining for acetylcholinesterase. The neuromuscular junctions are about 30 μm in length. The motor nerves are not stained but can just be seen arching over the surface of the muscle in the upper right quadrant. (B) Electron micrograph of a neruromuscular junction showing the motor nerve terminal (upper left quadrant) with many synaptic vesicles and two mitochondria. The opposing muscle surface is thrown into folds which are up to 1 μm in length. At the tops of the folds, opposite the nerve terminal, the folds are noticeably denser due to the very high concentration of acetylcholine receptors. (C) A diagram to represent the neuromuscular junction, illustrating the relative positions of the calcium channels on the motor nerve terminal and the acetylcholine receptors on the muscle surface. Voltage-gated sodium channels are thought to be located at the depths of the folds.
(A and B courtesy of Dr Clarke Slater, University of Newcastle Medical School.)

presynaptic membrane is freeze-fractured. When these channels open, there is a very transient and localized increase in intracellular calcium which results in the exocytosis of packets or quanta of acetylcholine. This process is similar to that which occurs in all neuronal cells (see Sudhof, 1995 for a review), but the subtype of VGCC, which is the P/Q-type at the NMJ, differs from the N-type that is present in many other peripheral nerve endings and also in neurosecretory cells. This P/Q-type

VGCC, however, is also present at many CNS synapses and was first identified in the Purkinje cells of the cerebellum (Llinas *et al.*, 1992).

ACh diffuses rapidly across the synaptic space (around 50 nm between the nerve and the muscle) and binds to the acetylcholine receptors (AChR). This results in opening of the AChR-associated ion channels (Figures 13.1C, 13.2A), and an influx of sodium and other cations leading to depolarization of the motor endplate. If this depolarization is sufficient, it opens the voltage-gated sodium channels that appear to be predominantly located at the bottom of the folds (Figure 13.1C). Opening of these channels produces a regenerative action potential in the muscle membrane that propagates along the entire muscle surface and leads to activation of the contractile mechanism. Meanwhile, the presynaptic VGCCs close, VGKCs open and the motor nerve terminal membrane potential is restored. The whole process takes place in a few milliseconds. An important point, not relevant to many other synapses in the CNS, is that under normal conditions neuromuscular transmission is all-or-none. If the endplate potential amplitude is sufficient to depolarize the post-synaptic membrane to the membrane potential required to open the voltage-gated sodium channels (the threshold potential), there will be successful transmission and the muscle will contract. If the endplate potential does not reach this threshold, there will be complete failure of transmission (see Wood and Slater, 1997).

Only about 50% of the ACh reaches the post-synaptic AChRs, the rest is destroyed by the enzyme acetylcholine esterase (AChE) that is attached by a collagen tail, called Col Q, to the basal lamina at the motor endplate. When ACh dissociates from the AChRs it is rapidly destroyed by AChE, ensuring that under normal conditions each nerve action potential produces only one muscle action potential. However, if AChE is absent or inhibited by drugs, if ACh release is excessive, or if there are repetitive action potentials in the motor nerve terminal (as is likely to be the case in acquired neuromyotonia; see Chapter 14), a single nerve action potential can lead to more than one muscle action potential. A similar consequence can result from prolongation of the AChR channel openings: this occurs in the genetic, slow channel syndrome, and may also be a feature of some autoimmune conditions (see below). The genetic disorders are discussed fully in Chapter 12.

The physiology of neuromuscular transmission can be examined both *in vivo* and *in vitro*. *In vivo* measurements include electromyography and single fibre measurements as discussed in Chapter 5. The *in vitro* observations include microelectrode measurements of miniature endplate potentials, which are the small post-synaptic potentials that result from the spontaneous release of a single packet of acetylcholine, and the larger endplate potentials that result when many packets or 'quanta' of ACh are released following a nerve impulse. The ratio in the amplitudes between the endplate potentials and the miniature endplate potentials gives a reasonably accurate assessment of the quantal content, that is the number of packets of ACh released per nerve impulse. Under most circumstances it is difficult to measure the quantal content because nerve stimulation leads to a muscle contraction with displacement of the microelectrode, but recently the use of a snail toxin, $\mu$-conotoxin, that specifically blocks the muscle action potentials so that the muscle fibre does not contract, has made it possible to measure both endplate potentials accurately at the same endplates (Hong and Chang, 1989). Using a patch-clamp technique it is also possible to measure single AChR openings at the NMJ. In human muscle, this has been done mainly by Milone *et al.* (1994) and the findings that are of particular relevance to genetic forms of myasthenia are discussed in Chapter 12.

It is important to realize that if the action of ACh is sustained, for instance by blocking AChE activity with anticholinesterase drugs, the AChRs may become desensitized, a state during which they fail to respond to ACh. This desensitized state recovers with quite a slow time course, during which, from time to time, individual AChRs will come out of the desensitized state and open repeatedly for brief periods before becoming desensitized again (Colquhoun, 1992).

## Development of the neuromuscular junction

During fetal development, myoblasts fuse to form myotubes and these express AChRs all over their surface. When the incoming motor nerves secrete ACh and factors such as agrin, the AChRs begin to cluster on the surface of the muscle, and the muscle itself sends signals to the nerves which begin to form synapses at the point of contact. Thereafter, the release of acetylcholine receptor inducing activity (ARIA) from the motor nerve terminal increases AChR expression by nuclei under the developing motor endplate, while at the same time muscle activity, induced by transmission at the developing NMJ, leads to down regulation of AChR expression by nuclei at other regions of the muscle fibre. Eventually, all but one of the motor nerve terminals are eliminated, the post-synaptic folds form, the voltage-gated sodium channels cluster at the bottom of the folds, and AChE expression becomes highly localized in the basal lamina. If the motor nerve is cut or damaged, the high density of AChRs and AChE at the NMJ are retained (they appear to be extremely stable, see below), but the lack of muscle activity

means that AChR is expressed once more throughout the muscle fibre, leading to denervation 'hypersensitivity'. These important features are discussed by Hall and Sanes (1993) and Sanes and Lichtman (1999).

The AChR is an oligomeric membrane protein consisting of five subunits (Figure 13.2A). The ACh binding sites are located at the interfaces between the two $\alpha$-subunits and their adjacent subunits. The snake toxin, $\alpha$-bungarotoxin, also binds to these sites (Karlin and Akabas, 1995; Lindstrom, 1997). The ion pore opens between the five subunits, but recent studies suggest that the

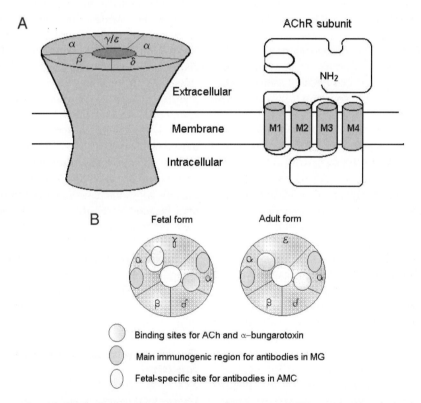

Figure 13.2 The acetylcholine receptor. (A) A diagram to illustrate the main features of the acetylcholine receptor as it sits in the membrane, and the topology of each of the AChR subunits. Each of the five subunits has a large extracellular domain of around 210 amino acids, four transmembrane sequences, and a large cytoplasmic loop between M3 and M4. There is a disulphide bond between aa 128 and 142 forming a loop in the extracellular domain. (B) The acetylcholine receptor viewed from above consists of two forms, the fetal and adult, differing by substitution of an $\varepsilon$-subunit for a $\gamma$-subunit. Many antibodies in myasthenia gravis bind to the main immunogenic regions on the $\alpha$-subunits that are distinct from the binding sites for ACh and $\alpha$-bungarotoxin. However, women with myasthenia whose babies have arthrogyrposis multiplex congenital have fetal-specific antibodies that bind to the $\gamma$-subunit (see Figure 13.3).

ions exit through transverse funnels in the channel walls rather than through a single pore on the intracellular surface (Miyazawa et al., 1999). During the early stages of development the fetal isoform, $\alpha, \beta, \gamma, \delta$, is expressed, whereas once the neuromuscular junction has formed, the adult isoform, $\alpha, \beta, \varepsilon, \delta$ takes over (Figure 13.2B). The replacement of the $\gamma$-subunit by an $\varepsilon$-subunit only happens at the maturing NMJ and is dependent on the up-regulation of AChR expression at the motor endplate nuclei that is induced by ARIA. In humans this takes place at some time during the last trimester of pregnancy (Hesselmans et al., 1993), but in rodents which have been studied in much more detail, it takes place during the first 10 postnatal days (see Sanes and Lichtman, 1999). The two isoforms differ in their conductance and single channel open-times (Missias et al., 1986). It appears that the longer open-times of the fetal isoform are beneficial during development, when opening frequency is probably low due to poor apposition between the nerve terminal and the muscle surface, whereas during adult life when ACh release is highly synchronized and precisely located, the shorter open-times of the adult form are necessary to prevent overactivity. Thus expression of fetal AChRs during adult life, resulting from genetic defects in the $\varepsilon$-subunit (see Chapter 12), or from denervation-like changes in the muscle, may in themselves be pathogenic.

The AChRs at the NMJ turnover at a very slow rate. The fetal isoform has a half-life of approximately 10 hours, due to its internalization and degradation, and there is a constant synthesis and replacement of existing AChRs. At the mature NMJ, by contrast, the AChRs are extremely stable with a half-life of over 10 days. It is not clear whether this is a feature of the subunit composition of the adult isoform or of the very rigid scaffold that anchors the AChRs at the NMJ (see Sanes and Lichtman, 1999).

## Use of neurotoxins to study neuromuscular transmission

Much of what we know about the ion channels at the neuromuscular junction depends on the action of certain drugs and neurotoxins. For instance, the importance of ACh release, and its action on the post-synaptic AChRs was inferred by classic experiments on the effects of curare and physostigmine, long before the concept of an acetylcholine 'receptor' could be confirmed by experiment. In particular, the ability to quantify, purify and characterize these receptors has depended on the use of certain neurotoxins, and their use in the characterization of voltage-gated calcium and potassium channels is proving to be equally important (Harvey, 1993).

$\alpha$-Bungarotoxin ($\alpha$-BuTx) is an 8000 kD polypeptide, one of many found in the venom of Bungarus multicinctus, the Taiwan banded krait. The toxin binds to sites on each of the $\alpha$-subunits, and directly inhibits the binding of ACh thus leading to muscle paralysis in animals, or humans, bitten by the snake. The toxin is easily labelled with radioactivity, usually by iodination with $^{125}$I. The $^{125}$I-toxin binds highly specifically to the muscle AChR (the neuronal forms of AChRs, that are encoded by different genes, mainly do not bind $^{125}$I-$\alpha$-BuTx, see Lindstrom, 1997), in a manner that is almost irreversible, making it a very useful reagent for measuring the number of AChRs in normal and diseased muscle, and for tagging the receptors after they have been extracted from the muscle membrane for use in immunological assays. Many other neurotoxins from different species of snake act similarly, including some that are somewhat smaller than $\alpha$-BuTx and have slightly lower affinities.

There are no useful snake toxins specific for voltage-gated calcium channels. However, a species of fish-eating snail, the Conus family, has developed a series of highly specific neurotoxins that not only inhibit VGCC function but distinguish between different subtypes of VGCC. In particular, the use of Conus geographus toxin, GIVA, and Conus magus toxin, MVIIC, has made it possible to define the role of N- and P/Q-type VGCCs in neuromuscular transmission (Olivera et al., 1994). $\omega$-Agatoxin is derived from the venom of the funnel-web spider, Agenolopsis apperta, and is highly specific for P-type VGCCs, but its use has been limited due to difficulties in obtaining an iodinated product that binds to purified VGCCs. These neurotoxins are only a few of those that are present in the animal kingdom, many of which have not yet been exploited for scientific or clinical use.

## Geometry of the NMJ

The very small volume of the synaptic space between the motor nerve terminal and the post-synaptic membrane, and the very high density of AChRs present on the post-synaptic surface (around $10\,000/\mu m^2$), means that the effective concentration of AChRs is very high. Thus the affinity of ACh for the AChRs does not need to be high in order for released ACh to have a high probability of binding to the AChR. At the same time, the NMJ is not protected by a 'blood–nerve barrier' and is accessible to circulating factors. Nevertheless, the efficacy of any circulating factor will be limited by its ability to diffuse out of the blood vessels, reach the synaptic space and to achieve a sufficient concentration within it.

## Antibody-mediated disorders

### Myasthenia gravis

Myasthenia gravis is a disease that is usually acquired in adult life, and is now known to be due to autoantibodies to the AChR. The patients complain of weakness and fatigue, limited to voluntary muscles. The symptoms commonly affect the muscles around the eye, causing drooping of the eyelids (ptosis) and double vision. Speech and facial muscles may be badly affected leading to communication difficulties, and weakness in the oesophageal muscles can interfere with nutrition. Involvement of respiratory muscles can lead to respiratory failure and be life-threatening. The condition is improved by administration of AChE inhibitors, that prolong the action of ACh at the NMJ, but these drugs must be used with care since excess ACh can result in a 'cholinergic crisis' due to AChR desensitization. Since the demonstration that MG is due to antibodies to the AChR, immunological treatments have been used with great effect. For a review see Drachman (1994).

MG occurs in several different forms. About 15% of MG patients with generalized disease do not have detectable anti-AChR antibodies (sero-negative MG) and they probably have antibodies to a different NMJ antigen (see below). Among the 85% of MG patients who do have anti-AChR antibodies, some only have ocular symptoms (ocular MG), but most have more generalized disease and these are usually divided into three subgroups (Compston et al., 1980). Early-onset MG patients develop the disease before 40 years of age (usually between 15 and 35), are frequently female and have a 'hyperplastic' thymus gland which contains germinal centres that secrete anti-AChR antibodies. These patients often improve when the thymus is removed. Elderly-onset MG patients develop the disease after 40 years of age, there is no sex bias, and the thymus is usually normal; they are most often treated with immunosuppression. Thymoma-associated MG patients have a thymic tumour which needs to be removed, but they are often difficult to treat even with immunosuppressive drugs and are liable to recurring problems (see Drachman, 1994).

## Antibodies to AChR in MG

The possibility that MG was an autoimmune disease was first formally proposed by Simpson in 1960. He noticed that it occurs frequently in young women, that they often have a personal or family history of autoimmune disease, that the thymus gland is abnormal, and that the disease can sometimes be transferred to the fetus, and suggested that it might be due to antibodies to an 'endplate' protein. But it was not until the 1970s that it was possible to demonstrate the presence of antibodies binding directly to AChRs in myasthenia gravis. The way in which this was done has provided experimental paradigms for the investigation of other antibody-mediated disorders.

The studies of Elmqvist et al. (1964) showed that the miniature endplate potentials were reduced in amplitude in muscle biopsies taken from patients with MG. Two possible causes were considered: a reduction in the amount of ACh in each packet or quantum, or a reduction in the number of AChRs on the muscle surface. Although the latter was perhaps more likely, it was not possible to demonstrate a loss of AChRs until the discovery of the highly specific and irreversible neurotoxins.

In 1973, Fambrough *et al.*, using $^{125}$I-$\alpha$-BuTx, found a marked decrease in the number of AChRs at the NMJs in biopsied muscle from MG patients. This finding was subsequently confirmed by Ito *et al.* (1978), and by others.

At much the same time, Patrick and Lindstrom (1973) were purifying AChRs from the *Torpedo* electric organ. The electric organ is a modified muscle-like tissue, and has a very high surface area of AChR-containing synapses, making it the best known source of the protein. Despite the evolutionary distance between *Torpedo* and mammals, rabbits immunized with the *Torpedo* AChR developed antibodies that cross-reacted with their own muscle AChRs leading to a myasthenia-like illness with marked weakness, loss of muscle tone, and respiratory failure. Importantly, injection of serum from these rabbits into normal animals induced similar symptoms, demonstrating that it was the antibodies, rather than any cellular immune response, that caused the disease.

It remained only to show that patients with MG had antibodies to AChRs in their serum. This was first clearly demonstrated by Lindstrom *et al.* (1976) using immunoprecipitation of $^{125}$I-$\alpha$-BuTx-labelled human AChRs. In this assay, which is now used for the diagnosis of MG on a routine basis, human muscle (or cell lines expressing human AChR; Beeson *et al.*, 1996) is extracted in detergent and the $^{125}$I-$\alpha$-BuTx added to label the AChRs. A small amount of test serum is added and the serum IgG antibodies are then precipitated by addition of an excess of an antiserum raised against human IgG. The precipitate is collected and washed and counted for radioactivity. The results of this test are quantitative and highly specific for MG. Healthy individuals or patients with other neurological or autoimmune diseases very infrequently have antibodies that bind to AChRs; but there is a subpopulation of patients that do not have anti-AChR antibodies (Vincent and Newsom-Davis, 1985; see below).

It is quite clear from the study of many other autoimmune disorders, that the presence of an antibody does not, *per se*, prove that the antibody causes the disorder. There are certain clues, however, that will help to define the pathogenic relevance. First, the antibodies must bind to antigenic determinants that will be accessible to circulating antibodies. For instance, antibodies to cytoplasmic antigens, or to cytoplasmic determinants of cell membrane components, are very unlikely to be pathogenic, and are often secondary to tissue destruction rather than the cause of it. In the case of antibodies to the AChR, the great majority bind to determinants on the extracellular aspect of the AChR, bind predominantly to the protein in its native form, and do not bind to the individual subunits when they have been denatured and separated by electrophoresis, strongly suggesting that these antibodies are induced against the native protein and are potentially pathogenic (see Vincent *et al.*, 1998).

Secondly, removal of antibodies from the patients by plasma exchange leads to clinical improvement (e.g. Newsom-Davis *et al.*, 1978). In this procedure, large volumes of plasma are removed over a period of several days and the blood cells returned to the patient with a substitute plasma. In this manner, the level of anti-AChR antibodies can be substantially reduced, and the patient almost invariably becomes better, beginning at around 48 hours after treatment commences.

Thirdly, and very importantly, the serum or purified IgG should be able to transfer disease. This crucial experiment is demonstrated in women with MG who have babies affected by neonatal MG (see below), due to placental transfer of anti-AChR antibodies, and was demonstrated experimentally by Toyka *et al.* (1977), who injected MG IgG into mice. Some of the mice became weak, and all showed reduced numbers of AChRs at their endplates and reduced amplitudes of MEPPs confirming that the anti-AChR antibodies (or theoretically some other IgG antibody) caused the disease.

In addition, it should be possible to show the effects of serum antibodies on the expression of the target antigen in *in vitro* studies. For instance, serum from patients with MG reduced the number of AChRs expressed on the cell surface of myotube cultures, and in cell lines expressing AChRs (Drachman *et al.*, 1982).

## Mechanisms of AChR loss

An important question that arises is, how do the antibodies affect the numbers of AChRs? Intuitively, one might expect them to block the binding of AChR (in a similar manner to $\alpha$-BuTx). However, the very fact that they can be detected by binding to AChR that already has $^{125}$I-$\alpha$-BuTx attached to it, indicates that most of the antibodies bind to determinants on the surface of the AChR that do not overlap with the ACh/$\alpha$-BuTx binding sites (see Figure 13.2B).

Experiments with serum and monoclonal antibodies derived from rats immunized against the *Torpedo* and other AChRs were very helpful in defining the sites for antibody binding on the AChR. Tzartos, Lindstrom and their colleagues found that the majority of anti-AChR antibodies in sera from immunized animals competed with monoclonal antibodies for a site on each of the AChR $\alpha$-subunits that they termed the Main Immunogenic Region (MIR; Tzartos *et al.*, 1980; 1982; 1991). These antibodies did not interfere with binding of $^{125}$I-$\alpha$-BuTx, confirming that the MIR was a distinct region (see Figure 13.2B). Moreover, using monoclonal antibodies against the MIR and density gradient separations, they could show that the anti-MIR antibodies were able to cross-link AChRs, forming multimeric complexes. By contrast, antibodies directed against the $\beta$-, $\gamma$- or $\delta$-subunits probably only form dimeric complexes (and sometimes not even those, if the binding sites are not situated appropriately).

Thus the MIR appears to be ideally situated for antibodies to cross-link between the subunits. This turns out to be very important in pathogenic terms, since cross-linking of AChRs in the membrane leads to an increase in their rate of internalization and degradation, as shown both in cultures of myotubes or cell lines (Drachman *et al.*, 1978), and in experimental animals *in vivo* (Drachman *et al.*, 1982). This modulation of AChR expression is potentially an important pathogenic mechanism, but an increase in AChR synthesis has been demonstrated both in culture systems, in mice *in vivo,* and in biopsied muscle suggesting that, by itself, increased degradation may not be sufficient to cause substantial loss of AChR (Wilson *et al.*, 1983; Guyon *et al.*, 1994).

Another mechanism that is of major importance is complement-dependent damage to the NMJ. Engel and his colleagues showed that IgG and complement components were present at the NMJ

in the great majority of MG patients' muscle biopsies, and that the terminal attack complex of complement was also present (Engel *et al.*, 1977; Engel and Arahata, 1987). Moreover, the greater the deposition of membrane attack complex, the less AChR that could be detected in parallel muscle sections. Thus, whereas the reduction in AChR numbers that occurs when divalent antibody modulates turnover will theoretically stop when numbers are reduced by about 40% (Wilson *et al.*, 1983), complement-induced damage to the AChR-containing post-synaptic membrane is probably only limited by the accessibility of the NMJ to circulating antibodies and complement factors (see above). There is no reason, or evidence, to suggest that antibodies directed against the MIR cannot induce complement-mediated damage as well as increasing AChR turnnover, although most of the studies have not tried to demonstrate the specificity of the antibodies involved.

Although anti-MIR antibodies are thought to dominate in many MG patients, there is ample evidence for the existence of antibodies to other sites on the AChR. In particular, some patients do have antibodies that interfere with $\alpha$-BuTx binding (Burges *et al.*, 1990), and others have antibodies that bind preferentially to the fetal isoform rather than to adult AChR (Vincent *et al.*, 1987). It is assumed that these antibodies bind to the $\gamma$-subunit, and indeed many compete with monoclonal antibodies that have subsequently been shown to be specific for the $\gamma$-subunit (Vincent *et al.*, 1987; Jacobson *et al.*, 1999). The $\gamma$-subunit is expressed on muscle-like cells in the thymus, providing one possible site of autosensitization in MG (Schluep *et al.*, 1987). The proportion of antibodies in any one human serum that bind to the MIR is quite variable, and it has not yet been shown directly that any $\alpha$-subunit sequence provides a major antigenic determinant in the human disease. Nevertheless, it does appear that patients have antibodies that bind to $\alpha$-subunit determinants, separate from the ACh binding site, and that other sites, with the exception of the $\gamma$- subunit, which should not contribute to the pathology of the disease in the adult, are less important.

One aspect of the NMJ that has recently come to notice is the importance of the post-synaptic folds (see Figure 13.1B) and the voltage-gated sodium channels that are located there (see Figure 13.1c; Wood and Slater, 1997). In MG, the folds are often absent or severely damaged by the complement-dependent lysis and one would expect the voltage-gated sodium channels to be reduced in number, and the threshold for activation of the action potential to rise. This has been demonstrated in MG and experimental autoimmune MG (EAMG) muscle (Ruff and Lennon, 1998). Interestingly, Plomp *et al.* (1995) showed that the number of AChR packets released per nerve impulse is increased at MG and EAMG endplates, probably as a compensatory mechanism. The increase in the threshold for activation (Ruff and Lennon, 1998) explains why the patients are weak despite the compensatory increase in release.

## Antibodies affecting AChR function

In general, therefore, it is thought that few antibodies directly interfere with AChR function, either by binding to the ACh binding site and competing with ACh, or by binding within the ion channel itself. However, in a few patients antibodies inhibiting function are very important.

A series of studies by Hall and colleagues, at a time when human AChR was less readily available, demonstrated that many patients with MG have antibodies that bind better to fetal rat AChR than to adult rat AChR, and that some of these antibodies inhibit the function of the rat fetal AChR (Weinberg and Hall, 1979). In particular, one serum contained a high proportion of antibodies that inhibited binding of $\alpha$-BuTx to one of its two binding sites on fetal AChR, and this serum inhibited fetal AChR function. This was expected, since it is thought that both ACh binding sites must be occupied by ACh for full AChR activation. Somewhat surprisingly, since this serum had very few antibodies to determinants on the rat adult AChR, the MG patient had severe disease. This paradox was reconciled when it was found that the patients' serum antibodies inhibited $\alpha$-BuTx binding to both sites on fetal *human* AChR, and to one on adult *human* AChR, and that this was accompanied by a marked reduction in AChR function in normal human muscle biopsies exposed to the serum (Burges *et al.*, 1990). These

observations illustrate how difficult it is to generalize concerning the actions of antibodies in MG, and how diverse and variable the specificities of the antibodies can be both within and between patients.

Antibodies inhibiting the function of fetal AChR have other implications. Patients with MG who become pregnant can transfer disease to their offspring via placental-transfer of anti-AChR antibodies. Only a proportion of babies born to MG mothers are affected, perhaps because complement activity is lower in the neonate and because the ability of the immature NMJ to synthesize AChRs protects them against loss of AChR. There is some evidence that mothers who transfer disease to their babies have more reactivity with fetal AChR than adult AChR (Vernet der Garabedian *et al.*, 1994), but this is certainly not the only determining feature. Neonatal MG usually lasts only weeks or months, and most babies make a full recovery with no persistent weakness.

However, some babies have persistent muscle changes, or deformities resulting from lack of fetal movement *in utero*. At its most severe, there may be multiple joint contractures with facial deformities and hypoplasia of the lungs resulting in stillbirth or fetal loss. This condition, which results from loss of movement *in utero*, is called arthrogryposis multiplex congenita (AMC). The importance of loss of fetal movement in causing AMC was clearly demonstrated by Drachman and Coulombre in 1962 when they showed that injection of curare into the chick embryo resulted in chicks with deformed joints. Moessinger (1983) obtained similar results with injections into rat embryos *in vivo*. Strikingly, a baby born to a woman who was treated with muscle relaxants for tetanus during her pregnancy, developed AMC (Jago, 1970). In each case, AMC appeared to be associated with paralysis during development.

Thus, AMC is caused by any condition that reduces fetal movement, and in many cases the actual aetiology is unknown. There are some cases in which a genetic inheritance can be shown, either recessive or dominant, and intrauterine factors such as multiple pregnancies can be important. However, it is now clear that maternal antibodies directed against the fetal AChR are an infrequent, but potentially treatable, cause of

AMC. Several women with histories of AMC in successive pregnancies have been identified who have high levels of antibodies to AChR in their serum. Importantly, several have no obvious symptoms of MG (Brueton *et al.*, 2000), or have not been diagnosed as having MG until after the birth of the affected babies (Barnes *et al.*, 1995). The antibodies bind preferentially to fetal AChR rather than to adult AChR, but this in itself does not distinguish them from anti-AChR antibodies in many other women with MG (see above). The most clear distinction that underlies the development of AMC is that there are high levels of serum antibodies inhibiting the function of the fetal AChR (Vincent *et al.*, 1995; Riemersma *et al.*, 1996; Figure 13.3A). These antibodies have no effect on the function of the adult AChR, partly explaining why the mothers may be completely symptom free (although they often do have some antibodies binding to other determinants on adult AChR, these do not appear to be pathogenic or the symptoms are subclinical).

The ability of these antibodies to cause AMC was demonstrated using a maternal-to-fetal transfer model (Jacobson *et al.*, 1999). Pregnant mice injected daily with serum or IgG from mothers of AMC babies gave birth to fetuses who were paralysed with fixed joint contractures, surprisingly

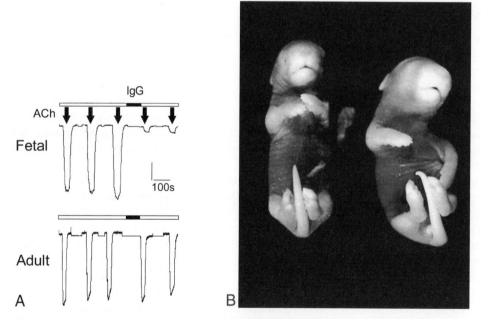

**Figure 13.3** Antibodies inhibiting fetal AChR function associated with arthrogyrposis multiplex congenita (AMC). (A) Inhibition of fetal AChR function by antibodies from a woman with antibodies directed at a fetal specific site. ACh-induced currents (arrows) were measured in *Xenopus* oocytes that had been injected with cloned RNA for the fetal (top) or adult (bottom) AChRs. At the bars, IgG purified from the serum of a woman with four babies, three of whom had died from arthrogryposis multiplex congenita was added. Currents through the fetal AChR almost disappeared, whereas those through the adult AChR were unaffected. (From Riemersma *et al.*, 1996 with permission of the publishers.) (B) Passive transfer of AMC. Pregnant mice were injected daily with serum from mothers of AMC babies. In about 50% of cases, the fetuses were born paralysed and did not survive. When removed under terminal anaesthesia just before term, the fetuses were found to show signs of arthrogryposis, similar to those in the human babies. A fetus removed at term from a mouse injected with healthy control serum (left) and one from a mouse injected with serum from the mother of AMC babies (right). (From Jacobson *et al.*, 1999 with permission of the publishers.)

similar to those exhibited by human babies (Figure 13.3B). Moreover, some of the mouse fetuses had internal abnormalities such as an Arnold Chiari malformation and an atrial-septal defect, suggesting that these or other maternal antibodies can cause internal deformities, and raising issues concerning the role of maternal antibodies in causing other neurodevelopmental disorders.

## Antibodies affecting AChR kinetics

Very few sera or IgG preparations have been shown to affect directly AChR function at the neuromuscular junction. This is largely because of the difficulty in obtaining normal human muscle biopsies for the studies, and perhaps also because of difficulties with accessibility of the serum antibodies to the NMJ *in vitro* (although the study by Burges *et al.*, (1990) clearly shows that serum antibodies can reach the NMJ *in vitro*). There is only one report of a patient in whom antibodies affecting the kinetics of the AChR function are suspected. In the muscle biopsy from this patient, both the endplate potentials and miniature endplate potentials showed marked prolongation of the decay phase, similar to that seen in the slow channel syndrome (see Chapter 12). Injection of her immunoglobulins into mice produced changes similar, though less marked, to those in her muscle. Antibodies in her serum were specific for adult AChR and did not bind appreciably to the fetal AchR, suggesting that they may be specific for a determinant on the $\varepsilon$-subunit that affects the duration of channel openings (Wintzen *et al.*, 1998).

## T cells in MG

The antibodies in MG are made by plasma cells, but their synthesis is also dependent on the presence of specific T-helper cells. Several groups have cloned T cells from the thymus or peripheral blood lymphocytes of MG patients, and shown specificity for different epitopes on the AChR subunits. These studies will not be discussed here, but the reader is referred to Vincent *et al.* (1998) for a recent review.

## Seronegative MG (SNMG)

About 15% of MG patients with typical generalized disease do not have antibodies to the AChR detectable by current methods, yet these patients improve with plasma exchange and their plasma or Ig antibodies can cause defects in neuromuscular transmission when injected into experimental animals (Mossman *et al.*, 1986) or reduce AChR function *in vitro* (Yamamoto *et al.*, 1991; Barrett-Jolley *et al.*, 1994). Moreover, there are reports of women with seronegative MG giving birth to babies with neonatal MG. Thus they appear to have serum antibodies that affect neuromuscular transmission but there is no evidence that these antibodies bind to AChRs (see Vincent *et al.*, 1998).

These antibodies are probably in both the IgG and IgM fractions, and bind to antigens expressed on muscle cells. Serum or plasma from SNMG patients inhibits the function of the AChR in a muscle-like cell line, TE671, but the inhibition is transient with full recovery occurring over a period of 60 minutes. This pattern of inhibition is very similar to that occurring in the presence of calcitonin-gene related peptide (CGRP); this peptide binds to G-protein-coupled CGRP receptors leading to an increase in the activity of protein kinase A (PKA). PKA can phosphorylate the AChR and increase the rate at which the AChR undergoes desensitization but, over time, dephosphorylation will take place and recovery occurs. Thus the similarity between the effects of SNMG plasmas and of CGRP suggest that the antibodies in SNMG bind to a surface receptor that is coupled to a second messenger system that leads to AChR phosphorylation. Some preliminary direct evidence for phosphorylation of the AChR in TE671 cells exposed to SNMG plasma has been obtained (see Vincent *et al.*, 1998).

Interestingly, the AChR inhibitory activity appears to be entirely due to IgM rather than IgG antibodies, raising questions as to how SNMG could be transferred to the fetus/neonate since IgM antibodies do not cross the placenta. In SNMG plasmas, however, there are also IgG antibodies that bind to the surface of TE671 cells (Blaes *et al.*, 2000). Importantly, these antibodies do not bind to human embryonic kidney (HEK) fibroblasts expressing human AChR, confirming that they bind to a surface protein that is expressed on the muscle-like TE671 cells but not on HEK cells or to AChR itself. It seems likely that these IgG antibodies are pathogenic *in vivo* by indirectly altering the function of the AChRs (as the IgM antibodies above) or by inducing complement-dependent destruction of the muscle surface, but they do not appear to activate second messengers *in vitro*. A recent report indicates that one target for these IgG antibodies is the muscle specific kinase, MuSK (Hoch *et al.*, 2001).

Further work is needed to try to define the nature of the antigens in SNMG, and to investigate the pathogenic mechanisms. Since some women with a history of several consecutive babies affected by AMC (see above) are negative for antibodies to AChR, it will be interesting to see whether SNMG IgG antibodies can affect fetal development using the maternal-to-fetal transfer model, and whether some anti-AChR negative mothers with recurrent AMC babies have antibodies to other muscle or neuronal antigens that cause fetal paralysis.

## The Lambert Eaton myasthenic syndrome

The Lambert Eaton myasthenic syndrome (LEMS) is a condition in which patients develop weakness, not unlike that in MG, but usually with a different distribution and characteristics. It is now known to be due to antibodies to VGCCs on the motor nerve terminal. The patients often present in middle age, and complain of weakness in trunk and limb muscles, whereas facial, ocular and bulbar involvement is less common than in MG. In MG, weakness is made worse by previous activation of the muscle, but in LEMS weakness can improve after sustained attempts to use the muscle. The basis for this difference lies in the pathophysiology of the two conditions and the all-or-none nature of neuromuscular transmission (see above). In MG, the endplate potentials become smaller during repetitive nerve impulses, perhaps because of a normal run-down in the number of quanta of ACh released. This leads to the endplate potential falling below the threshold for activation of the

voltage-gated sodium channels, resulting in failure of muscle contraction. In LEMS, there is a loss of VGCCs on the motor nerve terminal, and consequently a marked reduction in the number of packets of ACh released at rest; but during repetitive activity the number of released packets increases, probably due to accumulation of calcium in the presynaptic motor nerve terminal, and the endplate potential rises above the threshold for sodium channel activation (Elmqvist and Lambert, 1968; Lambert and Elmqvist, 1981). These differences in the behaviour of the NMJ in MG and LEMS are discussed more fully in Chapter 5.

LEMS is often associated with other autoimmune disorders, and can occur as a 'paraneoplastic' disorder since about 60% of patients have or develop a small cell lung cancer (O'Neill *et al.*, 1988). The role of antibodies to VGCCs in LEMS was established using the paradigms previously determined for defining the role of antibodies to AChRs in MG, but the sequence of observations was somewhat different. The first definitive evidence that LEMS was due to antibodies, was the marked clinical improvement that occurred after plasma exchange (Newsom-Davis and Murray, 1984; Lang *et al.*, 1981). Moreover, transfer of the plasma IgG fraction to mice resulted in a reduction in the quantal content of the endplate potential, similar to that seen in biopsies from LEMS patients (Lang *et al.*, 1983; Vincent *et al.*, 1989).

It was much more difficult to demonstrate the loss of VGCCs from the motor nerve terminals in LEMS cases, than it had been to demonstrate loss of AChRs in MG. Suitable neurotoxins were not available, and the number of VGCCs per NMJ is much lower than that of the AchRs, making quantitative experiments difficult. However, Engel and his colleagues used freeze fracture analysis of LEMS muscle and found a marked reduction in, and redistribution of, the active zone particles that are thought to represent VGCCs (Fukunaga *et al.*, 1982). Similar changes were found in mice after several days of injections of LEMS IgG (Fukunaga *et al.*, 1983) and this was preceded by a redistribution of active zone particles suggesting that they were clustered by divalent antibodies before they were lost from the nerve terminal surface (Nagel *et al.*, 1988). This did not occur if only monovalent IgG Fabs were injected suggesting that divalency of the antibodies is important for their pathogenicity. Finally, IgG was localized to the nerve terminals of mice injected with LEMS IgG (Fukuoka et al., 1987; Engel et al., 1989).

These observations were supported by *in vitro* experiments. VGCC numbers and function were measured in cultured cell lines by looking at $^{45}$calcium uptake following potassium-induced de-polarization. This uptake was sensitive to various non-specific calcium channel blockers. VGCCs were found to be expressed on the surface of SCLC cells (Roberts et al., 1985; De Azipurua et al., 1988), suggesting that the antigenic stimulus in paraneoplastic LEMS cases is the tumour itself. VGCC numbers were reduced when the cells were cultured for several days in LEMS IgG (Roberts et al., 1985), and again IgG monovalent Fabs were ineffectual.

However, none of the above observations proved without doubt that the antibodies were directed against VGCCs rather than some other cell surface molecule that could modulate their function (for instance as in the case of seronega-tive MG). Moreover, it was clear that VGCCs are a family of different channels, principally deter-mined by different $\alpha$-subunits of which there are at least five ($\alpha$1a, b, c, d, e; see Figure 13.4A). Following the use of $\alpha$-BuTx-labelled human AChR as an antigen in MG, several groups began to look for neurotoxins to use as a label for VGCCs. The breakthrough came from the work of Olivera and his colleagues (1994) who defined the specificity of the *Conus* snail toxins. A proportion of patients were found to have antibodies to N-type VGCCs extracted from human or rodent cerebellar tissue and labelled with $^{125}$I-*Conus geographus* GIVA toxin, but subsequently $> 90\%$ of LEMS patients were shown to have antibodies that bound VGCCs labelled with $^{125}$I-*Conus magus* MVII C neurotoxin, and this is now the routine diagnostic assay (Figure 13.4B; Motomura et al., 1995; Lennon et al., 1995).

The final proof would be in inducing an animal model of LEMS by immunization against VGCCs. This has not yet been proved possible, although some LEMS-like conditions have been induced by immunization with peptides representing synapto-tagmin or VGCC sequences (Takamori et al., 1994).

## Antibodies in LEMS patients define different subtypes of VGCCs

There is some evidence that antbodies to N-type VGCCs, as demonstrated by immunoprecipiation of $^{125}$I-GIVA-labelled cerebellar extracts, are more common in patients who have an associated cancer (Lennon et al., 1995). Some of the anti-bodies that recognize N-type VGCCs may be binding not to the extracellular surface but to cytoplasmic determinants on the $\beta$-subunit, sug-gesting that these determinants may be exposed to the immune system in the SCLC cells, but these antibodies to N-type VGCC are unlikely to be pathogenic.

To define the specificity of the antibodies more precisely, Johnston et al. (1994) used a SCLC cell line taken from a tumour removed from a woman with LEMS. They found that the VGCCs ex-pressed by the tumour were sensitive to MVIIC and aga-toxin, and not to GIVA, indicating that the VGCCs were of the P- or Q-type. Moreover, these VGCCs were reduced by culture in LEMS IgG, confirming that P- or Q-type VGCCs were the main target for the pathogenic antibodies. In addition, Pinto et al. (1998) used HEK cells transfected with different VGCC alpha subunits (with the appropriate beta subunits), and looked at calcium influx using photometric methods. They found that LEMS IgG only inhibited calcium influx through VGCCs encoded for by $\alpha$1a sub-units, and had no effect on VGCCs encoded by $\alpha$1b ,c or d subunits. Since the $\alpha$1a is thought to define the 'P/Q-type' VGCC, these results con-firmed that these are the target for the pathogenic antibodies.

The P-type and Q-type VGCCs appear to be both encoded by $\alpha$1a subunits, but have differ-ences in their electrophysiological characteristics. P-type VGCCs are characteristically found on Purkinje cells in the cerebellum, whereas Q-type VGCCs are found in the granular layer cells. To see whether both types were susceptible to LEMS antibodies, Pinto et al. (1998) cultured the two cell types separately and applied LEMS IgG. In both cases there was a highly significant reduction in the number of P- or Q-type VGCCs indicating that both are targets for LEMS antibodies. Thus LEMS antibodies have helped to establish that the P- and

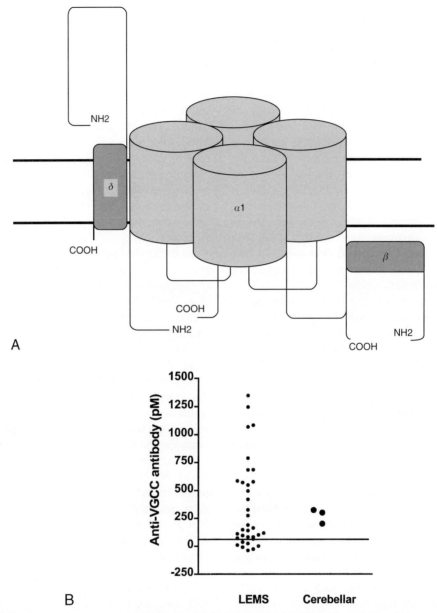

**Figure 13.4** The voltage-gated calcium channel and antibodies in the Lambert Eaton myasthenic syndrome and in some cases of cancer-associated cerebellar ataxia. (A) Diagram of the voltage-gated calcium channel illustrating the three main subunits. The $\alpha$1 subunit has at least eight different isofroms (A–H), is made up of four homologous domains (each with six transmembrane sequences), is the main determinant of sensitivity to different neurotoxins, and is thought to be the site of binding of antibodies to VGCCs in the Lambert Eaton myasthenic syndrome. The $\beta$-subunit (of which there are four known isoforms) is entirely intracellular. The $\delta$-subunit spans the membrane once and has a large extracellular domain. (B) Immunoprecipitation of VGCCs labelled with $^{125}$I-$\omega$-conotoxin MVIIC by serum from LEMS patients and from three patients who presented with cerebellar ataxia. This neurotoxin binds selectively to the $\alpha$1A isoform which defines the P/Q-type VGCC. The sera were the first available sample assayed in each case, but some had already received immunosuppressive treatment for some time. The three patients with cerebellar ataxia were identified from 280 cases sent for routine paraneoplastic antibody screening. Each of them was shown subsequently to have a lung tumour (probably small cell lung cancer). The cut off for healthy controls and other neurological diseases is shown by the horizontal line. Data by courtesy of Dr Bethan Lang.

Q-type VGCCs are indeed both encoded by $\alpha$1a subunits.

## Anti-VGCC antibodies and autonomic nervous system

An important feature of LEMS that distinguishes it from MG is the presence of autonomic symptoms. Typically, LEMS patients complain of dry mouth, constipation and often sexual impotence in males. Neurotransmitter release in the autonomic nervous system, however, is thought to be regulated mainly by N-type VGCC, raising questions concerning the role of the antibodies to P/Q-type VGCCs in causing these symptoms. However, Waterman (1996) showed that some of the nerve-induced muscle contraction in the bladder or vas deferens is sensitive to inhibitors of P-type VGCC such as agatoxin or conotoxin MVIIC. Moreover, when preparations were taken from mice injected for several days with LEMS IgG, although the nerve-induced muscle contraction was not substantially reduced, it was no longer sensitive to P-type VGCC channel blockers, indicating that LEMS IgG antibodies can alter the function in the autonomic nervous system (Waterman *et al.*, 1997).

## Anti-VGCC antibodies and cerebellar ataxia

Patients with SCLC have an increased chance of developing a range of neurological disorders including subacute sensory neuronopathy, limbic and brainstem encephalitis, and cerebellar ataxia. These disorders are often associated with the presence of an antibody to a neuronal nuclear antigen called 'Hu'. The antibodies are not pathogenic, since the antigen is intracellular, but their detection is important because it points to the presence of the SCLC (see Vincent, 1999).

Since LEMS is also associated with SCLC, it would not be surprising if some patients had antibodies to both Hu and VGCCs, and a range of symptoms involving both the central and peripheral nervous systems. Cerebellar ataxia is particularly interesting since it is due to progressive loss of Purkinje cells (that express VGCCs as discussed above). Mason *et al.* (1997) showed

that patients with cerebellar ataxia, associated with SCLC, can have either anti-Hu antibodies, anti-VGCC antibodies or both. When anti-VGCC antibodies are present, LEMS is likely to be a feature but may go unnoticed in the presence of severe cerebellar signs. Nevertheless, recognition of LEMS and anti-VGCC antibodies is important, because treatment of the peripheral LEMS symptoms can improve the patients' overall clinical state, and removal of anti-VGCC antibodies by plasma exchange or immunosuppression may also be able to slow progression of the Purkine cell loss. Although rare, this combination of LEMS and cerebellar ataxia with anti-VGCC antibodies suggests that in some situations circulating antibodies to neuronal antigens can cause CNS disease.

# Conclusions and further prospects

The existence of three clearly defined autoimmune disorders of neuromuscular transmission, each caused by an antibody to a distinct ion channel (see also Chapter 14), has not only thrown light on disease mechanisms but opened up many avenues for improved therapy. The questions arising, of course, are why do patients develop antibodies to these highly important ion channels, whether there are other peripheral disorders that are also caused by antibodies to ion channel proteins, or to other cell surface receptors, and in particular, whether central nervous system disorders can be caused by antibodies.

The analogy with the genetic 'channelopathies' suggests that one should look for antibodies to VGCCs, VGKCs and voltage-gated sodium channels in any acquired disorder of the central or peripheral nervous system, or of muscle. The possible role of anti-VGCC antibodies in some cases of cerebellar ataxia suggests that there should be further investigation of these cases looking for the existence of pathogenic antibodies. Recently, we found antibodies to VGCCs in three cases of cerebellar ataxia, all of which subsequently proved to have SCLC (see Figure 13.4B; Trivedi *et al.*, 2000), and to VGKCs in a number of individuals with symptoms resembling limbic encephalitis (Buckley *et al.*, 2001). Some of these have acquired neuromyotonia (see Chapter 14) but in others, no muscle symptoms were reported. In one particular case, a patient with a long history of MG who had had a thymoma removed many years previously had a single episode of limbic signs (confusion, memory loss, hallucinations) that coincided with a temporary but highly significant rise in antibodies to VGKC. These fell following plasma exchange, correlating with the patient's improvement (Buckley *et al.*, 2001). No antibodies to voltage-gated sodium channels have been demonstrated as of now.

In Rasmussen's encephalitis, a very severe childhood form of epilepsy, antibodies to the ligand-gated ion-channel, glutamate receptor GluR3, have been shown in a few cases, and there are reports of response to plasma exchange and intravenous immunoglobulin therapies (Whitney and McNamara, 1999). Whether all cases are associated with antibodies to GluR3 or antibodies to other neuronal receptors, or to antibodies at all is not yet clear. Recently, evidence for antibodies to GluR1 receptors has been shown in two cases of Hodgkin's-associated cerebellar ataxia (Silvius-Smit *et al.*, 2000).

Another possible role for antibodies to ion channels is in development. Transfer of antibodies across the placenta has been shown to be one cause of AMC, a rare but very disabling or fatal condition. Are there other antibodies to fetal-specific isoforms of ion channels, or are there other antibodies that can cross the placenta and cause CNS disorders in the fetus while not getting into the maternal CNS in sufficient amounts to affect the pregnant mother? The maternal-to-fetal transfer model that we have developed will allow us to test the role of maternal antibodies in causing neurodevelopmental abnormalities, and perhaps some of these will turn out to be due to antibodies to neuronal ion channels.

# References

Aidley, D. J. (1999). *The physiology of excitable cells.* Cambridge: Cambridge University Press.

Barnes, P. R. J., Kanabar, D. J., Brueton, L. *et al.* (1995). Recurrent congenital arthrogryposis leading to a diag-

nosis of myasthenia gravis in an initially asymptomatic mother. *Neuromusc Dis.*, **5**, 59–65.

Barrett-Jolley, R., Byrne, N., Vincent, A. and Newsom-Davis, J. (1994). Seronegative myasthenia gravis plasmas reduce acetylcholine-induced currents in TE671 cells. *Pflügers Arch.*, **428**, 492–8.

Beeson, D., Jacobson, L., Newsom-Davis, J. and Vincent, A. (1996). A transfected human muscle cell line expressing the adult subtype of the human muscle acetylcholine receptor for diagnostic assays in myasthenia gravis. *Neurology*, 47, 1552–5.

Blaes, F., Beeson, D., Plested, C. P., Lang, B. and Vincent, A. (2000). IgG from seronegative myasthenia gravis patients binds to Te671 cells but not to human AChR expressed in HEK cells. *Ann Neurol.*, 47, 504–10.

Brueton, L. A., Huson, S. M., Cox, P. M. *et al.* (2000). Asymptomatic maternal myasthenia as a cause of the Pena-Shokeir phenotype. *Am J Med Gen.*, **92**, 1–6.

Buckley, C., Oger, J., Carpenter, K., Jackson, M., Vincent, A. (2001). Potassium channel antibodies in two patients with reversible limbic encephalitis. *Ann Neurol.*, In Press.

Burges, J., Wray, D. W., Pizzighella, S., Hall, Z. and Vincent, A. (1990). A myasthenia gravis plasma immunoglobulin reduces miniature endplate potentials at human endplates *in vitro*. *Muscle Nerve*, **13**, 407–13.

Colquhoun, D. (1992). Agonists, antagonists and synaptic transmission at the neuromuscular junction. In *Neuromuscular transmission: basic and applied aspects* (eds Vincent, A. and Wray, D.), Studies in Neuroscience, 12. Manchester University Press, Manchester, pp. 132–156.

Compston, D. A. S., Vincent, A., Newsom-Davis, J., and Batchelor, J. R. (1980). Clinical, pathological, HLA antigen and immunological evidence for disease heterogeneity in myasthenia gravis. *Brain*, **103**, 579–601.

De Aizpurua, H. J., Lambert, E. H., Griesmann, G. E., Olivera, B. O. and Lennon, V. A. (1988). Antagonism of voltage-gated calcium channels in small cell carcinomas of patients with and without Lambert-Eaton myasthenic syndrome by autoantibodies, W-conotoxin and adenosine. *Cancer Res.*, **48**, 4719–24.

Drachman, D. B. (1994). Myasthenia gravis. *New Engl J Med.*, **330**, 1797–1810.

Drachman, D. B. and Coulombre, A. (1962). Experimental clubfoot and arthrogryposis multiplex congenita. *Lancet*, **2**, 523–6.

Drachman, D. B., Angus, D. W., Adams, R. N., Michelson, J. D. and Hoffman, G. J. (1978). Myasthenia antibodies cross-link acetylcholine receptors to accelerate degradation. *N Engl J Med.*, **198**, 1116–22.

Drachman, D. B., Adams, R. N., Josifek, L. F. and Self, S. G. (1982). Functional activities of autoantibodies to acetylcholine receptors and the clinical severity of myasthenia gravis. *N Engl J Med.*, **307**, 769–75.

Elmqvist, D., Hofmann, W. W., Kugelberg, J. and Quastel, D. M. J. (1964). An electrophysiological investigation of neuromuscular transmission in myasthenia gravis. *J Physiol (Lond.)*, **174**, 417–34.

Elmqvist, D. and Lambert, E. H. (1968). Detailed analysis of neuromuscular transmission in a patient with the myasthenic syndrome sometimes associated with bronchogenic carcinoma. *Mayo Clin Proc.*, **43**, 689–713.

Engel, A. G. and Arahata, K. (1987). The membrane attack complex of complement at the endplate in myasthenia gravis. *Ann NY Acad Sci.*, **505**, 326–32.

Engel, A. G., Lambert, E. H. and Howard, F. M. (1977). Immune complexes (IgG and C3) at the motor endplate in myasthenia gravis. Ultrastructural and light microscopic localization and electrophysiologic correlations. *Mayo Clin Proc.*, **52**, 267–80.

Engel, A. G., Nagel, A., Fukuoka, T. *et al.* (1989). Motor nerve terminal calcium channels in Lambert-Eaton myasthenic syndrome. Morphologic evidence for depletion and that the depletion is mediated by autoantibodies. *Ann N Y Acad Sci.*, **560**, 278–90.

Fambrough, D. M., Drachman, D. B. and Satyamurti, S. (1973). Neuromuscular junction in myasthenia gravis: decreased acetylcholine receptors. *Science*, **182**, 293–5.

Fukunaga, H., Engel, A. G., Osame, M. and Lambert, E. H. (1982). Paucity and disorganisation of presynaptic membrane active zones in the Lambert-Eaton myasthenic syndrome. *Muscle Nerve*, **5**, 686–97.

Fukunaga, H., Engel, A. G., Lang, B., Newsom-Davis, J. and Vincent, A. (1983). Passive transfer of Lambert-Eaton myasthenic syndrome with IgG from man to mouse depletes the presynaptic membrane active zones. *Proc Natl Acad Sci U SA*, **80**, 7636–40.

Fukuoka, T., Engel, A. G., Lang, B., Newsom-Davis, J. and Vincent, A. (1987). Lambert-Eaton myasthenic syndrome: II. Immunoelectron microscopy localization of IgG at the mouse motor end-plate. *Ann Neurol.*, **22**, 200–11.

Guyon, T., Lavasseru, P., Truffault, F., Cottin. C., Gaud. C. and Berrih Aknin, S. (1994). Regulation of acetylcholine receptor alpha subunit variants in human myasthenia gravis: Quantification of steady-state levels of messenger RNA in muscle biopsy using the polymerase chain reaction. *J Clin Invest.*, **94**, 16–24.

Hall, Z. W. and Sanes, J. R. (1993). Synaptic structure and development: the neuromuscular junction. *Cell*, **72**, 99–121.

Harvey, A. L. (ed). (1993). *Natural and Synthetic Neurotoxins*. Neuroscience Perspectives. Academic Press.

Hesselmans, L. F. G. M., Jennekens, F. G. I. , Van Den Oord, C. J. M., Veldman, H. and Vincent, A. (1993). Development of innervation of skeletal muscle fibres in man: relation to acetylcholine receptors. *Anat Rec.*, **236**, 553–62.

Hoch, W., McConville, J., Helms, S., Newsom-Davis, J.,

Melms, A., Vincent, A. (2001) Autoantibodies to the receptor tyrosine kinase MuSK in patients with myasthemia gravis without acetylcholine receptor antibodies. *Nat Med.*, **7**, In Press.

Hong, S. J. and Chang, C. C. (1989). Use of geographutoxin II (u-conotoxin) for the study of neuromuscular transmission in mouse. *Br J Pharmacol.*, **97**, 934–40.

Ito, Y., Miledi, R., Vincent, A. and Newsom-Davis, J. (1978). Acetylcholine receptors and end-plate electrophysiology in myasthenia gravis. *Brain*, **101**, 345–68.

Jacobson, L., Beeson, D., Tzartos, S. and Vincent, A. (1999a). Monoclonal antibodies raised against human acetylcholine receptor bind to all five subunits of the fetal isoform. *J Neuroimmunol.*, **98**, 112–20.

Jacobson, L., Beeson, D., Tzartos, S. and Vincent, A. (1999b). Plasma from human mothers of fetuses with severe arthrogryposis multiplex congenita causes deformities in mice. *J Clin Invest.*, **103**, 1031–8.

Jago, R. H. (1970). Arthrogryposis following treatment of maternal tetanus with muscle relaxants. *Arch Dis Child.*, **45**, 277–9.

Johnston, I., Lang, B., Leys, K. and Newsom-Davis, J. (1994). Heterogeneity of calcium channel autoantibodies detected using a small cell lung cancer line derived from a Lambert-Eaton syndrome patient. *Neurology*, **44**, 334–8.

Karlin, A. and Akabas, M. H. (1995). Toward a structural basis for the function of nicotinic acetylcholine receptors and their cousins. *Neuron*, **15**, 1231–44.

Komai, K., Iwasa, K., Takamori, M. Calcium channel peptide can cause an autoimmune-mediated model of Lambert-Eaton myasthenic syndrome in rats. *J Neurol Sci.*, 1999, **166**, 126–30.

Lambert, E. H. and Elmqvist, D. (1971). Quantal components of end-plate potentials in the myasthenic syndrome. *Ann NY Acad* Sci., **183**, 183–99.

Lang, B., Newsom-Davis, J., Prior, C. and Wray, D. (1983). Antibodies to motor nerve terminals: an electrophysiological study of a human myasthenic syndrome transferred to mouse. *J Physiol Lond.*, **344**, 335–45.

Lang, B., Newsom-Davis, J., Wray, D., Vincent, A. and Murray, N. M. F. (1981). Autoimmune aetiology for myasthenic (Eaton-Lambert) syndrome. *Lancet*, **ii**, 224–6.

Lennon, V. A., Kryzer, T. J., Griesmann, G. E. *et al.* (1995). Calcium channel antibodies in the Lambert Eaton myasthenic syndrome and other paraneoplastic syndromes. *New Eng J Med.*, **332**, 1467–74.

Lindstrom, J. M., Seybold, M. E., Lennon, V. A., Whittingham, S. and Duane, D. D. (1976). Antibody to acetylcholine receptor in myasthenia gravis. Prevalence, clinical correlates and diagnostic value. *Neurology*, **26**, 1054–9.

Lindstrom, J. (1997). Nicotinic acetylcholine receptors in health and disease. *Mol Neurobiol.*, **15**, 193–222.

Llinas, R., Sugimori, M., Hillman, D. E. and Cherksey, B. (1992). Distribution and functional significance of the P-type, voltage-dependent Ca2$^+$ channels in the mammalian central nervous system. *Trends Neurosci.*, **15**, 351–5.

Mason, W. P., Graus, F., Lang, B. *et al.* (1997). Small cell lung cancer: paraneoplastic cerebellar degeneration and the Lambert Eaton myasthenic syndrome. *Brain*, **120**, 1279–1300.

Milone, M., Hutchinson, D. and Engel, A. G. (1994). Patch clamp analysis of the properties of acetylcholine receptor channels at the normal human endplate. *Muscle Nerve*, **17**, 1364–9.

Missias, A. C., Chu, G. C., Klocke, B., Sanes, J. R. and Merlie, J. P. (1986). Maturation of the acetylcholine receptor in developing skeletal muscle: regulation of the AChR g to e switch. *Dev Biol.*, **179**, 223–38.

Miyazawa, A., Fujiyoshi, Y., Stowell, M. and Unwin, N. (1999). Nicotinic acetylcholine receptor at 4.6 A resolution: transverse funnels in the channel wall. *J Mol Biol.*, **288**, 765–86.

Motomura, M., Johnston, I., Lang B., Vincent, A. and Newsom-Davis, J. (1995). An improved diagnostic assay for Lambert-Eaton myasthenic syndrome. *J Neurol Neurosurg Psychiatr.*, **58**, 85–7.

Moessinger, A. (1983). Fetal akinesia deformation sequence; an animal model. *Pediatrics*, **72**, 857–63.

Mossman, S., Vincent, A. and Newsom-Davis, J. (1986). Myasthenia gravis without acetylcholine receptor antibody: a distinct disease entity. *Lancet*, **1**, 116–9.

Nagel, A., Engel, A. G., Lang B., Newsom-Davis, J. and Fukuoka, T. (1988). Lambert-Eaton myasthenic syndrome IgG depletes presynaptic membrane active zone particles by antigenic modulation. *Ann Neurol.*, **24**, 552–8.

Newsom-Davis, J. and Murray, N. M. (1984). Plasma exchange and immunosuppressive drug treatment in the Lambert-Eaton myasthenic syndrome. *Neurology*, **34**, 480–5.

Newsom-Davis, J., Pinching, A J., Vincent, A. and Wilson, S. G. (1978). Function of circulating antibody to acetylcholine receptor in myasthenia gravis: investigation by plasma exchange. *Neurology*, **28**, 266–72.

O'Neill, J. H., Murray, N. M. and Newsom-Davis, J. (1988). The Lambert-Eaton myasthenic syndrome. A review of 50 cases. *Brain*, **111**, 577–96.

Olivera, B. M., Miljanich, G. P., Ramachandran, J. and Adams, M E. (1994). Calcium channel diversity and neurotransmitter release: the w-conotoxins and w-Agatoxins. *Ann Rev Biochem.*, **63**, 823–67.

Patrick, J. and Lindstrom, J. (1973). Autoimmune response to acetylcholine receptor. *Science*, **180**, 871–2.

Pinto, A., Gillard, S., Moss, F. *et al.* (1998). Human autoantibodies specific for the a1A calcium channel subunit reduce both P-type and Q-type calcium currents in cerebellar neurons. *Proc Natl Acad Sci USA*, **95**, 8328–33.

Plomp, J. J., Van-Kempen, G. T. H., De Baets, M.,

Graus, Y. M. F., Kuks, J. B. M. and Molenaar, P. C. (1995). Acetylcholine release in myasthenia gravis: Regulation at single end-plate level. *Ann Neurol.*, **37**, 627–36.

Riemersma, S., Vincent, A., Beeson, D., Newland, C., Hawke, S., Vernet-der Garabedian, B. *et al.* (1996). Association of arthrogryposis multiplex congenita with maternal antibodies inhibiting fetal acetylcholine receptor function. *J Clin Invest.*, **98**, 2358–63.

Roberts, A., Perera S., Lang, B., Vincent, A. and Newsom-Davis, J. (1985). Paraneoplastic myasthenic syndrome IgG inhibits $^{45}$Ca$^{2+}$ flux in a human small cell carcinoma line. *Nature*, **317**, 737–9.

Ruff, R. L. and Lennon, V. A. (1998). End-plate voltage-gated sodium channels are lost in clinical and experimental myasthenia gravis. *Ann Neurol.*, **43**, 370–9.

Sanes, J. R. and Lichtman, J. W. (1999). Development of the vertebrate neuromuscular junction. *Ann Rev Neurosci.*, **22**, 389–442.

Schluep, M., Willcox, N., Vincent, A., Dhoot, G. K., Newsom-Davis, J. Acetylcholine receptors in human thymic myoid cells in situ: an immunohistological study. *Ann Neurol.*, 1987, **22**, 12–22.

Sillevis-Smitt, P., Kinoshita, A., De Leeuw, B., Moll, W., Coesmans, M., Jaarsma, D., Henzen-Logman, S., Vecht, C., DeZeeuw, C., Sekiyama, N., Nakanishi, S., Shigemoto, R. (2000). Paraneoplastic cerebellar ataxia due to autoantibodies against a glutamate receptor. *N Engl J Med.*, **342**, 21–7.

Simpson, J. A. (1960). Myasthenia gravis: a new hypothesis. *Scot Med J.*, **5**, 419–39.

Sudhof, T. C. (1995). The synaptic vesicle cycle: a cascade of protein-protein interactions. *Nature*, **375**, 645–53.

Takamori, M., Hamada, T., Komai, K., Takahashi, M. and Yoshida, A. (1994). Synaptotagmin can cause an immune-mediated model of Lambert Eaton myasthenic syndrome in rats. *Ann Neurol.*, **35**, 74–80.

Toyka, K. V., Drachman, D. B., Griffin, D. E. *et al.* (1977). Myasthenia gravis: study of humoral immune mechanisms by passive transfer to mice. *N Engl J Med.*, **296**, 125–31.

Trivedi, R., Mundanthanam, G., Amyes, E., Lang, B., Vincent, A. Autoantibody screening in subacute cerebellar ataxia. *Lancet*, 2000, **356**, 356–6.

Tzartos, S. J., Barkas, T., Cung, M. T. *et al.* (1991). The main immunogenic region of the acetylcholine receptor: structure and role in myasthenia gravis. *Autoimmunity*, **8**, 259–70.

Tzartos, S. J. and Lindstrom, J. M. (1980). Monoclonal antibodies used to probe acetylcholine receptor structure: localization of the main immunogenic region and detection of similarities between subunits. *Proc Natl Acad Sci USA*, **77**, 755–9.

Tzartos, S. J., Seybold, M. E. and Lindstrom, J. M. (1982). Specificities of antibodies to acetylcholine receptors in sera from myasthenia gravis patients measured by monoclonal antibodies. *Proc Natl Acad Sci USA*, **79**, 188–92.

Vernet der Garabedian, B., Lacokova, M., Eymard, B. *et al.* (1994). Association of neonatal myasthenia gravis with antibodies against the fetal acetylcholine receptor. *J Clin Invest.*, **94**. 555–9.

Vincent, A. (1999). Antibodies to ion channels in paraneoplastic disorders. *Brain Pathol.*, **9**, 285–91.

Vincent, A. and Wray, D. (eds) (1992). *Neuromuscular transmission: basic and applied aspects.* Oxford: Pergamon.

Vincent, A., Newland, C., Brueton, L. *et al.* (1995). Arthrogryposis multiplex congenita with maternal autoantibodies specific for a fetal antigen. *Lancet*, **346**, 24–5.

Vincent, A. and Newsom-Davis, J. (1985). Acetylcholine receptor antibody as a diagnostic test for myasthenia gravis: results in 153 validated cases and 2967 diagnostic assays. *J Neurol Neurosurg Psychiatr.*, **48**, 1246–52.

Vincent, A., Jacobson, L., Plested, P. *et al.* (1998). Antibodies affecting ion channel function in acquired neuromyotonia, in seropositive and seronegative myasthenia gravis, and in antibody-mediated arthrogryposis multiplex congenita. *Ann New York Acad Sci.*, **841**, 482–96.

Vincent, A., Lang, B. and Newsom-Davis, J. (1989). Autoimmunity to the voltage-gated calcium channel underlies the Lambert-Eaton myasthenic syndrome, a paraneoplastic disorder. *Trends Neurosci.*, **12**, 496–502.

Vincent, A., Whiting, P. J., Schluep, M. *et al.* (1987). Antibody heterogeneity and specificity in myasthenia gravis. *Ann NY Acad Sci.*, **505**, 326–32.

Vincent, A., Willcox, N., Hill, M., Curnow, J., MacLennan, C. and Beeson, D. (1998). Determinant spreading and immune responses to acetylcholine receptors in myasthenia gravis. *Immunol Rev.*, **164**, 157–68.

Waterman, S. A. (1996). Multiple subtypes of voltage-gated calcium channel mediate transmitter release from parasympathetic neurons in the mouse bladder. *J Neurosci.*, **16**, 4155–61.

Waterman, S. A., Lang, B. and Newsom-Davis, J. (1997). Effect of Lambert Eaton myasthenic syndrome antibodies on autonomic neurons in the mouse. *Ann Neurol.*, **42**, 147–56.

Weinberg, C. B. and Hall, Z. W. (1979). Antibodies from patients with myasthenia gravis recognise determinants unique to extrajunctional acetylcholine receptors. *Proc Natl Acad Sci.*, **76**, 504–8.

Whitney, K. D. and McNamara, J. O. (1999). Autoimmunity and neurological disease: antibody modulation of synaptic transmission. *Ann Rev Neurosci.*, **22**, 175–95.

Wilson, S., Vincent, A. and Newsom-Davis, J. (1983). Acetylcholine receptor turnover in mice with passively transferred myasthenia gravis. II. Receptor synthesis. *J Neurol Neurosurg Psychiatr.*, **46**, 383–7.

Wintzen, A. R., Plomp, J. J., Molenaar, P. C. *et al.* (1998). Acquired slow channel syndrome: a form of myasthenia gravis with prolonged open time of the acetylcholine receptor channel. *Ann Neurol.*, **44**, 657–64.

Wood, S. J. and Slater, C. R. (1997). The contribution of postsynaptic folds to the safety factor for neuromuscular transmission in rat fast and slow twitch muscles. *J Physiol.*, **500**, 165–76.

Wood, S. J. and Slater, C. R. (1998). b-Spectrin is colocalized with both voltage-gated sodium channels and ankyrinG at the adult rat neuromuscular junction. *J Cell Biol.*, **140**, 675–84.

Yamamoto, T., Vincent, A., Ciulla, T. A., Lang, B., Johnston, I. and Newsom-Davis, J. (1991). Seronegative myasthenia gravis: A plasma factor inhibiting agonist-induced acetylcholine receptor function co-purifies with IgM. *Ann Neurol.*, **30**, 550–7.

# 14 Autoimmune neuromyotonia

*I. K. Hart*

## Introduction

Neuromyotonia (NMT; Isaacs' syndrome) is a syndrome of nerve hyperexcitability that usually presents with clinical and electomyographic (EMG) features of continuous skeletal muscle overactivity. The syndrome is the common manifestation of nerve damage caused by several different pathogenic mechanisms. While some forms of NMT are inherited (Auger *et al.*, 1984) and occur in conditions such as hereditary motor polyneuropathies and familial episodic ataxia type 1 with myokymia, the great majority of cases are acquired. There is now compelling clinical and experimental evidence that many of the acquired cases are caused by autoantibodies that target nerve voltage-gated potassium channels (VGKC). This chapter reviews briefly the clinical features of the disorder and discusses the work that has defined the syndrome of autoimmune neuromyotonia (AINMT) and established it as an antibody-mediated potassium channelopathy.

## The clinical syndrome of AINMT

### Clinical features

Typically, the presenting features of the muscle overactivity in AINMT are myokymia (muscle twitching) and cramps (Denny-Brown and Foley, 1948; Gamstop and Wohlfart, 1959; Isaacs, 1961; Mertens and Zschoke, 1965). In the fully developed syndrome, these are associated with muscle stiffness, pseudomyotonia (delayed muscle relaxation after contraction), pseudotetany (for example Chvostek's and Trousseau's signs), weakness and increased sweating. Muscle contraction often provokes or exacerbates symptoms. The limb and trunk muscles are most commonly affected, although facial, bulbar and respiratory muscles can also be involved. The reflexes are usually normal but can be reduced or absent, especially when there is an accompanying neuropathy. Chronic cases can develop muscle hypertrophy.

About 10–20% of patients also have sensory symptoms such as paraesthesia and numbness that are usually unaccompanied by any other evidence of peripheral neuropathy, suggesting that sensory as well as motor nerves may be hyperexcitable (Lance *et al.*, 1979).

Central nervous system (CNS) symptoms ranging from personality change and insomnia to a psychotic-like state with delusions and hallucinations can occur. This association is called chorée fibrillaire, or maladie de Morvan (Morvan, 1890; Serratrice and Azulay, 1994). Autonomic dysfunction has been reported occasionally (Halbach *et al.*, 1987).

The severity of all the features of the syndrome range from the inconvenient to the incapacitating. The course is variably progressive, although spontaneous remissions can occur.

Good epidemiological data are lacking. Review of the published cases suggests that the syndrome can occur from the first to the ninth decade with median incidence between the ages of 30 to 40. In a survey of 44 patients from Oxford and Liverpool, the male to female ratio was 60:40. HLA typing of 12 patients showed no definite associations (unpublished data). The syndrome has been reported in most races.

## Electrophysiological features

The cardinal EMG feature of all variants of NMT is the spontaneous firing of single motor units as doublet, triplet or multiplet discharges (Denny-Brown and Foley, 1948; Gamstorp and Wohlfart, 1959; Isaacs, 1961). These neuromyotonic discharges have an intraburst frequency of 40 to 400 Hz and, in most patients, occur at irregular intervals of 1 to 30 seconds (Figure 14.1). They are usually found even when there is no visible muscle twitching. Voluntary or electrical activation of a peripheral nerve may trigger prolonged after-discharges that are similar in type. Fasciculation and fibrillation potentials can also occur.

Isaacs (1961, 1967) established that the motor unit activity arises in the peripheral motor nerves. In an elegant series of experiments, he demonstrated that the discharges were abolished by blockade of the neuromuscular junction by curare and persisted after proximal or distal nerve block by local anaesthesia. He concluded that the activity was generated in the terminal arborization of the motor axons. These findings have subsequently been reproduced in many other patients using the same methods. Furthermore, the application of botulinum toxin localized the origin of the neuromuscular discharges to the terminal regions of the peripheral nerves in patients where a proximal site of ectopic activity had been discounted (Deymeer

et al., 1998). Occasionally, however, the motor unit activity in AINMT patients has been reduced or stopped by either proximal nerve block (Irani et al., 1977; Partanen et al., 1980; Garciá-Merino et al., 1991) or epidural anaesthesia (Hosokawa et al., 1987). Thus, taken together, these findings suggest that the spontaneous activity can originate at different sites along the length of the nerve. In most patients the site is probably distal, although in a few patients the site may be proximal, perhaps even including the lower motor neuron cell body in the anterior horn of the spinal cord.

Sleep or general anaesthesia has no effect on NMT discharges (Isaacs, 1961), whereas they both abolish the centrally generated continuous motor unit activity that characterizes stiff man syndromes (Solimena et al., 1988). These features can be helpful in distinguishing these two syndromes, which can sometimes present in similar ways.

The observation that conventional nerve conduction studies are usually normal in AINMT led to the suggestion that the syndrome should be classed as an axonopathy, rather than a neuropathy (Gutmann and Gutmann, 1996). This assumes that all cases of AINMT are a manifestation of primary alterations in axon excitation, with normal axon structure and myelination. However, 5–10% of patients do have electrical evidence of an idiopathic axonal or demyelinating neuropathy that is typically mild, often subclinical, and non-progressive. The reason why this minority of AINMT patients have a neuropathy is unclear. In addition, AINMT patients with associated autoimmune diseases such as diabetes mellitus, rheumatoid disease, and systemic lupus erythematosus (SLE) can have a neuropathy with features typical of that disorder.

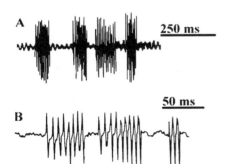

**Figure 14.1** Needle electromyograph recording from a small hand muscle of a patient with autoimmune neuromyotonia. (A) Four multiplet neuromyotonic discharges lasting 65 to 190 ms and occurring at irregular intervals. (B) Expanded view of one triplet and two multiplet discharges from a single motor unit with an intraburst firing frequency of up to 230 Hz.

## Serum and cerebrospinal fluid tests

Elevated titres of serum anti-VGKC antibodies are detected in 50–60% of AINMT patients by a radioimmunoprecipitation assay (RIA) (Hart et al., 1997). This assay uses an iodinated snake venom toxin ($^{125}$I-$\alpha$-dendrotoxin) that binds specifically to some subtypes of *Shaker*-related VGKCs (KCNA1, A2 and A6; see Table 14.2). A more sensitive molecular-immunohistochemical assay detects anti-VGKC antibodies to these channel subtypes in 80–90% of patients (Hart *et al.*, 1997). At present, however, it is not widely available (see later).

About 70% of patients have mild to moderate elevation of serum creatine kinase and other skeletal muscle proteins. These changes reflect muscle damage caused by overactivity and may be useful in monitoring an individual patient's response to therapy. Serum acid–base balance, calcium and magnesium are all normal. Cerebrospinal fluid (CSF) cell count and albumin are typically normal. CSF total IgG can be raised and oligoclonal bands are found in 5–10% of patients (Newsom-Davis and Mills, 1993).

## Associated autoimmune syndromes

AINMT occurs in association with a wide range of other autoimmune conditions. Of 44 patients with AINMT seen at Oxford or Liverpool, three had myasthenia gravis (MG) without thymoma, two had rheumatoid disease, two had SLE, two had diabetes mellitus without neuropathy at presenta-

tion, one had chronic inflammatory demyelinating polyneuropathy and another had vitiligo. Table 14.1 lists the other reported disorders, at least some of which may have been fortuitous (Harman and Richardson, 1954; Reeback *et al.*, 1979; Vilchez *et al.*, 1980; Vasilescu *et al.*, 1984; Newsom-Davis and Mills, 1993; Gutmann *et al.*, 1996; Hadjivassiliou *et al.*, 1997; Le Gars *et al.*, 1997; Benito-Leon *et al.*, 1999).

There is also strong clinical evidence that AINMT can be a paraneoplastic syndrome (Table 14.1) (Waerness, 1974; Walsh, 1976; Partanen *et al.*, 1980; Halbach *et al.*, 1987; Garciá-Merino *et al.*, 1991; Wakayama *et al.*, 1991; Ho *et al.*, 1993; Newsom-Davis and Mills 1993). Seven of the Oxford/Liverpool patients had a thymoma (six with and one without MG) before or at presentation, and three had or developed a small cell lung carcinoma (SCLC). The longest latency between onset of AINMT and diagnosis of SCLC was 4 years. Another patient had an adenocarcinoma of unknown origin. There are reports of AINMT occurring in a patient with a Hodgkin's lymphoma (Caress *et al.*, 1997) and another with a plasmacytoma and paraproteinaemia (Zifco *et al.*, 1994).

---

**Table 14.1 Autoimmune syndromes reported in association with AINMT**

*Paraneoplastic AINMT*
  Thymoma – benign or malignant; with or without myasthenia gravis
  Small cell lung carcinoma – with or without neuropathy
  Hodgkin's lymphoma
  Plasmacytoma with IgM paraproteinaemia
  Adenocarcinoma – primary unknown

*Other immune-mediated disorders*
  Myasthenia gravis – anti-AChR antibody positive or negative
  Rheumatoid disease – with or without neuropathy
  Systemic lupus erythematosus – with or without neuropathy
  Diabetes mellitus – with or without neuropathy
  Guillain-Barré syndrome
  Chronic inflammatory demyelinating polyneuropathy
  Hyperthyroidism
  Systemic sclerosis
  Addison's disease with demyelinating neuropathy
  Amyloidosis – primary with serum IgG kappa monoclonal band
  Penicillamine-induced in a patient with rheumatoid disease
  Vitiligo
  Coeliac disease

---

# The pathogenesis of AINMT

Advances in our knowledge of the electrophysiology, pharmacology, immunology and molecular biology of potassium channels provided the theoretical basis to implicate nerve *Shaker*-related VGKC dysfunction as a cause of the peripheral nerve hyperexcitability in neuromyotonia. These channels act as delayed rectifiers or type A rapid inactivators and are involved in the repolarization of the nerve membrane after passage of an action potential. They also provide accommodation and action potential frequency adaptation during periods of prolonged depolarization. Immunohistochemical studies (Sheng *et al.*, 1992; Wang *et al.*, 1993; Veh *et al.*, 1995), using antibodies raised against amino acid sequences unique to each channel subtype, and *in situ* hybridization studies (Drewe *et al.*, 1992) of rodent brain, localized the subcellular expression of VGKCs to the paranodal, juxtaparanodal and terminal regions of myelinated axons (see Table 14.2). Although the expression of these channels in human peripheral nerve is unknown, electrophysiological studies identified $K^+$ currents (K fast types 1 and 2) in human (Bostock and Baker, 1988) and isolated rat peripheral nerve (Roeper and Schwartz, 1989) that have similar electrical properties to those recorded from *Shaker*-related VGKC cRNAs expressed in *Xenopus* oocytes (Pongs, 1992; Wang *et al.*, 1993). When a drug such as 4-aminopyridine (4-AP) or a specific toxin such as $\alpha$-dendrotoxin blocks these currents, the axon membrane excitation threshold lowers and the cell membrane becomes hyperexcitable (Bostock and Baker, 1988; Kocsis *et al.*, 1988; Roeper and Schwartz, 1989). Spontaneous bursts of action potentials are generated, as happens in neuromyotonia.

Clinical neurophysiological studies suggested that in most AINMT patients the spontaneous activity originates from the terminal regions of the motor axons (Isaacs, 1961, 1967; Deymeer *et al.*, 1998). This region lies outwith the blood/nerve barrier that impedes the access of large molecules such as antibodies and, thus, it may be more susceptible to immune attack than the rest of the lower motor neuron. In mammalian motor axons, the membrane downstream to the last node of Ranvier expresses VGKC and voltage-gated calcium channels (VGCC) but not voltage-gated sodium channels (VGNC) (Boudier *et al.*, 1988). These VGCCs are the target of the autoantibodies that cause the Lambert–Eaton myasthenic syndrome (LEMS) by down-regulating channels and reducing transmitter release (see Chapter 13). By analogy, and by exclusion, the only other transmembrane voltage-gated channel expressed at the nerve terminal seemed the prime target for autoantibody attack in AINMT.

## Clinical evidence of a humoral factor in AINMT

The clinical features suggesting an autoimmune aetiology for NMT were supported by the response of several patients to intensive plasma exchange, a procedure that reduces the level of circulating immunoglobulins (Ig) (Newsom-Davis and Mills, 1993). In many patients, clinical improvement begins within 2 to 8 days and lasts for about one month. The response can be confirmed and quantified by comparing pre- with post-exchange EMG recordings of neuromyotonic discharge frequency from a resting muscle (Newsom-Davis, 1997).

## Pathophysiological effects of passive transfer of immunoglobulins

The VGKCs at the peripheral motor nerve terminal act to close the transmembrane VGCC by restoring the resting membrane potential. Thus, blocking these VGKCs with a drug such as 4-AP both prolongs $Ca^{2+}$ entry and depolarization at the nerve terminal and leads to an increase in the number of quanta of acetylcholine released by each action potential (quantal content). Passive transfer experiments have shown that AINMT plasma and purified IgG mimic these effects.

When AINMT plasma or IgG was intraperitoneally injected into mice daily for 10–12 days, the animals had neither clinical signs of muscle overactivity nor electrical evidence of spontaneous nerve activity (Sinha *et al.*, 1991; Shillito *et al.*, 1995). However, when neuromuscular transmission was studied *in vitro* using a preparation of the animals' phrenic nerve-diaphragm there was increased resistance to the neuromuscular blocking effects of d-tubocurarine (Sinha et al., 1991) and in further experiments, a statistically significant increase in quantal content compared with preparations from mice injected with control human plasma or IgG (Shillito et al., (1995). These findings implied that AINMT patient IgG prolonged the depolarization of the nerve terminals and were consistent with the hypothesis that circulating antibodies caused VGKC dysfunction. Complementary electrophysiological studies demonstrated that direct application of IgG from one AINMT patient to cultured dorsal root ganglion cells for 24 hours produced repetitive firing (Shillito et al., 1995). Low doses of 4-AP or its derivative 3,4 diaminopyridine (3,4-DAP) also produced all of these functional effects. Thus, these findings suggested that AINMT antibodies had the same effects on neuromuscular transmission as VGKC antagonists. A patch-clamp study using cultured PC12 cells confirmed that AINMT Ig suppresses voltage-dependent potassium currents (Sonoda et al., 1996). Taken together, these studies provided strong evidence that antibodies from AINMT patients can produce axonal hyperexcitability by reducing the number of functional nerve VGKCs.

## Voltage-gated potassium channels

Functional VGKCs consist of four $\alpha$-subunits, each of which has six transmembrane regions (S1–6) (Pongs, 1992). Together, S5 and S6 regions of the $\alpha$-subunits form the central ion pore. In humans, each Shaker-related VGKC $\alpha$-subunit is encoded by a different gene and, so far, eight mammalian cDNAs have been isolated (KCNA1 to A8; Table 14.2) (Ramaswami et al., 1990; Pongs, 1992; Street and Tempel, 1997; Kalman et al., 1998). The gene products combine as homomultimeric or heteromultimeric tetramers and associate with intracellular $\beta$-subunits that also function as a tetramer to modulate the gating properties and amplitudes of the channel (Rettig et al., 1994). Three $\beta$-subunit genes have been cloned (KCNAB1 to 3). Alternate splicing of KCNAB1 forms the $\beta3$ subunit.

## Anti-VGKC antibody detection by radioimmunoassay

Serum anti-VGKC antibodies were first looked for by a RIA using $^{125}$I-$\alpha$-dendrotoxin-labelled VGKCs extracted from human frontal cortex as the antigen (Hart et al., 1994, 1997; Shillito et al., 1995). Raised levels of antibodies were found in 50–60% of patients and the titres were generally low (200–300 picomoles of $\alpha$-dendrotoxin sites/l). Despite its relative insensitivity, this assay was able to demonstrate that in one AINMT patient the serum anti-VGKC antibody titre fell in response to plasma exchange and the level correlated with the clinical and EMG severity of the muscle overactivity (Shillito et al., 1995).

| Table 14.2 Mammalian *Shaker*-related voltage-gated potassium channel $\alpha$-subunit gene family | | | |
|---|---|---|---|
| *Gene* | | *Electrical properties* | *Expression* |
| KCNA1 | Kv1.1 | Delayed rectifier | CNS neurons – presynaptic and juxtanodal |
| KCNA2 | Kv1.2 | Delayed rectifier | CNS neurons – presynaptic and juxtanodal |
| KCNA3 | Kv1.3 | Delayed rectifier | CNS neurons – Juxtanodal. Skeletal muscle |
| KCNA4 | Kv1.4 | Type A rapid inactivator | CNS neurons – presynaptic and axonal. Fetal skeletal muscle |
| KCNA5 | Kv1.5 | Delayed rectifier | Brain. Heart. Insulinoma |
| KCNA6 | Kv1.6 | Delayed rectifier | CNS neurons |
| KCNA7 | Kv1.7 | Type A rapid inactivator | Brain. Skeletal muscle. Heart. Insulinoma |
| KCNA8 | Kv1.8 | Delayed rectifier | Heart. Intestine. Co-assembles with KCNE1 |

The specificity of the assay is yet to be established. Positive results have occasionally been found in patients with thymoma who have no clinical symptoms of muscle overactivity (Hart et al., 1994)

## Anti-VGKC antibody detection by molecular-immunohistochemical assay

This assay was developed in an attempt to improve the sensitivity of antibody detection. Compared with the RIA, it has several advantages. A ligand is not required to label the VGKC $\alpha$-subunit, the antigen – a single $\alpha$-subunit isoform – is expressed at high concentration in the oocyte cytoplasm and antibody binding can be studied without the need to extract and denature the antigen with detergent.

Three human VGKC $\alpha$-subunits (KCNA1, A2 and A6) were individually expressed in *Xenopus* oocytes injected with the relevant cRNA (Hart et al., 1997; Hart, 2000). Serial dilutions of serum from patients were applied to frozen oocyte sections, and binding to the VGKC $\alpha$-subunit in the oocyte cytoplasm detected by a biotin-conjugated anti-human IgG followed by streptavidin/horse radish peroxidase. In initial experiments, specific immunoreactivity to at least one of the three VGKC was found in all 12 AINMT sera studied at serum dilutions of 1:128 to 1:2500. Healthy and other autoimmune disease sera were negative. Table 14.3 shows the results from these and a further 18 AINMT patients. Twenty-six of the 30 patients tested positive (87%).

## Anti-VGKC antibody heterogeneity

The results in Table 14.3 also demonstrate the heterogeneity of anti-VGKC antibody binding in AINMT (Hart et al., 1997). Of the three VGKC $\alpha$-subunits studied in the molecular immunohistochemical assay, five sera bound to all three subunits, eleven sera bound to all the possible combinations of two subunits and ten sera bound to at least one subunit. This suggests both that individual patients have antibodies with a range of binding specificities and that the range varies between patients. This target heterogeneity is a feature shared with the other main antibody-mediated channelopathies of the peripheral nervous system. Antibodies from different patients can react with different acetylcholine receptor subunits in MG and with P, Q, L and N types of VGCC in LEMS (see Chapter 13).

In AINMT, antibodies with different target binding may explain at least some of the clinical diversity of the syndrome. Immunohistochemical and *in situ* hybridization studies of the rodent brain revealed that neurons differ in the types and combinations of VGKC $\alpha$-subunits that they synthesize and express, at both the cellular and subcellular level. In peripheral nerves, motor axons have $K^+$ currents with different characteristics to those in sensory axons (Kocsis et al., 1988; Applegate and Burke, 1989). Thus, this selective VGKC expression could be subject to antibody attack that is VGKC subtype-specific. For example, one patient may have antibodies that target only motor nerve VGKCs and others may also have antibodies to VGKCs on sensory nerves, CNS neurons or both.

**Table 14.3 Binding patterns of 30 AINMT sera on a molecular immunohistochemical assay**

| | Binding to expressed human VGKC $\alpha$-subunit subtype | | | | | | | |
|---|---|---|---|---|---|---|---|---|
| | KCNA1 KCNA2 KCNA6 | KCNA1 KCNA2 | KCNA1 KCNA6 | KCNA2 KCNA6 | KCNA1 | KCNA2 | KCNA6 | No binding |
| Number of sera | 5 | 1 | 5 | 5 | 1 | 5 | 4 | 4 |

In most AINMT patients, the anti-VGKC antibodies are IgG. However, one patient with a plasmacytoma and IgM monoclonal gammopathy developed NMT (Zifco et al., 1994). In addition, IgM but not IgG purified from another AINMT patient bound to an $\alpha$-dendrotoxin labelled protein on Western blotting and had immunoreactivity with both cultured PC12 cells and human intramuscular nerve axons (Arimura et al., 1997). These findings suggest that in some patients AINMT is IgM autoantibody-mediated.

## Mechanisms of anti-VGKC antibody action

In AINMT, autoantibodies probably reduce the number of functional VGKCs by downregulation. There is no evidence that anti-VGKC antibodies produce an acute block of channel function.

Electrophysiological studies of the effects of AINMT IgG on cultured dorsal root ganglion cells showed that repetitive firing was seen at 24 hours and not at 2 hours (Shillito et al., 1995). In patch-clamping studies, PC12 cells incubated with AINMT serum had reduced outward $K^+$ current only after 3–6 days (Sonida et al., 1996). In the human neuroblastoma cell line (NB–1), AINMT Ig suppressed $K^+$ currents after 3 days but not at one day (Nagado et al., 1999). Moreover, AINMT Ig did not alter the activation or inactivation kinetics of the $K^+$ currents. The simplest explanation for all these findings is that anti-VGKC antibodies act to increase VGKC uptake into cells. The pathogenicity of both anti-AChR antibodies in MG and anti-VGCC antibodies in LEMS involves similar mechanisms.

## Central abnormalities in AINMT

Although muscle overactivity caused by peripheral motor nerve hyperexcitability is the hallmark of AINMT, CNS abnormalities can also occur. The clinical association of neuromyotonia with hallucinations, delusions, insomnia and personality change was first recognized by Morvan, who called it chorée fibrillare (Morvan, 1890; Serratrice and Azulay, 1994). Some AINMT patients

have increased CSF total IgG or oligoclonal bands suggesting that there is intrathecal IgG synthesis (Hart et al., 1996; Newsom-Davis and Mills, 1997). Preliminary immunohistochemical studies demonstrated binding of both CSF and serum IgG from anti-VGKC antibody positive AINMT patients to neurons in the dentate nucleus of the human cerebellum (Hart et al., 1996; Hart, 2000). The staining pattern mimicked that of a polyclonal anti-VGKC antibody raised to a peptide encoding the S3–4 extracellular domain unique to KCNA1 (Ramaswami et al., 1990; Hart et al., 1997). This finding may suggest that the presence of central symptoms in some patients depends on whether there is CNS synthesis of anti-VGKC antibodies.

## Other antigens in AINMT

An excitotoxic antibody that increased the open time of voltage-gated sodium channels (VGNC) could also produce peripheral nerve hyperexcitability, and possibly clinical features of muscle overactivity, similar to that caused by antibodies that reduce VGKC function (Waxman, 1995; Gutmann and Gutmann, 1996). Most types of ciguatoxin (produced by the dinoflagellate Gambierdiscus toxicus associated with dead coral) prolong neuron VGNC activation and can produce repetitive firing of axons (Lombet et al., 1987). However, a patch-clamp study on NB-1 cells did not detect any effect of AINMT IgG on $Na^+$ currents (Nagado et al., 1999). In addition, the abnormal impulses in most AINMT patients are thought to be generated at the terminal regions of the motor axons, where the neuron membrane expresses VGKC but not VGNC (Boudier et al., 1988). Thus, as yet, there is no experimental evidence to support the idea that anti-VGNC antibodies contribute to the pathogenesis of AINMT.

An RIA using [125]I-labelled epibatidine (a specific agonist drug) identified autoantibodies to neuron nicotinic AChRs in sera from three of the six AINMT patients studied (Verino et al., 1998). This might suggest that some AINMT patients have antibodies acting at central nicotinic synapses, such as the recurrent spinal inhibitory synapse to Renshaw interneurons, which could mediate neuromuscular hyperexcitability. The pathogenicity of these antibodies has not yet been demonstrated (Verino *et al.*, 1999).

Neuromyotonia has been found in EMG studies of transgenic mice with a deficiency or overexpression of the peripheral myelin protein gene PMP22 (Toyka *et al.*, 1997; Zielasek and Toyka, 1999). In humans, different mutations of this gene lead to dysmyelination and are associated with hereditary motor sensory neuropathy type 1a (HMSN1a) and hereditary liability to pressure palsies. Neuromyotonia has been reported in several patients with HMSN1a (Lance *et al.*, 1979; Vasilescu *et al.*, 1984). Although the implications of these findings are most relevant to hereditary NMT syndromes, they are also an important and direct demonstration that alterations in a protein other than VGKCs can produce neuromyotonic nerve hyperexcitability. Moreover, PMP22 is expressed by Schwann cells reminding us that primary glial cell disorders can produce secondary changes in axons that can trigger peripheral nerve hyperexcitability.

## Studies of excitability of motor axons in AINMT patients

Threshold tracking and related techniques can be used to study axonal excitability and the generation of ectopic discharges *in situ* (Bostock *et al.*, 1998; Burke, 1999) (see Chapter 5). These methods require that the peripheral nerve under study receives submaximal stimuli, and use computer programs to adjust the stimulus intensity to a target size where the nerve is excited on about 40% of trials. The current intensity needed to achieve this is called the threshold for the nerve compound potential. Increased excitability requires a weaker stimulus to generate a test potential of constant size and decreased excitability requires a stronger stimulus. One of these measures is the strength-duration time constant (SDTC), which is a property of the nodal membrane determined by the passive membrane time constant and ion conductances active at the nerve threshold.

In one study, where the median nerve was stimulated at the wrist, the SDTC was prolonged in motor but not sensory axons in four of nine

AINMT patients when compared with control values (Maddison *et al.*, 1999). There are several possible ways that anti-VGKC antibodies could prolong SDTC in AINMT other than altering potassium conductance at all the nodes of Ranvier. For example, the antibodies could act to produce an ectopic focus that depolarizes the nerve nodal membrane directly at the site of the motor nerve stimulation or they could increase the size of nodes by immune-mediated demyelination.

However, motor axon SDTCs were normal in five of the nine AINMT patients studied. Another study using a more sensitive panel of measures of both motor and sensory axonal excitability in the median nerve at the wrist, including SDTC, recovery cycle after an impulse and threshold electrotonus (Bostock *et al.*, 1998), found that all excitability indices were normal in all eight AINMT patients examined (Kiernan *et al.*, 2001). These negative findings suggested that, at least at the time of the recordings, a generalized axonal membrane abnormality was not present in perhaps the majority of patients with AINMT. Moreover, they implied that the site of ectopic activity generation was remote from the stimulating electrodes and was, thus, probably focal or multifocal. The site(s) could be either proximal or distal to the midaxonal position of the electrode. In an EMG study, multiple generator sites were found in the same individual, including different loci along the intramuscular nerve tree (Torbergsen *et al.*, 1996).

Thus, these excitatory studies add to the evidence from histological and conventional electrophysiological studies that in most, but not all patients, the most likely locus for the generation of AINMT discharges seems to be distal at the motor nerve terminal or intramuscular arborization. At these sites, there are VGKCs producing fast $K^+$ currents unprotected by either a blood/nerve barrier or myelin sheath and, thus, potentially more vulnerable to immune attack.

## Inherited potassium channelopathies

Potassium channels are ubiquitous and involved in a myriad of cell regulatory processes. The growing list of hereditary channelopathies reflects their fundamental importance to the normal function of excitable cells, particularly in the nervous system and heart (Table 14.4).

Of particular interest to this discussion is episodic ataxia type1 (EA1) (Browne *et al.*, 1994). This syndrome is caused by a variety of point mutations in the KCNA1 gene and is associated with peripheral nerve hyperexcitability presenting as persistent myokymia. On EMG, the neuromyotonic discharges are regular, whereas in AINMT they are irregular. Nevertheless, this hereditary potassium channelopathy provides definitive evidence that decreased function of a single subtype of neuronal VGKC produces peripheral nerve hyperexcitability.

## Anti-VGKC antibodies in other diseases

The cramp, or muscular pain, fasciculation syndrome (CFS) is an acquired condition that presents with similar clinical features of muscle overactivity to AINMT (Tahmoush *et al.*, 1991). On EMG, there are fasciculation and fibrillation potentials, but unlike AINMT neuromyotonic discharges are absent. Immunoglobulins purified from two CFS patients suppressed outward $K^+$ currents of patch clamped NB-1 cells in culture in a manner similar to AINMT Ig (Nagado *et al.*, 1999). Moreover, three other CFS patients had raised anti-VGKC antibody titres on the molecular immunohisto-

chemical assay in patterns similar to those seen in AINMT (unpublished observation). These findings support the suggestion that at least some cases of CFS are probably mild variants of AINMT.

AINMT can occur in patients with GBS, an acute inflammatory demyelinating polyneuropathy (Lance *et al.*, 1979). Defects in myelination by themselves can induce nerve hyperexcitability, for example in humans and mice with PMP22 gene mutations, presumably by secondary effects on the regional expression of ion channels along the length of the axon (Toyka *et al.*, 1997; Zielasek and Toyka, 1999). In addition, however, purified Ig from two GBS patients reduced outward $K^+$ but not $Na^+$ currents of patch clamped NB-1 cells (Nagado *et al.*, 1999). Neither patient had clinical features of muscle overactivity. It has been suggested that anti-GM1 antibodies present in some patients with GBS produce conduction block by inhibiting nodal $Na^+$ channels (Waxman, 1995; Gutmann and Gutmann, 1996). The finding of antibodies with specific anti-$K^+$ current activity might suggest that both VGNC and VGKC dysfunction contribute to the clinical features of GBS.

So far, chorée fibrillaire de Morvan is the only CNS syndrome in which anti-VGKC antibodies have been implicated. However, the growing list of hereditary CNS potassium channelopathies (see Table 14.4) and the finding of IgG with anti-VGKC immunoreactivity in the CSF of some AINMT patients (Hart *et al.*, 1996; Hart, 2000), both suggest that the investigation of VGKC dys-

### Table 14.4 Potassium channelopathies

| Inherited | Gene |
|---|---|
| Episodic ataxia type 1 with myokymia | KCNA1 |
| Benign neonatal convulsions type 1 | KCNQ2 |
| Benign neonatal convulsions type 2 | KCNQ3 |
| Non-syndromic hearing loss | KCNQ4 |
| Long QT syndrome type 1 | KCNA8 |
| Long QT syndrome type 2 | KCNH2 |
| Long QT syndrome type 5 | KCNE1 |
| Long QT syndrome type 6 | KCNE2 |
| Bartter syndrome | KCNJ1 |
| *Acquired* | *Autoantibodies to* |
| Autoimmune neuromyotonia | KCNA6 > A2 > A1 |

function in other acquired PNS and CNS disorders where there is continuous or paroxysmal neuron hyperexcitability will be fruitful.

## Treatment of AINMT

The antiepilepsy drugs, carbamazepine and phenytoin, continue to be the first line symptomatic therapies for AINMT. They act probably by reducing axonal $Na^+$ conductance and, thus, counteract the effects of antibody-mediated loss of VGKC function. In most patients, one or other of these drugs improves symptoms of muscle overactivity and suppression of nerve excitability can be confirmed by quantifying the frequency of spontaneous discharges on EMG pre- and post-treatment. If necessary, these drugs are used together. Experience suggests that lamotrigine or sodium valproate can also be effective. A few patients find dantrolene or mexilitine useful. In general, baclofen, benzodiazepines, carbonic anhydrase inhibitors and quinine are unhelpful.

The linking of neuromyotonia with autoimmunity has prompted many attempts at immunomodulatory therapy. Plasma exchange often produces short-term relief (Newsom-Davis and Mills, 1993; Newsom-Davis, 1997; Hart, 2000). In difficult cases, a trial of plasma exchange may also help establish whether a patient's neuromyotonia is autoimmune. A positive response to plasma exchange has also been used, along with anti-VGKC antibody status, to help select those patients who may benefit from long-term immunosuppression. Experience suggests that human intravenous immunoglobulin can also be useful, despite reports that it worsened symptoms in one patient (Ishii *et al.*, 1994), and that its effect was inferior to plasma exchange in another (Van den Berg *et al.*, 1999).

Oral immunosuppressive therapy should be considered for patients with incapacitating AINMT who fail to respond to symptomatic therapy. Combinations of prednisolone with azathioprine or methotrexate have helped some patients (Newsom-Davis and Mills, 1993). Randomized control trials are needed to evaluate these therapies more fully.

## Summary

Encouraged by the clinical observation that NMT often clusters with recognized autoimmune disorders, experimental studies have provided three main strands of evidence that the motor neuron hyperexcitability that characterizes AINMT is mediated by autoantibodies that target peripheral nerve VGKCs. In many patients, the removal of circulating autoantibodies by plasma exchange was followed by clinical and EMG improvement. Serum anti-VGKC antibodies were found in up to 87% of patients. Passive transfer studies in mice and electrophysiological studies on cultured cells both demonstrated that Ig purified from AINMT patients reduces $K^+$ currents and increases neuron excitability. Although there is still much to learn about the molecular mechanisms that produce the clinical, immunological and *in situ* electrophysiological heterogeneity of the syndrome, the evidence is persuasive that AINMT is an autoantibody-mediated channelopathy.

## References

Applegate, C. and Burke, D. (1989). Changes in excitability of human cutaneous afferents following prolonged high frequency stimulation. *Brain*, **12**, 147–64.

Arimura, K., Watanabe, O., Kitajima, I. *et al.* (1997). Antibodies to potassium channels of PC12 in serum of Isaacs' syndrome: Western blot and immunohistochemical studies. *Muscle Nerve*, **20**, 299–305.

Auger, R. G., Daube, J. R., Gomez, M. R. and Lambert, E. H. (1984). Hereditary form of sustained muscle activity of peripheral nerve origin causing generalized myokymia and muscle stiffness. *Ann. Neurol.*, **5**, 13–21.

Benito-Leon, J., Miguelez, R., Vincent, A. *et al.* (1999). Neuromyotonia in association with systemic sclerosis. *J Neurol.*, **246**, 976–7.

Bostock, H. and Baker, M. (1988). Evidence for two types of potassium channel in human motor axons in vivo. *Brain Res.*, **462**, 354–8.

Bostock, H., Cikurel, K. and Burke, D. (1998). Threshold tracking techniques in the study of human peripheral nerve. *Muscle Nerve*, **21**, 137–58.

Boudier, J. L., Jover, E. and Cau, P. (1988). Autoradiographic localization of voltage-dependent sodium channels on the mouse neuromuscular junction using $^{125}I$-$\alpha$ scorpiontoxin. I. Preferential labeling of glial cells on the presynaptic side. *J. Neurosci.*, **8**, 1469–78.

Browne, D. L., Gancher, S. T., Nutt, J. G. *et al.* (1994). Episodic ataxia/myokymia syndrome is associated with point mutations in the human potassium channel gene KCNA1. *Nature Genet.*, **8**, 136–40.

Burke, D. (1999). Excitability of motor axons in neuromyotonia. *Muscle Nerve*, **22**, 797–9.

Caress, J. B., Abend, W. K., Preston, D. C. and Logigian, E. L. (1997). A case of Hodgkin's lymphoma producing neuromyotonia. *Neurology*, **49**, 258–9.

Denny-Brown, D. and Foley, D. M. (1948). Myokymia and the benign fasciculation of muscular cramps. *Trans Assoc Am Physicians*, **61**, 88–96.

Deymeer, F., Oge, A. E., Serdaroglu, P. *et al.* (1998). The use of botulinum toxin in localizing neuromyotonia to the terminal branches of the peripheral nerve. *Muscle Nerve*, **21**, 643–6.

Drewe, J. A., Verma, S., Frech, G. and Joho, R. H. (1992). Distinct spatial and temporal patterns of potassium channel mRNAs from different subfamilies. *J Neurosci.*, **12**, 538–48.

Gamstorp, I. and Wohlfart, G. (1959). A syndrome characterized by myokymia, myotonia, muscular wasting and increased perspiration. *Acta Psychiatr Scand.*, **34**, 181–94.

Garciá-Merino, A., Cabella, A., Mora, J.S. and Lianõ, H. (1991). Continuous muscle fiber activity, peripheral neuropathy, and thymoma. *Ann Neurol.*, **29**, 215–8.

Gutmann, L. and Gutmann, L. (1996). Axonal channelopathies: an evolving concept in the pathogenesis of peripheral nerve disorders. *Neurology*, **47**, 18–21.

Gutmann, L., Gutmann, L. and Schochet, S. S. (1996). Neuromyotonia and type 1 myofiber predominance in amyloidosis. *Muscle Nerve*, **19**, 1338–41.

Hadjivassiliou, M., Chattopadhyay, A. K., Davies-Jones, G. A. *et al.* (1997). Neuromuscular disorder as a presenting feature of coeliac disease. *J Neurol Neurosurg Psychiatr.*, **63**, 770–5.

Halbach, M., Homberg, V. and Freund, H.-J. (1987). Neuromuscular, autonomic and central cholinergic hyperactivity associated with thymoma and acetylcholine receptor-binding antibody. *J Neurol (Berlin)*, **234**, 433–6.

Harman, J. B. and Richardson, A. T. (1954). Generalized myokymia in thyrotoxicosis: report of a case. *Lancet*, **2**, 473–4.

Hart, I. K. (2000). Acquired neuromyotonia: A new autoantibody-mediated neuronal potassium channelopathy. *Am J Med Sci.*, **319**, 209–16.

Hart, I. K., Leys, K., Vincent, A. *et al.* (1994). Autoantibodies to voltage-gated potassium channels in acquired neuromyotonia. *Neuromusc Disord.*, **4**, 535(Abstr).

Hart, I. K., Waters, C. and Newsom-Davis, J. (1996). Cerebrospinal fluid and serum from acquired neuromyotonia patients seropositive for anti-potassium channel antibodies label dentate nucleus neurones. *Ann Neurol.*, **40**, 554–5.

Hart, I. K., Waters, C., Vincent, A. *et al.* (1997). Autoantibodies detected to expressed $K^+$ channels are implicated in neuromyotonia. *Ann Neurol.*, **41**, 238–46.

Ho, W. K. H. and Wilson, J. D. (1993). Hypothermia, hyperhidrosis, myokymia and increased urinary excretion of catecholamines associated with a thymoma. *Med J Aust.*, **158**, 787–8.

Hosokawa, S., Shinoda, H., Sakai, T., Kato, M. and Kuroiwa, Y. (1987). Electrophysiological study on limb myokymia in three women. *J Neurol Neurosurg Psychiatr.*, **50**, 877–81.

Irani, P. F., Purohit, A. V. and Wadia, H. H. (1977). The syndrome of continuous muscle fiber activity. *Acta Neuro. Scand.*, **55**, 273–88.

Isaacs, H. (1961). A syndrome of continuous muscle-fibre activity. *J Neurol Neurosurg Psychiatr.*, **24**, 319–25.

Isaacs, H. (1967). Continuous muscle fibre activity in an Indian male with additional evidence of terminal motor fibre abnormality. *J Neurol Neurosurg Psychiatr.*, **30**, 126–33.

Ishii, A., Hayashi, A., Ohkoshi, N. *et al.* (1994). Clinical evaluation of plasma exchange and high dose intravenous immunoglobulin in a patient with Isaacs' syndrome. *J Neurol Neurosurg Psychiatr.*, **57**, 840–2.

Kalman, K., Nguyen, A., Tseng-Crank, J. *et al.* (1998). Genomic organization, chromosomal localization, tissue distribution, and biophysical characterization of a novel mammalian Shaker-related voltage-gated potassium channel, Kv1.7. *J Biol Chem.*, **273**, 5851–7.

Kiernan, M. C., Hart, I. K. and Bostock, H. (2001). Excitability of motor axons in patients with spontaneous motor unit activity. *J Neurol Neurosurg Psychiatr.*, **70**, 56–64.

Kocsis, J. D., Bowe, C. M. and Waxman, S. G. (1988). Different effects of 4-aminopyridine on sensory and motor fibers: pathogenesis of paresthesias. *Neurology*, **36**, 117–20.

Lance, J. W., Burke, D. and Pollard, J. (1979). Hyperexcitability of motor and sensory neurons in neuromyotonia. *Ann Neurol.*, **5**, 523–32.

Le Gars, L., Clerc, D., Cariou, D. *et al.* (1997). Systemic juvenile rheumatoid arthritis and associated Isaacs' syndrome. *J Rheumatol.*, **24**, 178–80.

Lombet, A. J., Bidard, N. and Lazdunski, M. (1987). Ciguatoxin and brevetoxins share a common receptor site on the neuronal voltage-dependent $Na^+$ channel. *FEBS Lett.*, **219**, 355–9.

Maddison, P., Newsom-Davis, J. and Mills, K. R. (1999). Strength-duration properties of peripheral nerve in acquired neuromyotonia. *Muscle Nerve*, **22**, 823–30.

Mertens, H. G. and Zschoke, S. (1965). Neuromyotonie. *Klin Wochenscher.*, **43**, 917–25.

Morvan, A. (1890). De la chorée fibrillaire. *Gaz Hebdon de Med. Chirurg.*, **27**, 173–200.

Nagado, T., Arimura, K., Sonoda, Y. et al. (1999). Potassium current suppression in patients with peripheral nerve hyperexcitability. *Brain*, **122**, 2057–66.

Newsom-Davis, J. (1997). Autoimmune neuromyotonia (Isaacs' syndrome): An antibody-mediated potassium channelopathy. *Ann NY Acad Sci.*, **835**, 111–9.

Newsom-Davis, J. and Mills, K. R. (1993). Immunological associations of acquired neuromyotonia (Isaacs' syndrome). Report of five cases and literature review. *Brain*, **116**, 453–69.

Partanen, V. S. J., Soininen, H., Saksa, M. and Riekkinen, P. (1980). Electromyographic and nerve conduction findings in a patient with neuromyotonia, normocalcemic tetany and small-cell lung cancer. *Acta Neurol Scand.*, **61**, 216–26.

Pongs, O. (1992). Molecular biology of voltage-dependent potassium channels. *Physiol Rev.*, **72** (Suppl. 4), S69–S88.

Ramaswami, R., Gautam, M., Kamb, A. et al. (1990). Human potassium channel genes: molecular cloning and functional expression. *Mol Cell Neurosci.*, **1**, 214–23.

Reeback, J., Benton, S., Swash, M. and Schwartz, M. S. (1979). Penicillamine-induced neuromyotonia. *Br Med J.*, **279**, 1464–5.

Rettig, J., Heinemann, S. H., Wunder, F. et al. (1994). Inactivation properties of voltage-gated potassium channels altered by presence of $\beta$-subunit. *Nature*, **369**, 289–94.

Roeper, J. and Schwartz, J. R. (1989). Heterogeneous distribution of fast and slow potassium channels in myelinated rat nerve fibres. *J Physiol.*, **416**, 93–110.

Serratrice, G. and Azulay, J. P. (1994). Que reste-t-il de la chorée fibrillaire de Morvan? *Rev Neurol.*, **150**, 257–65.

Sheng, M., Tsaur, M.-L., Jan, Y. N. and Jan L. Y. (1992). Subcellular segregation of two A-type $K^+$ channel proteins in rat central neurons. *Neuron*, **9**, 271–84.

Shillito, P., Molenaar, P. C., Vincent, A. et al. (1995). Acquired neuromyotonia: Evidence for autoantibodies directed against $K^+$ channels of peripheral nerves. *Ann Neurol.*, **38**, 714–22.

Sinha, S., Newsom-Davis, J., Mills, K. et al. (1991). Autoimmune aetiology for acquired neuromyotonia (Isaacs' syndrome). *Lancet*, **338**, 75–7.

Solimena, M., Folli, F., Denis-Donini, S. et al. (1988). Autoantibodies to glutamic acid decarboxylase in a patient with the stiff-man syndrome, epilepsy, and type I diabetes mellitus. *N Engl J Med.*, **318**, 1012–20.

Sonoda, Y., Arimura, K., Kurono, A. et al. (1996). Serum of Isaacs' syndrome suppresses potassium channels in PC-12 cell lines. *Muscle Nerve*, **19**, 1439–46.

Street, V. A. and Tempel, B. L. (1997). Physical mapping of potassium channel gene clusters on mouse chromosomes three and six. *Genomics*, **44**, 110–7.

Tahmoush, A. J., Alonso, R. J., Tahmoush, G. P. et al.

(1991). Cramp-fasciculation syndrome: a treatable hyperexcitable peripheral nerve disorder. *Neurology*, **41**, 1021–4.

Torbergsen, T., Stalberg, E. and Brautaset, N. (1996). Generator sites for spontaneous activity in neuromyotonia. An EMG study. *Electroencephalogr Clin Neurophysiol.*, **101**, 69–78.

Toyka, K. V., Zielasek, J., Ricker, K. et al. (1997). Hereditary neuromyotonia: a mouse model associated with deficiency or increased gene dosage of the PMP22 gene. *J Neurol Neurosurg Psychiatr.*, **63**, 812–3.

Van den Berg, J. S., van Engelen, B. G., Boerman, R. H. and de Baets, M. H. (1999). Acquired neuromyotonia: superiority of plasma exchange over high-dose intravenous human immunoglobulin. *J Neurol.*, **246**, 623–5.

Vasilescu, C., Alexianu, M. and Dan, A. (1984). Muscle hypertrophy and a syndrome of continuous motor unit activity in prednisone-responsive Guillain-Barré polyneuropathy. *J Neurol (Berlin)*, **231**, 276–9.

Vasilescu, C., Alexianu, M. and Dan, A. (1984). Neuronal type of Charcot Marie-Tooth disease with a syndrome of continuous motor unit activity. *J Neurol Sci.*, **63**, 11–25.

Veh, R. W., Lichtinghagen, R., Sewing, S. et al. (1995). Immunohistochemical localization of five members of the Kv1 channel subunits: Contrasting subcellular locations and neurone-specific co-localizations in rat brain. *Eur J Neurosci.*, **7**, 2189–205.

Verino, S., Adamski, J., Kryzer, T. J. et al. (1998). Neuronal nicotinic ACh receptor antibody in subacute autonomic neuropathy and cancer-related syndromes. *Neurology*, **50**, 1806–13.

Verino, S., Auger, R. G., Emslie-Smith, A. M. et al. (1999). Myasthenia, thymoma, presynaptic antibodies, and a continuum of neuromuscular hyperexcitability. *Neurology*, **53**, 1233–9.

Vilchez, J. J., Cabello, A., Benedito, J. and Villarroya, T. (1980). Hyperkalaemic paralysis, neuropathy and persistent motor unit discharges at rest in Addison's disease. *J Neurol Neurosurg Psychiatr.*, **43**, 818–22.

Waerness, E. (1974). Neuromyotonia and bronchial carcinoma. *Electromyogr Clin Neurophysiol.*, **14**, 527–35.

Wakayama, Y., Ohbu, S. and Machida, H. (1991). Myasthenia gravis, muscle twitch, hyperhidrosis, and limb pain associated with thymoma: proposal of a possible new myasthenic syndrome. *Tohoku J Exp Med.*, **164**, 285–91.

Walsh, J. C. (1976). Neuromyotonia: an unusual presentation of intrathoracic malignancy. *J Neurol Neurosurg Psychiatr.*, **39**, 1086–91.

Wang, H., Kunkel, D. D., Martin, T. M. et al. (1993). Heteromultimeric potassium channels in terminal and juxtaparanodal regions of neurons. *Nature*, **365**, 75–9.

Waxman, S. G. (1995). Sodium channel blockade by

antibodies: a new mechanism of neurological disease? *Ann Neurol.*, **37**, 421–3.

Zielasek, J. and Toyka, K. V. (1999). Nerve conduction abnormalities and neuromyotonia in genetically engineered mouse models of human hereditary neuropathies. *Ann N Y Acad Sci.*, **883**, 310–20.

Zifko, U., Drlicek, M., Machacek, E. *et al.* (1994). Syndrome of continuous muscle fiber activity and plasmacytoma with IgM paraproteinemia. *Neurology*, **44**, 560–1.

# Central nervous system channel disorders

PART

6

# 15 Periodic and progressive ataxias

*Robert W. Baloh*

## Introduction

The familial episodic ataxias are rare, dominantly inherited diseases characterized by dramatic episodes of ataxia. Episodic ataxia type 1 (EA-1) has brief episodes of ataxia and interictal myokymia, while episodic ataxia type 2 (EA-2) is manifest by longer episodes of ataxia with interictal nystagmus. The episodes of ataxia are triggered by exercise and stress and often relieved by treatment with acetazolamide. These features are reminiscent of the periodic paralysis syndromes affecting muscle which suggested to early investigators that an ion channel mutation might be the cause.

Litt and colleagues (1994) mapped EA-1 to chromosome 12q13 near a cluster of three potassium channel genes. Two of the candidate genes, KCNA5 and KCNA6, were excluded by the genotype in one individual who later turned out to be a phenocopy. The remaining candidate, KCNA1, encodes for Kv1.1, a delayed rectifier potassium channel that is coded for by a single exon with 1488 base pairs. Browne *et al.* (1994) reported four different missense mutations in KCNA1 in four unrelated EA-1 pedigrees. This was the first report of a mutation in a human potassium channel and the first known ion channel mutation involving brain.

The disease locus for EA-2 was localized to a region on chromosome 19p (Kramer *et al.*, 1995; Vahedi *et al.*, 1995), previously shown to be the disease locus for familial hemiplegic migraine (FHM). FHM is a rare inherited type of migraine with aura characterized by recurrent episodes of headache and hemiparesis. Recovery between attacks is usually complete, but in some families, there is interictal nystagmus not unlike that seen

in EA-2. A calcium channel gene mapped to this locus on chromosome 19p and Ophoff and colleagues (1996) defined the complex structure of this gene, CACNA1A, which spans 300 000 base pairs and consists of 47 exons that encode the α1A subunit of the P/Q calcium channel. Analysis of the exons and flanking introns of CACNA1A identified point mutations that resulted in a premature stop codon or interfered with splicing in two families with EA-2 and missense mutations in four families with FHM. These findings confirmed that EA-2 and FHM were allelic disorders.

In 1996, Zhuchenko and colleagues (1997) were searching for CAG repeat expansions that might be associated with cerebellar ataxia syndromes when they found a CAG repeat expansion in CACNA1A. The CAG repeat expansion was in the open reading frame of a subset of splice variants expressed in the brain. They screened their large familial ataxia population for expansions in the CAG repeat in CACNA1A and found eight unrelated patients with late-onset ataxia that had alleles with repeat numbers (21 to 27) larger than the number of repeats seen in control subjects (4 to 16). This expanded CAG repeat segregated with the phenotype, a late-onset slowly progressive cerebellar ataxia. Subsequently there have been many reports of families around the world with the expanded CAG repeat in CACNA1A, all with a similar phenotype called spinocerebellar ataxia 6 (SCA-6).

## Epidemiology

The prevalence of inherited spinocerebellar ataxias in the general population is probably in the range of 1 to 2 per 100,000 in unselected populations but can be as high as 20 to 25 per 100,000 in isolated populations (Kurtze and Kurland, 1991). About a third of the inherited spinocerebellar ataxia syndromes are inherited in an autosomal dominant fashion.

The episodic ataxia syndromes (EA-1 and EA-2) are rare diseases representing less than 1% of the inherited ataxia syndromes. Age of onset is typically in childhood (age 2–15) for both conditions (Brunt and van Weerden, 1990; Baloh et al., 1997). Symptoms often attenuate after age 20 with EA-1 (Lubbers et al., 1995). There have been clear instances of non-penetrance with both syndromes. In a few families with EA-2, women have had milder symptoms and signs than men (Denier et al., 1999; Jen et al., 1999). Whether the type of missense mutation affects the age of onset or degree of penetrance awaits future studies of families with many different mutations.

The percentage of cases of dominantly inherited progressive ataxia with SCA-6 range from a low of 1% in France to a high of 31% in Japan (Geschwind et al., 1997; Matsumura et al., 1997; Sculs et al., 1997; Stevanin et al., 1997). The mean age of onset of SCA-6 is in the late 40s to early 50s with a wide range between 24 and 73 years of age. As with the other CAG repeat syndromes, there is an inverse relationship between the age of onset and the number of CAG repeats in CACNA1A. A few cases with expanded CAG repeats in CACNA1A have been reported without clinical symptoms or signs but these patients may develop the disorder with longer follow-up. There is no difference in the penetrance between men and women.

## Clinical features

### EA-1

EA-1 is characterized by sudden episodes of ataxia, typically triggered by exercise, startle, or emotional upset which lasts from seconds to a few minutes (Van Dyke et al., 1975; Brunt and van Weerden, 1990; Browne et al., 1994; Lubbers et al., 1995). Aura-like symptoms include a feeling of weakness or falling, dizziness and blurring of vision. During the episode, the ataxia involves the trunk and extremities and the speech is slurred. In between the episodes of ataxia, there is typically a continuous myokymia (muscle rippling), which may be either clinically evident or only detectable with EMG. The myokymia is most easily observed in the periorbital region and fingers. There appears to be an over-representation of epilepsy in family members with EA-1 compared to unaffected members (Zuberi et al., 1999). Many different seizure types have been reported including complex partial, partial with generalization, and generalized motor seizures (Zuberi et al., 1999). The episodes of ataxia typically diminish as the child becomes older and may completely disappear in the teens.

Examination during an attack reveals a generalized ataxia and dysarthria, but eye movements are normal. The interictal examination is typically normal except for myokymia.

### EA-2

Episodic ataxia type 2 is characterized by episodes of ataxia lasting hours and interictal nystagmus (Vahedi et al., 1995; Baloh et al., 1997; Denier et al., 1999; Jen et al., 1999). The episodes vary from pure ataxia to combinations of symptoms suggesting involvement of cerebellum and brainstem and even, occasionally, the cortex. Vertigo, nausea and vomiting are the most common associated symptoms, being present in more than 50% of patients. The episodes are typically triggered by exercise and emotional stress and often relieved by acetazolamide. Other known triggers include alcohol, phenytoin and caffeine. About half of the patients report headaches that meet the IHS criteria for migraine (Baloh et al., 1997).

On examination during acute episodes, the patients typically show severe ataxia and dysarthria. They may exhibit a spontaneous nystagmus not seen during the interictal examination. In between episodes, the most common finding is a gaze-evoked nystagmus with features typical of rebound nystagmus. Spontaneous vertical nystagmus, particularly downbeat nystagmus, is seen in about one-third of cases. This may begin with a positional downbeat nystagmus in the head-hanging position that, over time, becomes a spontaneous downbeat nystagmus (Jen et al., 1999). Later in the course, a mild truncal ataxia may be seen along with impaired smooth pursuit and saccade dysmetria similar to that seen in patients with SCA-6.

## SCA-6

The typical patient with SCA-6 presents with a slowly progressive truncal ataxia beginning in the late 40s to early 50s (Geschwind *et al.*, 1997; Ikecuhi *et al.*, 1997; Matsumura *et al.*, 1997; Sculs *et al.*, 1997; Stevanin *et al.*, 1997; Takiyama *et al.*, 1998). Dysarthria is the next most common symptom followed by dysphagia, vertigo and hypophonia. As noted earlier, there is an inverse relationship between the number of CAG repeats and the age of onset. Patients with small CAG repeat expansions may remain asymptomatic throughout life. Although the hallmark of SCA-6 is a slowly progressive ataxia, episodic features also occur. Patients may report fluctuations in the severity of ataxia related to stress and fatigue and other environmental factors. A small subset will have discrete episodes indistinguishable from episodes associated with EA-2. Jen *et al.* (1998) reported two families with SCA-6 who experienced episodes of positional vertigo more than 20 years before the onset of progressive ataxia. The episodes of positional vertigo were associated with a central type of positional nystagmus (downbeat). After late onset, the ataxia has an indolent course rarely progressing to severe disability within the first 10 years. Many patients remain ambulatory even 20 years after onset.

On neurological examination, gait ataxia and nystagmus are the most prominent findings. Horizontal gaze-evoked nystagmus is almost universally present while spontaneous vertical nystagmus (usually downbeat) is seen in more than half of cases. Other cerebellar oculomotor findings are also common, such as impaired smooth pursuit and dysmetric saccades. Corticospinal tract findings such as hyperreflexia and extensor plantar responses occur in a small minority of patients.

## Diagnostic tests

Magnetic resonance imaging (MRI) of the brain typically shows atrophy of the cerebellum, most pronounced in the midline, for both EA-2 and SCA-6 (Figure 15.1) (Baloh *et al.*, 1997; Geschwind *et al.*, 1997). The degree of atrophy is most prominent in patients with long-standing symptoms and signs. MRI and CT studies of the brain in patients with EA-1 have been normal. Nonspecific paroxysmal slowing on electroencephalography (EEG) has been reported with both EA-1 and EA-2 (Zasorin *et al.*, 1983; Feeney and Boyle, 1989; Zuberi *et al.*, 1999). Continuous muscle rippling (myokymia) can be detected in most patients with EA-1, particularly after provocation by limb ischaemia. Repetitive duplets, triplets or multiplets on electromyography (EMG) underlie the continuous muscle activity (Brunt and van Weerden, 1990; Zuberi *et al.*, 1999). The spontaneous muscle activity typically occurs at a frequency of about 10 per second and is often made more prominent with hyperventilation.

Eye movement recordings demonstrate a unique consistent oculomotor pattern in patients with EA-2 and SCA-6 (Baloh *et al.*, 1997; Buttner *et al.*, 1998). Saccade velocity remains normal but saccade dysmetria is common. Smooth pursuit and optokinetic responses are severely impaired and suppression of vestibular-induced nystagmus is severely impaired. On the other hand, the vestibulo-ocular reflex gain is either high normal or increased. This pattern of findings is highly localizing to the caudal midline cerebellum.

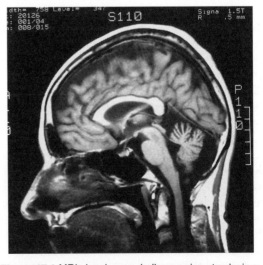

**Figure 15.1** MRI showing cerebellar vermian atrophy in a patient with EA-2. (Sagittal section, T1-weighted).

Genetic testing for the expanded CAG repeat in CACNA1A is now readily available in major laboratories around the USA and abroad. Identifying point mutations in KCNA1 and CACNA1A is a more difficult task and is currently available only in a small number of research laboratories. In the future, automated techniques will be available to screen these two genes rapidly for the known point mutations.

## Management

Since emotional stress is often a trigger for attacks of EA-1 and EA-2, stress management techniques such as biofeedback and meditation can be helpful in controlling symptoms in some patients. Alcohol and caffeine should be avoided and regular but modest exercise should be encouraged. Vigorous exercise often will trigger attacks of EA-1 and EA-2. Fluid and food intake should be regularly distributed throughout the day and binges should be avoided.

Acetazolamide can be dramatic in controlling episodes of ataxia with EA-2 (Griggs et al., 1978) and occasionally is also beneficial with EA-1 (Lubbers et al., 1995). There can be a variable response to acetazolamide even within a single family with a known mutation. Acetazolamide presumably works by altering the pH within the cerebellum, thus stabilizing the mutated ion channel (Bain et al., 1992). One typically begins with a low dose (125 mg a day) and then works up to an average effective dose between 500 and 750 mg a day. Most patients will experience paraesthesias of the extremities after taking the drug but these symptoms typically decrease over time. The main long-term side effect is development of kidney stones which can be markedly decreased if the patient regularly drinks citrus juices. Patients with known allergies to sulpha-containing drugs may have an allergic reaction to acetazolamide. There is relatively little experience with other carbonic anhydrase inhibitors, but these drugs are probably as effective as acetazolamide. Two children with EA-2 were reported to respond to the centrally active calcium channel blocker, flunarizine (Boel and Casaer, 1988). We have tried another centrally active calcium channel blocker, nimodipine, and

other peripheral calcium channel blockers including verapamil in multiple patients with EA-2 with little success.

## Genetics

### KCNA1

The KCNA1 gene codes for the six transmembrane segments (S1–S6) of the Kv1.1 potassium channel subunit (Figure 15.2A). Four of these subunits join together along with other auxiliary units to form the Kv1.1 potassium channel. The four subunits are believed to be arranged in a ring, like the staves of a barrel, around a central pore (Figure 15.2B). The four pore loops (between S5 and S6) reach into the barrel and confer the ion-conduction properties. The KCNA-1 protein is localized in a variety of brain and peripheral nerve regions. It is heavily expressed in Purkinje cells and basket and granular cells of the cerebellum and in the juxtaparanodal regions of nodes of Ranvier of peripheral nerves (Rhodes et al., 1997; Zhou et al., 1998).

A wide range of missense mutations in KCNA1 have been identified in families with EA-1 (Browne et al., 1994; Bretschneider et al., 1999) (Table 15.1). Most of the mutations involve either the transmembrane segments or the intracellular linkers affecting highly conserved amino acids. Otherwise there is no common pattern.

### CACNA1A

CACNA1A encodes for the α1A subunit of the P/Q calcium channel. Each of the four homologous domains of the α1A calcium channel subunit has six putative a-helical membrane-spanning segments (S1 to S6) similar to the six transmembrane segments of the potassium channel Kv1.1 (Figure 15.2C). CACNA1A is expressed throughout the brain but is particularly prominent in the cerebellum (Mori et al., 1991). It is also heavily expressed at the neuromuscular junction where it is tightly coupled with neurotransmitter release (Jen, 1999).

Ophoff et al. (1996) initially reported two muta-

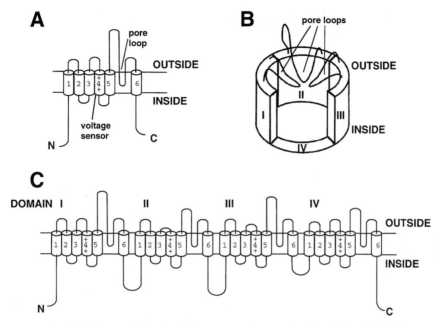

**Figure 15.2** (A) Schematic drawing of the transmembrane subunit coded for by KCNA1. The pore-forming region (pore loop)) is between segments 5 and 6. Segment 4 is the voltage-sensing region. (B) Illustration of how 4 of the subunits in A join together to form a potassium channel. The central pore is formed by the pore loops from each of the 4 subunits. (C) Schematic drawing of the transmembrane subunit coded for by CACNA1A. Each domain is equivalent to one of the subunits coded for by KCNA1.

**Table 15.1 Missense mutations in Kv1.1 a-subunit known to be associated with EA-1**

| Missense mutation | Protein location |
| --- | --- |
| F184C | S1 |
| I177N | S1 |
| V174F | S1 |
| T226M | S2 |
| T226A | S2 |
| R239S | S2 |
| F249I | S2–S3 |
| E325D | S4–S5 |
| V404I | S6 |
| V408A | S6 |

From Browne *et al.*, 1994; Comu *et al.*, 1996; Scheffer *et al.*, 1998.

tions disrupting the reading frame in CACNA1A and thus predicting truncated a1A subunits in two families with EA-2. Yue *et al.* (1997) identified a missense mutation in a family with a severe pro-gressive ataxia in some members and superimposed episodes of vertigo and ataxia in others. This mutation predicted a glycine to arginine substitution at codon 293, a highly conserved amino acid in the critical pore loop region of the $\alpha$1A transmembrane subunit. These same researchers also identified a patient with acetazolamide-responsive EA-2 and no family history that showed a *de novo* mutation in exon 23 that predicted a premature stop code and a truncated protein (Yue *et al.*, 1998). Subsequently several other families with mutations in CACNA1A and the EA-2 phenotype have been reported, most with nonsense mutations, although a few have critical missense mutations (Table 15.2) (Denier *et al.*, 1999; Jen *et al.*, 1999).

The CAG repeat expansion in CACNA1A responsible for SCA-6 is within the open reading frame and is predicted to encode a polyglutamine tract in a subset of isoforms of $\alpha$1A subunits expressed in the cerebellum (Zhuchenko *et al.*, 1997). Unlike the other CAG repeat expansion ataxia syndromes, SCA-6 results from a slight

| Table 15.2 Different mutations in CACNA1A associated with EA-2 | | | |
| --- | --- | --- | --- |
| *Mutation* | *Nucleotide shift* | *Domain* | *Effect on coding sequence* |
| Exon 22 | del C (4073) | III S1 | Stop 1294 |
| Intron 24 | G → A (4270+1) | Splice site | Aberrant splicing |
| Exon 6 | G → A (1152) | I S5–S6 | glycine → arginine 293 |
| Exon 23 | C → T (4410) | III S5–S6 | Stop 1279 |
| Exon 16 | del AG (2248) | II S6 | Stop 780 |
| Exon 27 | C → G (4332) | III S5–S6 | Stop 1443 |
| Exon 22 | del C (3798) | III S1 | Stop 1293 |
| Exon 29 | C → T (4639) | IV S1 | Stop 1546 |
| Intron 11 | G → A (1558+2) | Splice site | Aberrant splicing |
| Intron 26 | G → A (4256+2) | Splice site | Aberrant splicing |
| Exon 30 | del CTT (4781) | IV S2 | del tyrosine 1594 alamine → aspartate 1593 |
| Exon 29 | C → T (4914) | IV S1 | Stop 1547 |

From Ophoff *et al.*, 1996; Yue *et al.*, 1997, 1998; Denier *et al.*, 1999; Jen *et al.*, 1999.

expansion from an upper normal range of 19 to a disease-causing range of 21 and above. Also unlike the other CAG repeat expansion syndromes, the CAG repeat expansion causing SCA-6 is mostly stable when transmitted from one generation to another (anticipation has not been seen in clinical pedigrees). An exception to this general rule was a family reported by Jodice *et al.* (1997) in which a father with a 20 CAG repeat expansion passed on a 25 CAG repeat expansion to one of his five children. Three of the five children received the 20 CAG repeat expansion of the father. The offspring that received the 25 CAG repeat expansion passed it on unchanged to his two children. Interestingly, the phenotypes varied with the length of the CAG repeat expansion in this family. Family members with a 20 CAG repeat expansion exhibited episodic symptoms with minimal interictal findings while the members with the 25 CAG repeat expansion exhibited a progressive ataxia without episodic features. So far only one other intergenerational expansion in a CAG repeat with SCA-6 has been reported in about 100 meioses reported in families with SCA-6. Thus, although the expanded CAG repeat alleles with SCA-6 appear to be much more stable than that of the more typical CAG repeat expansions with more than 35 repeats, CAG repeat instability does occur in some families with SCA-6.

Although the great majority of patients with SCA-6 have only one allele with an expanded CAG repeat, individuals homozygous for an expanded CAG repeat have been reported. Several groups have found that individuals homozygous for the CAG repeat had an earlier age of onset and more severe clinical manifestations than other family members who had one normal and one expanded allele (Geschwind *et al.*, 1997; Ikecuhi *et al.*, 1997; Matsumura *et al.*, 1997). In contrast to this, Takiyama *et al.* (1998) identified three individuals homozygous for the expanded CAG repeat (21/21), only two of whom were symptomatic, and noted no apparent differences in the clinical phenotype between the individuals homozygous and those heterozygous for the expanded CAG repeat. Differences in the size of the CAG repeat expansion may explain the difference in the findings. Patients homozygous for large repeat sizes (greater than 21) probably have a more severe clinical course than heterozygous family members.

## Animal models

Sequencing of the shaker locus in *Drosophila* identified a potassium channel that was the first of a large number of homologous genes in the shaker family. KCNA1, the gene for EA-1, is a shaker homologue in humans. There are no known natural mutants of the shaker homologue in mice but Kv1.1 null mice generated by gene targeting in embryonic stem cells results in an epileptic phenotype but no ataxia (Smart *et al.*, 1998). Kv1.1 null mice show a striking temperature-sensitive excitability change localized to the nerve terminals that can explain the myokymia seen with this disorder (Zhou *et al.*, 1998).

Mutations in genes encoding for various calcium channel subunits have been identified in a number of recessive mouse mutants. Homozygous point mutations in the $\alpha$1A gene (P1802L, domain 2P region) cause epilepsy and ataxia in the mutant mouse tottering (tg) (Fletcher *et al.*, 1996). Novel sequences in the intercellular carboxy terminus of the $\alpha$1A subunit also result in a mutant mouse phenotype leaner (tgla) with ataxia and epilepsy (Fletcher *et al.*, 1996). Burgess and colleagues (1997) found a mutation in a calcium channel gene with a predicted deletion of the highly conserved $\alpha$1 binding motif of the b4 subunit in the mutant mouse lethargic exhibiting both ataxia and seizures. Characterization of the genetic defects in the stargazer and waggler mutants led to the identification of a new neuronal calcium channel subunit $\gamma$ (Letts *et al.*, 1998). Stargazer mice have epilepsy, ataxia and unusual head posturing suggesting inner ear vestibular damage.

# Molecular pathogenesis

## EA-1

KCNA1 encodes for a subunit of a delayed rectifier potassium channel Kv1.1. The delayed rectifier potassium channels are a family of potassium channels that allow sustained $K^+$ efflux with a delay after membrane depolarization. The outflow of potassium ions rapidly repolarizes the membrane. Kv1.1 channels play a key role in neurotransmitter release, action potential generation and axonal impulse conduction (Zhou *et al.*, 1998). Studies of the biophysical properties of mutant Kv1.1 channels in *Xenopus* oocytes or mammalian cell lines demonstrate physiological consequences of the genetic mutations, although

no consistent pattern has emerged (Adelman *et al.*, 1995; Letts *et al.*, 1998; Bretschneider *et al.*, 1999). Boland *et al.* (1999) introduced seven different episodic ataxia type 1 mutations and studied the effect on the expressed channels in *Xenopus* oocytes. The voltage range of steady state inactivation was altered in all cases and most changes were also associated with changes in activation gating. They concluded that the EA-1 mutations altered potassium channel function by two mechanisms: (1) reduced channel expression; and (2) altered channel gating. Bretschneider *et al.* (1999) studied the functional consequences of two EA-1 mutations by injecting cRNA coding for the mutations into mammalian cells and comparing currents with a patch-clamp technique in the mutant and wild-type channels. One of the mutant channels deactivated and inactivated faster compared to the wild-type, while the other showed no change in maximum open probability, suggesting that its effect was due to a reduced number of functional channels on the cell surface. Interestingly, acetazolamide had no measurable effect on either the wild-type or mutant channels.

## CACNA1A

Kraus *et al.* (1998) introduced the four missense mutations, reported in families with FHM by Ophoff *et al.* (1996), into *Xenopus laevis* oocytes and investigated possible changes in channel function after functional expression of the mutant subunits. Changes in channel gating were observed in three out of four of the mutants, but the time course of recovery from the channel inactivation was accelerated in two and slower in the third compared to wild-type. Hans *et al.* (1999) introduced the four missense mutations causing FHM into human $\alpha$1A subunits and investigated their functional consequences after expression in human kidney cells. They also found a range of effects from shifts in the voltage range of activation toward more negative voltages, increases in both the open probability and the rate of recovery from inactivation, and decreases in the density of functional channels in the membrane. Interestingly, the reduction in single channel conductance induced by two of the mutations was not observed in some patches or periods of activity, suggesting that the abnormal channel may switch on and off due to some unknown factor. So far the physiological effects of the truncating mutations associated with EA-2 have not been reported, but one might well expect that these major mutations would lead to non-functional channels. Furthermore, alterations in calcium channel function might lead to altered function and expression of other membrane ion channels (Ruff, 1999).

Matsuyama *et al.* (1999) studied the effects of polyglutamine expansion on channel properties by analysing currents flowing through the P/Q-type calcium channels with an expanded stretch of 24, 30, or 40 polyglutamines, recombinantly expressed in baby hamster kidney cells. Calcium channels with 30 or 40 polyglutamines showed an 8 mV hyperpolarizing shift in the voltage dependence of inactivation compared with calcium channels having 24 or fewer polyglutamines. These changes seen in the larger polyglutamine expansions reduced the available channel population at a resting membrane potential suggesting that the polyglutamine expansion in SCA-6 could lead to neuronal death and cerebellar atrophy by reducing calcium influx into Purkinje cells and in other neurons. The expanded CAG repeats did not affect the expression level of the functional calcium channels based on the unaltered current densities. The authors concluded that the calcium channel proteins with a pathologically expanded polyglutamine stretch are transported to the plasma membrane in a normal manner, unlike the case in the mouse mutants leaner and tottering where the mutant recombinant channels show a decreased expression in baby hamster kidney cells.

The mechanism by which the CAG repeat expansion in CACNA1A leads to a predominant Purkinje cell degeneration is a mystery since the gene is expressed widely throughout the brain with expression levels in many neurons equal to that of Purkinje cells. In their original description of SCA-6, Zhuchenko *et al.* (1997) noted that only a small subset of splice variants of CACNA1A were predicted to express the polyglutamine tract on the carboxyl end of the protein. The splice variant with a 5-base GGCAG insertion in the 5′ terminus of exon 47 was predicted to translate the expanded polyglutamine tract. Ishikawa and colleagues

(1999a, b) examined the differences in the levels of messenger RNAs spanning the GGCAG insertion site and the CAG repeat by semiquantitative reverse transcriptase PCR analysis. Splice variants with the GGCAG insertion were predominantly amplified from cerebellar messenger RNA, suggesting that the isoform with the polyglutamine tract is the one predominantly expressed in the human cerebellum. *In situ* hybridization showed that cellular expression of CACNA1A messenger RNA containing the CAG repeat was highest in cell bodies of Purkinje cells, with other neurons throughout the brain showing less intense signals. They then examined the expression of the $\alpha$1A calcium channel protein using antibodies raised against synthetic peptides corresponding to the region between domains II and III and to the C-terminal region of the protein containing the expanded polyglutamine tract. In control brains, the immunoreactivity of the two antibodies was essentially the same with the most intense immunoreaction seen in the cell bodies of Purkinje cells. In the brains from SCA-6 patients, they found densely immunoreactive oval or rod-shaped structures in the cytoplasm of Purkinje cells. These cytoplasmic aggregates were not positive for ubiquitin and were not seen in the nuclei of Purkinje cells. In cultured cells, expressed channel protein with an expanded polyglutamine tract formed dense accumulations in the perinuclear and internuclear spaces which was associated with apoptotic cell death. The authors concluded that aggregation of $\alpha$1A calcium channel protein is associated with the pathogenic mechanism of SCA-6.

## Animal models

Lau and colleagues (1998) studied the expression of $\alpha$1A messenger RNA and $\alpha$1A protein in the cerebellum from 20-day-old homozygous leaner mice and control mice using *in situ* hybridization, histochemistry and immunocytochemistry. They found no difference in the messenger RNA or protein expression in the mutated $\alpha$1A subunit in the leaner mice compared to controls. Thus they showed that the $\alpha$1A subunit splice donor consensus sequence mutation carried by leaner mice does not result in any significant quantitative changes in either messenger RNA or protein expression. The data suggest that the leaner phenotype results from abnormal calcium channels that contain the altered $\alpha$1A subunits.

## Pathology

The main pathological finding in SCA-6 is a prominent drop-out of Purkinje cells in the cerebellum with the greatest loss in the vermis and flocculonodular region and milder loss in the cerebellar hemispheres (Gomez et al., 1997; Ishikawa et al., 1999a). Granular neurons are relatively spared and afferents to the cerebellum are uninvolved with the exception of the inferior olives. Gliosis identified in the inferior olives, the deep cerebellar nuclei and vestibular nuclei may be secondary to the loss of Purkinje cell efferents because there is little evidence of neuronal degeneration in these structures. One patient with SCA-6 showed axonal degeneration in the corticospinal tracts below the level of the medullary pyramids (Gomez et al., 1997). This correlated with the clinical finding of hyperreflexia and extensor plantar responses, findings infrequently seen but reported with SCA-6. So far there have been no studies reporting pathological findings in patients with documented EA-1 or EA-2.

## References

Adelman, J. P., Bond, C. T., Pessia, M. and Maylie, J. (1995). Episodic ataxia results from voltage-dependent potassium channels with altered functions. *Neuron*, **15**, 1449–54.

Bain, P. G., O'Brien, M. D., Keevil, S. F. and Porter, D. A. (1992). Familial periodic cerebellar ataxia: a problem of molecular pH homeostasis. *Ann Neurol.*, **31**, 146–54.

Baloh, R. W., Yue, Q., Furman, J. M. and Nelson, S. F. (1997). Familial episodic ataxia: clinical heterogeneity in four families linked to chromosome 19p. *Ann Neurol.*, **41**, 8–16.

Boel, M. and Casaer, P. (1988). Familial periodic ataxia responsive to flunarizine. *Neuropediatrics*, **19**, 218–20.

Boland, L. M., Price, D. L. and Jackson, K. A. (1999). Episodic ataxia/myokymia mutations functionally expressed in the shaker potassium channel. *Neuroscience*, **91**, 1557–64.

Bretschneider, F., Wrisch, A., Lehmann-Horn, F., and Grissmar, S. (1999). Expression in mammalian cells and electrophysiological characterization of two mutant Kv1.1 channels causing episodic ataxia type 1 (EA-1). *Eur J Neurosci.*, **11**, 2403–12.

Browne, D. L., Gancher, S. T, Nutt, J. G. et al. (1994). Episodic ataxia/myokymia syndrome is associated with point mutations in the human potassium channel gene, KCNA1. *Nat Genet.*, **8**, 136–40.

Brunt, E. R. and van Weerden, T. W. (1990). Familial paroxysmal kinesigenic ataxia and continuous myokymia. *Brain*, **113**, 1361–82.

Burgess, D. L., Jones, J. M., Meisler, M. H. and Noebels, J. L. (1997). Mutation in the $Ca2^{+}$ channel beta subunit gene Cchb4 is associated with ataxia and seizures in the lethargic (lh) mouse. *Cell*, **88**, 185–2.

Buttner, N., Geschwind, D., Jen, J. C. et al. (1998). Oculomotor phenotypes in autosomal dominant ataxias. *Arch Neurol.*, **55**, 1353–7.

Comu, S., Giuliani, M. and Narayanan, V. (1996). Episodic ataxia and myokymia syndrome: a new mutation of potassium channel gene Kv1.1. *Ann Neurol.*, **40**, 684–7.

Denier, C., Ducros, A., Vahedi, K. et al. (1999). High prevalence of CACNA1A truncations and broader clinical spectrum in episodic ataxia type 2. *Neurology*, **52**, 1816–21.

Feeney, G. F. X. and Boyle, R. S. (1989). Paroxysmal cerebellar ataxia. *Aust NZ J Med.*, **19**, 113–7.

Fletcher, C. F., Lutz, C. M., O'Sullivan, T. N. et al. (1996). Absence epilepsy in tottering mutant mice is associated with calcium channel defects. *Cell*, **87**, 607–17.

Geschwind, D. H., Perlman, S., Figueroa, K. P. et al. (1997). Spinocerebellar ataxia type 6. Frequency of the mutation and genotype-phenotype correlations. *Neurology*, **49**, 1247–51.

Gomez, C. M., Thompson, R. M., Gammack, J. T. et al. (1997). Spinocerebellar ataxia type 6: gaze-evoked and vertical nsytagmus, Purkinje cell degeneration and variable age of onset. *Ann Neurol.*, **42**, 933–50.

Griggs, R. C., Moxley, R. T., Lafrance, R. A. and McQuillen, J. (1978). Hereditary paroxysmal ataxia: response to acetazolamide. *Neurology*, **28**, 1259–64.

Hans, M., Luvisetto, S., Williams, M. E. et al. (1999). Functional consequences of mutations in the human a1A calcium channel subunit linked to familial hemiplegic migraine. *J Neurosci.*, **19**, 1610–9.

Ikecuhi, T., Takano, H., Koide, R. et al. (1997). Spinocerebellar ataxia type 6: CAG repeat expansion in a1A voltage-dependent calcium channel gene and clinical variations in Japanese population. *Ann Neurol.*, **42**, 879–84.

Ishikawa, K., Fujigasaki, H., Saegusa, H. et al. (1999). Abundant expression and cytoplasmic aggregations of a1A voltage-dependent calcium channel protein associated with neurodegeneration in spinocerebellar ataxia type 6. *Hum Molec Genet.*, **8**, 1185–93.

Ishikawa, K., Watanabe, M., Yoshikawa, K. et al.

(1999). Clinical, neuropathological, and molecular study in two families with spinocerebellar ataxia type 6 (SCA6). *J Neurol Neurosurg Psychiatr.*, **67**, 86–89.

Jen, J. (1999). Calcium channelopathies in the central nervous system. *Curr Opin Neurobiol.*, **9**, 274–80.

Jen, J., Yue, Q., Nelson, S. F. *et al.*(1999). A novel nonsense mutation in CACNA1A causes episodic ataxia and hemiplegia. *Neurology*, **53**, 34–7.

Jen, J. C., Yue, Q., Karrim, J. *et al.* (1998). Spinocerebellar ataxia type 6 with positional vertigo and acetazolamide-responsive episodic ataxia. *J Neurol Neurosurg Psychiatr.*, **65**, 565–8.

Jodice, C., Mantuano, E., Veneziano, L. *et al.* (1997). Episodic ataxia type 2 (EA2) and spinocerebellar ataxia type 6 (SCA6) due to CAG repeat expansion in the CACNA1A gene on chromosome 19p. *Hum Molec Genet.*, **6**, 1973–8.

Kramer, P. L., Yue, Q., Gancher, S. T. *et al.* (1995). A locus for the nystagmus-associated form of episodic ataxia maps to an 11-cM region on chromosome 19p. *Am J Hum Genet.*, **57**, 182–5.

Kraus, R. L., Sinnegger, M. J., Glossman, H. *et al.* (1998). Familial hemiplegic migraine mutations change a1A Ca$^{2+}$ channel kinetics. *J Biol Chem.*, **273**, 5586–90.

Kurtzke, J. F. and Kurland, L. T. (1991). The epidemiology of neurologic disease. In *Clinical Neurology* (ed. Joynt, R. D.) pp. 66–8. J.B. Lippincott, Philadelphia.

Lau, F. C., Abbott, L. C., Rhyu, I. J. *et al.* (1998). Expression of calcium channel a1A mRNA and protein in the leaner mouse (tgla/tgla) cerebellum. *Molec Brain Res.*, **59**, 93–9.

Letts, V. A., Felix, R., Biddlecome, G. H. *et al.* (1998). The mouse stargazer gene encodes a neuronal Ca2$^+$-channel g subunit. *Nature Genet.*, **19**, 340–7.

Litt, M., Kramer, P., Browne, D. *et al.* (1994). A gene for episodic ataxia/myokymia maps to chromosome 12p13. *Am J Hum Genet.*, **55**, 702–9.

Lubbers, W. J., Brunt, E. R., Scheffer, H. *et al.* (1995). Hereditary myokymia and paroxysmal ataxia linked to chromosome 12 is responsive to acetazolamide. *J Neurol Neurosurg Psychiatr.*, **59**, 400–5.

Matsumura, R., Futamura, N., Fujimoto, Y. *et al.* (1997). Molecular and clinical features of 35 Japanese patients including one homozygous for the CAG repeat expansion. *Neurology*, **39**, 1238–43.

Matsuyama, Z., Wakamori, M., Mori, Y. *et al.* (1999). Direct alteration of the P/Q-type Ca2$^+$ channel property by polyglutamine expansion in spinocerebellar ataxia 6. *J Neurosci.*, **19**, 1–5.

Mori, Y., Friedrich, I., Kim, M. S. *et al.* (1991). Primary structure and functional expression from complementary DNA of a brain calcium channel. *Nature*, **350**, 398–402.

Ophoff, R. A., Terwindt, G. M., Vergouwe, M. N. *et al.* (1996). Familial hemiplegic migraine and episodic ataxia type-2 are caused by mutations in the Ca2$^+$ channel gene CACNA1A. *Cell*, **87**, 543–52.

Rhodes, K. J, Strassle, B. W., Monaghan, M. M. *et al.* (1997). Association and colocalization of the Kvb1- and Kvb2- subunits with Kv1 a-subunits in mammalian K$^+$ channel complexes. *J Neurosci.*, **17**, 8246–58.

Ruff, R. (1999). Insulin acts in hypokalemic periodic paralysis by reducing inward rectifier K$^+$ current. *Neurology*, **53**, 1556–63.

Scheffer, H., Brunt, E. R. P., Mol, G. J. J. *et al.* (1998). Three novel KCNA1 mutations in episodic ataxia type I families. *Hum Genet.*, **102**, 464–6.

Schüls, L., Amoiridis, G., Büttner, T. *et al.* (1997). Autosomal dominant cerebellar ataxia: phenotypic differences in genetically defined subtypes. *Ann Neurol.*, **42**, 924–32.

Smart, S. L., Lopantsev, V., Zhang, C. L. *et al.* (1998). Deletion of the Kv1.1 potassium channel causes epilepsy in mice. *Neuron*, **20**, 809–19.

Stevanin, G., Dürr, A., David, G. *et al.* (1997). Clinical and molecular features of spinocerebellar ataxia type 6. *Neurology*, **49**, 1243–6.

Takiyama, Y., Sakoe, K., Namekawa, M. *et al.* (1998). A Japanese with a spinocerebellar ataxia type 6 which includes three individuals homozygous for an expanded CAG repeat in the SCA6/CACNL1A4 gene. *J Neurol Sci.*, **158**, 141–7.

Vahedi, K., Joutel, A., Van Bogaert, P., *et al.* (1995). A gene for hereditary paroxysmal cerebellar ataxia maps to chromosome 19p. *Ann Neurol.*, **37**, 289–93.

Van Dyke, D. H., Griggs, R. C., Murphy, M. J. and Goldstein, M. N. (1975). Hereditary myokymia and periodic ataxia. *J Neurol Sci.*, **25**, 109–18.

Yue, Q., Jen, J. C., Nelson, S. F. and Baloh, R. W. (1997). Progressive ataxia due to a missense mutation in a calcium-channel gene. *Am J Hum Genet.*, **61**, 1078–87.

Yue, Q., Jen, J. C., Thwe, M. M. *et al.* (1998). De novo mutation in CACNA1A caused acetazolamide-responsive episodic ataxia. *Am J Med Genet.*, **77**, 298–301.

Zasorin, N. L., Baloh, R. W. and Myers, L. B. (1983). Acetazolamide-responsive episodic ataxia syndrome. *Neurology*, **33**, 1212–4.

Zhou, L., Zhang, C.-L., Messing, A. and Chiu, S.Y. (1998). Temperature-sensitive neuromuscular transmission in Kv1.1 null mice: role of potassium channels under the myelin sheath in young nerves. *J Neurosci.*, **18**, 7200–15.

Zhuchenko, O., Bailey, J., Bonnen, P. *et al.* (1997). Autosomal dominant cerebellar ataxia (SCA6) associated with small polyglutamine expansions in the a1A-voltage-dependent calcium channel. *Nature Genet.*, **15**, 62–9.

Zuberi, S. M., Eunson, L. H., Spauschus, A. *et al.* (1999). A novel mutation in the human voltage-gated potassium channel gene (Kv1.1) associates with episodic ataxia type 1 and sometimes with partial epilepsy. *Brain*, **122**, 817–25.

# 16 Epilepsies

## Samuel F Berkovic

## Introduction

The epilepsies, defined as disorders with recurrent afebrile seizures, affect at least 2% of the population at some time in life. In addition, approximately 3% of children experience febrile seizures (Hauser *et al.*, 1993). The epilepsies comprise a heterogeneous group of syndromes that are broadly divided into generalized and focal (partial) types. These broad groups are subdivided into numerous identifiable clinical forms of epilepsy (probably more than 50) although some are very rare (Commission, 1989). The classification is evolving, and this evolution is being driven by basic biological discoveries in genetics and neuroimaging, in addition to traditional analysis based on clinical features and EEG.

## Aetiology of the epilepsies

The biological bases of the various clinical syndromes are different. Since the time of Hippocrates, it has been known that epilepsies have an inherited component (see below). It has also been well recognized that major acquired brain lesions have an aetiological role in the epilepsies. Accepted and undisputed acquired causes include serious prenatal events (e.g. periventricular haemorrhage), major perinatal trauma, serious head injury (e.g. penetrating brain injury or non-penetrating injury with significant coma), encephalitis, bacterial meningitis, and tumours (Hesdorffer and Verity, 1997).

It used to be assumed that 'minor' acquired factors are also important causative factors in epilepsy. These include prenatal events (minor antepartum haemorrhage, maternal illness during pregnancy), minor perinatal factors (e.g. breech birth, prolonged labour, forceps extraction), and head injury without prolonged loss of consciousness (Nielsen and Courville, 1951; Lilienfeld and Pasamanick, 1954). It is clear that the role of perinatal factors in the aetiology of epilepsies has been overemphasized in the past, but a role for such 'minor' factors, at least in certain cases, cannot be entirely discounted (Deymeer and Leviton, 1985; Nelson and Ellenberg, 1984).

The view that such minor events 'cause' epilepsies is simplistic. If and when they have a role, the effects may be additive and, particularly if occurring in an individual with a genetic predisposition, might increase the probability of epilepsy in that individual. This view was first suggested in a scientific sense by William Lennox approximately 40 years ago, who suggested that there is a general genetic predisposition to seizures. Individuals with this predisposition who acquire additional minor risk factors are more likely to have epileptic seizures (Lennox and Lennox, 1960). In contrast, those who did not have a genetic predisposition, might require a more severe acquired lesion ever to have seizures, although all humans can have epileptic seizures given a sufficiently severe brain insult. This remains an attractive concept and has been developed further. Rather than viewing an individual's epilepsy as either genetic or acquired, assessment from a neurobiological viewpoint is helpful, incorporating all known genetic and acquired factors that can be elucidated by clinical evaluation and investigation (Gloor *et al.*, 1982; Berkovic *et al.*, 1987).

The original view of Lennox clearly needs modification. There is no single genetic predisposition or 'epileptic diathesis'. It is now quite clear that there are many genes that cause or predispose an individual to develop epilepsy and that a multi-factorial aetiology, with an interaction of genetic and acquired factors may underlie many epilepsies. The fundamental biology of the interaction of genetic and acquired factors is not presently understood.

## Genetics of the epilepsies

Many and perhaps most epilepsies have an inherited component. It is common to find a family history of febrile seizures or epilepsy in patients being routinely evaluated for a seizure disorder. It is unusual, however, to encounter examples where epilepsy is inherited in a simple (Mendelian) fashion; that is with autosomal dominant, recessive or X-linked inheritance (Berkovic and Scheffer, 1997).

There are, in fact, hundreds of conditions with simple inheritance where seizures are part of the phenotype and most of these disorders are rare. Most are associated with significant neurological impairment, and seizures are symptomatic of severe neuronal dysfunction due to a wide variety of processes. Some examples of recent interest include progressive myoclonus epilepsies such as Unverricht-Lundborg disease (cystatin B gene mutations) (Pennacchio et al., 1996) and Lafora disease (tyrosine phosphatase mutations) (Minassian et al., 1998; Serratosa et al., 1999) and the inherited developmental cortical malformations such as familial subcortical band heterotopia (doublecortin mutations) (des Portes et al., 1998; Gleeson et al., 1998) and familial periventricular heterotopia (filamin 1 mutations) etc. (Fox et al., 1998). These genetic defects are unlikely to be relevant to the causation of the majority of people with epilepsies and are not considered further here.

Most patients with a genetic component to their epilepsy show complex inheritance, where more than one gene, probably with the influence of acquired factors (multifactorial), leads to the particular epilepsy syndrome. In most families with a complex trait, few or even only one individual may be clinically affected, whereas in some families there will be many affected subjects scat-

tered through a number of generations. For any given individual within such a family, the closer their relationship to the proband, the more likely he or she will be affected.

The distinction between simple and complex inheritance is extremely important for molecular genetic studies. Nearly all the recent successes in finding genes for human disease have been in conditions with simple inheritance, which are uncommon or rare. It is much more difficult to perform linkage analysis and find genes in diseases with complex inheritance; very few have been found to date and some of the molecular findings remain controversial (Risch and Merikangas, 1996). A successful strategy for finding genes for common diseases with complex inheritance has been to start with rare families where the trait has simple inheritance. Once the gene or genes are identified in such rare families, the question can be asked if those genes are relevant to the majority of cases where inheritance is complex. This strategy has been successful in Alzheimer's disease, breast cancer, diabetes etc.

This strategy is now being applied to the common idiopathic epilepsies. A surprising number of 'new' single gene epilepsies have been described in the last few years and linkage analysis has led to localization of the genes for many of these (Table 16.1). To date, five genes, causing three of these syndromes, have been identified and all code for ion channel subunits, either ligand gated or voltage-gated. The clinical and molecular features of these syndromes are described below.

## Benign familial neonatal convulsions (BFNC)

BFNC was the first idiopathic epilepsy where linkage analysis was successful. Seizures characteristically occur from about day 3 of life. Seizures in the neonatal period often indicate the presence of serious pre- or perinatal damage or a significant metabolic derrangement. These infants are, however, otherwise healthy and family history is the key to diagnosis. Inheritance is autosomal dominant with a penetrance of about 90%, but a careful history must be taken from mothers and usually

**Table 16.1 Molecular genetic progress in idiopathic epilepsies with simple inheritance**

| Syndrome | Locus | Gene | References |
|---|---|---|---|
| Benign familial neonatal convulsions | 20q | KCNQ2 | (Leppert *et al* 1989, Singh *et al* 1998, Bievert *et al* 1998) |
| | 8q | KCNQ3 | (Lewis *et al* 1983; Charlier *et al* 1998) |
| X-linked infantile spasms | Xp11 | ? | (Claes *et al* 1997) |
| Benign familial infantile convulsions | 19q | ? | (Guipponi *et al* 1997) |
| | 16 | ? | (Szeptowski *et al* 1997) |
| AR rolandic epilepsy with paroxysmal dystonia | 16 | ? | (Guerrini *et al* 1999) |
| AD nocturnal frontal lobe epilepsy | 20q | CHRNA4 | (Phillips *et al* 1995, Steinlein *et al* 1995) |
| | 15q | ? | (Phillips *et al* 1998) |
| Partial epilepsy with auditory features | 10q | ? | (Ottman *et al* 1995) |
| Partial epilepsy with variable foci | 22q | ? | (Xiong *et al* 1999) |
| Generalized epilepsy with febrile seizures plus | 2q | SCN1A | (Baulac *et al* 1999; Moulard *et al* 1999; Lopes-Cendes *et al* 2000; Escayg *et al* 2000) |
| | 19q | SCN1B | (Wallace *et al* 1998) |
| Familial adult myoclonic epilepsy | 8q | ? | (Mikami *et al* 1999) |

*Table lists linkages and genes described for idiopathic epilepsies with simple inheritance and for GEFS⁺ which usually has complex inheritance. All the findings listed are regarded as secure. Linkages that are not confirmed, where lod scores are marginal or there is controversy are not listed.

grandmothers to establish the familial pattern (Quattlebaum, 1979; Plouin, 1994).

The seizures in BFNC comprise clonic jerking sometimes with apnoea and last 1–3 minutes. In rare instances where seizures have been recorded on EEG, they appear to have a focal onset. Seizures may recur frequently over the first week of life but cease completely over the following weeks. About 11% of affected individuals have rare seizures in later childhood or adult life. There is no associated neurological or intellectual impairment (Plouin, 1994).

## Molecular genetics

Linkage to chromosome 20q was identified in 1989 by Leppert *et al.* and subsequently genetic heterogeneity was shown by discovery of a second linkage at 8q (Lewis *et al.*, 1993). Many families with BFNC map to the chromosome 20q locus, whereas the 8q locus is a rare cause of BFNC. It is probable that a third locus also exists.

Discovery of the responsible genes was reported in 1998; two novel potassium channel genes, KCNQ2 and KCNQ3 were found at the 20q and 8q loci respectively (Biervert *et al.*, 1998; Charlier *et al.*, 1998; Singh *et al.*, 1998). These genes are homologous to KCNQ1, which is expressed in the heart and ear and is mutated in some families with the long QT syndrome.

## Functional effects of the mutations

KCNQ2 and KCNQ3 are expressed in the brain and contribute to the physiologically defined M current (Biervert *et al.*, 1998; Wang *et al.*, 1998). This current, which is regulated by several receptor systems, is critically involved in subthreshold electrical excitability of neurons, thus determining their firing properties. The mutations in BFNC families are heterogeneous but include large truncation mutations suggesting that there is a major change in the expressed protein. *In vitro* expression studies suggest complete loss of function of

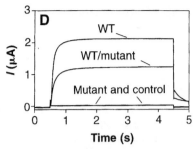

**Figure 16.1** *In vitro* studies of KCNQ2 studied in *Xenopus* oocytes. The wild-type (WT) gene was expressed and from a holding potential of −80 mV, the voltage was clamped for 4 seconds to +20 mV resulting in a robust current. Injection of mutant KCNQ2 from a family with benign familial neonatal convulsions showed no current. Injection of a 1:1 ratio of wild type and mutant showed half the current of the wild type alone (from Biervert *et al.*, 1998).

the mutant subunits, without a dominant negative effect (Biervert *et al.*, 1998; Schroeder *et al.*, 1998; Schwake *et al.*, 2000) (Figure 16.1).

Seizures in BFNC are presumably caused by neuronal hyperexcitability as a consequence of impairment of the membrane stabilizing effect of the M current. Watanabe *et al.* (2000) recently created KCNQ2 knock-out mice. Homozygotes died due to pulmonary atelectasis without observed seizures. Heterozygotes (which mimic human BFNC) had increased sensitivity to the convulsant pentylenetetrazol, although spontaneous seizures were not observed. The reason for remarkable age-dependence of BFNC may be due to specific developmental expression of these and perhaps other potassium channel genes (Tinel *et al.*, 1998).

## Autosomal dominant nocturnal frontal lobe epilepsy (ADNFLE)

ADNFLE is the prototype of the newly discovered group of inherited partial epilepsies and was described in 1994. Unlike BFNC, where seizures occur in a very restricted epoch of life, seizure onset in ADNFLE can be from infancy to adult life, although onset around age 10 years is typical (Scheffer *et al.*, 1994, 1995).

Seizures occur in sleep, often in clusters, and are brief, each seizure typically lasting less than a minute. Seizures often occur during dozing or before awakening, but can occur throughout the night. Patients frequently awaken with non-specific auras and have brief motor seizures consisting of tonic spasms or hyperkinetic motor seizures. Retained awareness throughout the attacks is often described. Partial seizures sometimes evolve into secondarily generalized tonic-clonic seizures. The interictal EEG is usually normal but ictal recordings show that these events are frontal lobe seizures (Scheffer *et al.*, 1994, 1995).

Misdiagnosis as normal sleep, parasomnias or hysteria is common. Previously some families were regarded as having paroxysmal nocturnal dystonia. Indeed, the so-called brief form of paroxysmal nocturnal dystonia probably does not exist and familial cases are almost certainly examples of autosomal dominant nocturnal frontal lobe epilepsy. In children the distinction from night terrors is most important. In contrast to the seizures of this epilepsy, night terrors occur once per night, typically a few hours after going to sleep, they last more than 5 minutes and are associated with amnesia (Scheffer *et al.*, 1994, 1995).

In most patients autosomal dominant nocturnal frontal lobe epilepsy is mild and responds well to antiepileptic drugs such as carbamazepine. Occasional patients are refractory, although seizures are usually confined to sleep. The penetrance of ADNFLE is 70% with a marked variation in severity among family members. This makes the familial nature easy to overlook as relatives may be only mildly affected (Scheffer *et al.*, 1994, 1995).

### Molecular genetics

ADNFLE was mapped to chromosome 20q13.2-q13.3 by Phillips *et al.* (1995) and the genetic defect was subsequently isolated to the $\alpha4$ subunit gene of the neuronal nicotinic acetylcholine receptor (nAChR) by a positional candidate approach. A missense mutation of a highly conserved amino acid residue in the M2 domain (C743T effecting a Ser248Phe substitution) was detected in a large Australian ADNFLE family (Steinlein *et al.*, 1995). The M2 domain forms the wall of the pore of the nAChR ion channel which is permeable to small cations (Galzi *et al.*, 1991). Subsequently the identical mutation was found in unrelated Norwegian and Spanish families (Saenz *et al.*, 1999; Steinlein *et al.*, 2000). Two other mutations in the M2 domain have been identified in Norwegian (776insGCT causing a 259insLeu insertion mutation) and Japanese (Ser252Leu) families (Steinlein *et al.*, 1997; Hirose *et al.*, 1999). Recently we found the Ser252Leu mutation in a sporadic patient with nocturnal frontal lobe epilepsy (Phillips *et al.*, 2000). Most families with ADNFLE, however, do not have the 20q locus and a second locus on 15q, where there is a cluster of other neuronal nicotinic subunits has been reported, and in yet other families there is evidence of a third locus (Phillips *et al.*, 1998).

## Functional effects of the mutations

Neuronal nicotinic receptors are believed to be almost exclusively presynaptic, regulating the release of a number of neurotransmitters including glutamate, dopamine etc. They are widely dispersed in the cortex. These receptors are comprised of five subunits and the most abundant receptor in the brain consists of $\alpha4$ and $\beta2$ subunits (Galzi *et al.*, 1991; Sargent, 1993; McGehee *et al.*, 1995). Two of the mutations, which affect the $\alpha4$ subunit (Ser248Phe, 259insLeu) have been shown to have functional consequences by *in vitro* studies in *Xenopus* oocytes when co-expressed with $\beta2$ subunits (Weiland *et al.*,. 1996; Kuryatov *et al.*, 1997; Steinlein *et al.*, 1997; Bertrand *et al.*, 1998; Figl *et al.*, 1998; Picard *et al.*, 1999).

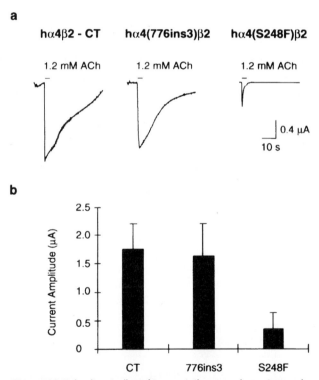

**Figure 16.2** *In vitro* studies of two mutations causing autosomal dominant nocturnal frontal lobe epilepsy. (a) Typical currents from *Xenopus* oocytes expressing normal control (CT) $\alpha4/\beta2$ neuronal nicotinic channels, and channels created using mutant 259insLeu (776ins3) and Ser248Phe (S248F) $\alpha$-subunits. Currents were evoked by a saturating pulse of acetylcholine for 3 seconds (horizontal bars). (b) Mean current amplitudes recorded in several oocytes using the same conditions (from Bertrand *et al.*, 1998).

Surprisingly, the *in vitro* effects of the two mutations show a number of differences, even though the clinical syndrome they cause is identical (Figure 16.2; Table 16.2). Compared to normal $\alpha 4\beta 2$ receptors, the mutant $\alpha 4(\text{Ser248Phe})\beta 2$ receptors showed a shift to the right of the dose-response curve to acetylcholine, became inactivated or desensitized upon exposure to agonists at a significantly faster rate, showed a reduced maximal current and reduced calcium entry. These observations suggest receptor hypofunction. The $\alpha 4(259\text{insLeu})\beta 2$ receptors showed a shift to the left of the dose-response curve to acetylcholine, became desensitized upon exposure to agonists at a similar rate to controls, showed a similar maximal current, and reduced calcium entry was inferred (Weiland *et al.*, 1996; Kuryatov *et al.*, 1997; Steinlein *et al.*, 1997; Bertrand *et al.*, 1998; Picard *et al.*, 1999). Overall these observations suggested hypofunction of mutant receptors, perhaps with reduced calcium entry being the common critical effect. Experiments in another laboratory largely confirmed these findings, but an additional observation of use-dependent potentiation, not seen in controls, was suggested as a critical finding to explain seizures in patients with these mutations (Figl *et al.*, 1998).

Many questions about the biology of ADNFLE remain unanswered. Why is the epilepsy focal? Why do seizures arise in the frontal lobes? Why are the seizures almost exclusively in sleep? Assuming the defect is largely a presynaptic one, which post-synaptic neurotransmitter system/s are affected? It is known that the ascending cholinergic system, which projects heavily to the frontal lobes, is involved in regulation of sleep giving a clue as to why the seizures may be frontal and

nocturnal. *In vitro* studies will give further insights, but it is likely that a more complete understanding will come from study of transgenic animals with these mutations.

## Generalized epilepsy with febrile seizures plus (GEFS⁺)

The two syndromes described above, BFNC and ADNFLE, are clear-cut autosomal dominant disorders and affected individuals with each syndrome have very similar phenotypes, although the severity may vary. In GEFS⁺, there is a remarkable heterogeneity of phenotypes. We described the condition in 1997 in a large family with autosomal dominant inheritance of epilepsy (Berkovic and Scheffer, 1997). It was the inheritance pattern in that family that led us to deduce that heterogeneous epilepsy phenotypes could be largely determined by a major autosomal dominant gene. Subsequently many families have been described and it appears that GEFS⁺ is a reasonably common form of childhood epilepsy (Baulac *et al.*, 1999; Moulard *et al.*, 1999; Singh *et al.*, 1999).

The common phenotypes in families with GEFS⁺ are typical febrile seizures, and febrile seizures plus (FS⁺). Individuals with the FS⁺ phenotype have febrile seizures that extend outside the classical age-related definition of FS occurring between 3 months and 6 years or they have additional *afebrile* seizures. Less common phenotypes include FS⁺ associated with absence, myoclonic or atonic seizures. These children are otherwise clinically normal, their EEG may show irregular generalized spike-wave discharges and

---

**Table 16.2 *In vitro* effects of two mutations causing ADNFLE**

|  | Ser248Phe | 259insLeu |
|---|---|---|
| Acetylcholine affinity | Decreased X 7 | Increased X 10 |
| Desensitization | Major decrease | Minor decrease |
| Maximal current | Decreased X 5 | No change |
| Calcium permeability | Decreased | Decreased |
| Use dependent potentiation | Increased X 3 | Increased X 2 |

seizures generally cease by adolescence. Rarer phenotypes include FS[+] associated with complex partial seizures and more severe epilepsy phenotypes including myoclonic-astatic epilepsy and severe myoclonic epilepsy of infancy (Berkovic and Scheffer, 1997; Baulac *et al.*, 1999; Singh *et al.*, 1999)

## Molecular genetics

In many families the inheritance of GEFS[+] is complex, sometimes with bilineal transmission (Singh *et al.*, 1999). In some pedigrees, however, there is obvious autosomal dominant inheritance and a number of such families have been successfully mapped. Two loci have been identified, on chromosomes 19q and 2q and the genes responsible are sodium channel subunits (Wallace *et al.*, 1998; Baulac *et al.*, 1999; Moulard *et al.*, 1999; Lopes-Cendes *et al.*, 2000).

The responsible gene at the 19q locus is the $\beta1$ subunit of the neuronal sodium channel (*SCN1B*). *SCN1B* is expressed in brain, peripheral nerves, muscle and heart. Neuronal sodium channels are composed of a large pore-forming $\alpha$-subunit and the regulatory subunits $\beta1$ and $\beta2$, plus the recently described $\beta3$. The $\beta1$ subunit exerts significant modulatory effects on gating behaviour of the $\alpha$-subunits. These modulatory effects are principally dependent on the extracellular domain of the $\beta1$ subunit which contains a single immunoglobulin-like fold motif. This fold is maintained by a single disulphide bridge between two highly conserved cysteine residues. One of these cysteines is mutated (Cys121Trp) in a least two Australian GEFS[+] families (Wallace *et al.*, 1998).

Recently, the responsible gene at the 2q locus in two French GEFS[+] families was found to be *SCN1A*, one of three $\alpha$-subunit genes in that chromosomal region. The two families have different missense mutations in the S4 transmembrane segments of that subunit (Thr875Met, Arg1648His) (Escayg *et al.*, 2000a). The 2q locus appears to be more common than the 19q locus. There are a number of other families mapping to 2q where mutations in *SCN1A* have not been found raising the possibility that the other two $\alpha$-subunit genes in that region *SCN2A* and *SCN3A* might be responsible.

## Functional effects of the mutations

*In vitro* studies of the *SCN1B* mutant subunit with the wild-type pore-forming $\alpha$-subunit showed that the mutation interferes with the ability of the $\beta1$ subunit to modulate sodium channel gating (Figure 16.3). Normally the $\beta1$ subunit hastens the time course of inactivation compared to currents

*a*

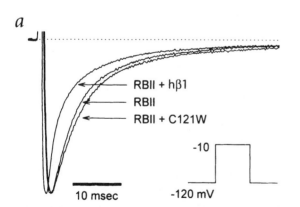

*b*

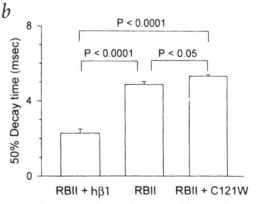

**Figure 16.3** *In vitro* studies of an *SCN1B* mutation causing generalized epilepsy with febrile seizures plus. Voltage-clamp recording from *Xenopus* oocytes expressing normal rat brain sodium channel $\alpha$-subunits (RBII) alone or in combination with normal $\beta1$ subunits (h$\beta1$) or $\beta1$ subunits with the Cys121Trp mutation (C121W). (a) Single traces recorded during a test depolarization to $-10$ mV from a holding potential of $-120$ mV shown superimposed after peak current amplitudes were normalized. (b) Comparison of time required to achieve 50% inactivation (from Wallace *et al.*, 1998).

observed with expression of the $\alpha$-subunit alone. With the mutant subunit, this effect of speedier inactivation is lost suggesting a loss of function of the mutant protein. The *in vitro* results suggest more persistent inward sodium currents with more prolonged depolarization of the membrane, with consequent increased excitability.

## Other ion channel mutations in inherited human epilepsies

The three above mentioned syndromes, BFNC, ADNFLE, and GEFS[+], are the only human epilepsies where the strategy of linkage mapping followed by identification of a mutant gene has given definitive evidence for the causative role of ion channel abnormalities. However, there have been a number of observations suggesting that channel mutations may contribute to other forms of epilepsy, both common and rare.

The syndrome of episodic ataxia type 1 (EA1) is due to mutations in the potassium channel Kv1.1 (also known as KCNA1), which is distinct from the potassium channels involved with BFNC. EA1 is associated with seizures in about 10% of cases, and the mutations in Kv1.1 have been demonstrated in a few patients with seizures combined with the episodic ataxia (Zuberi *et al.*, 1999). This suggests that Kv1.1 may contribute to seizures in EA1. Mice where Kv1.1 is knocked out have a severe epilepsy phenotype (Smart *et al.*, 1998). The large family of potassium channel genes are thus emerging as major candidate genes for other forms of human epilepsy.

Calcium channel mutations cause a number of mouse models of human epilepsy (see below), but definitive evidence for the involvement of calcium channels in human epilepsy is lacking to date. Two different mutations in the coding regions of the calcium channel *CACNB4* were recently detected in a screen of 90 families with idiopathic generalized epilepsy. It is not yet clear whether these mutations are related to the associated epilepsy syndrome as the functional alterations are subtle (Escayg *et al.*, 2000b).

## Ion channel dysfunction in inherited murine epilepsies

A large number of inbred or knockout mice phenotypes include seizures, often with other significant neurological impairment (McNamara and Puranam, 1988). In a small number of these mice the phenotype appears to be seizures alone, with or without some ataxia, thus being models for idiopathic epilepsies. Where identification of the responsible gene has occurred for such mice models, they have almost invariably been due to ion channel mutations, particularly in the calcium channel system. Specifically, mice that are the models for generalized absence epilepsy (tottering, lethargic, stargazer and ducky) are due to mutations in the $\alpha 1a$, $\beta 4$, $\gamma 2$ and $\alpha 2\delta$-subunits of neuronal calcium channels (Fletcher *et al.*, 1996; Burgess *et al.*, 1997; Letts *et al.*, 1998; Steinlein and Noebels, 2000).

## Ion channel changes in acquired epilepsies

A number of lines of evidence suggest that ion channels may be altered in epilepsies with a predominantly acquired aetiology. For example, in tissue from patients with chronic epilepsy, alterations in the distribution of regulatory beta subunits of neuronal calcium channels has been reported (Lie *et al.*, 1999). From these observations, however, it is difficult to know if the changes are a cause or result of the seizures.

Experimental studies of acquired models of epilepsy including kindling, kainate-induced focal epilepsy and chronic epilepsy induced by pilocarpine, have shown changes in neuronal ion channels that could be crucial to epileptogenesis (Brooks-Kayal *et al.*, 1998; Mody, 1998, 1999). In the pilocarpine model, where the development of epileptogenesis can be followed, the number of GABA channels and stoichiometry of the GABA subunits are altered before the expression of chronic epilepsy (Brooks-Kayal *et al.*, 1998).

# Conclusions

Evidence from family studies in humans and from experimental familial epilepsies in mice is now converging to suggest that the idiopathic epilepsies are a family of ligand-gated and voltage-gated channelopathies. Moreover, the observation of alteration in ion channel number and subunit stoichiometry in acquired epilepsies raises the tantalizing possibility that ion channels are the neurobiological substrate of the interaction between inherited and acquired factors that underlies many human epilepsies.

# References

Baulac, S., Gourfinkel-An, I., Picard, F. *et al.* (1999). A second locus for familial generalized epilepsy with febrile seizures plus maps to chromosome 2q21-q33. *Am J Hum Genet.*, **65**, 1078–85.

Berkovic, S. F., Andermann, F., Andermann, E. and Gloor, P. (1987). Concepts of absence epilepsies: discrete syndromes or biological continuum? *Neurology*, **37**, 993–1000.

Berkovic, S. F. and Scheffer, I. E (1997). Epilepsies with single gene inheritance. *Brain Dev.*, **19**, 13–18.

Bertrand, S., Weiland, S., Berkovic, S. F. *et al.* (1998). Properties of neuronal nicotinic acetylcholine receptor mutants from humans suffering from autosomal dominant nocturnal frontal lobe epilepsy. *Br J Pharmacol.*, **125**, 751–60.

Biervert, C., Schroeder, B. C. and Kubisch, C. (1998). A potassium channel mutation in neonatal human epilepsy. *Science*, **279**, 403–6.

Brooks-Kayal, A. R., Shumate, M. D., Jin, H. *et al.* (1998). Selective changes in single cell GABA(A) receptor subunit expression and function in temporal lobe epielpsy. *Nat Med.*, **4**, 1166–72.

Burgess, D. L., Jones, J. M., Meisler, M. H. and Noebels, J. L. (1997). Mutation of the $Ca^{2+}$ channel $\beta$-subunit gene *Cchb4* is associated with ataxia and seizures in the lethargic (*lh*) mouse. *Cell*, **88**, 385–92.

Charlier, C., Singh, N. A. and Ryan, S. G. (1998). A pore mutation in a novel KQT-like potassium channel gene in an idiopathic epilepsy family. *Nature Genet.*, **18**, 53–5.

Claes, S., Devriendt, K., Lagae, L. *et al.* (1997). The X-linked infantile spasms syndrome (MIM 308350) maps to Xp11.4-Xpter in two pedigrees. *Ann Neurol.*, **42**, 360–4.

Commission on Classification and Terminology of the International League against Epilepsy (1989). Proposal for revised classification of epilepsies and epileptic syndromes. *Epilepsia*, **30**, 389–99.

des Portes, V., Pinard, J.-M., Billuart, P. *et al.* (1998). A novel CNS gene required for neuronal migration and involved in X-linked subcortical laminar heterotopia and lissencephaly syndrome. *Cell*, **92**, 51–61.

Deymeer, F. and Leviton, A. (1985). Perinatal factors and seizure disorders: an epidemiological review. *Epilepsia*, **26**, 287–98.

Escayg, A., Macdonald, B. T., Baulac, S., *et al.* (2000a). Mutations of *SCN1A*, encoding a neuronal sodium channel, in two families with GEFS + 2. *Nature Genet.*, **24**, 343–5.

Escayg, A., De Waard, M., Lee, D. D. *et al.* (2000b). Coding and noncoding variations of the human calcium-channel $\beta$4-subunit gene *CACNB4* in patients with idiopathic generalized epilepsy and episodic ataxia. *Am J Hum Genet.*, **66**, 1531–9.

Figl, A., Viseshakul, N., Shafaee, N. *et al.* (1998). Two mutations linked to nocturnal frontal lobe epilepsy cause use-dependent potentiation of the nicotinic ACh response. *J Physiol (Lond).*, **513**, 655–70.

Fletcher, C. F., Lutz, C. M., O'Sullivan, T. N. *et al.* (1996). Absence epilepsy in tottering mice is associated with calcium channel defects. *Cell*, **87**, 607–17.

Fox, J. W., Lamperti, E., Eksioglu, Y. Z. *et al.* (1998). Mutations in filamin 1 prevent migration of cerebral cortical neurons in human periventricular heterotopia. *Neuron*, **21**, 1315–25.

Galzi, J. L., Revah, F., Bessis, A. and Changeux, J.-P. (1991). Functional architecture of the nicotinic acetylcholine receptor: from electric organ to brain. *Ann Rev Pharmacol.*, **31**, 37–72.

Gleeson, J. G., Allen, K. M., Fox, J. W. *et al.* (1998). *doublecortin*, a brain specific gene mutated in human X-linked lissencephaly and double cortex syndrome, encodes a putative signalling protein. *Cell*, **92**, 63–72.

Gloor, P., Metrakos, J., Metrakos, K., Andermann, E. and Van Gelder, N. (1982). Neurophysiological, genetic and biochemical nature of the epileptic diathesis. *Electroencephalogr Clin Neurophysiol.*, Suppl. 35, 45–56.

Guerrini, R., Bonanni, P., Nardocci, N. *et al.* (1999). Autosomal recessive rolandic epilepsy with paroxysmal exercise-induced dystonia and writer's cramp: delineation of the syndrome and gene mapping to chromosome 16p12-11.2. *Ann Neurol.*, **45**, 344–52.

Guipponi, M., Rivier, F., Vigevano, F. *et al.* (1997). Linkage mapping of benign familial infantile convulsions (BFIC) to chromosome 19q. *Hum Mol Genet.*, **6**, 473–7.

Hauser, W. A., Annegers, J. F., Kurland, L. T. (1993). Incidence of epilepsy and unprovoked seizures in Rochester, Minnesota: 1935–1984. *Epilepsia*, **34**, 453–68.

Hesdorffer, D. C. and Verity, C. M. (1997). Risk factors. In *Epilepsy: a comprehensive textbook* (eds Engel, J.

Jr and Pedley, T. A.) pp 59–67. Philadelphia: Lippin-cott-Raven.

Hirose, S., Iwati, H., Akiyoshi, H. *et al.* (1999). A novel point mutation of CHRNA4 responsible for autosomal dominant nocturnal frontal lobe epilepsy. *Neurology*, **53**, 1749–53.

Kuryatov, A., Gerzanich, V., Nelson, M. *et al.* (1997). Mutation causing autosomal dominant nocturnal frontal lobe epilepsy alters Ca2+ permeability, conductance, and gating of human alpha4beta2 nicotinic acetylcholine receptors. *J Neurosci.*, **17**, 9035–47.

Lennox, W. G. and Lennox, M. A. (1960). *Epilepsy and related disorders.* pp 518–574. Boston: Little Brown.

Leppert, M., Anderson, V. E., Quattlebaum, T. G. *et al.* (1989). Benign familial neonatal convulsions linked to genetic markers on chromosome 20. *Nature*, **337**, 647–8.

Letts, V. A., Felix, R., Biddlecome, G. H. *et al.* (1998). The mouse stargazer gene encodes a neuronal Ca$^{2+}$-channel $\gamma$ subunit. *Nature Genet.*, **19**, 340–7.

Lewis, T. B., Leach, R. J., Ward, K. *et al.* (1993). Genetic heterogeneity in benign familial neonatal convulsions: identification of a new locus on chromosome 8q. *Am J Hum Genet.*, **53**, 670–6.

Lie, A. A., Blumcke, I., Volsen, S. G. *et al.* (1999). Distribution of voltage dependent calcium channel beta subunits in the hippocampus of patients with temporal lobe epilepsy. *Neuroscience*, **93**, 449–56.

Lilienfeld, A. M. and Pasamanick, B. (1954). Association of maternal and fetal factors with the development of epilepsy. *JAMA*, **155**, 719–24.

Lopes-Cendes, I., Scheffer, I. E. and Berkovic, S. F. (2000). A new locus for generalized epilepsy with febrile seizures plus maps to chromosome 2. *Am J Hum Genet.*, **66**, 698–701.

McGehee, D. S., Heath, M. J. S., Gelber, S. *et al.* (1995). Nicotine enhancement of fast excitatory synaptic transmission in CNS by presynaptic receptors. *Science*, **269**, 1692–6.

McNamara, J. O. and Puranam, R. S. (1988). Epilepsy genetics: an abundance of riches for biologists. *Curr Biol.*, **8**, 168–70.

Mikami, M., Yasudo, T., Terao, A. *et al.* (1999). Localization of a gene for benign adult familial myoclonic epilepsy to chromosome 8q23.3-q24.1. *Am J Hum Genet.*, **65**, 745–51.

Minassian, B. A., Lee, J. R., Herbrick, J. A. *et al.* (1998). Mutations in a gene encoding a novel protein tyrosine phosphatase cause progressive myoclonus epilepsy. *Nat Genet.*, **20**, 171–4.

Mody, I. (1998). Ion channels in epilepsy. *Int Rev Neurobiol.*, **42**, 199–226.

Mody, I. (1999). Synaptic plasticity in kindling. *Adv Neurol.*, **79**, 631–43.

Moulard, B., Guipponi, M. and Chaigne, D. (1999). Identification of a new locus for generalized epilepsy with febrile seizures plus (GEFS+) on chromosome 2q24-q33. *Am J Hum Genet.*, **65**, 1396–400.

Nelson, K. B. and Ellenberg, J. H. (1984). Obstetric complications as risk factors for cerebral palsy or seizure disorders. *JAMA*, **251**, 1843–8.

Nielsen, J. M. and Courville, C. B. (1951). Role of birth injury and asphyxia in idiopathic epilepsy. *Neurology*, **1**, 48–52.

Ottman, R., Risch, N., Hauser, W. A. *et al.* (1995). Localization of a gene for partial epilepsy to chromosome 10q. *Nat Genet.*, **10**, 56–60.

Peiffer, A., Thompson, J., Charlier, C. *et al.* (1999). A locus for febrile seizures (FEB3) maps to chromosome 2q23-24. *Ann Neurol.*, **46**, 671–8.

Pennacchio, L. A., Lehesjoki, A. E., Stone, N. E. *et al.* (1996). Mutations in the gene encoding cystatin B in progressive myoclonus epilepsy (EPM1). *Science*, **271**, 1731–4.

Phillips, H. A., Marini, C., Scheffer, I. E. *et al.* (2000). A de novo mutation in sporadic nocturnal frontal lobe epilepsy. *Ann Neurol.*, **48**, 264–7.

Phillips, H. A., Scheffer, I. E., Berkovic, S. F. (1995). Localization of a gene for autosomal dominant nocturnal frontal lobe epilepsy to chromosome 20q13.2. *Nature Genet.*, **10**, 117–8.

Phillips, H. A., Scheffer, I. E., Crossland, K. M. *et al.* (1998). Autosomal dominant nocturnal frontal lobe epilepsy: genetic heterogeneity and evidence for a second locus at 15q24. *Am J Hum Genet.*, **63**, 1108–16.

Picard, F., Bertrand, S., Steinlein, O. K. and Bertrand, D. (1999). Mutated nicotinic receptors responsible for autosomal dominant nocturnal frontal lobe epilepsy are more sensitive to carbamazepine. *Epilepsia*, **40**, 1198–209.

Plouin, P. (1994). Benign familial neonatal convulsions. In *Idiopathic generalized epilepsies: clinical, experimental and genetic aspects* (eds Malafosse, A., Genton, P., Hirsch, E., Marescaux, C., Broglin, D. and Bernasconi, R.) pp 39–44. London: John Libbey.

Quattlebaum, T. G. (1979). Benign familial convulsions in the neonatal period and early infancy. *J Pediatr.*, **95**, 257–9.

Risch, N. and Merikangas, K. (1996). The future of genetic studies of complex human diseases. *Science*, **273**, 1516–7.

Saenz, A., Galan, J. and Caloustian, C. (1999). Autosomal dominant nocturnal frontal lobe epilepsy in a Spanish family with a Ser252Phe mutation in the CHRNA4 gene. *Arch Neurol.*, **56**, 1004–9.

Sargent, P. B. (1993). The diversity of neuronal nicotinic acetylcholine receptors. *Ann Rev Neurosci.*, **16**, 403–43.

Scheffer, I. E., Bhatia, K. P., Lopes-Cendes, I. *et al.* (1995). Autosomal dominant nocturnal frontal epilepsy: a distinctive clinical disorder. *Brain*, **118**, 61–73.

Scheffer, I. E., Bhatia, K. P., Lopes-Cendes, I. *et al.* (1994). Autosomal dominant frontal epilepsy misdiagnosed as sleep disorder. *Lancet*, **343**, 515–7.

Schroeder, B. C., Kubisch, C., Stein, V. and Jentsch, T. J. (1998). Moderate loss of function of cyclic-AMP-modulated KCNQ2/KCNQ3 K$^+$ channels causes epilepsy. *Nature*, **396**, 687–90.

Schwake, M., Pusch, M., Kharkovets, T. and Jentsch, T. J. (2000). Surface expression and single channel properties of KCNQ2/KCNQ3, M-type K$^+$ channels involved in epilepsy. *J Biol Chem.*, **275**, 13343–8.

Serratosa, J. M., Gomez-Garre, P., Gallardo, M. E. *et al.* (1999). A novel protein tyrosine phosphatase gene is mutated in progressive myoclonus epilepsy of the Lafora type (EPM2). *Hum Mol Genet.*, **8**, 345–52.

Singh, N. A., Charlier, C., Stauffer, D. *et al.* (1998). A novel potassium channel gene, KCNQ2, is mutated in an inherited epilepsy of newborns. *Nature Genet.*, **18**, 25–9.

Singh, R., Scheffer, I. E., Crossland, K. and Berkovic, S. F. (1999). Generalised epilepsy with febrile seizures plus (GEFS$^+$): a common, childhood onset, genetic epilepsy syndrome. *Ann Neurol.*, **45**, 75–81.

Smart, S. L., Lopantsev, V., Zhang, C. L. *et al.* (1998). Deletion of the K(V)1.1 potassium channel causes epilepsy in mice. *Neuron*, **20**, 809–19.

Steinlein, O. K., Magnusson, A., Stoodt, J. *et al.* (1997). An insertion mutation of the CHRNA4 gene in a family with autosomal dominant nocturnal frontal lobe epilepsy. *Hum Mol Genet.*, **6**, 943–8.

Steinlein, O. K., Mulley, J. C., Propping, P. *et al.* (1995). A missense mutation in the neuronal nicotinic acetylcholine receptor $\alpha$4 subunit is associated with autosomal dominant nocturnal frontal lobe epilepsy. *Nature Genet.*, **11**: 201–3.

Steinlein, O. K., Stoodt, J., Mulley, J. *et al.* (2000). Independent occurrence of the CHRNA4 Ser248Phe mutation in a Norwegian family with nocturnal frontal lobe epilepsy. *Epilepsia*, **41**, 529–35.

Steinlein, O. K. and Noebels, J. L. (2000). Ion channels and epilepsy in man and mouse. *Curr Opin Genet Dev.*, **10**, 286–91.

Szepetowski, P., Rochette, J., Berquin, P. *et al.* (1997). Familial infantile convulsions and paroxysmal choreoathetosis: a new neurological syndrome linked to the pericentromeric region of human chromosome 16. *Am J Hum Genet.*, **61**, 889–98.

Tinel, N., Lauritzen, I., Choabe, C. *et al.* (1998). The KCNQ2 potassium channel: splice variants, functional and developmental expression. Brain localization and comparison with KCNQ3. *FEBS Lett.*, **438**, 171–6.

Wallace, R. H., Wang, D. W., Singh, R. *et al.* (1998). Febrile seizures and generalised epilepsy associated with a mutation in the Na$^+$- channel $\beta$1 subunit gene SCN1B. *Nat Genet.*, **19**, 366–70.

Wang, H. S., Pan, Z., Shi, W. *et al.* (1998). KCNQ2 and KCNQ3 potassium channel subunits: molecular correlates of the M-channel. *Science*, **282**, 1890–3.

Watanabe, H., Nagata, E. and Kosakai, A. (2000). Disruption of the epilepsy KCNQ2 gene results in neural hyperexcitability. *J Neurochem.*, **75**, 28–33.

Weiland, S., Witzemann, V., Villarroel, A. *et al.* (1996). An amino acid exchange in the second transmembrane segment of a neuronal nicotinic receptor causes partial epilepsy by altering its desensitization kinetics. *FEBS Lett.*, **398**, 91–6.

Xiong, L., Labuda, M., Li, D.-S. *et al.* (1999). Mapping of a gene determining familial partial epilepsy with variable foci to chromosome 22q11-q12. *Am J Hum Genet.*, **65**, 1698–710.

Zuberi, S. M., Eunson, L. H., Spauschus, A. *et al.* (1999). A novel mutation in the human voltage-gated potassium channel gene (Kv1.1) associates with episodic ataxia type 1 and sometimes with partial epilepsy. *Brain*, **122**, 817–25.

# 17 Paroxysmal movement disorders as channelopathies

## Kailash P Bhatia and Enza Maria Valente

## Introduction

Paroxysmal dyskinesias are a heterogeneous group of disorders characterized by recurrent brief episodes of abnormal involuntary movements. Gowers (1885) probably gave the first description of paroxysmal involuntary movements, but called it epilepsy. Mount and Reback (1940) were the first to introduce the term *paroxysmal dystonic choreoathetosis* (PDC) to describe episodes of dystonia in a 23-year-old man with a familial disorder. These attacks were precipitated by drinking alcohol, coffee or tea, and fatigue and smoking and could last hours but, between attacks, the patient was entirely normal. More than 20 other family members were also affected with a clear autosomal dominant pattern of inheritance. Soon, other families with a similar disorder were also reported (Forssman, 1961; Lance, 1963; Richards and Barnett, 1968). Subsequently, another type of paroxysmal dyskinesia, in which brief dyskinetic episodes were induced by sudden movement, i.e. *kinesigenic*, was described by Kertesz (1967). This type termed *paroxysmal kinesigenic choreoathetosis* (PKC) responded well to antiepileptic medications (Kato and Araki, 1969; Houser *et al.*, 1999). Lance (1977) described a third variety which he called the intermediate form (between PKC and PDC) of *paroxysmal exercise- induced dyskinesia* (PED). In this variety the affected family members had dyskinetic episodes lasting between 5 and 30 minutes provoked by prolonged exercise such as walking or running. Lance, therefore, classified the paroxysmal dyskinesias into three main varieties based on the precipitating event and the duration of episodes. Added to these three forms was a disorder in which dyskinetic attacks occurred only at night during sleep, called *paroxysmal hypnogenic dyskinesia* (PHD) (Lugaresi and Cirignotti, 1981; Fahn, 1994).

Recently, Demirkirin and Jankovic (1995) modified the earlier classification into two main categories, classifying patients as having paroxysmal kinesigenic dyskinesia (PKD) if the disorder was induced by sudden movement, or paroxysmal non-kinesigenic dyskinesia (PNKD) if it was not. Patients in whom exercise was the precipitating cause were described as having paroxysmal exercise-induced dyskinesia (PED). These terms broadly correlate to PKC, PDC and the intermediate variety of the old classification.

The paroxysmal dyskinesias are thus a clinically heterogeneous group of disorders that have a shared feature of episodic hyperkinetic movement disorder. These conditions can be either idiopathic (usually familial), or acquired due to a variety of causes (Demirkirin and Jankovic, 1995; Bhatia, 1999). This chapter will focus on the 'idiopathic' (familial) varieties.

## Clinical descriptions of the four main types of idiopathic paroxysmal dyskinesias

### Paroxysmal kinesigenic dyskinesia (PKD) (previously known as PKC)

In PKD, the episodes of hyperkinetic movements are initiated by a sudden movement or change in movement velocity. The attacks in these patients frequently manifest as dystonia or choreodystonia induced by a sudden change in position, classically from a sitting to standing position; however, startle, hyperventilation and continuous exercise can also trigger them (Houser et al., 1999). Even changes in velocity (from slow walking to walking more quickly) can initiate an episode. Many patients report variable 'aura like' sensations preceding an attack. Attacks commonly involve the hemibody, in some almost always on the same side or alternating sides (Houser et al., 1999). Speech can be affected but consciousness is not lost. PKD occurs from early childhood and attack frequency often decreases in adult life.

Patients with PKD may have dozens of attacks per day and respond dramatically to low doses of carbamazepine. Although there are reports of symptomatic PKD (Berger et al., 1984; Camac et al., 1990), the majority of cases of PKD are 'idiopathic', often with a family history of autosomal dominant inheritance. In a recent review of 26 cases with idiopathic PKC by Houser et al. (1999), there was a notable predominance of males (23 males, 3 females). Twenty-six per cent of patients had other affected family members, with an autosomal dominant inheritance pattern in most (Houser et al., 1999).

## The infantile convulsions and choreoathetosis (ICCA) syndrome

Until recently an association of PKD/PKC with epilepsy in affected patients (or other family members) was not recognized. However, two papers have now described families with infantile convulsions and later onset of episodes of paroxysmal choreoathetosis (called infantile convulsions and choreoathetosis- ICCA syndrome) linked to chromosome 16p12-q12 (Szepetowski et al., 1997; Lee et al., 1998). In both these reports, attacks of paroxysmal choreoathetosis in the affected members were very brief, frequent and induced by sudden exertion and therefore similar to PKD. Not surprisingly, a recent report of eight Japanese families with typical PKD attacks also localized the genetic abnormality to the pericentromic region of chromosome 16 (Tomita et al., 1999).

## Paroxysmal non-kinesigenic dyskinesia (PNKD) (previously known as PDC)

PNKD is characterized by spontaneous attacks which tend to be more dystonic than those seen in PKD. Attacks are frequently precipitated by alcohol, caffeine, stress or fatigue. Patients with PNKD have longer (10 minutes to 6 hours) and less frequent attacks as compared to PKD, with long attack-free intervals. As in PKD more males than females are affected (1.4:1) (Fahn, 1994), and onset is in childhood with a tendency for the attacks to diminish with age.

The initial PDC cases reported were familial with an autosomal dominant pattern of inheritance (Mount and Reback, 1940; Richards and Barnett, 1968). Subsequently, sporadic cases were reported (Bressman et al., 1988). Generally PDC cases have no detectable abnormalities between attacks, although there has been one report of patient with PDC who also had some interictal dystonia (Bressman et al., 1988). There has also been a family with PDC with additional myokimia (Byrne et al., 1991).

PNKD is more difficult to treat than PKD. Patients do not benefit from antiepileptics like carbamazepine, although some patients may respond to levodopa (Fink et al., 1997; Jarman et al., 2000).

Recently, two groups independently linked families with PNKD to chromosome 2q, although the gene has not yet been identified (Fink et al., 1996; Fouad et al., 1996).

### PNKD plus syndrome

The above mentioned families with PNKD/PDC usually have no abnormal clinical signs between episodes. Auburger et al. (1996) reported a large German family in whom affected members had dyskinetic attacks (choreodystonic) induced by alcohol, fatigue and exercise and thus similar to typical PNKD. However, in addition these patients also had perioral paraesthesias, double vision, headache and generalized myoclonic jerks often culminating in a seizure with unconsciousness. Some affected also had marked spastic paraparesis. This syndrome therefore is clearly different from typical PNKD. Not surprisingly this family was linked to a different locus designated *CSE* (choreoathetosis/spasticity, episodic) on chromosome 1p (Auburger *et al.*, 1996).

## Paroxysmal exercise-induced dyskinesia (PED)

PED is distinct from paroxysmal kinesigenic dyskinesia (PKD) in that the attacks come on after 10 or 15 minutes of continuing exercise rather than at the initiation of movement (Bhatia *et al.*, 1997). The attacks are usually dystonic and appear in the body part involved in the exercise, most commonly the legs after prolonged walking or running. Focal dystonia of the jaw after chewing gum has been reported (Munchau *et al.*, 2000). The dystonic episodes usually cease in 10–15 minutes after stopping the exercise. Anticonvulsants are generally not useful treatment, but one case showed some benefit with acetazolamide (Bhatia *et al.*, 1997).

There has been debate as to whether familial PED is a forme-fruste of PNKD (Lance, 1977; Kurlan *et al.*, 1987). However, in one family with classical PED, linkage to the PNKD locus on chromosome 2q was excluded, although a genome-wide search to detect a novel locus could not be performed due to the small size of this family (Munchau *et al.*, 2000). PED is a rare disorder and only a few families have been described mostly with an autosomal dominant pattern of inheritance (Bhatia *et al.*, 1997)

### PED plus syndrome

Recently, a family with an apparently recessive disorder characterized by rolandic epilepsy, episodes of exercise-induced dystonia and writers cramp (RE-PED-WC syndrome) affecting three members of the same generation has been linked to chromosome 16p 12-11.2 (Guerrini *et al.*, 1999).

## Paroxysmal hypnogenic dyskinesia (PHD)

Paroxysmal hypnogenic dyskinesia occurs at night during sleep and is often misdiagnosed as night terrors or other forms of sleep disorders (Scheffer *et al.*, 1994). Lugaresi and Cirignotta (1981) first described this condition in five patients who had attacks in sleep almost every night. In a typical attack the patient would awaken with a cry and have involuntary dystonic and ballistic thrashing movements lasting up to 45 seconds, with no detectable concurrent EEG abnormalities. Several attacks could occur each night. Carbamazepine was found to be very effective in most cases. Lee *et al.* (1985) and others described similar familial cases. Recently, it has become clear that, in a large proportion of these cases, especially the familial variety, these nocturnal dyskinesias are due to mesial frontal lobe seizures which are often difficult to pick up on surface EEG recordings (Tinuper *et al.*, 1990, Scheffer *et al*, 1995). The eponym autosomal dominant nocturnal frontal lobe epilepsy (ADNFLE) has recently been given to describe this condition in six families in whom affected members had typical PHD attacks (Scheffer *et al.*, 1995).

## Pathophysiology of paroxysmal dyskinesias

Since the outset there has been much controversy regarding the pathophysiology of these disorders. The debate so far has been whether these conditions are a form of reflex epilepsy or a basal ganglia disorder (Lishman *et al.*, 1962; Falconer *et al.*, 1963). In the case of PKD arguments favouring an epileptic aetiology include the paroxysmal, non-progressive and remitting character of the disorder as well as the excellent response to anticonvulsants (Kinast *et al.*, 1980). The absence of seizure discharges on EEG in the majority of cases and the lack of an associated alteration of consciousness, or of amnesia is said to be due to a subcortical focus. Indeed, support for a subcortical focus includes depth electrode recordings showing a focus in the supplementary motor cortex in one patient during an episode (Lombroso, 1995) and from the patient reported by Falconer *et al.* (1963) whose 'seizures induced by movement' stopped after excision of a cortical scar from the left supplementary motor cortex.

Conversely, others have suggested that these

are basal ganglia disorders in view of the clinical characteristics of the involuntary movements, the absence of EEG abnormalities during attacks, and the occurrence of similar attacks caused by symptomatic lesions affecting the basal ganglia. Additional support for the extrapyramidal theory comes from abnormalities seen with specialized electrophysiological studies, including contingent negative variation (Franssen *et al.*, 1983), reciprocal inhibition (Lee *et al.*, 1999) and the Bereitschaftspotential (Houser *et al.*, 1999), in patients with PKD suggesting a possible functional disturbance of the prefrontal basal ganglia circuit.

However, as discussed below, it is clear that the paroxysmal dyskinesias have similarities to other episodic disorders of the nervous system, many of which are now known to be due to disorders of ion channels, and therefore may have a common pathophysiology.

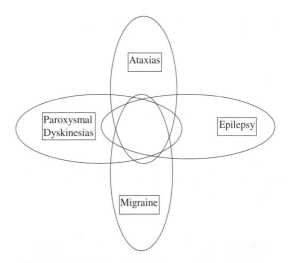

**Figure 17.1** Episodic ataxia, paroxysmal dyskinesias, epilepsy and migraine are all episodic phenomena. Patients may have more than one of these disorders. Episodic ataxias are known to be channelopathies and as the other episodic disorders have many similarities with them they may also have a similar pathophysiology. (Adapted from Bhatia *et al.* 2000)

## Similarities between the paroxysmal dyskinesias and other episodic disorders

The paroxysmal dyskinesias have many features in common with other episodic nervous system disorders, many of which are known to be due to mutations of genes regulating ion channels, i.e. channelopathies (Griggs and Nutt, 1995; Hanna *et al.*, 1998). Clinically the episodic ataxias, the paroxysmal dyskinesias, periodic paralysis and other episodic disorders including migraine and epilepsy syndromes, share the common feature of episodic attacks on a normal interictal background (Bhatia *et al.*, 2000) (Figure 17.1). Many of these disorders have similar precipitating factors like stress, fatigue, diet. There is also an overlap for many of these disorders with regard to drug treatment. Carbamazepine, for example, prevents epileptic seizures and is also very effective in patients with paroxysmal kinesigenic dyskinesia. Acetazolamide is helpful not only for patients with periodic paralysis, but also for myotonia, episodic ataxias, and some paroxysmal dyskinesias. There are also reports of families with multiple episodic disorders, for example paroxysmal dyskinesia in a family with episodic ataxia and association of

episodic problems like migraine and epilepsy in families with paroxysmal dyskinesias (Szeptowski *et al.*, 1997; Munchau *et al.*, 2000). These similarities suggest a common pathophysiological process.

In this context it is interesting to observe the similarities between PKD and episodic ataxia type 1 (EA1), which is caused by mutations of the potassium channel KCNA1 gene ( Browne *et al.*, 1994). Both conditions begin early in life, and both tend to abate in adulthood. Like PKD, episodes of ataxia in patients with EA1 can be provoked by kinesigenic stimuli, and tend to be brief and frequent (Brunt and Van Weerden, 1990). Although EA1 typically responds to acetazolamide like PKD, anticonvulsants may reduce EA1 attacks in some patients and also help the interiactal myokymia seen in this disorder (Griggs *et al.*, 1978; Brunt and Van Weerden, 1990).

It is therefore suspected that the familial paroxysmal dyskinesias may also be due to defects in genes regulating ion channels. The section below deals with the advances in the genetics of these disorders so far.

# The genes/loci associated with different paroxysmal dyskinesias

## Paroxysmal non-kinesigenic dyskinesia (PNKD)

Fink and co-workers performed a genome-wide search in a large American kindred of Polish descent, with 28 affected members, and mapped PNKD on chromosome 2q33-q35 (Fink *et al.*, 1996). In a five-generation Italian family with 20 affected members, Fouad and co-workers also showed tight linkage between PNKD and microsatellite markers on distal 2q (2q31-q36) (Fouad *et al.*, 1996). The smallest region of overlap of the candidate intervals identified by the two groups placed the PNKD locus in a 6-cM interval. In a six-generation British family, Jarman and co-workers confirmed linkage to distal chromosome 2q and narrowed the candidate region to a 4-cM interval (Jarman *et al.*, 1997). Linkage to the same genetic location, designated FPD1 (familial paroxysmal dyskinesia type 1) was further confirmed by Hofele *et al.*, (1997) in a German family originally described by Przuntek and Monninger (1983) as classical of Mount and Reback type of PNKD. Also linked to the same locus are two other typical PNKD families, one North American of German descent (Raskind *et al.*, 1998) and a Japanese family (Matsuo *et al.*, 1999). This suggests that there is *genetic homogeneity* for classical familial PNKD/PDC.

With regard mapping of ion channel genes within the linked interval, a possible candidate gene is SLC4A3. This gene is the third member of a family of anion exchangers and encodes a membrane-bound protein which functions as a chloride/bicarbonate exchanger and an alkali extruder. It plays a role in the regulation of intracellular pH, intracellular chloride concentration and maintenance of cell volume (Kopito, 1990). The protein isoform is widely expressed throughout the brain, namely in the deep pontine grey matter, the substantia nigra and the caudal medulla (Alper, 1991). Jarman and colleagues (1997) analysed polymorphic tandem repeat sequences within the gene, and found no recombinations between

PNKD and the intragenic polymorphism. Linkage of PNKD with the SLC4A3 gene was also confirmed in the two other families described by Raskind *et al.* (1998) and by Matsuo *et al.* (1999) respectively. A mildly positive lod score was obtained in both cases, as the polymorphism was not fully informative in the two families. These results suggest a putative role of the SLC4A3 gene in the pathogenesis of PNKD, but further confirmation is required by means of mutation analysis of the SLC4A3 gene.

## PNKD plus syndome: paroxysmal choreoathetosis/spasticity (CSE)

As mentioned earlier, this condition was described in a large German family with an autosomal dominant inheritance pattern by Auburger and co-workers (1996). Linkage analysis in this family placed the disease locus in a 12-cM interval on chromosome 1p21. There is a cluster of several potassium channel genes mapped to this region but further investigations are needed to determine the gene responsible for this disease.

## Paroxysmal kinesigenic choreoathetosis (PKD/PKC), familial infantile convulsions and choreoathetosis (ICCA syndrome) and Rolandic epilepsy, paroxysmal exercise-induced dystonia and writers cramp (RE-PED-WC syndrome)

It is necessary to consider the above three entities together given the linkage of all three to pericentromic region of chromosome 16. Szepetowski and colleagues (1997) described four French families with the 'ICCA syndrome' and linked this to the pericentromeric region of chromosome 16. Critical recombinants narrowed the region of interest to a 10-cM interval around the centromere. Linkage to the same locus was further confirmed in a Chinese family with a similar syndrome (Lee *et al.*, 1998), supporting genetic homogeneity for this condition. The clinical characteristics of some of the paroxysmal dyskinetic episodes in families with the ICCA syndrome were very similar to those described for PKD in terms of their brevity, frequency and onset by kinesigenic stimulus in some episodes. It was therefore not surprising that in one report of eight Japanese families (Tomita *et al.*, 1999) and in a subsequent report of a three-generation African-American kindred (Bennett *et al.*, 2000) with typical PKC attacks, the disease locus was mapped by linkage analysis to the pericentromeric region of chromosome 16. The PKC region in the Japanese families spans 12.4 cM and overlaps the ICCA region by 6.0 cM (see below). As there was an increased prevalence of afebrile infantile convulsions in the Japanese families with PKC, it has been postulated that one gene may be responsible for both PKC and ICCA (Tomita *et al.*, 1999). The PKC interval identified in the African-American family in which individuals have PKC alone (and no infantile seizures), spans 16.7 cM (between flanking markers D16S3100 and D16S771), and overlaps by 3.4 cM with the ICCA region and by 9.8 cM with the PKC region identified in Japanese families. The three regions overlap by 3.4 cM between markers D16S3100 and D16S517. At the moment it is unclear whether there are two genes or a single gene in this interval which could give rise to both ICCA and PKC (Figure 17.2).

Making the situation more interesting (and perhaps complicated) is the family with an autosomal recessive inheritance pattern described to have rolandic epilepsy, paroxysmal exercise-induced dyskinesia and writers cramp (RE-PED-WC) syndrome which has *also* been linked on chromosome 16 within the ICCA region, but outside the 3.4 cM overlap between ICCA and PKC. Thus, RE-PED-WC might be allelic to ICCA but is probably not allelic to PKC. Furthermore, epilepsy is the most striking feature of both the ICCA and RE-PED-WC syndromes and some of the ICCA attacks were induced by exercise, which perhaps suggests a common underlying gene/s for these two conditions which may be different from that giving rise to PKC.

A recent linkage study by our group (unpublished data) in a large Indian PKC family with 13 affected individuals allowed us to map a second PKC locus to chromosome 16q13-q22.1. This locus appears to be in close proximity to, but distinct from, the PKC locus identified in the Japanese families reported by Tomita *et al.* (1999). The localization of PKC in the African-

## Table 17.1 Mapped loci/genes for familial paroxysmal dyskinesia conditions

| Condition | Chromosome | Gene | Ion channel |
|---|---|---|---|
| **PNKD** | | | |
| Familial paroxysmal non-kinesiogenic dyskinesia (PNKD) | 2q33-35 | nk | nk |
| Paroxysmal choreoathetosis/spasticity | 1p | nk | nk |
| **PKD/ICCA** | | | |
| Infantile convulsions and paroxysmal choreoathetosis (ICCA) | 16p12-q12 | nk | nk |
| Familial paroxysmal kinesigenic dyskinesias (PKD) | 16p11.2-q12.1 | nk | nk |
| **PED** | | | |
| Autosomal recessive RE-WC-PED syndrome | 16p12-11.2 | nk | nk |
| **HPD** | | | |
| Autosomal dominant nocturnal frontal lobe epilepsy (ADNFLE) | 20q13 | *CHRNA4* | Ach receptor |
| Autosomal dominant nocturnal frontal lobe epilepsy (ADNFLE) | 15q24 | ?*CHRNA3* | Ach receptor |

nk = not known; RE-WC-PED = Rolandic epilepsy, writers cramp and paroxysmal exercise induced dystonia syndrome; Achp = acetylcholine receptor.

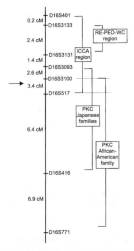

**Figure 17.2** Schematic representation of the genetic map of part of chromosome 16 showing the ICCA region (flanking markers: D16S401 and D16S517), the RE-PED-WC region (flanking markers: D16S3133 and D16S3131), the PKC region as determined by Tomita *et al.* (1999) (flanking markers: D16S3093 and D16S416) and as determined by Bennet *et al.* (2000) (flanking markers: D16S53100 and D16S5771). The arrow indicates the position of the centromere, the dashed lines indicate the region of overlap between ICCA and PKC loci. Marker location and intermarker distances are taken from the Genetic Location Database consensus map.

American family (Bennett *et al.*, 2000) overlaps with both these regions. The African-American PKC locus may thus be allelic with either the Japanese or the Indian PKC locus or represent a third gene (Figure 17.2). These results demonstrate *genetic heterogeneity* of PKC. The identification of at least two PKC loci lying in close vicinity on chromosome 16 raises the intriguing possibility that a family of genes in the pericentromeric region of chromosome 16 are responsible for multiple paroxysmal disorders (PKC, ICCA, RE-PED-WC). The identification of several duplicated regions and frequent chromosomal rearrangements in the pericentromeric region of human chromosome 16 supports this hypothesis (Loftus *et al.*, 1999). Clusters of genes causing similar but distinct phenotypes, which map in close proximity, have previously been reported, e.g. two hereditary non-chromaffin paraganglioma loci on the long arm of chromosome 11 (Heutink *et al.*, 1992; Mariman *et al.*, 1993), two loci for familial benign hypercalcaemia on the pericentromeric region of

chromosome 19 (Heath *et al.*, 1993; Lloyd *et al.*, 1999), and several epilepsy genes causing phenotypically different epilepsy syndromes on the long arm of human chromosome 8 (Steinlein *et al.*, 1995; Zara *et al.*, 1995; Wallace *et al.*, 1996; Fong *et al.*, 1998; Mikami *et al.*, 1999).

A group of ion channel genes such as the g subunit of a sodium channel (SCNN1G), a sodium-glucose co-transporter (SLC5A2) and an ATPase calcium transporter gene lie in the pericentromeric region of chromosome 16, within the ICCA and PKC intervals and represent excellent candidates for these paroxysmal disorders. However, the causative gene/genes is yet to be discovered.

## Summary and conclusions

In summary, the paroxysmal movement disorders have many shared aspects with other episodic disorders of the nervous system, many of which are known to be channelopathies. The list of linked gene loci causing the paroxysmal dyskinesia phenotypes is growing rapidly (Table 17.1), although the genes for most of these conditions (apart from ADNFLE) are still to be identified. One expects that in the near future one should know whether the paroxysmal dyskinesias like other episodic movement disorders are the result of ion channel mutations. Another possibility is that these disorders could result from mutations in genes that encode proteins that modulate ion channel function. Finding the genes will result in better understanding of the pathophysiology of these curious disorders. For example why do coffee, tea and alcohol precipitate attacks of PNKD? The knowledge about the genes will also lead to better diagnosis, classification and also treatment of the paroxysmal movement disorders.

## References

Alper, S. L. (1991). The band 3-related anion exchanger (AE) gene family. *Annu Rev Physiol.*, **53**, 549–64.
Auburger, G., Ratzlaff, T., Lunkes, A. *et al.* (1996). A gene for autosomal dominant paroxysmal choreoathetosis/spasticity (CSE) maps to the vicinity of a potassium channel gene cluster on chromosome 1p,

probably within 2cM between D1S443 and D1S197. *Genomics*, **31**, 90–4.

Bennett, L. B., Roach, E. S. and Bowcock, A. M. (2000). A locus for paroxysmal kinesigenic dyskinesia maps to human chromosome 16. *Neurology*, **54**, 125–30.

Berger, J. R., Sheremata, W. A. and Melamed, E. (1984). Paroxysmal dystonia as the initial manifestation of multiple sclerosis. *Arch Neurol.*, **41**, 747–50.

Bhatia, K. P., Soland, V. L., Bhatt, M. H., Quinn, N. P. and Marsden, C. D. (1997). Paroxysmal exercise induced dystonia: eight new sporadic cases and a review of the literature. *Mov Disord.*, **12**, 1007–12.

Bhatia, K. P. (1999). The paroxysmal dyskinesias. *J Neurol.*, **246**, 149–55.

Bhatia, K. P., Griggs, R. C. and Ptacek, L. J. (2000). Episodic movement disorders as channelopathies. *Mov Disord.*, **15**, 429–33.

Bressman, S. B., Fahn, S. and Burke, R. E. (1988). Paroxysmal non-kinesigenic dystonia. *Adv Neurol.*, **50**, 403–13.

Browne, D. L., Gancher, S. T., Nutt, J. G. *et al.* (1994). Episodic ataxia myokimia syndrome is associated with point mutations in the human potassium channel gene, KCNA1. *Nature Genet.*, **8**, 136–40.

Brunt, E. R. P. and Van Weerden, T. W. (1990). Familial paroxysmal kinesigenic ataxia and continuous myokimia. *Brain*, **113**, 1361–82.

Byrne, E., White, O. and Cook, M. (1991). Familial dystonic choreoathetosis with myokimia; a sleep responsive disorder. *J Neurol Neurosurg Psychiatr.*, **54**, 1090–2.

Camac, A., Greene, P. and Khandji, A. (1990). Paroxysmal kinesigenic dystonic choreoathetosis associated with a thalamic infarct. *Mov Disord.*, **5**, 235–8.

Demirkirin, M. and Jankovic, J. (1995). Paroxysmal dyskinesias: clinical features and classification. *Ann Neurol.*, **38**, 571–9.

Fahn, S. (1994). The paroxysmal dyskinesias. In *Movement Disorders 3* (eds Marsden, C. D. and Fahn, S.) pp 310–45. Oxford: Butterworth-Heinemann.

Falconer, M., Driver, M. and Serafetinides, E. (1963). Seizures induced by movement: report of case relieved by operation. *J Neurol Neurosurg Psychiatr.*, **26**, 300–7.

Fink, J. K., Rainier, S., Wilkowski, J. *et al.* (1996). Paroxysmal dystonic choreoathetosis: tight linkage to chromosome 2q. *Am J Hum Genet.*, **59**, 140–5.

Fink, J. K., Hedera, P., Mathay, J. G. and Albin, R. (1997). Paroxysmal dystonic choreoathetosis linked to chromosome 2q: clinical analysis and proposed pathophysiology. *Neurology*, **49**, 177–83.

Fong, G. C., Shah, P. U., Gee, M. N. *et al.* (1998). Childhood absence epilepsy with tonic-clonic seizures and electroencephalogram 3-4Hz spike and multi-spike-slow wave complexes: linkage to chromosome 8q24. *Am J Hum Genet.*, **63**, 1117–29.

Forssman, H. (1961). Hereditary disorder characterized by attacks of muscular contractions, induced by alcohol amongst other factors. *Acta Med Scand.*, **170**, 517–33.

Fouad, G. T., Servidei, S., Durcan, S., Bertini, E. and Ptacek, L. J. (1996). A gene for familial dyskinesia (FPD1) maps to chromosome 2q. *Am J Hum Genet.*, **59**, 135–9.

Franssen, H., Fortgens, C., Wattendorff, A. E. and Van Woerom, T. C. A. M. (1983). Paroxysmal kinesigenic choreoathetosis and abnormal contingent negative variation. A case report. *Arch Neurol.*, **40**, 381–5.

Gowers, W. R. (1885). *Epilepsy and other chronic convulsive diseases. Their causes, symptoms and treatment* pp 75–6. New York: Dover (Reprint of 1885 edition); 1964.

Griggs, R. C., Moxley, R. T. III, Lafralane, R. A. and McQuillen, J. (1978). Hereditary paroxysmal ataxia, response to acetazolamide. *Neurology*, **28**, 1259–64.

Griggs, R. C. and Nutt, J. G. (1995). Episodic ataxias as channelopathies (editorial; comment). *Ann Neurol.*, **37**, 285–7.

Guerrini, R., Bonanni, P., Nardocci, N. *et al.* (1999). Autosomal recessive rolandic epilepsy with paroxysmal exercise-induced dystonia and writers cramp: delineation of the syndrome and gene mapping to chromosome 16p12-11.2. *Ann Neurol.*, **45**, 344–52.

Hanna, M. G., Wood, N. W. and Kullmann, D. (1998). Ion channel and neurological disease: DNA based diagnosis is now possible, and ion channels may be important in common paroxysmal disorders. *J Neurol Neurosurg Psychiatr.*, **65**, 427–41.

Heath, H., Jackson, C. E., Otterud, B. and Leppert, M. F. (1993). Genetic linkage analysis in familial benign (hypocalciuric) hypercalcemia: evidence for locus heterogeneity. *Am J Hum Genet.*, **53**, 193–200.

Heutink, P., van der Mey, A. G., Sandkuijl, L. A. *et al.* (1992) A gene subject to genomic imprinting and responsible for hereditary paragangliomas maps to chromosome 11q23-qter. *Hum Mol Genet.*, **1**, 7–10.

Hofele, K., Benecke, R. and Auburger, G. (1997). Gene locus FPD1 of the dystonic Mount-Reback type of autosomal-dominant paroxysmal choreoathetosis. *Neurology*, **49**, 1252–7.

Houser, M. K., Soland, V. L., Bhatia, K. P., Quinn, N. P. and Marsden, C. D. (1999). Paroxysmal kinesigenic choreoathetosis: a report of 26 cases. *J Neurol.*, **246**, 120–6.

Jarman, P. R., Davis, M. B., Hodgson, S. V., Marsden, C. D. and Wood, N. W. (1997). Paroxysmal dystonic choreoathetosis. Genetic linkage studies in a British family. *Brain*, **120**, 2125–30.

Jarman, P. R., Bhatia, K. P., Davie, C. *et al.* (2000). Paroxysmal dystonic choreoathetosis: clinical features and investigation of pathophysiology in a large family. *Mov Disord.*, **15**, 648–57.

Kato, M. and Araki, S. (1969). Paroxysmal kinesigenic choreoathetosis. Report of a case relieved by carbamazepine. *Arch Neurol.*, **20**, 508–13.

Kertesz, A. (1967). Paroxysmal kinesigenic choreoathetosis. An entity within the paroxysmal choreoathetosis syndrome. Description of 10 cases, including 1 autopsied. *Neurology*, **17**, 680–90.

Kinast, M., Erenberg, G. and Rothner, A. D. (1980). Paroxysmal choreoathetosis, report of five cases and review of the literature. *Pediatrics*, **65**, 74–7.

Kopito, R. R. (1990). Molecular biology of the anion exchanger gene family. *Int Rev Cytol.* **123**, 177–99.

Kurlan, R., Behr, J., Medved, L. and Shoulson, I. (1987). Familial paroxysmal dystonic choreoathetosis: a family study. *Mov Disord.*, **2**, 187–92.

Lance, J. W. (1963). Sporadic and familial varieties of tonic seizures. *J Neurol Neurosurg Psychiatr.*, **26**, 51–9.

Lance, J. W. (1977). Familial paroxysmal dystonic choreoathetosis and its differentiation from related syndromes. *Ann Neurol.*, **2**, 285–93.

Lee, B. I., Lesser, R. P., Pippenger, C. E. *et al.* (1985). Familial paroxysmal hypnogenic dystonia. *Neurology*, **35**, 1357–60.

Lee, W. L., Tay, A., Ong, H. T., Goh, L. M., Monaco, A. P. and Szepetowski, P. (1998). Association of infantile convulsions with paroxysmal dyskinesias (ICCA syndrome): confirmaton of linkage to human chromosome 16p12-q12 in a Chinese family. *Hum Genet.*, **103**, 608–12.

Lee, M. S., Kim, W. C., Lyoo, C. H. and Lee, H. J. (1999). Reciprocal inhibition between the forearm muscles in patients with paroxysmal kinesigenic dyskinesia. *J Neurol Sci.*, **168**, 57–61.

Lishman, W. A., Symonds, C. D., Whitty, C. W. and Wilson, R. G. (1962). Seizures induced by movement. *Brain*, **85**, 93–108.

Lloyd, S. E., Pannett, A. A., Dixon, P. H., Whyte, M. P. and Thakker, R. V. (1999). Localization of familiar benign hypercalcemia, Oklahoma variant (FBHOk) to chromosome 19q13. *Am J Hum Genet.*, **64**, 189–95.

Loftus, B. J., Kim, U. J., Sneddon, V. P. *et al.* (1999). Genome duplications and other features in 12 Mb of DNA sequence from human chromosome 16p and 16q. *Genomics*, **6**, 295–308.

Lombroso, C. T. (1995). Paroxysmal choreoathetosis: an epileptic or non-epileptic disorder? *Ital J Neurol Sci.*, **16**, 271–7.

Lugaresi, E. and Cirignotta, F. (1981). Hypnogenic paroxysmal dystonia: epileptic seizure or a new syndrome? *Sleep*, **4**, 129–38.

Mariman, E. C., van Beersum, S. E., Cremers, C. W., van Baars, F. M. and Ropers, H. H. (1993). Analysis of a second family with hereditary non-chromaffin paragangliomas locates the underlying gene at the proximal region of chromosome 11q. *Hum Genet.*, **91**, 357–61.

Matsuo, H., Kamakura, K., Saito, M. *et al.* (1999). Familial paroxysmal dystonic choreoathetosis: clinical findings in a large Japanese family and genetic linkage to 2q. *Arch Neurol.*, **56**, 721–6.

Mikami, M., Yasuda, T., Terao, A. *et al.* (1999). Localization of a gene for benign adult familial myoclonic epilepsy to chromosome 8q23.3-q24.1. *Am J Hum Genet.*, **65**, 745–51.

Mount, L. A. and Reback, S. (1940). Familial paroxysmal choreoathetosis. *Arch Neurol Psychiatr.*, **44**, 841–7.

Munchau, A., Valente, E. M., Shahidi, G. A. *et al.* (2000). A new family with paroxysmal exercise-induced dystonia and migraine: a clinical and genetic study. *J Neurol Neurosurg Psychiatr.*, **68**, 609–14.

Przuntek, H. and Monninger, P. (1983). Therapeutic aspects of kinesiogenic paroxysmal choreoathetosis and familial paroxysmal choreoathetosis of the Mount and Reback type. *J Neurol.*, **230**, 163–9.

Raskind, W. H., Bolin, T., Wolff, J. *et al.* (1998). Further localization of a gene for paroxysmal dystonic choreoathetosis to a 5-cM region on chromosome 2q34. *Hum Genet.*, **102**, 93–7.

Richards, R. N. and Barnett, H. J. (1968). Paroxysmal dystonic choreoathetosis. A family study and review of the literature. *Neurology*, **18**, 461–9.

Scheffer, I. E., Bhatia, K. P., Lopes-Cendes, I. *et al.* (1994). Autosomal dominant frontal lobe epilepsy misdiagnosed as a sleep disorder. *Lancet*, **343**, 515–7.

Scheffer, I. E., Bhatia, K. P., Lopes-Cendes, I. *et al.* (1995). Autosomal dominant nocturnal frontal lobe epilepsy. A distinctive clinical disorder. *Brain*, **118**, 61–73.

Steinlein, O., Schuster, V., Fischer, C. and Haussler, M. (1995). Benign familial neonatal convulsions: confirmation of genetic heterogeneity and further evidence for a second locus on chromosome 8q. *Hum Genet.*, **95**, 411–5.

Szepetowski, P., Rochette, J., Berquin, P., Piussan, C., Lathrop, G. M. and Monaco, A. P. (1997). Familial infantile convulsions and paroxysmal choreoathetosis: a new neurological syndrome linked to the pericentromic region of human chromosome 16. *Am J Hum Genet.*, **61**, 889–98.

Tinuper, P., Cerullo, A., Cirignotta, F., Cortelli, P., Lugaresi, E. and Montagna, P. (1990). Nocturnal paroxysmal dystonia with short lasting attacks: three cases with evidence for an epileptic frontal lobe origin of seizures. *Epilepsia*, **31**, 549–56.

Tomita, H., Nagamitsu, S., Wakui, K. *et al.* (1999). A gene for paroxysmal kinesigenic choreoathetosis mapped to chromosome 16p11.2-q12.1. *Am J Hum Genet.*, **65**, 1688–97.

Wallace, R. H., Berkovic, S. F., Howell, R. A., Sutherland, G. R., Mulley, J. C. (1996). Suggestions of a major gene for familial febrile convensions mapping to 8913-21. *J Med Genet.*, **33**, 308–12.

Zara, F., Bianchi, A., Avanzini, G., *et al.* (1995). Mapping of genes predisposing to idiopathic generalized epilepsy. *Hum Mol Genet.*, **4**, 1201–7.

*Marina A. J. Tijssen and Peter Brown*

## Introduction

Hyperekplexia, or Startle Disease is a neurological disorder characterized by continuous generalized stiffness during the first years of life, excessive startle with unexpected stimuli, and short periods of generalized stiffness following the startle reflex (Suhren *et al.*, 1966). This momentary stiffness causes severe falls during standing and walking, as it is impossible to stretch out the arms (Suhren *et al.*, 1966). Tapping on the nose induces an exaggerated head-retraction reflex in most patients (Suhren *et al.*, 1966). Clonazepam may provide symptomatic relief (Ryan *et al.*, 1992b). The disorder was first described in 1958 (Kirstein and Silfverskiold, 1958), followed by a detailed description in a large Dutch family in 1966 (Suhren *et al.*, 1966). Further reports have since been published (Morley *et al.*, 1982; Kurczynski, 1983; Markand *et al.*, 1984; Saenz *et al.*, 1984b; Brown *et al.*, 1991b; Hayashi *et al.*, 1991; Shahar *et al.*, 1991; Ryan *et al.*, 1992b; Bernasconi *et al.*, 1996).

Linkage analysis mapped a major gene for this disorder to chromosome 5q33-35 (Ryan *et al.*, 1992a). Different missense mutations in the $\alpha 1$ subunit of the glycine receptor (human) (GLRA1) gene, Pro250Thr (Saul *et al.*, 1999), Gln266His (Milani *et al.*, 1996), Arg271Leu (Shiang *et al.*, 1993), Arg271Gln (Tijssen *et al.*, 1995; Shiang *et al.*, 1993, 1995; Rees *et al.*, 1994; Schorderet *et al.*, 1994; Elmslie *et al.*, 1996; Bernasconi *et al.*, 1996), Lys276Glu (Seri *et al.*, 1997), and Tyr279Cys (Shiang *et al.*, 1995), have been identified in families with the autosomal dominant form of hyperekplexia (Baxter *et al.*, 1996). In addition to the dominant form of hyperekplexia, two recessive cases, both offspring of consanguineous parents, have been described (Rees *et al.*, 1994; Brune *et al.*, 1996). In one patient a recessive point mutation, Ile244Asn (Rees *et al.*, 1994), was detected, while the other patient carried a homozygous deletion encompassing exon 1 to 6 of the GLRA1 gene (Brune *et al.*, 1996). In one family, two patients compound heterozygous for two mutations, Arg252His and Arg392His, showed the hyperekplexia phenotype (Vergouwe *et al.*, 1999).

Glycine is an inhibitory neurotransmitter and the glycine receptor is a hetero-oligomeric ligand-gated chloride channel, mainly located in post-synaptic membranes in vertebrate brainstem and spinal cord (Betz, 1991; Rajendra and Schofield, 1995). A high concentration of glycine receptors is found in the interneurons; Renshaw cells and Ia inhibitory interneurons (Fyffe, 1991). The receptor consists of five subunits ($3\alpha$ and $2\beta$) forming a ring with a central ion-conducting pore. The glycine receptor has different isoforms, comprising different variants of the ligand-binding $\alpha$-subunits. The mutations described in hyperekplexia are located in the alpha-1 subunit. The glycine receptor alpha-1 subunit consists of a large extracellular N-terminal domain, four transmembrane segments (M1–M4) and a short extracellular C terminus (Rajendra *et al.*, 1995; Grenningloh *et al.*, 1990). Autosomal dominant mutations in the GLRA1 gene, located within the intracellular M1–M2 loop, M2 domain or the extracellular M2–M3 loop, disrupt the signal transduction. Normally, the chloride influx through the channel antagonizes membrane depolarization. Decreased chloride permeability of the neuronal membrane results in diminished inhibition of neuronal firing.

Electrophysiological studies in hereditary hyperekplexia show increased spinal motor excitability, as the reciprocal inhibition of H-reflexes was disinhibited (Floeter *et al.*, 1996). The main focus of research in these patients has been the excessive motor response to unexpected stimuli. This response has been identified as an exaggerated startle reflex, which is generated in the lower brainstem, probably in the medial bulbopontine reticular formation (Brown *et al.*, 1991b). The startle reflex in hyperekplexia is identical to that in normals, although the magnitude of the motor response is larger compared to normal controls (Brown *et al.*, 1991b; Tijssen *et al.*, 1997a).

In conclusion, hyperekplexia is a paroxysmal disorder triggered by unexpected external stimuli. The excessive startle reflex and startle-induced stiffness are a result of a lack of inhibition in the brainstem and spinal cord interneurons due to a reduced chloride permeability of the glycine receptor.

# Clinical aspects

## Clinical forms of hyperekplexia

### Hereditary major form

Hyperekplexia, or startle disease, derives from the Greek word 'εκ-πλησσω' which means 'to startle excessively' (Suhren *et al.*, 1966). The clinical picture is characterized by three clinical features (Tijssen *et al.*, 1995). The first is a generalized stiffness immediately after birth, normalizing during the first years of life. The stiffness increases with handling and disappears during sleep. Secondly, patients suffer from an excessive startle reflex, to unexpected, particularly auditory, stimuli, which is present from birth. The third feature is a temporary generalized stiffness following the startle response, causing patients to fall 'as stiff as a stick' (Suhren *et al.*, 1966). Consciousness remains clear during these falls. Several reports have been published on hereditary hyperekplexia (Andermann *et al.*, 1980; Morley *et al.*, 1982; Kurczynski, 1983; Markand *et al.*, 1984; Saenz *et al.*, 1984b; Brown *et al.*, 1991b; Hayashi *et al.*, 1991; Shahar *et al.*, 1991; Ryan *et al.*, 1992b; Bernasconi *et al.*, 1996). In a few reports, a

congenital form of stiff-man syndrome, the 'hereditary stiff-baby syndrome', has been described (Klein *et al.*, 1972; Sander *et al.*, 1980). The resemblance with the major form of hyperekplexia is so striking, that this disorder is now considered to be hyperekplexia (Lingam *et al.*, 1981; Weaver *et al.*, 1982).

The severity and frequency of the excessive startle reflexes can increase due to emotional tension, nervousness, fatigue, and the expectation of being frightened (Suhren *et al.*, 1966). The severity decreases with holding objects or drinking alcohol (Suhren *et al.*, 1966). The frequency of startle responses varies considerably, not only between subjects, but also over the course of time (Suhren *et al.*, 1966). Several additional clinical features have been described in patients with hyperekplexia, which are not obligatory for the diagnosis. Periodic limb movements in sleep (PLMS) and hypnagogic myoclonus are frequently mentioned (Kirstein and Silfverskiold, 1958; Gastaut and Villeneuve, 1967; Andermann *et al.*, 1980; Morley *et al.*, 1982; Kurczynski, 1983; Saenz *et al.*, 1984; Brown *et al.*, 1991b; Hayashi *et al.*, 1991; Shahar *et al.*, 1991; Matsumoto *et al.*, 1992; Pascotto and Coppola, 1992). Other associated features are inguinal, umbilical or epigastric herniations (Suhren *et al.*, 1966; Klein *et al.*, 1972; Lingam *et al.*, 1981), congenital dislocations of the hip (Hayashi *et al.*, 1991), epilepsy (Suhren *et al.*, 1966; Saenz *et al.*, 1984), feeding and breathing problems in newborns (Shahar *et al.*, 1991; Giacoia and Ryan, 1994), and sudden infant death (Suhren *et al.*, 1966; Giacoia and Ryan, 1994). Most patients show normal intelligence, but some mildly retarded patients have been reported (Shahar *et al.*, 1991; Ryan *et al.*, 1992b).

On neurological examination, newborns have a markedly increased muscle tone. Held horizontally the baby is as 'stiff as a stick' (Suhren *et al.*, 1966; Tijssen and Brouwer, 2000). The startle reflex is not the most prominent sign during the first years. The baby is alert, but shows marked hypokinesia (Tijssen and Brouwer, 2000). Adults with the major form of hyperekplexia often walk with a stiff-legged, mildly wide-based gait without signs of ataxia (Suhren *et al.*, 1966). Tendon reflexes and tone are normal, or slightly increased, without clear evidence of a pyramidal syndrome (Suhren *et al*., 1966). Tapping the nose induces an exaggerated head-retraction reflex (HRR) in most patients with hyperekplexia (Suhren *et al*., 1966; Andermann *et al*., 1980; Kurczynski, 1983; Shahar *et al*., 1991; Matsumoto *et al*., 1992). This reflex movement, consisting of a brisk, involuntary backward jerk of the head, occurs when the root of the nose is tapped in a downward direction with the percussion hammer. HRR occurs infrequently in normal subjects (Wartenberg, 1941). Shahar considered it a hallmark of hyperekplexia in stiff newborns (Shahar *et al*., 1991).

Standard tests of serum and cerebrospinal fluid (CSF) did not show any abnormalities (Sander *et al*., 1980; Kurczynski, 1983; Saenz *et al*., 1984; Dubowitz *et al*., 1992; Stephenson, 1992; Berthier *et al*., 1994). Computerized tomography and magnetic resonance imaging of the brain are normal (Tijssen, unpublished observations in three cases). Magnetic resonance spectroscopy (MRS) showed frontal dysfunction in four patients with hyperekplexia, but these patients did not show a point mutation in the gene encoding the $\alpha1$ subunit (Bernasconi *et al*., 1998). A study in four patients with a genetically proven point mutation in the GLRA1 gene did not reveal abnormalities upon MRS (Tijssen and Brown, unpublished data).

## Hereditary minor form

In the original Dutch family, described in 1966, two clinical forms of the disorder were recognized (Suhren *et al*., 1966). These two forms have also been described in a Canadian family and named the major and minor form of hyperekplexia (Andermann *et al*., 1980). The major form consists of the classical description of hyperekplexia described above. The minor form consists of excessive startle responses without any signs of stiffness, neither in relation to the startle response, nor in the neonatal period. Exaggerated startle responses in the hereditary minor form begin during childhood, rather than in the neonatal period (Suhren *et al*., 1966). The two forms were believed to reflect variations in expression of the same gene defect disease. The occasional occurrence of the minor form has been confirmed in other families (Brown *et al*., 1991b; Pascotto and

Coppola, 1992). Recently, a large pedigree with 10 affected patients has been described, suffering from both major and minor forms of hyperekplexia. Unfortunately, the clinical features have not been described in detail for each individual (Saul *et al*., 1999).

On neurological examination, patients with the minor form of hyperekplexia have no abnormalities, except for an exaggerated startle response and the frequent occurrence of an exaggerated head-retraction reflex (Suhren *et al*., 1966).

## Sporadic patients

Several patients with a non-familial, sporadic form of hyperekplexia have been described, representing both the major and minor clinical forms (Andermann *et al*., 1980; Saenz *et al*., 1984; Melki *et al*., 1988; Stephenson, 1992; Berthier *et al*., 1994; Rees *et al*., 1994; McAbee *et al*., 1995; Shiang *et al*., 1995; Vergouwe *et al*., 1997; Scarcella and Coppola, 1997). Many of these patients had additional abnormalities, not encountered in hereditary hyperekplexia.

# Differential diagnosis

The triad of excessive startle reflexes, stiffness related to the startle response and continuous stiffness in the neonatal period leads to the clinical diagnosis of hyperekplexia. If only one or two of these features occur the following differential diagnosis may be considered.

## Excessive responses to startling stimuli without intercurrent stiffness

### Symptomatic hyperekplexia

Occasionally, symptomatic hyperekplexia (defined as excessive startle responses) has been described in patients with brainstem lesions (Duensing, 1952; Kohara *et al*., 1988; Shibasaki *et al*., 1988; Kimber and Thompson, 1997; Kellett *et al*., 1998), cervicomedullar compression (Winston, 1983), multiple sclerosis (Duensing, 1952; Brown *et al*., 1991b), sarcoidosis (Brown *et al*., 1991b), post-anoxic encephalopathy (Brown *et al.*, 1991b), post-traumatic (Duensing, 1952), paraneoplastic (Duensing, 1952), cerebral abscess with encephalitis (Duensing, 1952), occlusion of the posterior thalamic arteries (Fariello *et al.*, 1983), and obstructive sleep apnoea (Hochman *et al.*, 1994).

## Startle-induced epilepsy

In startle epilepsy, seizures are precipitated by an unexpected stimulus (Saenz *et al.*, 1984). Clinically, the seizures consist of asymmetric tonic posturing following the startle response (Manford *et al.*, 1996). In most cases patients are young and many, but not all, have suffered from infantile cerebral hemiplegia. (Manford *et al.*, 1996). If there is a positive family history of startle epilepsy, familial frontal lobe epilepsy should be considered (Oldani *et al.*, 1998).

## Reflex myoclonus

Reticular and propriospinal myoclonus can resemble hyperekplexia. In order to discriminate between myoclonus and hyperekplexia, EMG-reflex tests are necessary (Hallett *et al.*, 1977; Brown *et al.*, 1991a).

## Culturally related syndromes

The 'Jumping Frenchmen of Maine', (Stevens, 1965; Howard and Ford, 1992), Latah (Yap, 1951), and Myriachit (Yap, 1951) are culturally related syndromes which include excessive startle responses, echolalia, and echopraxia. Stiffness has not been described in these patients.

## Gilles de la Tourette syndrome

In Gilles de la Tourette syndrome excessive startling has occasionally been described (Stell *et al.*, 1995) but, more frequently, a normal startle reflex induces motor tics and obsessive compulsive behaviour (Lees *et al.*, 1984; Eapen *et al.*, 1994; Tijssen *et al.*, 1999).

## Excessive responses to startling stimuli with intercurrent stiffness

### Strychnine poisoning

Many features of strychnine poisoning (Tohier *et al.*, 1991) closely resemble hyperekplexia, but it is very rare.

### Stiff-man syndrome

Stiff-man syndrome (Gordon *et al.*, 1967) is characterized by progressive intermittent spasms and stiffness of the axial muscles. The spasms can be induced by unexpected stimuli. The axial stiffness is continuous. Antibodies against gamma-aminobutyric acid (GABA)-ergic neurons, especially antiglutamic acid decarboxylase (GAD), occur in many patients (Barker *et al.*, 1998). In the jerking stiff-man syndrome the stiffness is accompanied by reflex myoclonus (Leigh *et al.*, 1980). Progressive encephalomyelitis with rigidity (Whiteley *et al.*, 1976) may initially resemble stiff-man syndrome, but is distinguished from it by a relentlessly progressive course (Thompson, 1993).

### Tetanus

Tetanus can be distinguished from stiff-man syndrome by its quick onset and rapid progression (Alfrey and Rauscher, 1979). In addition, pronounced trismus is present in acute tetanus.

## Continuous stiffness in the neonatal period

The most important differential diagnosis is perinatal asphyxia (Aicardi, 1992). In these babies pyramidal signs and irritability are essential features, discriminating it from hyperekplexia. Congenital generalized muscle hypertonia as an autosomal recessive disorder was described in a Mexican family (Cantu and Cuellar, 1974). These children also suffered from cardiopulmonary distress. Extrapyramidal signs, including stiffness, may occur in a child born to a mother using phenothiazine (Hill *et al.*, 1966) or cocaine (Chiriboga *et al.*, 1995).

# Treatment

Several drugs have been used to treat hyperekplexia, including diazepam (Klein *et al.*, 1972; Morley *et al.*, 1982), clobazepam (Brown *et al.*, 1991b), chlordiazepoxide (Suhren *et al.* 1966), carbamazepine (Brown *et al.*, 1991b), phenytoin (Brown *et al.*, 1991b), valproate (Saenz *et al.*, 1984; Dooley and Andermann, 1989; Dubowitz *et al.*, 1992; McAbee *et al.*, 1995), 5-hydroxytryptophan (Saenz *et al.*, 1984), piracetam (Saenz *et al.*, 1984) and phenobarbital (Andermann *et al.*, 1980; Dubowitz *et al.*, 1992). The most effective drug, both clinically and neurophysiologically, is clonazepam (Andermann *et al.*, 1980; Morley *et al.*, 1982; Markand *et al.*, 1984; Kelts and Harrison J, 1988; Saenz *et al.*, 1984; Pascotto and Coppola, 1992; Ryan *et al.*, 1992b; Tijssen *et al.*, 1997b). Clonazepam binds to specific high affinity binding sites for benzodiazepines on brain membranes (Browne, 1976; Dreifuss and Sato, 1982; Sato, 1989) and potentiates the inhibitory neurotransmitter gamma-aminobutyric acid (Dreifuss and Sato, 1982; Mumford and Lewis, 1991). In two open label studies a beneficial effect of vigabatrin has been reported supporting the GABA hypothesis (Stephenson, 1992). However, in a double-blind placebo-controlled study in four patients with hereditary hyperekplexia, the startle responses were not diminished by vigabatrine (Tijssen *et al.*, 1997b). The effect of clonazepam may be due to a direct effect of clonazepam on the modified $\alpha$1 subunit of the glycine receptor.

# Glycine receptor

The amino acid glycine is an essential intermediate in many metabolic processes throughout the body (Kikuchi, 1973). In the CNS it is one of the major inhibitory neurotransmitters (Betz, 1991). It also has an excitatory function at the N-methyl-D-aspartate (NMDA) receptor (Johnson and Ascher, 1987), but only the inhibitory neurotransmitter function will be discussed. The glycine receptor is a member of the ligand-gated ion-channel superfamily (Betz, 1990), which also includes the GABA-A receptor, serotonin receptors, and the excitatory nicotinic acetylcholine receptor family (Schofield *et al.*, 1987). These receptors mediate fast synaptic neurotransmission in the mammalian central nervous system and share a similar structure with five subunits forming a ring with a central ion-conducting pore. The subunits each comprise an N-terminal extracellular domain that contains the ligand-binding sites and four membrane-spanning domains (Schofield *et al.*, 1987).

The glycine receptor is a ligand-gated chloride channel (Langosch *et al.*, 1990). The chloride influx through the channel antagonizes membrane depolarization. By increasing chloride permeability of the neuronal membrane, inhibition of neuronal firing is effected (Grenningloh *et al.*, 1990). The function of this inhibition is to achieve sensible transduction of signals by accomplishing concerted action of excitatory and inhibitory receptors (Langosch *et al.*, 1990). In the mammalian CNS, the glycine receptors are mostly found in the brainstem and spinal cord (Zarbin *et al.*, 1981; Frostholm and Rotter, 1985; Probst *et al.*, 1986; White *et al.*, 1990). A high concentration of glycine receptors was found in the interneurons which mediate recurrent and reciprocal inhibition, Renshaw cells and Ia inhibitory interneurons respectively (Fyffe, 1991).

The mammalian glycine receptor has two homologous polypeptides, $\alpha$ (48 kDa) and $\beta$ (58 kDa), as subunits of the receptor (Rajendra and Schofield, 1995). Each receptor consists of 3 $\alpha$- and 2 $\beta$-subunits. The $\alpha$1 subunit has four transmembrane domains (M1–M4) with a short cytoplasmic loop between M1 and M2, a short extracellular domain between M2 and M3, and a long cytoplasmic loop between M3 and M4 (Langosch *et al.*, 1990). The M2 domain is thought to line the chloride channel and the extracellular loops are believed to form the mouth of the channel (Langosch *et al.*, 1990; Devillers *et al.*, 1993). The ligand-binding site of the receptor was mapped to the $\alpha$-subunit (Grenningloh *et al.*, 1990). The agonist binding site is located in the amino-terminal end of the protein. The agonists described were glycine, $\beta$-alanine and taurine, while the main antagonist was strychnine (Langosch *et al.*, 1990). The $\beta$-subunit plays a more structural rather than ligand binding role (Handford *et al.*, 1996).

## Alpha subunit

Different isoforms of the glycine receptor have been described, comprising different variants of the ligand-binding $\alpha$-subunits: the original $\alpha$-subunit (now termed $\alpha 1$) (Langosch et al., 1990), two different $\alpha 2$ subunits, an $\alpha 3$, and an $\alpha 4$ subunit (Grenningloh et al., 1990; Kuhse et al., 1990a, b, 1991).

During development in mice a receptor consisting of $\alpha 2$ subunits in the neonatal period changed to one using $\alpha 1$ subunits (Kuhse et al., 1990a, b, 1991; Becker et al., 1992). The replacement of the neonatal type with the adult type occurs within 2–3 weeks after birth (Becker et al., 1988). Subtype variants can be detected in different parts of the rat CNS. The $\alpha 1$ transcripts were found in the spinal cord, brainstem and colliculi (Matzenbach et al., 1994). The variants $\alpha 1$, $\alpha 2$, and 3 were also detected in man (Kuhse et al., 1990a, b, 1991). In man the genes encoding the $\alpha 1$, $\alpha 2$, and $\alpha$- subunits were mapped to chromosome 5q (Shiang et al. 1993), the short arm of the human X chromosome (Sheffield et al., 1989) and chromosome 4q33-q34 (Nikolic et al., 1998) respectively.

## Beta subunit

The $\beta$-subunits were found throughout the entire brain and spinal cord (Rajendra and Schofield, 1995; Zafra et al., 1997). The gene encoding the $\beta$-subunit of the glycine receptor in man has been located on chromosome 4q31.3 $\beta$-subunit of the glycine receptor (human) (GLRB) (Handford et al., 1996; Milani et al., 1998). The $\beta$-subunit appears to play a structural rather than ligand-binding role in the glycine receptor function (Handford et al., 1996).

## Genetic and biochemical aspects

### Autosomal dominant mutations

In 1992 a hyperekplexia locus was mapped to chromosome 5q33-q35 in four families with the major form of hyperekplexia (Ryan et al., 1992a, b). The gene encoding the $\alpha 1$ subunit of the glycine receptor (GLRA1) was located in this area and different missense mutations in this gene have been identified in families with the autosomal dominant form of hyperekplexia: Pro250Thr (Saul et al., 1999), Arg271Leu (Shiang et al., 1993), Arg271Gln ( Shiang et al., 1993, 1995; Rees et al., 1994; Schorderet et al., 1994; Tijssen et al., 1995a; Bernasconi et al., 1996; Elmslie et al., 1996), Lys276Glu (Seri et al., 1997), and Tyr279Cys (Shiang et al., 1995) (Figure 18.1).

## M2–M3 loop

The mutations at Arg271 (Arg271Leu; Arg271Gln) (Shiang et al., 1993; Tijssen et al., 1995; Bernasconi et al., 1996) are located in a part of the extracellular loop linking the second and third membrane-spanning domains (the M2–M3 loop). The physiological effect of the mutations is reduced potency of glycine with decreased single chloride-channel conductance. (Langosch et al., 1994). Apart from these effects, both mutations converted $\beta$-alanine and taurine from agonists into competitive antagonists, while the binding affinities were almost unchanged (Rajendra et al., 1995). The sensitivity of glycine currents to strychnine were unchanged (Langosch et al., 1994; Rajendra et al., 1994). It appears that the Arg271 residue is crucial for transducing the allosteric coupling from ligand binding to channel activation.

Mutations of amino acid 276 (Lys276Glu) (Elmslie et al., 1996; Seri et al., 1997) and Tyr279 (Tyr279Cys) (Shiang et al., 1995) are also located at the short extracellular domain between M2 and M3. These mutations resulted similarly, in decreased glycine sensitivity effects and they also converted $\beta$-alanine and taurine from agonists into competitive antagonists, with little changing in the binding affinities (Lynch et al., 1997). Functional studies of the Lys276Glu mutation showed impairment of channel-gating kinetics without effects on ligand binding or conductance (Lewis et al., 1998), also suggesting an uncoupling of the agonist binding process from the channel activation gate.

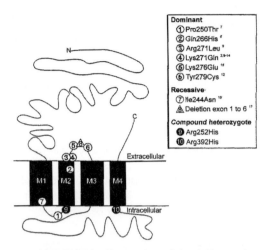

Dominant
① Pro250Thr [7]
② Gln266His [6]
③ Arg271Leu [9]
④ Lys271Gln [2,9-14]
⑤ Lys276Glu [15]
⑥ Tyr279Cys [12]

Recessive
⑦ Ile244Asn [19]
Ⓐ Deletion exon 1 to 6 [17]

Compound heterozygote
⑨ Arg252His
⑩ Arg392His

**Figure 18.1** GLRA1 with mutations. Schematic overview of dominant, recessive and compound heterozygous mutations present in the alpha-1 subunit of the human glycine receptor. (From Vergouwe *et al*, Hyperekplexia phenotype due to compound heterozygosity for GLRA1 gene mutations. *Ann Neurol.*, 1999 Oct; **46**(4): 634–8. Reprinted with permission of Lippincott Williams & Wilkins.)

The phenotype of patients with autosomal dominant mutations in the M2–M3 loop is the 'classical' major form of hyperekplexia (Suhren *et al.*, 1966). Interestingly, in one family carrying the Lys276Glu mutation hyperekplexia co-segregated with spastic paraparesis (Baxter *et al.*, 1996; Elmslie *et al.*, 1996), while Italian patients with a similar mutation only showed hyperekplexia (Seri *et al.*, 1997).

A point of interest is that molecular genetic evaluation of the Dutch hyperekplexia family demonstrated that the major form, but not the minor form, showed an Arg271Gln mutation in GLRA1-gene (Tijssen *et al.*, 1995). This disproved the hypothesis that the major and minor hyperekplexia in this pedigree are variations in expression of the same gene defect disease. In the Dutch pedigree there was only one example of a patient with the minor form passing on the major form (Suhren *et al.*, 1966) and re-evaluation resulted in reclassification of this patient (major form) (Tijssen *et al.*, 1995). The genetic cause of the minor form in this pedigree remains unclear. One might suppose that another gene elsewhere in the genome is responsible for the minor form, but the rarity of the disease makes the presence of two mutations in one pedigree very unlikely. The absence of mutations in patients with the minor form was confirmed in small pedigrees (Turecki *et al.*, 1996; Bernasconi *et al.*, 1998). In those pedigrees with both major and minor forms neither form showed a mutation in the GLRA1 gene.

## M2 membrane spanning segment

In an Italian pedigree an autosomal dominant mutation Gln266His has been described (Milani *et al.*, 1996). The affected amino acid is located in the M2 membrane spanning segment of the glycine receptor. Functional tests of this mutation revealed a reduced ability of glycine and taurine to open the channel, while agonist displacement of strychnine binding was unchanged (Moorhouse *et al.*, 1999). Taurine was converted to a weak partial agonist, antagonizing glycine. Single-channel recordings showed normal conductance, but a significant reduction in open times in the mutant receptors, consistent with a less stable open state of the channel (Moorhouse *et al.*, 1999). The phenotype of the major form of hyperekplexia associated with this particular mutation was different from the 'classical' description (Suhren *et al.*, 1966) in that patients had additional features of myoclonic fits and a persistent flexed posture (Milani *et al.*, 1996). This mutation is variably expressed as it was detected in a patient with the minor form of hyperekplexia as well as in two asymptomatic sibs. The severity of the disease worsened over the three generations reported suggesting anticipation which has not been described in other hyperekplexia pedigrees.

## M1 and M2 cytoplasmatic loop

The autosomal dominant Pro250Thr mutation is located at the cytoplasmic loop linking transmembrane regions M1 and M2 (Saul *et al.*, 1999). Functional tests of the recombinant receptors displayed moderate changes in agonist affinity but a strong reduction of maximum whole-cell chloride currents with a prolonged recovery from desensitization. This mutation in the M1–M2 loop destabilized open channel conformations (Saul *et al.*, 1999).

The phenotype in this pedigree was variable, consisting of both major and minor forms (Saul *et al.*, 1999). Unfortunately, the clinical characteristics of the individuals were not given.

## Recessive mutations

Two recessive cases, both offspring of consanguineous parents, have been described (Rees *et al.*, 1994; Brune *et al.*, 1996). In one patient a recessive point mutation, Ile244Asn (Rees *et al.*, 1994) was detected while the other patient carried a homozygous deletion encompassing exon 1 to 6 of the GLRA1 gene (Brune *et al.*, 1996).

The recessive mutation at amino acid Ile244 (Ile244Asn) was located three amino acids before the end of the predicted first transmembrane domain (Rees *et al.*, 1994), in the intracellular M1–M2 loop. This mutation resulted in a decreased glycine sensitivity and a large reduction in taurine efficacy (Lynch *et al.*, 1997). The displayed properties were similar to the autosomal dominant mutation at position 271 (Lynch *et al.*, 1997).

The homozygous deletion encompassing exons 1–6 of the GLRA1 gene (Brune *et al.*, 1996) spans segments of the gene indispensable for glycine receptor α1 subunit expression and function. This homozygous deletion in mice (oscillator mouse) has a lethal effect (Buckwalter *et al.*, 1994; Kling *et al.*, 1997). In man, the loss of the α1 subunit of the glycine receptor is effectively compensated (Buckwalter *et al.*, 1994; Kling *et al.*, 1997).

Clinically, both children had symptoms identical to those of the classical hereditary major form of hyperekplexia (Brune *et al.*, 1996).

## Compound heterozygosity

Recently, a compound heterozygosity was described (Vergouwe *et al.*, 1999). Mutation analysis revealed different missense mutations on the two haplotypes, changing an arginine to a histidine at amino acid positions 252 and 392 respectively. Amino acid Arg252 is the last residue of the intracellular M1–M2 loop and located directly before the M2 domain and the Arg392 residue is located at the end of the M3–M4 intracellular loop right before the M4 transmembrane domain (Grenningloh *et al.*, 1990). The 'classical' major form hyperekplexia phenotype was only seen in individuals compound heterozygous for the two mutations, whereas family members carrying either one of the two mutations were healthy (Vergouwe *et al.*, 1999). The physiological effects of these mutations have not yet been studied.

## Sporadic patients

In 10 sporadic cases of hyperekplexia, nine with atypical features and one with classical features, no mutations were detected in the GLRA1-gene (Shiang *et al.*, 1995; Elmslie *et al.*, 1996; Vergouwe *et al.*, 1997). It has been suggested that such cases of hyperekplexia might be due to mutations of genes encoding the β-subunit (GLRB) or other subtypes of the α-subunits. In a further series of 30 sporadic hyperekplexia no mutations of either the GLRA1 or GLAB genes were found (Milani *et al.*, 1998).

## Conclusions

Mutations in the GLRA1 gene, encoding the α1 subunit of the glycine receptor, have given insight in the function of the glycine receptor. In the closed state the M2 domains are bent inwards to narrow the channel pore. Following ligand binding, to receptor sites present in the large N-terminal extracellular domain, the M2 domains are twisted sideways to create an open passage with the M1–M2 and M2–M3 loops acting as hinges to facilitate this rotation (Lynch *et al.*, 1997). Mutations in the GLRA1 gene, located within the intracellular M1–M2 loop, M2 domain or the extracellular M2–M3 loop, prevent this rotation and disrupt the transduction process between ligand binding and channel activation (Lynch *et al.*, 1997). Agonists interact with the external M2–M3 loop to activate the channel, while the M1–M2 loop contributes to glycine receptor desensitization properties (Lewis and Schofield, 1999). In addition, the described mutations reduce or eliminate the agonist function of taurine and alanine without changing their ligand binding affinities, indicating that agonist or antagonist behaviour is determined by channel-gating efficacy. The finding of the Arg392His mutation, located in the intracellular M3–M4 loop, implies a possible role for this loop in the signal transduction pathway.

## Animal models

The spasmodic mouse (*spd*) shows the best phenotypical resemblance to human hyperekplexia. They suffer from an exaggerated acoustic startle reflex with prolonged righting reflex, fine motor tremor, leg clasping, and stiffness. S*pd* mice are most severely affected by the third to fifth week of life, with lessened symptoms in adulthood (Simon, 1997). Analogous to human hyperekplexia, the *spd* mouse possesses a point mutation in the gene encoding the $\alpha$1 subunit of the glycine receptor (GLRA1), localized on mouse chromosome 11 (Buckwalter *et al.*, 1993). In contrast to most mutations in man, the mutation in the mouse is recessive in nature. The mutation was identified as substitution of alanine by serine at amino acid 52 (*Ala52Ser*) (Ryan *et al.*, 1994). The *spd* mutation leads to a 60% reduction in sensitivity of the glycine-activated current (Ryan *et al.*, 1994). In contrast to human hyperekplexia where the stiffness is present at birth, the *spd* mice are normal during the first two weeks of life, in keeping with the replacement of normal neonatal type glycine receptors with the adult type (Becker *et al.*, 1992). The reason for this discrepancy is unknown.

An extreme example of hyperekplexia in the mouse is the oscillator mouse (*spd*[ot]). These mice appear normal until postnatal day 11 but then develop a spastic gait with reduced spontaneous movements, stimulus-induced myoclonic jerks, rigidity, and tremor. Death occurs at day 21 (Simon, 1997; Kling *et al.*, 1997). In this mouse a microdeletion was identified within the GLA1 gene (Buckwalter *et al.*, 1994). Biochemical analysis revealed that the spinal cord of homozygous mutants is totally devoid of the glycine $\alpha$1 polypeptide, characterizing the *spd*[ot] gene as the functional null allele of the $\alpha$1 subunit of the glycine receptor (Brune *et al.*, 1996; Kling *et al.*, 1997).

The gene encoding the $\beta$-subunit of the glycine receptor in the mouse was mapped to the spastic (*spa*) mouse locus on mouse chromosome 3 (Kingsmore *et al.*, 1994; Handford *et al.*, 1996). Systemic administration of strychnine, a selective glycine receptor antagonist, to normal animals showed a clinical picture similar to the *spa* mouse. These mice suffer from an exaggerated acoustic startle reflex with impaired righting response, tremor and stiffness (Simon, 1997). These mice are, like the *spd* mice, most severely affected by the third to fifth week of life with lessening of symptoms in adulthood (Simon, 1997). The mutation leads to markedly reduced levels of functional $\beta$-subunit. Increasing the amount of $\beta$-subunits to 25% of normal in the *spa* mouse ameliorates the symptoms (Hartenstein *et al.*, 1996). One could therefore infer that mutations in the human glycine receptor $\beta$-subunit gene (GLRB) might cause inherited disorders of the startle response, inherited myoclonus, or spastic paraparesis.

## Electrophysiology

Hyperekplexia is characterized by three abnormal motor responses: the continuous stiffness in the neonatal period, the temporary tonic spasm and the briefer pathological startle reflex. The last two occur in response to unexpected auditory, visual and somaesthetic stimuli. The transient tonic spasms consist of a generalized stiffening, lasting a few seconds, during which patients are unable to take any protective action and, if erect, fall stiffly to the ground, without losing consciousness. It is during these tonic attacks that patients suffer the repeated injuries that occur in hyperekplexia. These transient tonic episodes are different to the brief, generalized startle reflexes seen in these patients and are less common. The tonic spasms, unlike the startle response, tend to improve with clonazepam (Tijssen *et al.*, 1997b).

## Stiffness

There are, as yet, no reported electrophysiological studies performed on the stiffness occurring during the neonatal period. In adults with GLRA1 mutations and hyperekplexia of the major form, spinal motor excitability as measured by reciprocal inhibition of H-reflexes, is increased (Floeter et al., 1996; personal observation). Bisynaptic reciprocal Ia inhibition mediated by spinal interneurons has been shown in the cat to be glycinergic. Thus increased spinal motor excitability may well account for the stiffness seen in hyperekplexia. Further electrophysiological studies are necessary to give more insight in the pathophysiology of this stiffness. In the Dutch pedigree, patients with the minor form of hyperekplexia without a mutation in the GLRA1 gene, the reciprocal inhibition of H-reflexes was normal (Tijssen, personal observation in three patients). It would be of interest to evaluate whether glycinergic inhibition is deficient in patients with the GLRA1 positive minor form of the disease (Milani et al., 1996; Saul et al., 1999).

## Startle reflexes

There is now general agreement that the startle response in the hereditary major form of hyperekplexia is a pathological exaggeration of the normal startle reflex (Brown et al., 1991b; Matsumoto et al., 1992; Tijssen et al., 1997a). The reflex jerks to auditory, somaesthetic or visual stimuli involve many muscles, both proximal and distal, bilaterally and synchronously to produce a sudden shock-like movement usually involving a grimace, abduction of the arms, and flexion of the neck, trunk, elbows, hips and knees. As in the normal startle reflex the auditory blink reflex may not be an integral part of the auditory startle response (Colebatch et al., 1990; Brown et al., 1991a; Chokroverty et al., 1992). Assuming that the blink reflex in orbicularis oculi is a separate physiological process, then the earliest muscle activity in the true generalized startle response is recorded in sternocleidomastoid (Brown et al., 1991a). EMG activity in mentalis, masseter and in trunk and limb muscles follows later. The responses re-

corded in the intrinsic hand and foot muscles are particularly delayed relative to more proximal limb muscles (Brown et al., 1991b; Matsumoto et al., 1992; Tijssen et al., 1997a).

The pattern of muscle activity in the reflex responses to auditory and somaesthetic stimulation in both normals and patients with the major form of hyperekplexia implicates the lower brainstem as the generator for the observed reflex responses. Motor activity begins in the caudal brainstem and then spreads rostrally up the brainstem and caudally down the spinal cord. It is of little surprise, therefore, that many of the previously reported cases of acquired startle disease have involved brainstem pathology. The similarity of the response following different types of stimuli suggests that within the lower brainstem, the pathological startle response may originate in the medial bulbopontine reticular formation, which receives afferents from multiple modalities.

Within a single pedigree family members with the minor form of hyperekplexia, without a mutation in the GLRA1 gene, had startle responses which were different from those seen in family members with the GLRA1 positive major form of hyperekplexia (Tijssen et al., 1996). In both the motor responses were excessive, but in those with the minor form EMG responses were delayed compared to the major form, and startle responses did not habituate (Tijssen et al., 1996). The cause of the excessive startle responses, and the differences seen in these two groups of patients remains unexplained. One possible explanation is that the startle response seen in those with the minor form may represent a learned psychogenic startle response. However, the jerks do not share all the characteristics of the psychogenic startle response (Thompson et al., 1992). An alternative explanation is that an excessive startle response, caused by an autosomal dominant or sporadic trait, may be much more common than previously thought (Gastaut and Villeneuve, 1967) in which case the minor form of hyperekplexia represents a normal variant. As neither explanation is very convincing, the cause of the minor form of hyperekplexia in this pedigree must remain uncertain. It would be of interest to study the startle reflexes in those patients with the minor form of hyperekplexia who do show a mutation in the

GLRA1 gene (Milani *et al.*, 1996; Saul *et al.*, 1999).

# References

Aicardi, J. (ed.) (1992). Neurological diseases in the perinatal period. In *Diseases of the nervous system in childhood*, pp. 47–105. Suffolk: Lavenham Press Ltd.

Alfrey, D. D. and Rauscher, L. A. (1979). Tetanus: a review. *Crit Care Med.*, **7**, 176–81.

Andermann, F., Keene, D. L., Andermann, E. and Quesney, L. F. (1980). Startle disease or hyperekplexia: further delineation of the syndrome. *Brain*, **103**, 985–97.

Barker, R. A., Revesz, T., Thom, M., Marsden, C. D. and Brown, P. (1998). Review of 23 patients affected by the stiff man syndrome: clinical subdivision into stiff trunk (man) syndrome, stiff limb syndrome, and progressive encephalomyelitis with rigidity (see comments). *J Neurol Neurosurg Psychiatr.*, **65**, 633–40.

Baxter, P., Connolly, S., Curtis, A. *et al.* (1996). Codominant inheritance of hyperekplexia and spastic paraparesis. *Dev Med Child Neurol.*, **38**, 739–43.

Becker, C. M., Hoch, W. and Betz, H. (1988). Glycine receptor heterogeneity in rat spinal cord during postnatal development. *EMBO J.*, **7**, 3717–26.

Becker, C. M., Schmieden, V., Tarroni, P., Strasser, U. and Betz, H. (1992). Isoform-selective deficit of glycine receptors in the mouse mutant spastic. *Neuron*, **8**, 283–9.

Bernasconi, A., Cendes, F., Shoubridge, E. A. *et al.* (1998). Spectroscopic imaging of frontal neuronal dysfunction in hyperekplexia. *Brain*, **121**, 1507–12.

Bernasconi, A., Regli, F., Schorderet, D. F. and Pescia, G. (1996). Familial hyperekplexia: startle disease. Clinical, electrophysiological and genetic study of a family. *Rev Neurol Paris*, **152**, 447–50.

Berthier, M., Bonneau, D., Desbordes, J. M. *et al.* (1994). Possible involvement of a gamma-hydroxybutyric acid receptor in startle disease. *Acta Paediatr.*, **83**, 678–80.

Betz, H. (1990). Homology and analogy in transmembrane channel design: lessons from synaptic membrane proteins. *Biochemistry*, **29**, 3591–9.

Betz, H. (1991). Glycine receptors: heterogeneous and widespread in the mammalian brain. *Trends Neurosci.*, **14**, 458–61.

Brown, P., Rothwell, J. C., Thompson, P. D., Britton, T. C., Day, B. L. and Marsden, C. D. (1991a). New observations on the normal auditory startle reflex in man. *Brain*, **114**, 1891–902.

Brown, P., Rothwell, J. C., Thompson, P. D., Britton, T. C., Day, B. L. and Marsden, C. D. (1991b). The hyperekplexias and their relationship to the normal startle reflex. *Brain*, **114**, 1903–28.

Browne, T. R. (1976). Clonazepam. A review of a new anticonvulsant drug. *Arch Neurol.*, **33**, 326–32.

Brune, W., Weber, R. G., Saul, B. *et al.* (1996). A GLRA1 null mutation in recessive hyperekplexia challenges the functional role of glycine receptors. *Am J Hum Genet.*, **58**, 989–97.

Buckwalter, M. S., Cook, S. A., Davisson, M. T., White, W. F. and Camper, S.A. (1994). A frameshift mutation in the mouse alpha 1 glycine receptor gene (Glra1) results in progressive neurological symptoms and juvenile death. *Hum Mol Genet.*, **3**, 2025–30.

Buckwalter, M. S., Testa, C. M., Noebels, J. L. and Camper, S. A. (1993). Genetic mapping and evaluation of candidate genes for spasmodic, a neurological mouse mutation with abnormal startle response. *Genomics*, **17**, 279–86.

Cantu, J. M. and Cuellar, A. (1974). Congenital severe generalized muscle hypertonia during wakefulness: a distinct autosomal recessive disorder. *Clin Genet.*, **6**, 32–5.

Chiriboga, C. A., Vibbert, M., Malouf, R. *et al.* (1995). Neurological correlates of fetal cocaine exposure: transient hypertonia of infancy and early childhood. *Pediatrics*, **96**, 1070–7.

Chokroverty, S., Walczak, T. and Hening, W. (1992). Human startle reflex: technique and criteria for abnormal response. *Electroencephalogr Clin Neurophysiol.*, **85**, 236–42.

Colebatch, J. G., Barrett, G. and Lees, A. J. (1990). Exaggerated startle reflexes in an elderly woman. *Mov Disord.*, **5**, 167–9.

Devillers, T. A., Galzi, J. L., Eisele, J. L., Bertrand, S., Bertrand, D. and Changeux, J. P. (1993). Functional architecture of the nicotinic acetylcholine receptor: a prototype of ligand-gated ion channels. *J Membr Biol.*, **136**, 97–112.

Dooley, J. M. and Andermann, F. (1989). Startle disease or hyperekplexia: adolescent onset and response to valproate. *Pediatr Neurol.*, **5**, 126–7.

Dreifuss, F. E. and Sato, S. (1982). Benzodiazepines, Clonazepam. In *Antiepileptic Drugs* 2nd edn. (eds Woodbury DM *et al.*), pp 737–752. New York: Raven Press.

Dubowitz, L. M., Bouza, H., Hird, M. F. and Jaeken, J. (1992). Low cerebrospinal fluid concentration of free gamma-aminobutyric acid in startle disease (see comments). *Lancet*, **340**, 80–1.

Duensing, F. (1952). Schreckreflex und schreckreaktion als hirnorganische zeichen. *Arch Psychiatr Nervenkr.*, **188**, 162–92.

Eapen, V., Moriarty, J. and Robertson, M. M. (1994). Stimulus induced behaviours in Tourette's syndrome. *J Neurol Neurosurg Psychiatr.*, **57**, 853–5.

Elmslie, F. V., Hutchings, S. M., Spencer, V. *et al.* (1996). Analysis of GLRA1 in hereditary and sporadic hyperekplexia: a novel mutation in a family cosegregating for hyperekplexia and spastic paraparesis. *J Med Genet.*, **33**, 435–6.

Fariello, R. G., Schwartzman, R. J. and Beall, S. S. (1983). Hyperekplexia exacerbated by occlusion of posterior thalamic arteries. *Arch Neurol.*, **40**, 244–6.

Floeter, M. K., Andermann, F., Andermann, E., Nigro, M. and Hallett, M. (1996). Physiological studies of spinal inhibitory pathways in patients with hereditary hyperekplexia. *Neurology*, **46**, 766–72.

Frostholm, A. and Rotter, A. (1985). Glycine receptor distribution in mouse CNS: autoradiographic localization of [³H]strychnine binding sites. *Brain Res Bull.*, **15**, 473–86.

Fyffe, R. E. (1991). Glycine-like immunoreactivity in synaptic boutons of identified inhibitory interneurons in the mammalian spinal cord. *Brain Res.*, **547**, 175–9.

Gastaut, H. and Villeneuve, A. (1967). The startle disease or hyperekplexia. Pathological surprise reaction. *J Neurol Sci.*, **5**, 523–42.

Giacoia, G. P. and Ryan, S. G. (1994). Hyperekplexia associated with apnea and sudden infant death syndrome (letter). *Arch Pediatr Adolesc Med.*, **148**, 540–3.

Gordon, E. E., Januszko, D. M. and Kaufman, L. (1967). A critical survey of stiff-man syndrome. *Am J Med.*, **42**, 582–99.

Grenningloh, G., Schmieden, V., Schofield, P. R. *et al.* (1990). Alpha subunit variants of the human glycine receptor: primary structures, functional expression and chromosomal localization of the corresponding genes. *EMBO J.*, **9**, 771–6.

Hallett, M., Chadwick, D., Adam, J. and Marsden, C. D. (1977). Reticular reflex myoclonus: a physiological type of human post-hypoxic myoclonus. *J Neurol Neurosurg Psychiatr.*, **40**, 253–64.

Handford, C. A., Lynch, J. W., Baker, E. *et al.* (1996). The human glycine receptor beta subunit: primary structure, functional characterisation and chromosomal localisation of the human and murine genes. *Brain Res Mol Brain Res.*, **35**, 211–9.

Hartenstein, B., Schenkel, J., Kuhse, J. *et al.* (1996). Low level expression of glycine receptor beta subunit transgene is sufficient for phenotype correction in spastic mice. *EMBO J.*, **15**, 1275–82.

Hayashi, T., Tachibana, H. and Kajii, T. (1991). Hyperekplexia: pedigree studies in two families. *Am J Med Genet.*, **40**, 138–43.

Hill, R. M., Desmond, M. M. and Kay, J. L. (1966). Extrapyramidal dysfunction in an infant of a schizophrenic mother. *J Pediatr.*, **69**, 589–95.

Hochman, M. S., Chediak, A. D. and Ziffer, J. A. (1994). Hyperekplexia: report of a nonfamilial adult onset case associated with obstructive sleep apnea and abnormal brain nuclear tomography. *Sleep*, **17**, 280–3.

Howard, R. and Ford, R. (1992). From the jumping Frenchmen of Maine to post-traumatic stress disorder: the startle response in neuropsychiatry. *Psychol Med.*, **22**, 695–707.

Johnson, J. W. and Ascher, P. (1987). Glycine potentiates the NMDA response in cultured mouse brain neurons. *Nature*, **325**, 529–31.

Kellett, M. W., Humphrey, P. R., Tedman, B. M. and Steiger, M. J. (1998). Hyperekplexia and trismus due to brainstem encephalopathy. *J Neurol Neurosurg Psychiatr.*, **65**, 122–5.

Kelts, K. A. and Harrison, J. (1988). Hyperekplexia: Effective treatment with clonazepam. *Ann Neurol.*, **24**, 309.

Kikuchi, G. (1973). The glycine cleavage system: composition, reaction mechanism, and physiological significance. *Mol Cell Biochem.*, **1**, 169–87.

Kimber, T. E. and Thompson, P. D. (1997). Symptomatic hyperekplexia occurring as a result of pontine infarction. *Mov Disord.*, **12**, 814–6.

Kingsmore, S. F., Giros, B., Suh, D., Bieniarz, M., Caron, M. G. and Seldin, M. F. (1994). Glycine receptor beta-subunit gene mutation in spastic mouse associated with LINE-1 element insertion. *Nat Genet.*, **7**, 136–41.

Kirstein, L. and Silfverskiold, B. P. (1958). A family with emotionally precipitated 'drop seizures'. *Acta Psychiatr Neurol Scand.*, **33**, 471–6.

Klein, R., Haddow, J. E. and DeLuca, C. (1972). Familial congenital disorder resembling stiff-man syndrome. *Am J Dis Child.*, **124**, 730–1.

Kling, C., Koch, M., Saul, B. and Becker, C. M. (1997). The frameshift mutation oscillator (Glra1(spd-ot)) produces a complete loss of glycine receptor alpha1-polypeptide in mouse central nervous system. *Neuroscience*, **78**, 411–7.

Kohara, N., Ugawa, Y., Kuzuhara, S. and Yamanouchi, H. (1988). (An electrophysiological study on spinobulbospinal reflex in three brainstem stroke patients.) *Rinsho Shinkeigaku.*, **28**, 137–46.

Kuhse, J., Kuryatov, A., Maulet, Y., Malosio, M. L., Schmieden, V. and Betz, H. (1991). Alternative splicing generates two isoforms of the alpha 2 subunit of the inhibitory glycine receptor. *FEBS Lett.*, **283**, 73–7.

Kuhse, J., Schmieden, V. and Betz, H. (1990a). A single amino acid exchange alters the pharmacology of neonatal rat glycine receptor subunit. *Neuron*, **5**, 867–73.

Kuhse, J., Schmieden, V. and Betz, H. (1990b). Identification and functional expression of a novel ligand binding subunit of the inhibitory glycine receptor. *J Biol Chem.*, **265**, 22317–20.

Kurczynski, T. W. (1983). Hyperekplexia. *Arch Neurol.*, **40**, 246–8.

Langosch, D., Becker, C. M. and Betz, H. (1990). The inhibitory glycine receptor: a ligand-gated chloride channel of the central nervous system. *Eur J Biochem.*, **194**, 1–8.

Langosch, D., Laube, B., Rundstrom, N., Schmieden, V., Bormann, J. and Betz, H. (1994). Decreased agonist affinity and chloride conductance of mutant glycine receptors associated with human hereditary hyperekplexia. *EMBO J.*, **13**, 4223–8.

Lees, A. J., Robertson, M., Trimble, M. R. and Murray, N. M. (1984). A clinical study of Gilles de la Tourette syndrome in the United Kingdom. *J Neurol Neurosurg Psychiatr.*, **47**, 1–8.

Leigh, P. N., Rothwell, J. C., Traub, M. and Marsden, C. D. (1980). A patient with reflex myoclonus and muscle rigidity: 'jerking stiff-man syndrome'. *J Neurol Neurosurg Psychiatr.*, **43**, 1125–31.

Lewis, T. M. and Schofield, P. R. (1999). Structure-function relationships of the human glycine receptor: insights from hyperekplexia mutations. *Ann NY Acad Sci.*, **868**, 681–4.

Lewis, T. M., Sivilotti, L. G., Colquhoun, D., Gardiner, R. M., Schoepfer, R. and Rees, M. (1998). Properties of human glycine receptors containing the hyperekplexia mutation alpha1(K276E), expressed in Xenopus oocytes. *J Physiol Lond.*, **507**, 25–40.

Lingam, S., Wilson, J. and Hart, E. W. (1981). Hereditary stiff-baby syndrome. *Am J Dis Child.*, **135**, 909–11.

Lynch, J. W., Rajendra, S., Pierce, K. D., Handford, C. A., Barry, P. H. and Schofield, P. R. (1997). Identification of intracellular and extracellular domains mediating signal transduction in the inhibitory glycine receptor chloride channel. *EMBO J.*, **16**, 110–20.

Manford, M. R., Fish, D. R. and Shorvon, S. D. (1996). Startle provoked epileptic seizures: features in 19 patients. *J Neurol Neurosurg Psychiatr.*, **61**, 151–6.

Markand, O. N., Garg, B. P. and Weaver, D. D. (1984). Familial startle disease (hyperexplexia). Electrophysiologic studies. *Arch Neurol.*, **41**, 71–4.

Matsumoto, J., Fuhr, P., Nigro, M. and Hallett, M. (1992). Physiological abnormalities in hereditary hyperekplexia. *Ann Neurol.*, **32**, 41–50.

Matzenbach, B., Maulet, Y., Sefton, L. *et al.* (1994). Structural analysis of mouse glycine receptor alpha subunit genes. Identification and chromosomal localization of a novel variant. *J Biol Chem.*, **269**, 2607–12.

McAbee, G. N., Kadakia, S. K., Sisley, K. C. and Delfiner, J. S. (1995). Complete heart block in nonfamilial hyperekplexia. *Pediatr Neurol.*, **12**, 149–51.

Melki, I., Rizkallah, E. and Akatcherian, C. (1988). (Hyperexplexia: the startle disease.) *Pediatrie*, **43**, 35–7.

Milani, N., Dalpra, L., del, P. A., Zanini, R. and Larizza, L. (1996). A novel mutation (Gln266→His) in the alpha 1 subunit of the inhibitory glycine-receptor gene (GLRA1) in hereditary hyperekplexia (letter). *Am J Hum Genet.*, **58**, 420–2.

Milani, N., Mulhardt, C., Weber, R. G. *et al.* (1998). The human glycine receptor beta subunit gene (GLRB): structure, refined chromosomal localization, and population polymorphism. *Genomics*, **50**, 341–5.

Moorhouse, A. J., Jacques, P., Barry, P. H. and Schofield,

P. R. (1999). The startle disease mutation Q266H, in the second transmembrane domain of the human glycine receptor, impairs channel gating. *Mol Pharmacol.*, **55**, 386–95.

Morley, D. J., Weaver, D. D., Garg, B. P. and Markand, O. (1982). Hyperekplexia: an inherited disorder of the startle response. *Clin Genet.*, **21**, 388–96.

Mumford, J. P. and Lewis, P. J. (1991). New antiepileptic drugs; *Vigabatrin*. Amsterdam.: Elsevier Science Publishers.

Nikolic, Z., Laube, B., Weber, R. G. *et al.* (1998). The human glycine receptor subunit alpha3. Glra3 gene structure, chromosomal localization, and functional characterization of alternative transcripts. *J Biol Chem.*, **273**, 19708–14.

Oldani, A., Zucconi, M., Asselta, R. *et al.* (1998). Autosomal dominant nocturnal frontal lobe epilepsy. A video-polysomnographic and genetic appraisal of 40 patients and delineation of the epileptic syndrome. *Brain*, **121**, 205–23.

Pascotto, A. and Coppola, G. (1992). Neonatal hyperekplexia: a case report. *Epilepsia*, **33**, 817–20.

Probst, A., Cortes, R. and P. J. (1986). The distribution of glycine receptors in the human brain. A light microscopic autoradiographic study using [$^3$H]strychnine. *Neuroscience*, **17**, 11–35.

Rajendra, S., Lynch, J. W., Pierce, K. D., French, C. P., Barry, P. H. and Schofield, P. R. (1994). Startle disease mutations reduce the agonist sensitivity of the human inhibitory glycine receptor. *J Biol Chem.*, **269**, 18739–42.

Rajendra, S., Lynch, J. W., Pierce, K. D., French, C. R., Barry, P. H. and Schofield, P. R. (1995). Mutation of an arginine residue in the human glycine receptor transforms beta-alanine and taurine from agonists into competitive antagonists. *Neuron*, **14**, 169–75.

Rajendra, S. and Schofield, P. R. (1995). Molecular mechanisms of inherited startle syndromes. *Trends Neurosci.*, **18**, 80–2.

Rees, M. I., Andrew, M., Jawad, S. and Owen, M. J. (1994). Evidence for recessive as well as dominant forms of startle disease (hyperekplexia) caused by mutations in the alpha 1 subunit of the inhibitory glycine receptor. *Hum Mol Genet.*, **3**, 2175–9.

Ryan, S. G., Buckwalter, M. S., Lynch, J. W. *et al.* (1994). A missense mutation in the gene encoding the alpha 1 subunit of the inhibitory glycine receptor in the spasmodic mouse. *Nat Genet.*, **7**, 131–5.

Ryan, S. G., Dixon, M. J., Nigro, M. A. *et al.* (1992a). Genetic and radiation hybrid mapping of the hyperekplexia region on chromosome 5q. *Am J Hum Genet.*, **51**, 1334–43.

Ryan, S. G., Sherman, S. L., Terry, J. C., Sparkes, R. S., Torres, M. C. and Mackey, R. W. (1992b). Startle disease, or hyperekplexia: response to clonazepam and assignment of the gene (STHE) to chromosome 5q by linkage analysis. *Ann Neurol.*, **31**, 663–8.

Saenz, L. E., Herranz, F. J. and Masdeu, J. C. (1984a).

Startle epilepsy: a clinical study. *Ann Neurol.*, **16**, 78–81.

Saenz, L. E., Herranz, T. F., Masdeu, J. C. and Chacon, P. J. (1984b). Hyperekplexia: a syndrome of pathological startle responses. *Ann Neurol.*, **15**, 36–41.

Sander, J. E., Layzer, R. B. and Goldsobel, A. B. (1980). Congenital stiff-man syndrome. *Ann Neurol.*, **8**, 195–7.

Sato, S. (1989). Benzodiazepines, Clonazepam. In *Antiepileptic Drugs*, 3rd edn. (eds Levy, R. H. *et al.*) pp.765–784. New York: Raven Press.

Saul, B., Kuner, T., Sobetzko, D. *et al.* (1999). Novel GLRA1 missense mutation (P250T) in dominant hyperekplexia defines an intracellular determinant of glycine receptor channel gating. *J Neurosci.*, **19**, 869–77.

Scarcella, A. and Coppola, G. (1997). Neonatal sporadic hyperekplexia: a rare and often unrecognized entity. *Brain Dev.*, **19**, 226–8.

Schofield, P. R., Darlison, M. G., Fujita, N. *et al.* (1987). Sequence and functional expression of the GABA A receptor shows a ligand-gated receptor super-family. *Nature*, **328**, 221–7.

Schorderet, D. F., Pescia, G., Bernasconi, A. and Regli, F. (1994). An additional family with Startle disease and a G1192A mutation at the alpha 1 subunit of the inhibitory glycine receptor gene. *Hum Mol Genet.*, **3**, 1201.

Seri, M., Bolino, A., Galietta, L. J., Lerone, M., Silengo, M. and Romeo, G. (1997). Startle disease in an Italian family by mutation (K276E): The alpha-subunit of the inhibiting glycine receptor. *Hum Mutat.*, **9**, 185–7.

Shahar, E., Brand, N., Uziel, Y. and Barak, Y. (1991). Nose tapping test inducing a generalized flexor spasm: a hallmark of hyperekplexia. *Acta Paed Scand.*, **80**, 1073–7.

Sheffield, V. C., Cox, D. R., Lerman, L. S. and Myers, R. M. (1989). Attachment of a 40-base-pair G + C-rich sequence (GC-clamp) to genomic DNA fragments by the polymerase chain reaction results in improved detection of single-base changes. *Proc Natl Acad Sci USA*, **86**, 232–6.

Shiang, R., Ryan, S. G., Zhu, Y. Z. *et al.* (1995). Mutational analysis of familial and sporadic hyperekplexia. *Ann .Neurol.*, **38**, 85–91.

Shiang, R., Ryan, S. G., Zhu, Y. Z., Hahn, A. F., O'Connell, P. and Wasmuth, J. J. (1993). Mutations in the alpha 1 subunit of the inhibitory glycine receptor cause the dominant neurologic disorder, hyperekplexia. *Nat Genet.*, **5**, 351–8.

Shibasaki, H., Kakigi, R., Oda, K. and Masukawa, S. (1988). Somatosensory and acoustic brain stem reflex myoclonus. *J Neurol Neurosurg Psychiatr.*, **51**, 572–5.

Simon, E. S. (1997). Phenotypic heterogeneity and disease course in three murine strains with mutations in genes encoding for alpha 1 and beta glycine receptor subunits. *Mov Disord.*, **12**, 221–8.

Stell, R., Thickbroom, G. W. and Mastaglia, F. L. (1995). The audiogenic startle response in Tourette's syndrome. *Mov Disord.*, **10**, 723–30.

Stephenson, J. B. (1992). Vigabatrin for startle-disease with altered cerebrospinal-fluid free gamma-aminobutyric acid (letter; comment). *Lancet*, **340**, 430–1.

Stevens, H. (1965). 'Jumping frenchman of Maine': myarichit. *Arch Neurol.*, **12**, 311–4.

Suhren, Bruyn, G. W. and Tuynman, A. (1966). Hyperexplexia, a hereditary startle syndrome. *J Neurol Sci.*, **3**, 577–605.

Thompson, P. D. (1993). Stiff muscles (editorial). *J Neurol Neurosurg Psychiatr.*, **56**, 121–4.

Thompson, P. D., Colebatch, J. G., Brown, P. *et al.* (1992). Voluntary stimulus-sensitive jerks and jumps mimicking myoclonus or pathological startle syndromes. *Mov Disord.*, **7**, 257–62.

Tijssen, M. A. J. and Brouwer, O. F. (2000). Hyperekplexia in the first year of life. *Mov Disord.*, **15**, 1293–6.

Tijssen, M. A., Shiang, R., van Deutekom, J. *et al.* (1995). Molecular genetic reevaluation of the Dutch hyperekplexia family. *Arch Neurol.*, **52**, 578–82.

Tijssen, M. A., Padberg, G. W. and van Dijk, J. G. (1996). The startle pattern in the minor form of hyperekplexia. *Arch Neurol.*, **53**, 608–13.

Tijssen, M. A., Voorkamp, L. M., Padberg, G. W. and van Dijk, J. G. (1997a). Startle responses in hereditary hyperekplexia. *Arch Neurol.*, **54**, 388–93.

Tijssen, M. A., Schoemaker, H. C., Edelbroek, P. J., Roos, R. A., Cohen, A. F. and van, D. J. (1997b). The effects of clonazepam and vigabatrin in hyperekplexia. *J Neurol Sci.*, **149**, 63–7.

Tijssen, M. A., Brown, P., Morris, H. R. and Lees, A. (1999). Late onset startle induced tics. *J Neurol Neurosurg Psychiatr.*, **67**, 782–4.

Tohier, C., Roze, J. C., David, A., Veccierini, M. F., Renaud, P. and Mouzard, A. (1991). Hyperexplexia or stiff baby syndrome (editorial). *Arch Dis Child.*, **66**, 460–1.

Turecki, G., Grand'Maison, F., Lemieux, B. and Rouleau, G. (1996). Hyperekplexia and the alpha1 subunit glycine receptor gene (GLRA1) (letter). *Arch Neurol.*, **53**, 836–7.

Vergouwe, M. N., Tijssen, M. A., Peters, A. C., Wielaard, R. and Frants, R. (1999). Hyperekplexia phenotype due to compound heterozygosity for GLRA1 gene mutations. *Ann Neurol.*, **46**, 634–8.

Vergouwe, M. N., Tijssen, M. A., Shiang, R., van, D. J., al, S. S., Ophoff, R. A. and Frants, R. R. (1997). Hyperekplexia-like syndromes without mutations in the GLRA1 gene. *Clin Neurol Neurosurg.*, **99**, 172–8.

Wartenberg, R. (1941). Head retraction reflex. *Am J Med Sci.*, **201**, 553–61.

Weaver, D. D., Morley, D. J., Garg, B. P. and Markand, O. (1982). Hyperexplexia: not hereditary stiff-baby syndrome (letter). *Am J Dis Child.*, **136**, 562.

White, W. F., O'Gorman, S. and Roe, A. W. (1990). Three-dimensional autoradiographic localization of quench-corrected glycine receptor specific activity in the mouse brain using $^3$H-strychnine as the ligand. *J Neurosci.*, **10**, 795–813.

Whiteley, A. M., Swash, M. and Urich, H. (1976). Progressive encephalomyelitis with rigidity. *Brain*, **99**, 27–42.

Winston, K. (1983). Hyperekplexia relieved by surgical decompression of the cervicomedullary region. *Neurosurgery*, **13**, 708–10.

Yap, P. M. (1951). Mental diseases peculiar to certain cultures. *J Ment Sci.*, **97**, 313–27.

Zafra, F., Aragon, C. and Gimenez, C. (1997). Molecular biology of glycinergic neurotransmission. (Review) (187 refs). *Mol Neurobiol.*, **14**, 117–42.

Zarbin, M. A., Wamsley, J. K. and Kuhar, M. J. (1981). Glycine receptor: light microscopic autoradiographic localization with [3H[strychnine. *J Neurosci.*, **1**, 532–47.

# Migraine: a multifactorial, neurovascular episodic channelopathy?

*Peter J. Goadsby and Michel D. Ferrari*

## Introduction

Migraine has come under particular focus as a common (Stewart *et al.*, 1992), disabling condition (Menken *et al.*, 2000) whose horizons were limited until the last 10 years. A model of migraine pathophysiology needs to explain several features: the mechanism of the pain and nausea, the centrally determined sensory sensitivity and behavioural aspects of migraine, and the episodic nature of the attacks. It is the episodic nature of migraine that is likely to be related to ion channel dysfunction as evidenced by known calcium channel gene abnormalities associated with some types of migraine. It is useful to review the overall pathophysiology of migraine before reviewing the recent discoveries concerning the role of calcium channel gene mutations in migraine (see Table 19.1). The role of the same calcium channel gene

in other diseases, some of which show overlap features with migraine, will be mentioned. Although the discovery of a proven calcium channel gene disorder in some types of migraine is exciting, it is appropriate to appreciate that migraine research has highlighted other possible genetic influences which will also be reviewed.

## Pathophysiology of migraine

### Anatomical considerations

Surrounding the large cerebral vessels, pial vessels, large venous sinuses and dura mater is a plexus of largely unmyelinated fibres that arise from the ophthalmic division of the trigeminal ganglion (McNaughton, 1938, 1966; Penfield and McNaughton, 1940) and in the posterior fossa

**Table 19.1 Bedside pathophysiology**

| Clinical feature | Possible pathophysiological substrate |
|---|---|
| *Pain*<br>  throbbing<br>  unilateral | Trigeminovascular system<br>pain-producing innervation of the large cranial vessels<br>trigeminal nerve/nucleus processing |
| *Nausea* | Trigeminal connections with caudal medial NTS |
| *Sensory sensitivity*<br>  head movement<br>  light<br>  sound<br>  smells | Abnormal brainstem modulation of sensory input, e.g. locus coeruleus |
| *Episodic attacks* | Channelopathic dysfunction in brainstem aminergic nociceptive control systems influencing trigeminovascular connections |

from the upper cervical dorsal roots (Arbab *et al.*, 1986, 1988). Trigeminal fibres innervating cerebral vessels arise from neurons in the trigeminal ganglion that contain substance P and calcitonin gene-related peptide (CGRP) (Uddman *et al.*, 1985), both of which can be released when the trigeminal ganglion is stimulated either in humans or cat (Goadsby *et al.*, 1988). Stimulation of the cranial vessels, such as the superior sagittal sinus (SSS), is certainly painful in humans (Feindel *et al.*, 1960). Human dural nerves that innervate the cranial vessels largely consist of small diameter myelinated and unmyelinated fibres that almost certainly subserve a nociceptive function (McNaughton and Feindel, 1977).

## Mechanisms of pain production

The source of pain in migraine is likely to be a combination of direct factors, such as activation of the nociceptors of pain-producing intracranial structures, and indirect factors, such as a reduction in the function of the endogenous pain control pathways (Goadsby *et al.*, 1991).

### Vascular mechanisms of pain

Distension of major cerebral vessels by balloon dilatation leads to pain referred to the ophthalmic division of the trigeminal nerve (Martins *et al.*, 1993; Nichols *et al.*, 1990, 1993). However, if the carotid artery is occluded ipsilateral to the side of headache in migraineurs then two-thirds will experience relief, yet the other one-third continue to have pain (Drummond and Lance, 1983). PET studies performed following injection of capsaicin into the forehead of volunteers without headache (May *et al.*, 1998b) resulted in a bilateral activation pattern that anatomically corresponds to intracranial arteries and the cavernous sinus. Similarly, in the cluster headache study there is a strong activation observed in the cavernous sinus during acute attacks of pain (May *et al.*, 1998a). Since vasodilatation is a feature of both cluster headache and capsaicin injection-induced headache, the vascular changes seem to occur whatever the trigger to the pain. These vascular changes could be due to either increased venous inflow from the superior ophthalmic vein draining the ophthalmic artery (Waldenlind *et al.*, 1993), or a longer transit time for the tracer in this region possibly due to an impeded venous drainage. Magnetic resonance angiography performed during NTG inhalation induced cluster headache shows dilatation of the internal carotid arteries bilaterally compared to the rest state (May *et al.*, 1999b). Bilateral dilation of the internal carotid artery suggests a neurally driven vasodilatation mediated by the ophthalmic division of the trigeminovascular system. In contrast studies of cerebral blood flow using both SPECT (Olesen *et al.*, 1990) and perfusion-weighted MRI (Cutrer *et al.*, 1998) have shown reduced blood flow persisting into the headache phase of migraine with aura.

Electrical stimulation of the trigeminal ganglion in both humans and the cat leads not only to increases in cerebral (Tran-Dinh *et al.*, 1992) and extracerebral blood flow (Drummond *et al.*, 1983), but also to local release of both calcitonin gene-related peptide (CGRP) and substance P (SP) (Goadsby *et al.*, 1988). In the cat trigeminal ganglion, stimulation also increases cerebral blood flow by a pathway traversing the greater superficial petrosal branch of the facial nerve (Goadsby and Duckworth, 1987) releasing a powerful vasodilator peptide, vasoactive intestinal polypeptide (VIP) (Goadsby *et al.*, 1984). Stimulation of the more specifically vascular pain-producing superior sagittal sinus increases cerebral blood flow (Lambert *et al.*, 1988) and jugular vein CGRP levels (Zagami *et al.*, 1990).

In humans CGRP is elevated in the headache phase of migraine (Goadsby *et al.*, 1990; Gallai *et al.*, 1995), cluster headache (Goadsby and Edvinsson, 1994; Fanciullacci *et al.*, 1995) and chronic paroxysmal hemicrania (Goadsby and Edvinsson, 1996). Furthermore, CGRP infusion will trigger headache, some clearly migrainous, in humans (Lassen *et al.*, 1998).

The vascular changes are likely to be an epiphenomenon of activation of the trigeminovascular system (Goadsby and Duckworth, 1987). The data suggest that activation of the trigeminal system triggers either impeded venous drainage or increase in arterial flow in the region of these vessels. Headache does not, therefore, require vasodilatation. At a physiological level the common link in primary neurovascular headache and experimental headache is the involvement of the ophthalmic division of the trigeminal nerve by a neurally driven dilatation of the carotid vessels.

## Plasma protein extravasation in pain production

Neurogenic plasma protein extravasation (PPE) can be seen during electrical stimulation of the trigeminal ganglion in the rat (Markowitz *et al.*, 1987). PPE can be blocked by ergot alkaloids (Markowitz *et al.*, 1988), indomethacin, acetylsalicylic acid (Buzzi *et al.*, 1989), and the serotonin, $5-HT_{1B/1D}$, agonist, sumatriptan (Moskowitz and Cutrer, 1993). In addition, trigeminal ganglion stimulation can result in dural mast cell degranulation (Dimitriadou *et al.*, 1991) and platelet aggregation in post-capillary venules (Dimitriadou *et al.*, 1992). These changes and the initiation of a sterile inflammatory response would cause pain (Strassman *et al.*, 1996; Burstein *et al.*, 1998), but it is not clear whether this is sufficient on its own or requires other stimulators or promoters. Blockade of neurogenic PPE is not completely predictive of antimigraine efficacy in humans as evidenced by the failure in clinical trials of substance P, neurokinin-1 antagonists (Diener, 1996; Goldstein *et al.*, 1997; Connor *et al.*, 1998; Norman *et al.*, 1998), specific PPE blockers, CP122,288 (Roon *et al.*, 2000) and 4991w93 (Earl *et al.*, 1999), an endothelin antagonist, bosentan (May *et al.*, 1996) and a neurosteriod, ganaxolone (Data *et al.*, 1998). Moreover, although plasma extravasation in the retina that is blocked by sumatriptan is seen after trigeminal ganglion stimulation in rat, no changes are seen with retinal angiography during acute attacks of migraine or cluster headache (May *et al.*, 1998c).

## Central processing in migraine

Using Fos immunohistochemistry as a method for anatomically defining activated neurons shows that stimulation of the superior sagittal sinus induces Fos-like immunoreactivity in the trigeminal nucleus caudalis and in the dorsal horn at the $C_1$ and $C_2$ levels in the cat (Kaube *et al.*, 1993) and monkey (Goadsby and Hoskin, 1997). Using 2-deoxyglucose measurements after superior sagittal sinus stimulation it has also been shown that neuronal activity is increased in the trigeminal nucleus caudalis and in the dorsal horn at the $C_1$ and $C_2$ levels (Goadsby and Zagami, 1991). These findings suggest that the trigeminal nucleus extends beyond the traditional nucleus caudalis to the dorsal horn of the high cervical region in a functional continuum that could be regarded as a *trigeminocervical complex*. This structure provides second order neurons for the entire set of intracranial pain-producing structures. This arrangement explains why patients with primary headache complain of pain in the head that does not respect the cutaneous distribution of either the trigeminal or cervical nerves. Moreover, stimulation of a lateralized structure, the middle meningeal artery, produces Fos expression bilaterally in both cat and monkey brain (Hoskin *et al.*, 1999), a finding that is consistent with the fact that up to one-third of patients complain of bilateral pain.

Following transmission in the caudal brainstem and high cervical spinal cord information is relayed in a group of fibres (the quintothalamic tract) to the thalamus. Processing of vascular pain in experimental animals in the thalamus occurs in the ventroposteromedial thalamus, medial nucleus of the posterior complex and in the intralaminar thalamus (Zagami and Goadsby, 1991). Zagami and Lambert (1991) have shown, by application of capsaicin to the superior sagittal sinus, that trigeminal projections with a high degree of nociceptive input are processed in neurons particularly in the ventroposteromedial thalamus and in its ventral periphery. Human imaging studies have confirmed activation of thalamus contralateral to pain in acute cluster headache (May *et al.*, 1998a) and in SUNCT (short-lasting unilateral neuralgiform headache with conjunctival injection and tearing) (May *et al.*, 1999a). The properties and further higher centre connections of these neurons are the subject of ongoing studies that will allow us to build up a more complete picture of the trigeminovascular pain pathways (Table 19.2).

Activation of the rostral brainstem has been seen using PET during acute migraine without

**Table 19.2 Neuroanatomical processing of vascular head pain**

| | Structure | Comments |
|---|---|---|
| *Target innervation*: cranial vessels dura mater | Ophthalmic branch of trigeminal nerve | |
| 1st | Trigeminal ganglion | Middle cranial fossa |
| 2nd | Trigeminal nucleus (*quintothalamic tract*) | Trigeminal n. caudalis and C1/C2 dorsal horns |
| 3rd | Thalamus | Ventrobasal complex Medial n. of posterior group Intralaminar complex |
| Final | Cortex | Insulae Frontal cortex Anterior cingulate cortex Basal ganglia |

aura (Weiller *et al.*, 1995). The brainstem areas were active during headache and immediately after successful treatment of the headache, but are not active interictally, whereas cingulate cortex and visual and auditory association cortex were only active during headache and not after treatment. This differentiation suggests that the brainstem activation represented some fundamental part of the disorder not simply a response to pain. The activation corresponds with the brain region that Raskin (1987) initially reported, and Veloso confirmed (Veloso *et al.*, 1998), to cause migraine-like headache when stimulated in patients with electrodes implanted for pain control.

It has been shown in the experimental animal that stimulation of a discrete nucleus in the brainstem, nucleus locus coeruleus (the main central noradrenergic nucleus) reduces cerebral blood flow in a frequency-dependent manner (Goadsby *et al.*, 1982) through an $\alpha_2$-adrenoceptor-linked mechanism (Goadsby *et al.*, 1985). This reduction is maximal in the occipital cortex (Goadsby and Duckworth, 1989). While a 25% overall reduction in cerebral blood flow is seen, extracerebral vasodilatation occurs in parallel (Goadsby *et al.*, 1982). In addition, the main serotonin-containing nucleus in the brainstem, the midbrain dorsal raphe nucleus, can increase cerebral blood flow

when activated (Goadsby *et al.*, 1991). Most recently it has been shown that stimulation of this ventrolateral periaqueductal grey region will inhibit sagittal sinus evoked trigeminal neuronal activity in cat (Knight and Goadsby, 1999). It seems that rostral brainstem areas play a pivotal, if not defining role, in migraine and may be considered the generator for migraine.

## The migraine threshold: role of genetics

Transmission of migraine from parents to children has been reported as early as the seventeenth century (Willis, 1682). Since then, numerous studies have reported a positive family history of migraine (Russell, 1997). Many of these reports were imprecise and, because the relatives were usually not directly interviewed, information on their exact migraine subtype is lacking (Leone *et al.*, 1994; Rasmussen *et al.*, 1991; Russell *et al.*, 1996a). Direct clinical interviews by physicians are indispensable in family studies of migraine.

Multiple genetic factors are believed to be involved in migraine and attacks appear to involve physiological mechanisms initiated by migraine-specific triggers. Genetic factors seem to set the individual threshold and both endogenous and exogenous factors modulate this set point (Ferrari, 1998). The search for genetic risk factors for multifactorial paroxysmal diseases, such as migraine, is complicated by a number of clinical, genetic and statistical problems. Major clinical issues are how to determine whether or not a person is affected and how to distinguish likely gene carriers from possible phenocopies. While early onset and severe clinical course are traditionally regarded as indicators for a genetic background, it is unclear how one should deal with episodic disorders. Are the number of attacks or their severity indicators of the presence of genetic risk factors, or are these merely a consequence of the frequency and intensity of the exposure to environmental triggers?

## Population studies

Clinical, epidemiological, pathophysiological and genetic differences suggest that migraine without aura and migraine with aura may be, in part, distinct entities (Olesen et al., 1981a, b; Rasmussen and Olesen, 1992; Russell and Olesen, 1995; Russell et al., 1996b). An argument against this notion, however, is that both types of migraine frequently coexist in patients, or may occur after each other over a lifetime (Ferrari, 1998; Launer et al., 1999). Nevertheless, for scientific purposes it may be wise to analyse the two subtypes of migraine separately.

## Migraine without aura

### Genetic epidemiological surveys

Table 19.3 shows the relative risk (odds ratio) or population relative risk of migraine without aura in different genetic epidemiological surveys (Mochi et al., 1993; Russell and Olesen, 1995; Stewart et al., 1997). First degree relatives of probands with migraine without aura had increased risks of migraine with aura and migraine without aura, both compared to first degree relatives of probands without migraine (relative risk), and compared to the risk of migraine without aura in the general population (population relative risk).

## Twin studies

Studies of twin pairs are the classical method to investigate the relative importance of genetic and environmental factors. A Danish study included 1013 monozygotic and 1667 dizygotic twin pairs of the same gender, from a population based twin register (Ulrich et al., 1999). Table 19.4 shows the number of concordant and discordant twin pairs. The pairwise concordance rate was significantly higher among monozygotic than dizygotic twin pairs ($P < 0.05$).

Both twin studies and population-based epidemiological surveys strongly suggest that migraine without aura is a multifactorial disorder, caused by a combination of genetic and environmental factors.

## Migraine with aura

### Genetic epidemiological surveys

Table 19.3 shows the relative risk (odds ratio) or population relative risk of migraine with aura in different genetic epidemiological surveys (Mochi et al., 1993; Kalfakis et al., 1996; Russell et al., 1996b; Stewart et al., 1997). All the studies except the American one showed an increased risk of migraine with aura among first-degree relatives. In the US study (Stewart et al., 1997), the family members were only asked about their most severe type of headache. The International Headache Society's criteria for migraine with aura were adjusted in such a way that the requirements of the headache characteristics were similar to those of migraine without aura (Headache Classification Committee of The International Headache Society, 1988). This may have caused an underestimation of migraine with aura since the headache in that type is often less severe than it is in migraine without aura (Rasmussen and Olesen, 1992; Russell and Olesen, 1995). Furthermore, for an unerring diagnosis of migraine with aura, interviews by physicians are to be preferred. Thus, the US survey seems inconclusive for the family risk of migraine with aura.

### Twin studies

In a large Danish population-based twin survey, the pair-wise concordance rate was significantly

**Table 19.3 Participants in genetic epidemiological surveys of migraine without aura (MO) and migraine with aura (MA)**

| Disease in probands | Study population | Disease in first degree relatives | No. of probands | First degree relatives | | Relative risk[1] | Population relative risk[2] | 95% Confidence intervals |
|---|---|---|---|---|---|---|---|---|
| | | | | No. of affected | No. of total | | | |
| *Migraine without aura* | | | | | | | | |
| Mochi et al. (1993) | Clinic | MO | 34 | 64 | 171 | 3.62 | | 1.10–6.14 |
| | | MO | | 102 | 354 | | 1.86 | 1.56–2.16 |
| Russell and Olesen (1995) | General | MA | 126 | 42 | | | 1.44 | 1.03–1.85 |
| | | MO | | 30 | | 1.43 | | 0.83–2.47 |
| Stewart et al.(1997)* | General | MA | 45 | 10 | 156 | 2.36 | | 0.87–6.38 |
| *Migraine with aura* | | | | | | | | |
| Mochi et al. (1993) | Clinic | MA | 35 | 13 | 144 | 6.95 | | 3.15–10.75 |
| | | MA | | 111 | | | 3.79 | 3.21–4.38 |
| Russell and Olesen (1995) | General | MO | 127 | 56 | 359 | | 1.02 | 0.77–1.26 |
| Kalfakis et al. (1996) | Clinic | MA | 60 | 58 | 328 | 11.85 | | 7.00–16.70 |
| | | MA | | 3 | | 1.24 | | 0.28–5.47 |
| Stewart et al. (1997)* | General | MO | 28 | 17 | 87 | 1.41 | | 0.71–2.77 |

[1] First degree relatives of probands with migraine compared with first degree relatives of probands who had never had migraine.
[2] First degree relatives of probands with migraine compared with the risk of migraine in the general population.
* Probands were interviewed by a physician, while first degree relatives were interviewed by lay interviewers.

higher among monozygotic than dizygotic twin pairs ($P < 0.001$; Table 19.4) (Gervil et al., 1998; Ulrich et al., 1999). Analysing each gender separately showed a significant difference in women and a similar trend in men ($P = 0.002$ and $P = 0.07$).

Both twin studies and population-based epidemiological surveys strongly suggest that migraine with aura is also a multifactorial disorder, caused by a combination of genetic and environmental factors.

It is possible that migraine aura may require separate *aura genes* which may not be sufficient to cause aura or headache without the *headache genes*.

## Migraine as a cerebral calcium channelopathy

### Migraine as a channelopathy: clinical arguments

Migraine has many general clinical characteristics in common with established neurological channelopathies. These include a paroxysmal presentation with attacks that can be provoked by both endogenous and exogenous stimuli, which may last from minutes to hours or days, and which may come in a frequency ranging from once in a lifetime to one per day. Onset is usually at puberty, amelioration and complete remission may occur after age 40, and penetrance and expression is gender-related (F. Lehman-Horn 1997; personal communication).

Hormones are likely to be of importance in migraine. There is a female preponderance among migraine patients and in females attacks may be triggered by menstruation and temporarily prevented by pregnancy. An influence of hormones on ion channels has been considered in hypokalaemic and hyperkalaemic periodic paralysis, primarily mediated via an effect on calcium rather than potassium channels (Joels and Karst, 1995; Lehmann-Horn and Rudel, 1996).

### Familial hemiplegic migraine: clinical features and linkage data

Familial hemiplegic migraine (FHM) is a rare autosomal dominantly inherited subtype of migraine with aura (Headache Classification Committee of The International Headache Society, 1988). Patients with FHM have attacks of migraine with aura which, in addition to the typical migraine aura and headache symptoms, are associated with hemiparesis. In some FHM families

**Table 19.4 The numbers of concordant and discordant monozygotic (MZ) and dizygotic (DZ) twin pairs of the same gender. Concordance rates are in percentages**

|  | Men | | Women | | Overall | |
|---|---|---|---|---|---|---|
|  | MZ | DZ | MZ | DZ | MZ | DZ |
| *Migraine without aura* | | | | | | |
| Concordant pairs | 8 | 6 | 30 | 41 | 38 | 47 |
| Discordant pairs | 39 | 69 | 60 | 141 | 99 | 210 |
| Pairwise concordance rate | 17 | 8 | 33 | 23 | 28 | 18* |
| Probandwise concordance rate | 29 | 15 | 50 | 37 | 43 | 31 |
| *Migraine with aura* | | | | | | |
| Concordant pairs | 12 | 10 | 14 | 6 | 26 | 16 |
| Discordant pairs | 21 | 48 | 30 | 70 | 51 | 118 |
| Pairwise concordance rate | 36 | 17 | 32 | 8 | 34 | 12+ |
| Probandwise concordance rate | 53 | 29 | 48 | 15 | 50 | 21 |

*$P = 0.04$.
+$P = 0.004$.

there may be associated progressive cerebellar ataxia and cerebellar atrophy on MRI scan. Patients may also have attacks of 'non-hemiplegic' typical migraine with or without aura. In FHM families there may be individuals with FHM and with 'non-hemiplegic' typical migraine. This strongly suggests that FHM is part of the migraine spectrum, and that genes involved in FHM are candidate genes for 'non-hemiplegic' typical migraine with and without aura.

In approximately 50% of the reported families, FHM has been linked to chromosome 19p13 (Joutel et al., 1994; Ophoff et al., 1994). Recently, two groups also found linkage to chromosome 1 (Ducros et al., 1997; Gardner et al., 1997). The North-American group showed, in one large family, a lod score of 3.04 at $\lambda = 0.09$ with marker D1S249 on chromosome 1q31 (Gardner et al., 1997), whereas the French group showed linkage to chromosome 1q21-q23 in three FHM families (Ducros et al., 1997). Further analysis may determine whether chromosome 1q harbours one or two FHM genes. There remain some FHM families that could not be linked to either chromosome 19 or 1, indicating that at least a third gene must be involved in FHM (Ducros et al., 1997).

Only few clinical differences have been found between chromosome 19-linked and unlinked FHM families. The most striking exception is cerebellar ataxia, which occurs in approximately 50% of the chromosome 19-linked, but in none of the unlinked families (Joutel et al., 1993, 1994; Haan et al., 1994; Ophoff et al., 1994; Teh et al., 1995). Other less striking differences include the observation that patients from chromosome 19-linked families are more likely to have attacks which can be triggered by minor head trauma or which are associated with coma (Terwindt et al., 1996).

## Mutations in the P/Q type calcium channel $\alpha_{1A}$-subunit gene in FHM

Using exon trapping, a human cDNA highly homologous to a brain-specific rabbit and rat voltage gated P/Q type calcium channel $\alpha_{1A}$-subunit gene was identified at the 10p13 locus (Mori et al., 1991; Starr et al., 1991). The human gene was originally designated CACNL1A4 (Diriong et al., 1995), but subsequently renamed CACNA1A (Lory et al., 1997).

Initially, four different missense mutations were identified in five unrelated FHM families (see Figure 19.1) (Ophoff et al., 1996).

A transition from G to A was identified resulting in an arginine to glutamine substitution (R192Q) within the fourth segment of the first membrane-spanning domain (IS4). The highly conserved S4 segment is thought to be part of the voltage sensor.

The second mutation occurred within the pore-forming (P) hairpin loop of the second domain replacing a threonine residue for methionine (T666M). These conserved P-segments, located between each S5 and S6, are involved in the ion-selectivity of ion channels and present binding sited for toxins (Dunlap et al., 1995).

Two other mutations were located in the sixth transmembrane spanning segment of repeats II and IV. The IIS6 mutation was a T-to-C transition at codon 714, resulting in a valine-to-alanine substitution (V714A). The IVS6 mutation was an A-to-C transversion at codon 1811 that resulted in a substitution of isoleucine for leucine (I1811L) and was found in two independent FHM families. The S6 mutations do not actually change the neutral-polar nature of the amino acid residues, but the original residues are conserved in all calcium channel $\alpha_1$ subunit genes described (Stea et al., 1995). Residues in the S6 transmembrane segments may be of influence in the inactivation of the calcium channel (Hering et al., 1996).

Subsequently, 10 more missense mutations have been found, making a total of 14 known missense mutations associated with FHM (See Figure 19.2). Six of these cause pure FHM and the other eight have been associated with FHM plus cerebellar ataxia; two of these latter mutations were also found in a few sporadic patients with hemiplegic migraine.

## FHM mutations alter the calcium channel function

Kraus and colleagues (1998) introduced FHM mutations into rabbit $\alpha_{1A}$-subunits, which show a 94% sequence identity with the human gene, and

# FHM mutations in the $\alpha_{1A}$ Ca$^{2+}$ channel subunit gene (CACNA1A)

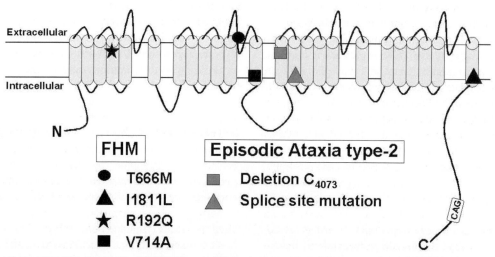

**Figure 19.1** Mutations in the CACNA1A $\alpha_{1A}$ calcium channel subunit gene responsible for familial hemiplegic migraine (FHM) and episodic ataxia type (EA-2) as originally described by Ophoff *et al.* 1996.

# FHM mutations in the $\alpha_{1A}$ Ca$^{2+}$ channel subunit gene (CACNA1A)

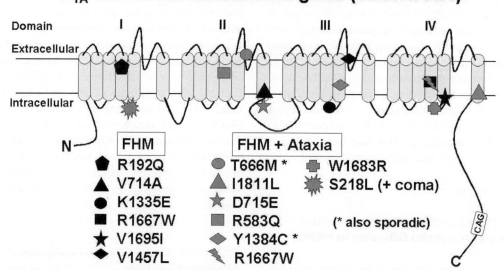

**Figure 19.2** Additional mutations in the CACNA1A $\alpha_{1A}$ calcium channel subunit gene causing familial hemiplegic migraine in either 'pure' form or in association with cerebellar ataxia. Two of the mutations (indicated with an asterix) were found in a few cases of 'sporadic' migraine. Other mutations in this gene (not illustrated) cause progressive ataxia, spino-cerebellar ataxia type 6, and tottering/leaner mice (see chapters 15 and 16).

functionally expressed the mutant subunits in *Xenopus laevis* oocytes without other calcium channel subunits. They found that all but one of the FHM mutations (R192Q) altered the inactivation gating of the calcium channels, increasing or decreasing their functional availability. Hans and colleagues (1999) introduced FHM mutations into human $\alpha_{1A}$ calcium channel subunits and co-expressed them in HEK-293 cells with other regulatory subunits. They also found both loss- and gain-of-function effects, depending on the specific mutation. Further studies are needed to establish fully the functional consequences of these mutations in human $\alpha_{1A}$-subunits and calcium channels.

Abnormalities in the 19p13 calcium channel gene also cause, depending on the site and nature of the mutations, other episodic and chronic cerebral and cerebellar disorders. These disorders include Episodic Ataxia type 2 (EA-2) and Spinocerebellar Ataxia type 6 (SCA-6) in human, and epilepsy and episodic ataxia in the leaner and tottering mice (see Chapters 16 and 17). The tottering mouse may be considered a possible animal model for migraine. Tottering mutations have mutations affecting $\alpha_{1A}$ calcium channel subunits which lead to profound effects on the function of calcium channels. They reduce the calcium influx and current density, are associated with apoptosis and cerebellar atrophy (Wakamori *et al.*, 1998; Caddick *et al.*, 1999), reduce the thalamic and cortical release of glutamate (Caddick *et al.*, 1999), increase (10-fold) the resistance to, and slow down the spread of cortical spreading depression (Ayata *et al.*, 2000), and increase spontaneous release of acetylcholine at the neuromuscular junction (Plomp *et al.*, 2000). This latter finding is in line with a preliminary observation that some migraine patients may show subclinical single fibre EMG abnormalities (Ambrosini *et al.*, 1999).

## Expression of the CACNA1A gene

Preliminary investigations have shown that the CACNA1A gene is primarily expressed in the human cerebellar and occipital cortex, the hippocampus, and the upper brainstem. The latter location is of particular interest because of the apparent overlap with the postulated site of the migraine generator (Weiller *et al.*, 1995). Thus, abnormalities in calcium channel function can be topographically correlated to the area in the brain believed to be involved with the onset of migraine attacks. The hypothesis of a calcium channel dysfunction-mediated reduced local threshold for migraine onset seems possible but remains unproven.

## Involvement of the CACNA1A gene in 'non-hemiplegic' typical migraine

Two independent affected sib-pair analysis studies (May *et al.*, 1995) and one classical linkage study (Nyholt *et al.*, 1998b) have demonstrated the likely involvement of the chromosome 19 calcium channel gene in typical 'non-hemiplegic' migraine. In a first, limited sib-pair analysis study in 28 mainly German families with migraine with and without aura, tentative evidence was found that the FHM locus on chromosome 19p13 is involved in 'non-hemiplegic' typical migraine with and without aura (May *et al.*, 1995). The results, however, were inconclusive as to the magnitude of the involvement and the relative importance of migraine with or without aura. Subsequently, in a larger second and independent affected sib-pair analysis involving 36 extended Dutch families with migraine with and without aura, significant increased sharing of the marker alleles in sibs with migraine with aura (maximum multipoint lod score MLS = 1.29 corresponding with $P < 0.013$) was confirmed (Terwindt *et al.*, 1996). No such increased sharing was found for migraine without aura. A combined analysis for both migraine types, including sib pairs in which one had migraine with aura and the other migraine without aura, resulted in a higher increased allele sharing (MLS = 1.69 corresponding with $P < 0.005$). The relative risk ratio for a sib ($\lambda_s$) to suffer from migraine with aura, defined as the increase in risk of the trait attributable to the 19p13 locus, was $\lambda_s = 2.4$. When combining migraine with and without aura, $\lambda_s$ was 1.25. When the results of both studies were combined, the maximum multipoint lod score increased to 2.27 ($P < 0.001$).

In a classical linkage study in one large multi-generational family including 17 available affected members with migraine with or without aura, linkage was demonstrated with the chromosome 19 FHM locus (Nyholt *et al.*, 1998b). In addition, evidence was found for heterogeneity, since linkage to the chromosome 19 FHM locus could be excluded in three other migraine families.

Finally, in a genotype-phenotype relation study the I1811L FHM mutation was found to occur both in patients with FHM and in two family members with 'non-hemiplegic' typical migraine (Terwindt *et al.*, 1998c). This supports the notion that FHM is part of the migraine spectrum and that other, as yet unknown factors modulate the clinical expression of the gene defect.

## Possible role of calcium channels in migraine pathophysiology

Indirect evidence supports a possible role for calcium channels in migraine pathophysiology, both at the onset of attacks and in the aura- and headache-phases. Calcium acts as an intracellular second messenger by initiating or regulating numerous biochemical and electrical events in the cell. Calcium ions are implicated in the regulation of several enzymes and for the control of the activity of several other ion channels (de Waard *et al.*, 1996). They also control many neuronal events such as neurotransmitter release (Gaur *et al.*, 1994; Dunlap *et al.*, 1995; Uchitel *et al.*, 1997), synaptogenesis, and neurite outgrowth (de Waard *et al.*, 1996). P/Q type calcium channels seem to be more effective in modulating neurotransmitter release than other channel types (Mintz *et al.*, 1995). P-type neuronal $Ca^{2+}$ channels mediate neurotransmitter release including 5-HT (Codignola *et al.*, 1993; Frittoli *et al.*, 1994). Conversely, serotonin acts at $5-HT_{2c}$ receptors to increase intracellular calcium activity in choroid plexus epithelial cells, both by liberating $Ca^{2+}$ from intracellular stores and by activating a $Ca^{2+}$ influx pathway (Watson *et al.*, 1995). In rat, motoneurons serotonin inhibits N- and P-type calcium currents (Bayliss *et al.*, 1995).

Calcium and other ion channels are also pivotal to the mechanism of cortical spreading depression (CSD) (Lauritzen, 1994). Thus, impaired function of cerebral calcium channels could alter the susceptibility for CSD and consequently the migraine aura. $Mg^{2+}$ is also known to interfere with $Ca^{2+}$ channels (Altura, 1985; Zhang *et al.*, 1992). Magnetic resonance spectroscopy studies suggest that intracellular brain magnesium is reduced in migraine patients and that the regional distribution of brain magnesium is altered in patients with FHM (Ramadan *et al.*, 1996).

## Other CACNA1A gene disorders

Episodic ataxia 2 (EA-2) (see Chapter 15) has been linked to the same interval on chromosome 19p as FHM (Teh *et al.*, 1995), and mutation analysis revealed two different truncating mutations in the CACNA1A calcium channel gene in two unrelated EA-2 families (see Figure 19.1) (Ophoff *et al.*, 1996). Patients with episodic ataxia 2 may have migraine-like symptoms, both between and during the attacks of ataxia (Hawkes, 1992; Moon and Koller, 1991; Vahedi *et al.*, 1995). Magnetic resonance imaging may show cerebellar atrophy in EA-2 (Vighetto *et al.*, 1988; Joutel *et al.*, 1993; Haan *et al.*, 1994). Mutations of the CACNA1A gene can also result in a progressive spinocerebellar ataxia type 6 (see Chapter 15), in this case consisting of small triplet expansions of the intragenic CAG repeat ranging from 21 to 30 repeat units as compared with the normal 4 to 20 repeats (Matsuyama *et al.*, 1997; Riess *et al.*, 1997; Zhuchenko *et al.*, 1997).

As both chromosome 19-linked FHM families and EA-2 families may develop progressive cerebellar ataxia and atrophy (Joutel *et al.*, 1993, 1994; Haan *et al.*, 1994; Ophoff *et al.*, 1994) screening for CAG repeat expansion in FHM and EA-2 families with chronic cerebellar ataxia has been performed to answer the question whether the FHM or EA-2 mutations are capable of causing chronic progressive cerebellar ataxia independent of the number of CAG repeats. So far, in the investigated FHM families with associated ataxia, no evidence for CAG repeat expansions has been obtained, suggesting that the FHM point mutations (e.g. the I1811L mutation) suffice to cause both FHM and cerebellar atrophy and ataxia.

# Other possible migraine susceptibility genes

## Associations of migraine and other hereditary disorders

A number of hereditary disorders may be associated with migraine. These include epilepsy, cluster headache, dyslipoproteinaemias, hereditary haemorrhagic telangiectasia, Tourette's syndrome, autosomal dominant alternating hemiplegia of childhood, several psychiatric disorders, the Stormorken syndrome, hereditary essential tremor, mitochondrial disorders, cerebral cavernous malformations, hereditary cerebral amyloid angiopathy, and a recently described combination of migraine, vascular retinopathy and Raynaud's disease (Terwindt et al., 1998a). Such associations may provide candidate genes for migraine when the causative gene for the disorder is known. In the next paragraphs some of the most interesting and promising associations will be discussed.

## CADASIL

In cerebral autosomal dominant arteriopathy with subcortical infarcts and leukoencephalopathy (CADASIL), affected individuals exhibit a variety of symptoms, including recurrent subcortical ischaemic strokes, progressive vascular dementia, and mood disorders with severe depression (Chabriat et al., 1995b). Remarkably, migraine with aura occurs in up to one-third of patients in CADASIL pedigrees (Chabriat et al., 1995b; Jung et al., 1995; Verin et al., 1995). One CADASIL family has been described with typical FHM attacks (Hutchinson et al., 1995), and a family, linked to the CADASIL locus, has been reported with migraine and CADASIL-like white matter lesions on magnetic resonance imaging (Chabriat et al., 1995a). All these observations contributed to the clinical spectrum of migraine-FHM-CADASIL. The CADASIL locus was mapped to chromosome 19 (Tournier-Lasserve et al., 1993) and initially CADASIL and FHM were considered to be allelic (Joutel et al., 1993). However, further linkage studies narrowed the CADASIL gene region and argued against allelism of CADASIL and FHM

(Dichgans et al., 1996; Ducros et al., 1996). Recently, a Notch3 gene was identified in the CADASIL critical region (Joutel et al., 1996). Fifty-one unrelated CADASIL patients were screened for mutations in the Notch3 gene. Twenty-three distinct mutations were identified in 39 unrelated patients; seven mutations were recurrent without signs of a founder effect. All 23 mutations were located within the extracellular domain of the gene which contains 34 epidermal growth factor repeats (EGF). Twenty-one are missense mutations, predicted to create or delete a cysteine residue, the last two are splice sites mutations (Joutel et al., 1997). Notch codes for a glycosylated transmembrane receptor, which is involved in intercellular signalling essential for proper embryonic development in Drosophila (Artavanis-Tsakonas et al., 1995; de Celis and Garcia-Bellido, 1994). The Notch gene has closely related homologues in the nematode Caenorhabditis elegans, Xenopus, mouse and humans suggesting that the Notch function has been widely conserved throughout evolution (de Celis and Garcia-Bellido, 1994). Another Notch family receptor in C. elegans, called the sel-12 gene (Levitan and Greenwald, 1995), is highly homologous to the mammalian presenilin genes, PS-1 and PS-2, that are involved in Alzheimer's disease (Cruts et al., 1996). Thus, the Notch-receptor genes are important in age-related dementia syndromes. The finding of separate genes for CADASIL and FHM show that these diseases are genetically unrelated. The question remains, however, why migraine with aura occurs so frequently in CADASIL. In the above described family with migraine and CADASIL-like white matter abnormalities (Chabriat et al., 1995a), Notch3 splice site mutations were recently found to be responsible, clearly supporting the notion that defects in this gene can cause migraine.

## Mitochondrial disorders

Mitochondrial function is encoded by two physically separate genomes, the mitochondrial and the nuclear genome. Diseases caused by alterations of the mitochondrial genome have a maternal inheritance, because mitochondrial DNA is transmitted exclusively from mothers to their children. As many migraine families show a predominant maternal inheritance pattern, migraine could be associated with mitochondrial dysfunction. Associations between migraine and possible mitochondrial disorders have been reviewed by Haan and colleagues (1994). The most prominent association is with MELAS; many patients with MELAS, and their relatives suffer from migraine. Screening for mitochondrial DNA mutations in migraine patients has been inconclusive (Haan *et al.*, 1997).

## X-Linked migraine genes

There is a strong preponderance of females among migraineurs. Nyholt and colleagues (1998a) therefore studied three large multigenerational typical migraine pedigrees and found evidence of significant excess allele sharing to chromosome Xq markers in two families. This could indicate that X-linked genetic factors are associated with an increased risk of migraine with and without aura.

## Dopamine D2 receptor genes

There are several arguments to implicate the dopaminergic system in the onset of migraine attacks. In an association study, increased frequency of the dopamine DRD2 receptor NcoI alleles was observed among patients with migraine with aura (Peroutka *et al.*, 1997). These results should, however, be regarded as preliminary evidence and independent confirmation is needed.

## Genes implicated in the serotonin system

Serotonin (5-HT) is clearly implicated in migraine pathophysiology (Goadsby, 1998). In an association study, Ogilvie and colleagues (1998) found some preliminary evidence of involvement of the serotonin transporter gene in migraine patients, but this finding clearly needs further confirmation. The 5-HT$_{2A}$ receptor gene has been assigned to chromosome 13q14-q21. No evidence for linkage to migraine without aura was found in three large

multigenerational pedigrees using the classical linkage approach (Nyholt *et al.*, 1996). Since such an approach presumes one gene to be involved in the disease under investigation, linkage cannot be excluded, although this was stated as such in the publication.

## Nitric oxide synthase genes

Nitric oxide (NO) has been implicated in the pathophysiology of migraine (Olesen *et al.*, 1994). In a small association study, no evidence was found for an association between migraine and the endothelial NO synthase (NOS3) gene (Griffiths *et al.*, 1997). No data are available on a possible association between migraine and the other NOS genes.

## Vascular retinopathy, Raynaud and migraine

Terwindt and colleagues (1998a) described an extended Dutch family with autosomal dominant vascular retinopathy, migraine and Raynaud's phenomenon. Retinopathy occurred in 20 family members, migraine in 65, and Raynaud in 50. A combination of all three symptoms was found in 11 subjects. Thus far 75% of the genome, including the CACNA1A gene, has been excluded and further genome search is underway. Identification of the responsible gene will certainly improve the further understanding of genes involved in vascular disorders including migraine.

## Familial migraine with vertigo and essential tremor

Baloh and colleagues (1996) excluded the involvement of the CACAN1A calcium channel gene in a family with acetozolamide-responsive migraine, vertigo and essential tremor. Because of the response to acetozolamide, other ion channel genes might be involved and further investigations should clarify this possibility.

Clearly, further analysis is necessary to unravel fully the genetic basis of migraine. This will ultimately lead to a better understanding of the onset of migraine attacks and thus hopefully in the development of more specific and better prophylactic antimigraine drugs.

# References

Altura, B. M. (1985). Calcium antagonist properties of magnesium: implications for antimigraine actions. *Magnesium*, **4**, 169–75.

Ambrosini, A., de Noordhout, A. M., Alagona, G., Dalpozzo, F. and Schoenen, J. (1999). Impairment of neuromuscular transmission in a subgroup of migraine patients. *Neurosci Lett.*, **276**, 201–3.

Arbab, M. A.-R., Delgado, T., Wiklund, L. and Svendgaard, N. A. (1988). Brain stem terminations of the trigeminal and upper spinal ganglia innervation of the cerebrovascular system: WGA-HRP transganglionic study. *J Cereb Blood Flow Metabol.*, **8**, 54–63.

Arbab, M. A.-R., Wiklund, L. and Svendgaard, N. A. (1986). Origin and distribution of cerebral vascular innervation from superior cervical, trigeminal and spinal ganglia investigated with retrograde and anterograde WGA-HRP tracing in the rat. *Neuroscience*, **19**, 695–708.

Artavanis-Tsakonas, S., Matsuno, K. and Fortini, M. E. (1995). Notch signalling. *Science*, **268**, 225–32.

Ayata, C., Shimizu-Sasamata, M., Lo, E. H., Noebels, J. L. and Moskowitz, M. A. (2000). Impaired neurotransmitter release and elevated threshold for cortical spreading depression in mice with mutations in the alpha 1A subunit of P/Q type calcium channels. *Neuroscience*, **95**, 639–45.

Baloh, R. W., Foster, C. A., Qing Yue, M. D. and Nelson, S. F. (1996). Familial migraine with vertigo and essential tremor. *Neurology*, **46**, 458–60.

Bayliss, D. A., Umemiya, M. and Berger, A. J. (1995). Inhibition of N- and P-type calcium currents and the after-hyperpolarization in rat motoneurones by serotonin. *J Physiol.*, **485**, 635–47.

Burstein, R., Yamamura, H., Malick, A. and Strassman, A. M. (1998). Chemical stimulation of the intracranial dura induces enhanced responses to facial stimulation in brain stem trigeminal neurons. *J Neurophysiol.*, **79**, 964–82.

Buzzi, M. G., Sakas, D. E. and Moskowitz, M. A. (1989). Indomethacin and acetylsalicylic acid block neurogenic plasma protein extravasation in rat dura mater. *Eur J Pharmacol.*, **165**, 251–8.

Caddick, S. J., Wang, C., Fletcher, C. F., Jenkins, N. A., Copeland, N. G. and Hosford, D. A. (1999). Excitatory but Not Inhibitory Synaptic Transmission Is Reduced in Lethargic (Cacnb4(Lh)) and Tottering (Cacna1atg) Mouse Thalami. *J Neurophysiol.*, **81**, 2066–74.

Chabriat, H., Tournier-Lasserve, E., Vahedi, K. *et al.* (1995a). Autosomal dominant migraine with MRI white-matter abnormalities mapping to the CADASIL locus. *Neurology*, **45**, 1086–91.

Chabriat, H., Vahedi, K., Iba-Zizen, M. T. *et al.* (1995b). Clinical spectrum of CADASIL: a study of 7 families. *Lancet*, **346**, 934–9.

Codignola, A., Tarroni, P., Clementi, F. *et al.* (1993). Calcium channel subtypes controlling serotonin release from human small cell lung carcinoma cell lines. *J Biol Chem.*, **268**, 26240–7.

Connor, H. E., Bertin, L., Gillies, S., Beattie, D. T., Ward, P. (1998). The GR205171 Clinical Study Group. Clinical evaluation of a novel, potent, CNS penetrating NK$_1$ receptor antagonist in the acute treatment of migraine. *Cephalalgia*, **18**, 392.

Cruts, M., Hendriks, L. and van Broeckhoven, C. (1996). The presenilin genes: a new gene family involved in Alzheimer disease pathology. *Hum Mol Genet.*, **5**, 1449–55.

Cutrer, F. M., Sorensen, A. G., Weisskoff, R. M. *et al.* (1998). Perfusion-weighted imaging defects during spontaneous migrainous aura. *Ann Neurol.*, **43**, 25–31.

Data, J., Britch, K., Westergaard, N. *et al.* (1998). A double-blind study of ganaxolone in the acute treatment of migraine headaches with or without an aura in premenopausal females. *Headache*, **38**, 380.

de Celis, J. F. and Garcia-Bellido, A. (1994). Modifications of the Notch function by Abruptex mutations in Drosophila melanogaster. *Genetics*, **136**, 183–94.

de Waard, M., Gurnett, C. A. and Campbell, K. P. (1996). Structural and functional diversity of voltage-activated calcium channels. In *Ion Channels* (ed. Narahashi, T.) pp. 41–87. New York: Plenum Press.

Dichgans, M., Mayer, M., Muller-Myhsok, B., Straube, A. and Gasser, T. (1996). Identification of a key recombinant narrows the CADASIL gene region to 8 cM and argues against allelism of CADASIL and Familial Hemiplegic Migraine. *Genomics*, **32**, 151–4.

Diener, H. C. (1996). Substance-P antagonist RPR100893-201 is not effective in human migraine attacks. In *Proceedings of the VIth International Headache Seminar* (eds Olesen, J. and Tfelt-Hansen, P.). New York: Lippincott-Raven.

Dimitriadou, V., Buzzi, M.G., Moskowitz, M. A. and Theoharides, T. C. (1991). Trigeminal sensory fiber stimulation induces morphological changes reflecting secretion in rat dura mater mast cells. *Neuroscience*, **44**, 97–112.

Dimitriadou, V., Buzzi, M. G., Theoharides, T. C. and Moskowitz, M. A. (1992). Ultrastructural evidence for neurogenically mediated changes in blood vessels of the rat dura mater and tongue following antidromic trigeminal stimulation. *Neuroscience*, **48**, 187–203.

Diriong, S., Lory, P., Williams, M. E., Ellis, S. B., Harpold, M. M. and Taviaux, S. (1995). Chromosomal localization of the human genes for $\alpha$1A, $\alpha$1B, and

$\alpha$1E voltage-dependent $Ca^{2+}$ channel subunits. *Genomics*, **30**, 605–9.

Drummond, P. D., Gonski, A. and Lance, J. W. (1983). Facial flushing after thermocoagulation of the gasserian ganglion. *J Neurol Neurosurg Psychiatr.*, **46**, 611–6.

Drummond, P. D. and Lance, J. W. (1983). Extracranial vascular changes and the source of pain in migraine headache. *Ann Neurol.*, **13**, 32–7.

Ducros, A., Joutel, A., Vahedi, K. *et al.* (1997). Mapping of a second locus for familial hemiplegic migraine to 1q21-q23 and evidence of further heterogeneity. *Ann Neurol.*, **42**, 885–90.

Ducros, A., Nagy, T., Alamowitch, S. *et al.* (1996). Cerebral autosomal dominant arteriopathy with subcortical infarcts and leukoencephalopathy, genetic homogeneity, and mapping of the locus within a 2-cM interval. *Am J Hum Genet.*, **58**, 171–81.

Dunlap, K., Luebke, J. I. and Turner, T. J. (1995). Exocytotic Ca2+ channels in mammalian central neurons. *Trend Neurosci.*, **18**, 89–98.

Earl, N. L., McDonald, S. A. and Lowy, M. T. 4991W93 Investigator Group. (1999). Efficacy and tolerability of the neurogenic inflammation inhibitor, 4991W93, in the acute treatment of migraine. *Cephalalgia*, **19**, 357.

Fanciullacci, M., Alessandri, M., Figini, M., Geppetti, P. and Michelacci, S. (1995). Increases in plasma calcitonin gene-related peptide from extracerebral circulation during nitroglycerin-induced cluster headache attack. *Pain*, **60**, 119–23.

Feindel, W., Penfield, W. and McNaughton, F. (1960). The tentorial nerves and localisation of intracranial pain in man. *Neurology*, **10**, 555–63.

Ferrari, M. D. (1998). Migraine. *Lancet*, **351**, 1043–51.

Frittoli, E., Gobbi, M. and Mennini, T. (1994). Involvement of P-type $Ca^{2+}$ channels in $K^+$ and D-fenfluramine-induced [$^3$H]5-HT release from rat hippocampal synaptosomes. *Neuropharmacology*, **33**, 833–5.

Gallai, V., Sarchielli, P., Floridi, A. *et al.* (1995). Vasoactive peptides levels in the plasma of young migraine patients with and without aura assessed both interictally and ictally. *Cephalalgia*, **15**, 384–90.

Gardner, K., Barmada, M., Ptacek, L. J. and Hoffman, E. P. (1997). A new locus for hemiplegic migraine maps to chromosome 1q31. *Neurology*, **49**, 1231–8.

Gaur, S., Newcomb, R., Rivnay, B. *et al.* (1994). Calcium channel antagonist peptides define several components of transmitter release in the hippocampus. *Neuropharmacology*, **33**, 1211–9.

Gervil, M., Ulrich, V., Olesen, J. and Russell, M. B. (1998). Screening for migraine in the general population: validation of a simple questionnaire. *Cephalalgia*, **18**, 342–8.

Goadsby, P. J. (1998). Serotonin and the acute attack of migraine. *Clin Neurosci.*, **5**, 18–23.

Goadsby, P. J. and Duckworth, J. W. (1987). Effect of stimulation of trigeminal ganglion on regional cerebral blood flow in cats. *Am J Physiol.*, **253**, R270–R4.

Goadsby, P. J. and Duckworth, J. W. (1989). Low frequency stimulation of the locus coeruleus reduces regional cerebral blood flow in the spinalized cat. *Brain Res.*, **476**, 71–7.

Goadsby, P. J. and Edvinsson, L. (1994). Human *in vivo* evidence for trigeminovascular activation in cluster headache. *Brain*, **117**, 427–34.

Goadsby, P. J. and Edvinsson, L. (1996). Neuropeptide changes in a case of chronic paroxysmal hemicrania – evidence for trigemino-parasympathetic activation. *Cephalalgia*, **16**, 448–50.

Goadsby, P. J., Edvinsson, L. and Ekman, R. (1988). Release of vasoactive peptides in the extracerebral circulation of man and the cat during activation of the trigeminovascular system. *Ann Neurol.*, **23**, 193–6.

Goadsby, P. J., Edvinsson, L. and Ekman, R. (1990). Vasoactive peptide release in the extracerebral circulation of humans during migraine headache. *Ann Neurol.*, **28**, 183–7.

Goadsby, P. J. and Hoskin, K. L. (1997). The distribution of trigeminovascular afferents in the non-human primate brain *macaca nemestrina*: a c-fos immunocytochemical study. *J Anat.*, **190**, 367–75.

Goadsby, P. J. , Knight, Y. E., Hoskin, K. L. and Butler, P. (1997). Stimulation of an intracranial trigeminally-innervated structure selectively increases cerebral blood flow. *Brain Res.*, **751**, 247–52.

Goadsby, P. J., Lambert, G. A. and Lance, J. W. (1982). Differential effects on the internal and external carotid circulation of the monkey evoked by locus coeruleus stimulation. *Brain Res.*, **249**, 247–54.

Goadsby, P. J., Lambert, G. A. and Lance, J. W. (1984). The peripheral pathway for extracranial vasodilatation in the cat. *J Auto. Nerv Syst.*, **10**, 145–55.

Goadsby, P. J., Lambert, G. A. and Lance, J. W. (1985). The mechanism of cerebrovascular vasoconstriction in response to locus coeruleus stimulation. *Brain Res.*, **326**, 213–7.

Goadsby, P. J. and Zagami, A. S. (1991). Stimulation of the superior sagittal sinus increases metabolic activity and blood flow in certain regions of the brainstem and upper cervical spinal cord of the cat. *Brain*, **114**, 1001–11.

Goadsby, P. J., Zagami, A. S. and Lambert, G. A. (1991). Neural processing of craniovascular pain: a synthesis of the central structures involved in migraine. *Headache*, **31**, 365–71.

Goldstein, D. J., Wang, O., Saper, J. R., Stoltz, R., Silberstein, S. D., Mathew, N. T. (1997). Ineffectiveness of neurokinin-1 antagonist in acute migraine: a crossover study. *Cephalalgia,* **17**, 785–90.

Griffiths, L. R., Nyholt, D. R., Curtain, R. P., Goadsby, P. J., Brimage, P. J. (1997). Migraine association and linkage studies of an endothelial nitric oxide synthase (NOS3) gene polymorphism. *Neurology*, **49**, 614–7.

Haan, J., Terwindt, G. and Ferrari, M. D. (1997). Genetics of Migraine. *Neurol Clin.*, **15**, 43–60.

Haan, J., Terwindt, G. M., Bos, P. L., Ophoff, R. A., Frants, R. R. and Ferrari, M. D. The Dutch Migraine Genetics Group. (1994). Familial hemiplegic migraine in The Netherlands. *Clin Neurol Neurosurg.*, **96**, 244–9.

Hans, M., Luvisetto, S., Williams, M. E. *et al.* (1999). Functional consequences of mutations in the human alpha(1A) calcium channel subunit linked to familial hemiplegic migraine. *J Neurosci.*, **19**, 1610–9.

Hawkes, C. H. (1992). Familial *paroxysmal ataxia: report of a family. J Neurol Neurosurg Psychiatr.*, **55**, 212–3.

Hering, S., Aczel, S., Grabner, M. *et al.* (1996). Transfer of high sensitivity for benzothiazepines from L-type to class A (BI) calcium channels. *J Biol Chem.*, **271**, 24471–5.

Hoskin, K. L., Zagami, A. and Goadsby, P. J. (1999). Stimulation of the middle meningeal artery leads to bilateral Fos expression in the trigeminocervical nucleus: a comparative study of monkey and cat. *J Anat.*, **194**, 579–88.

Hutchinson, M., O'Riordan, J., Javed, M. *et al.* (1995). Familial hemiplegic migraine and autosomal dominant arteriopathy with leukoencephalopathy (CADASIL). *Ann Neurol.*, **38**, 817–24.

Joels, M. and Karst, H. (1995). Effects of estradiol and progesterone on voltage-gated calcium and potassium conductances in rat CA1 hippocampal neurons. *J Neurosci.*, **15**, 289–97.

Joutel, A., Bousser, M. G., Biousse, V. *et al.* (1993). A gene for familial hemiplegic migraine maps to chromosome 19. *Nat Genet.*, **5**, 40–5.

Joutel, A., Corpechot, C., Ducros, A. *et al.* (1996). Notch3 mutations in CADASIL, a hereditary adult-onset condition causing stroke and dementia. *Nature*, **383**, 707–10.

Joutel, A., Corpechot, C., Vayssière, C. and *et al.* (1997). Characterization of Notch3 mutations in CADASIL patients. *Neurology*, **48**, 1729–30.

Joutel, A., Ducros, A., Vahedi, K. *et al.* (1994). Genetic heterogeneity of familial hemiplegic migraine. *Am J Hum Genet.*, **55**, 1166–72.

Jung, H. H., Bassetti, C., Tournier-Lasserve, E. *et al.* (1995). Cerebral autosomal dominant arteriopathy with subcortical infarcts and leukoencephalopathy: a clinicopathological and genetic study of a Swiss family. *J Neurol Neurosurg Psychiatr.*, **59**, 138–43.

Kalfakis, N., Panas, M., Vassilopoulo, D., Malliara Loulakaki, S. (1996). Migraine with aura: segregation analysis and heritability estimation. *Headache*, **36**, 320–2.

Kaube, H., Keay, K., Hoskin, K. L., Bandler, R. and Goadsby, P. J. (1993). Expression of c-fos-like immunoreactivity in the trigeminal nucleus caudalis and high cervical cord following stimulation of the sagittal sinus in the cat. *Brain Res.*, **629**, 95–102.

Knight, Y. E. and Goadsby, P. J. (1999). Brainstem stimulation inhibits trigeminal neurons in the cat. *Cephalalgia*, **19**, 315.

Kraus, R. L., Sinnegger, M. J., Glossmann, H., Hering, S. and Striessnig, J. (1998). Familial hemiplegic migraine mutations change alpha(1A) $Ca^{2+}$ channel kinetics. *J Biol Chem.*, **273**, 5586–90.

Lambert, G. A., Goadsby, P. J., Zagami, A. S. and Duckworth, J. W. (1988). Comparative effects of stimulation of the trigeminal ganglion and the superior sagittal sinus on cerebral blood flow and evoked potentials in the cat. *Brain Res.*, **453**, 143–9.

Lassen, L. H., Jacobsen, V. B., Petersen, P., Sperling, B., Iversen, H. K. and Olesen, J. (1998). Human calcitonin gene-related peptide (hCGRP)-induced headache in migraineurs. *Eur J Neurol.*, **5**(Suppl. 3), S63.

Launer, L. J., Terwindt, G. M. and Ferrari, M. D. (1999). The prevalence and characteristics of migraine in a population-based cohort. The GEM study. *Neurology*, **53**, 537—42.

Lauritzen, M. (1994). Pathophysiology of the migraine aura. The spreading depression theory. *Brain*, **117**, 199–210.

Lehmann-Horn, F. and Rudel, R. (1996). Molecular pathophysiology of voltage-gated ion channels. *Rev Physiol Biochem Pharmacol.*, **128**, 195–268.

Leone, M., Filippini, G., D'Amico, D., Farinotti, M. and Bussone, G. (1994). Assessment of International Headache Society diagnostic criteria: a reliability study. *Cephalalgia*, **14**, 280–4.

Levitan, D. and Greenwald, I. (1995). Facilitation of lin-12-mediated signalling by sel-12, a Caenorhabditis elegans S182 Alzheimer's disease gene. *Nature*, **377**, 351–4.

Lory, P., Ophoff, R. A. and Nahmias, L. (1997). Towards a unified nomenclature describing voltage-gated calcium channel genes. *Hum Genet.*, **100**, 149–50.

Markowitz, S., Saito, K. and Moskowitz, M. A. (1987). Neurogenically mediated leakage of plasma proteins occurs from blood vessels in dura mater but not brain. *J Neurosci.*, **7**, 4129–36.

Markowitz, S., Saito, K. and Moskowitz, M. A. (1988). Neurogenically mediated plasma extravasation in dura mater: effect of ergot alkaloids. A possible mechanism of action in vascular headache. *Cephalalgia*, **8**, 83–91.

Martins, I. P., Baeta, E., Paiva, T., Campo, T. and Gomes, L. (1993). Headaches during intracranial endovascular procedures: a possible model of vascular headache. *Headache*, **33**, 227–33.

Matsuyama, Z., Kawakami, H., Maruyama, H., Izumi, Y., Komure, O., Udaka, F., *et al.* (1997). Molecular features of the CAG repeats of spinocerebellar ataxia 6 (SCA6). *Human Molecular Genetics*, **6**, 1283–7.

May, A., Bahra, A., Buchel, C., Frackowiak, R. S. J. and Goadsby, P. J. (1998a). Hypothalamic activation in cluster headache attacks. *Lancet*, **351**, 275–8.

May, A., Bahra, A., Buchel, C., Turner, R. and Goadsby,

P. J. (1999a). Functional MRI in spontaneous attacks of SUNCT: short-lasting neuralgiform headache with conjunctival injection and tearing. *Ann Neurol.*, **46**, 791–3.

May, A., Buchel, C., Bahra, A., Goadsby, P. J. and Frackowiak, R. S. J. (1999b). Intra-cranial vessels in trigeminal transmitted pain: a PET Study. *Neuro-Image*, **9**, 453–60.

May, A., Gijsman, H. J., Wallnoefer, A., Jones, R., Diener, H. C. and Ferrari, M. D. (1996). Endothelin antagonist bosentan blocks neurogenic inflammation, but is not effective in aborting migraine attacks. *Pain*, **67**, 375–8.

May, A., Kaube, H., Buechel, C. *et al.* (1998b). Experimental cranial pain elicited by capsaicin: a PET-study. *Pain*, **74**, 61–6.

May, A., Ophoff, R. A., Terwindt, G. M. *et al.* (1995). Familial hemiplegic migraine locus on chromosome 19p13 is involved in common forms of migraine with and without aura. *Hum Genet.*, **96**, 604–8.

May, A., Shepheard, S., Wessing, A., Hargreaves, R. J., Goadsby, P. J. and Diener, H. C. (1998c), Retinal plasma extravasation can be evoked by trigeminal stimulation in rat but does not occur during migraine attacks. *Brain*, **121**, 1231–7.

McNaughton, F. L. (1938). The innervation of the intracranial blood vessels and dural sinuses. *Proc Assoc Res Nerv Ment Dis.*, **18**, 178–200.

McNaughton, F. L. (1966). The innervation of the intracranial blood vessels and the dural sinuses. In *The Circulation of the Brain and Spinal Cord* (eds Cobb, S., Frantz, A. M., Penfield, W. and Riley, H. A.) pp.178–200. New York: Hafner Publishing Co. Inc.

McNaughton, F. L. and Feindel, W. H. (1977). Innervation of intracranial structures: a reappraisal. In *Physiological aspects of Clinical Neurology.* (ed. Rose, F. C.) pp 279–93. Oxford: Blackwell Scientific Publications.

Menken, M., Munsat, T. L. and Toole, J. F. (2000). The global burden of disease study – implications for neurology. *Arch Neurol.*, **57**, 418–20.

Mintz, I. M., Sabatini, B. L. and Regehr, W. G. (1995). Calcium control of transmitter release at a cerebellar synapse. *Neuron*, **15**, 675–88.

Mochi, M., Sangiorgi, S., Cortelli, P., Carelli, V., Scapoli, C., Crisci, M. *et al.* (1993). Testing models for genetic determination in migraine. *Cephalalgia*, **13**, 389–94.

Moon, S. L. and Koller, W. C. (1991). Hereditary Periodic Ataxias. In *Hereditary Neuropathies and Spinocerebellar Ataxias* (ed. de Jong, J. M. B. V.) pp 433–43. Amsterdam: Elsevier Science. Handbook of Clinical Neurology.

Mori, Y., Friedrich, T., Kim, M. S. *et al.* (1991). Primary structure and functional expression from complementary DNA of a brain calcium channel. *Nature*, **350**, 398–402.

Moskowitz, M. A. and Cutrer, F. M. (1993). Sumatrip-

tan: a receptor-targeted treatment for migraine. *Ann Rev Med.*, **44**, 145–54.

Nichols, F. T., Mawad, M., Mohr, J. P., Hilal, S. and Adams, R. J. (1993). Focal headache during balloon inflation in the vertebral and basilar arteries. *Headache*, **33**, 87–9.

Nichols, F. T., Mawad, M., Mohr, J. P., Hilal, S., Stein, B. and Michelson, J. (1990). Focal headache during balloon inflation in the internal carotid and middle cerebral arteries. *Stroke*, **21**, 555–9.

Norman, B., Panebianco, D. and Block, G. A. (1998). A placebo-controlled, in-clinic study to explore the preliminary safety and efficacy of intravenous L-758,298 (a prodrug of the NK1 receptor antagonist L-754,030) in the acute treatment of migraine. *Cephalalgia*, **18**, 407.

Nyholt, D. R., Curtain, R. P., Gaffney, P. T., Brimage, P., Goadsby, P. J. and Griffiths, L. R. (1996). Migraine association and linkage analyses of the human 5-hydroxytryptamine (5HT$_{2A}$) receptor gene. *Cephalalgia*, **16**, 463–7.

Nyholt, D. R., Dawkins, J. L., Brimage, P. J., Goadsby, P. J., Nicholson, G. A. and Griffiths, L. R. (1998a). Evidence for an X-linked genetic component in familial typical migraine. *Hum Mol Genet.*, **7**, 459–63.

Nyholt, D. R., Lea, R. A., Goadsby, P. J., Brimage, P. J. and Griffiths, L. R. (1998b). Familial typical migraine: linkage to chromosome 19p13 and evidence for genetic heterogeneity. *Neurology*, **50**, 1428–32.

Ogilvie, A. D., Russell, M. B., Dhall, P. *et al.* (1998). Altered allelic distributions of the serotonin transporter gene in migraine without aura and migraine with aura. *Cephalalgia*, **18**, 23–6.

Olesen, J., Friberg, L., Skyhoj-Olsen, T. *et al.* (1990). Timing and topography of cerebral blood flow, aura and headache during migraine attacks. *Ann Neurol.*, **28**, 791–8.

Olesen, J., Larsen, B. and Lauritzen M. (1981a). Focal hyperemia followed by spreading oligemia and impaired activation of rCBF in classic migraine. *Ann Neurol.*, **9**, 344–52.

Olesen, J., Tfelt-Hansen, P., Henriksen, L. and Larsen, B. (1981b).The common migraine attack may not be initiated by cerebral ischemia. *Lancet*, **2**, 438–40.

Olesen, J., Thomsen, L. L. and Iversen, H. K. (1994). Nitric oxide is a key molecule in migraine and other vascular headaches. *Trend Pharmacol Sci.*, **15**, 149–53.

Ophoff, R. A., Eijk, R., Sandkuijl, L. A. *et al.* (1994). Genetic heterogeneity of familial hemiplegic migraine. *Genomics*, **22**, 21–6.

Ophoff, R. A., Terwindt, G. M., Vergouwe, M. N. *et al.* (1996). Familial hemiplegic migraine and episodic ataxia type-2 are caused by mutations in the Ca$^{2+}$ channel gene CACNLA4. *Cell*, **87**, 543–52.

Penfield, W. and McNaughton, F. L. (1940). Dural headache and the innervation of the dura mater. *Arch Neurol Psychiatr.*, **44**, 43–75.

Peroutka, S. J., Wilhoit, T. and Jones, K. (1997). Clinical susceptibility to migraine aura is modified by dopamine D2 receptor (DRD2) NcoI alleles. *Neurology*, **49**, 201–6.

Plomp, J. J., Vergouwe, M. N., Van den Maagdenberg, A. M., Ferrari, M. D., Frants, R. R. and Molenaar, P. C. (2000). Abnormal Transmitter Release at Neuromuscular Junctions of Mice Carrying the *Tottering* Alpha-1-A Ca$^{2+}$ Channel Mutation. *Brain*, **123**, 463–71.

Ramadan, N. M., Barker, P., Boska, M. D. *et al.* (1996). Selective occipital cortex magnesium Mg$^{2+}$ deficiency reduction in familial hemiplegic migraine may reflect an ion channel disorder. *Neurology*, A168.

Raskin, N. H., Hosobuchi, Y. and Lamb, S. (1987). Headache may arise from perturbation of brain. *Headache*, **27**, 416–20.

Rasmussen, B. K., Jensen, R. and Olesen, J. (1991). Questionnaire versus clinical interview diagnosis of headache. *Headache*, **31**, 290–5.

Rasmussen, B. K. and Olesen, J. (1992). Migraine with aura and migraine without aura: an epidemiological study. *Cephalalgia*, **12**, 221–8.

Riess, O., Schöls, L., Böttger, H., Nolte, D., Menezes Vieira-Saecker, A. M., Schimming, C., *et al.* (1997). SCA6 is caused by moderate CAG expansion in the α1A-voltage-dependent calcium channel gene. *Human Molecular Genetics*, **6**, 1289–93.

Roon, K. I., Olesen, J., Diener, H. C. *et al.* (2000). No acute antimigraine efficacy of CP-122,288, a highly potent inhibitor of neurogenic inflammation: results of two randomized double-blind placebo-controlled clinical trials. *Ann Neurol.*, **47**, 238–41.

Russell, M. B. (1997). Genetic epidemiology of migraine and cluster headache. *Cephalalgia*, **17**, 683–701.

Russell, M. B., Fenger, K. and Olesen, J. (1996a). The family history of migraine. Direct versus indirect information. *Cephalalgia*, **16**, 156–60.

Russell, M. B. and Olesen, J. (1995). Increased familial risk and evidence of genetic factor in migraine. *BMJ*, **311**, 541–4.

Russell, M. B., Rassmussen, B. K., Fenger, K. and Olesen, J. (1996b). Migraine without aura and migraine with aura are distinct clinical entities: a study of four hundred and eight-four male and female migraineurs from the general population. *Cephalalgia*, **16**, 239–45.

Starr, T. V., Prystay, W. and Snutch, T. P. (1991). Primary structure of a calcium channel that is highly expressed in the rat cerebellum. *Proc Natl Acad Sci USA*, **88**, 5621–5.

Stea, A., Soong, T. W. and Snutch, T. P. (1995). Voltage-gated calcium channels. In *Handbook of Receptors and Channels. Ligand and Voltage-gated Ion Channels* (ed. North, R. A.). pp. 113–53. CRC Press.

Stewart, W. F., Lipton, R. B., Celentano, D. D. and Reed, M. L. (1992). Prevalence of migraine headache in the United States: relation to age, income, race and other sociodemographic factors. *J Am Med. Assoc.*, **267**, 64–9.

Stewart, W. F., Staffa, J., Lipton, R. B. and Ottman, R. (1997). Familial risk of migraine: a population-based study. *Ann Neurol.*, **41**, 166–72.

Strassman, A. M., Raymond, S. A. and Burstein, R. (1996). Sensitization of meningeal sensory neurons and the origin of headaches. *Nature*, **384**, 560–3.

Teh, B. T., Silburn, P., Lindblad, K. *et al.* (1995). Familial cerebellar periodic ataxia without myokymia maps to a 19-cM region on 19p13. *Am J Hum Genet.*, **56**, 1443–9.

Terwindt, G. M., Haan, J., Ophoff, R. A. *et al.* (1998a). Clinical and genetic analysis of a large Dutch family with autosomal dominant vascular retinopathy, migraine and Raynaud's phenomenon. *Brain*, **121**, 303–16.

Terwindt, G. M., Ophoff, R. A., Haan, J. and Ferrari, M. D. The Dutch Migraine Genetics Research Group. (1996). Familial hemiplegic migraine: a clinical comparison of families linked and unlinked to chromosome 19. *Cephalalgia*, **16**, 153–5.

Terwindt, G. M., Ophoff, R. A., Haan, J., Sandkuijl, L. A., Frants, R. R. and Ferrari, M. D. (1998b). Migraine, ataxia and epilepsy: a challenging spectrum of genetically determined calcium channelopathies. *Eur J Hum Genet.*, **6**, 297–307.

Terwindt, G. M., Ophoff, R. A., Haan, J. *et al.* (1998c). Variable clinical expression of mutations in the P/Q-type calcium channel gene in familial hemiplegic migraine. *Neurology*, **50**, 1105–10.

Tournier-Lasserve, E., Joutel, A., Melki, J. *et al.* (1993). Cerebral autosomal dominant arteriopathy with subcortical infarcts and leukoencephalopathy maps to chromosome 19p12. *Nat Genet.*, **3**, 256–9.

Tran-Dinh, Y. R., Thurel, C., Cunin, G., Serrie, A. and Seylaz, J. (1992). Cerebral vasodilation after the thermocoagulation of the trigeminal ganglion in humans. *Neurosurgery*, **31**, 658–62.

Uchitel, O. D., Protti, D. A., Sanchez, V., Cherksey, B. D., Sugimori, M. and Llinas, R. (1997). P-type voltage-dependent calcium channel mediates presynaptic calcium influx and transmitter release in mammalian synapses. *Proc Natl Acad Sci USA*, **89**, 3330–3.

Uddman, R., Edvinsson, L., Ekman, R., Kingman, T. and McCulloch, J. (1985). Innervation of the feline cerebral vasculature by nerve fibers containing calcitonin gene-related peptide: trigeminal origin and coexistence with substance P. *Neurosci. Lett.*, **62**, 131–6.

Ulrich, V., Gervil, M., Kyvik, K. O., Olesen, J. and Russell, M. B. (1999). Evidence of a genetic factor in migraine with aura: a population based Danish twin study. *Ann Neurol.*, **45**, 242–6.

Vahedi, K., Joutel, A., van Bogaert, P. *et al.* (1995). A gene for hereditary paroxysmal cerebellar ataxia maps to chromosome 19p. *Ann Neurol.*, **37**, 289–93.

Veloso, F., Kumar, K. and Toth, C. (1998). Headache secondary to deep brain implantation. *Headache*, **38**, 507–15.

Verin, M., Rolland, Y., Landgraf, F. *et al.* (1995). New phenotype of the cerebral autosomal dominant arteriopathy mapped to chromosome 19: migraine as the prominent clinical feature. *J Neurol Neurosurg Psychiatr.*, **59**, 579–85.

Vighetto, A., Froment, J. C., Trillet, M. and Aimard, G. (1988). Magnetic resonance imaging in familial paroxysmal ataxia. *Arch Neurol.*, **45**, 547–9.

Wakamori, M., Yamazaki, K., Matsunodaira, H. *et al.* (1998). Single Tottering Mutations Responsible for the Neuropathic Phenotype of the P-Type Calcium Channel. *J Biol Chem.*, **273**, 34857–67.

Waldenlind, E., Ekbom, K. and Torhall, J. (1993). MR-Angiography during spontaneous attacks of cluster headache: a case report. *Headache*, **33**, 291–5.

Watson, J. A., Elliot, A. C. and Brown, P. D. (1995). Serotonin elevates intracellular $Ca^{2+}$ in rat choroid plexus epithelial cells by acting on 5-HT$_{2C}$ receptors. *Cell Calcium*, **17**, 120–8.

Weiller, C., May, A., Limmroth, V. *et al.* (1995). Brain stem activation in spontaneous human migraine attacks. *Nat Med.*, **1**, 658–60.

Willis, T. (1682). *Opera Omnia*. Amstelaedami: Henricum Wetstenium.

Zagami, A. S. and Goadsby, P. J. (1991). Stimulation of the superior sagittal sinus increases metabolic activity in cat thalamus. In *New Advances in Headache Research: 2* (ed. Rose, F. C.) pp. 169–71. London: Smith-Gordon and Co Ltd.

Zagami, A. S., Goadsby, P. J. and Edvinsson, L. (1990). Stimulation of the superior sagittal sinus in the cat causes release of vasoactive peptides. *Neuropeptides*, **16**, 69–75.

Zagami, A. S. and Lambert, G. A. (1991). Craniovascular application of capsaicin activates nociceptive thalamic neurons in the cat. *Neurosci. Lett.*, **121**, 187–90.

Zhang, A., Cheng, P. T. O. and Altura, B. M. (1992). Magnesium regulates intracellular free ionized calcium concentration and cell geometry in vascular smooth muscle cell. *Biophys Acta*, **1134**, 25–9.

Zhuchenko, O., Bailey, J., Donnen, P. *et al.* (1997). Autosomal dominant cerebellar ataxia (SCA6) associated with small polyglutamine expansions in the $\alpha$1A-voltage-dependent calcium channel. *Nat Genet.*, **15**, 62–9.

# Ciguatera (fish poisoning)

*Peter Fenner and Richard Lewis*

## Introduction

Ciguatera is an illness caused by the consumption of fish contaminated with orally effective levels of polyether sodium channel activator toxins (ciguatoxins), and is characterized by neurological, gastrointestinal and cardiovascular disorders. The syndrome only occurs after eating species of tropical and subtropical fish. Ciguatera is arguably the most common fish food poisoning encountered in man, with approximately 25 000 cases annually, but is rarely fatal. With increased travel to and from the tropics and increasing imports of tropical fish, ciguatera will continue to grow in importance, even in non-tropical areas (Sanner *et al.*, 1997). Ciguatera is currently the most common fish poisoning in many countries, including the USA (Calvert *et al.*, 1987).

The ciguatoxins arise from blooms of certain strains of the benthic dinoflagellate, *Gambierdiscus toxicus*. Environmental degradation may play a role in the increased incidence of ciguatera, although the precise factors involved remain to be elucidated (Lewis and Holmes, 1993). The role played by other marine toxins in ciguatera, including those produced by other toxic benthic dinoflagellates, has not been clearly demonstrated, although mild cases of palytoxin poisoning may be mistaken for ciguatera.

The name ciguatera was coined in the 15th century, when it was used to describe poisonings from marine snail *Turbo pica* (known as 'cigua' in Spanish), a staple food in the Caribbean in the 18th century. The name later became associated with what was believed to be related poisoning caused by fish in the region (Lewis and King, 1996). More than 200 species of fish have been implicated in ciguatera, the most common of which include grouper (Epinephelids), snapper (Lutjanids), barracuda (Sphyraenids), moray eel (Muraenids), mackerels (Scombrids), amberjack (*Seriola* spp.), surgeonfish (Acanthurids), and parrot fish (Scarids). The particular species or families of fish involved varies across ciguatera-endemic regions. The high-risk species in the Caribbean Sea, and Pacific and Indian Oceans vary widely. Toxin contaminated fish may be found in tropical areas extending approximately 35 degrees latitude on both sides of the equator, but for reasons discussed above, both travellers and people living outside those areas may be affected. Ciguatera has its greatest impact in the atoll island countries of the Pacific Ocean, where fish is the primary source of protein (Lewis, 1992).

## Epidemiology

Incidences of ciguatera are common, although highly unpredictable and variable throughout tropical and subtropical waters. The highest incidences occur in atoll island countries, where the annual rate of reported cases often exceeds 1% of the population, e.g. Republic of Kiribati, Tokelau and Tuvalu (Lewis, 1992). This incidence is increased at least a further 10-fold in particular atolls such as Marakei in Kiribati, where there are few alternatives to reef fish as a source of protein. Queensland (Australia) and Tonga (0.16 cases per 10 000 population) have similarly low levels of ciguatera, yet the problem in developed countries is perceived to be more severe (Lewis, 1992).

Under-reporting and misdiagnosis is common

and the recorded incidence figures may represent only 20% of the true incidence of ciguatera (Lewis, 1992; Lewis and King, 1996). In major endemic areas, including the Caribbean and the South Pacific islands, the incidence of ciguatera poisoning ranges from 50 to 500 cases annually per 10 000 population, making it one of the more common illnesses in those areas (Lewis, 1992; Rakita, 1995). Selected reports on the incidence of ciguatera are outlined below.

In French Polynesia during 1991, 551 cases were assessed (notification rate 276 per 100 000) (Glaziou and Martin, 1992). The mean age was 36.6 years (SD 15.6) and the largest age group was the 30–39 age class (138 cases, notification rate 970 per 100 000). Sex ratio (M/F) was 1.6. A clinical score was calculated to assess the outcome for each case. The adjusted odds ratio (OR) for a severe disease (33.2% with a score $>5$) were significantly increased when the fish ingested was carnivorous (OR $= 1.62$, 95% confidence interval (CI): 1.07–2.45) and when a history of a previous attack was reported (OR $= 1.71$, 95% CI: 1.17–2.5). This later finding could be related to an accumulation of toxin in the human organism (Glaziou and Martin, 1992). Men aged 30–39 years are at a higher risk of ciguatera fish poisoning, whatever its severity.

In another study of ciguatera (Katz et al., 1993), 10 of the 15 cases demonstrated bradycardia; seven were hospitalized, including two requiring placement in intensive care. Bradycardia was associated with increasing age and body weight ($P < 0.01$ and $< 0.05$, respectively) as well as the amount of toxic fish consumed ($P < 0.01$). Duration of illness ranged from 2 to 132 days. Increasing duration of illness was correlated with both increasing age and weight (rs $= 0.64$ and rs $= 0.72$, respectively, both $P < 0.01$) and was independent of amount and components of toxic fish consumed. The correlation between increasing age and weight with duration and severity of symptoms may be explained by prior subclinical toxin exposure and is consistent with the observation that repeated ciguatoxin exposures are associated with more severe illness. The association between amount of toxic fish consumed and bradycardia is consistent with an increased dose of ciguatoxin (Katz et al., 1993).

One hundred and fifty-nine ichtyosarcotoxic outbreaks, comprising 477 people, were recorded for the Reunion Islands, Indian Ocean (Quod and Turquet, 1996). Ciguatera annual incidence rate was estimated to be 0.78/10 000 between 1986 and 1994. Hallucinations were reported in 16% of the patients (Quod and Turquet, 1996).

Ciguatera outbreaks have been reported from widely dispersed locations. For example, a southern California outbreak was traced to fish caught off the coast of Baja California, Mexico (Barton et al., 1995). A group of Canadian adults ingested grouper imported from Florida, two required hospitalization (Ho et al., 1986). Putative ciguatera has been reported on at least three occasions from Israel. One causative fish was identified as Sarpa salpa, caught in the Mediterranean coastal waters of Israel, although mullet and rabbitfish caught at the same site caused no harm (Raighlin-Eisenkraft et al., 1988).

## Signs and symptoms

The time between the ingestion of contaminated fish and symptoms varied from 20 minutes to over 24 hours. Patients with this illness usually became symptomatic less than 24 hours after ingestion of the fish and most patients (76.8%) developed symptoms in less than 12 hours (Bagnis et al., 1979). Studies suggest that the amount of toxic fish eaten, or the previous ingestion of contaminated fish, even at a subtoxic level, will affect the severity of the symptoms (Bagnis et al., 1979; Glaziou and Martin, 1992; Fenner et al., 1997), although one recent study did not find this correlation (Arcila-Herrera et al., 1998). Symptoms may last for weeks, months and, rarely, years (Gillespie et al., 1986; Lewis and King, 1996).

Common symptoms can be categorized into four main areas: gastrointestinal, neurological, non-specific and cardiovascular, and are listed in Table 20.1.

Paradoxical reversal of temperature perception is often reported in ciguatera. The tingling, burning, and 'electric' impulses described are generated in C-polymodal nociceptor fibres in skin and deep structures. Cameron and Capra (1993) suggested that the paradoxical sensory discomfort

---

**Table 20.1 Signs and symptoms of ciguatera in the Pacific Ocean**

*Gastrointestinal*
- Diarrhoea (>60 % of patients)
- Abdominal pain, nausea (>50%)
- Actual vomiting (>30%)

*Neurological*
- Myalgia (muscle aching) (>80%)
- Paradoxical reversal of temperature perception, pruritus (itching), arthralgia (>70%)
- Paraesthesiae (tingling and numbness) of hands, feet, mouth and lips, headache (>60%)
- Mood disorders (depression, irritability, anxiety) (50%)
- Ataxia (unsteadiness), or vertigo (sensation of spinning), sweating, eye pain (>40%)
- Dental pain, tremor (>30%)
- Neck stiffness, demonstrable paresis (decreased power in specific muscle groups)(>20%)
- Salivation or hypersalivation (10%)

*Non-specific*
- Fatigue and lassitude (90%)
- Chills (40%)
- Skin rash, shortness of breath (including exertional), pain on urination (20%)

*Cardiovascular effects (variable in incidence)*
- Hypotension (Geller and Benowitz, 1992)
- Bradycardia (Katz *et al.*, 1993)
- Tachycardia (Levine, 1995)
- Transient hypertension or heart failure (Legrand *et al.*, 1982)

---

Reproduced from Lewis and King, *Venomous and Poisonous Marine Animals: a Medical and Biological Handbook*, NSW University Press, Sydney, 1996.

---

experienced is probably from exaggerated and intense nerve depolarization occurring in peripheral small A-delta myelinated fibres, particularly the C-polymodal nociceptor fibres. However, they also showed that actual reversal of temperature does not occur and that overall, gross temperature perception was found to be intact in ciguatera poisoning (Cameron and Capra, 1993).

Significant differences in some symptoms occur between Melanesian and Polynesian ethnic groups, suggesting a susceptibility difference, or a difference in the nature of the toxin found in different areas of the Pacific (Bagnis *et al.*, 1979).

## Rare and unusual symptoms

One person in Rhode Island, USA, developed an acute gastrointestinal and neurological syndrome and then became comatose after ingestion of fish soup made locally. Laboratory studies confirmed the clinical diagnosis of ciguatera poisoning (DeFusco *et al.*, 1993).

- Prolonged and symptomatic orthostatic hypotension from ciguatera occurred after eating barracuda. Volume depletion was excluded with the patient having low plasma catecholamine levels and marked pressor hypersensitivity to noradrenaline infusion. The hypotension and bradycardia could be reversed by atropine infusion. These results suggest that the orthostatic hypotension was caused by both parasympathetic excess and sympathetic failure (Geller and Benowitz, 1992).
- Left retrobulbar eye pain occurred in a 57-year-old woman, taking 3 months to resolve completely (Hamburger, 1986).
- Painful ejaculation in an affected male and dyspareunia in an unaffected female following her partner's ejaculation suggest the sexual transfer of ciguatoxin (Lange *et al.*, 1989). In two Australian cases symptoms were also transmitted sexually, one male to female and one female to male (Lewis and King, 1996).
- Severe demyelinating polyneuropathy mainly in motor fibres occurred in ciguatera with the

clinical pattern, electromyography, cerebro-spinal fluid test and sural nerve biopsy confirming the diagnosis (Sozzi et al., 1988).

- Polymyositis proven by biopsy and histological confirmation has also occurred (Stommel et al., 1991, 1993).
- Symptoms of ciguatera may be exacerbated by consumption of alcohol, which may also cause irritation and itching of the skin, particularly the forearms, palms and the soles of the feet (Gillespie et al., 1986; Lewis and King, 1996).
- A rare 'allergy-like' syndrome may occur in some cases where typical symptoms of ciguatera may recur in victims when they eat non-reef fish (Lewis and King, 1996).

### Ciguatera in pregnancy

Ciguatera in pregnancy has been reported (Pearn et al., 1982). Three case studies are given below.

1. The whole family and their two cats suffered ciguatera after consuming a toxic meal. The mother, in the first trimester of pregnancy suffered moderate symptoms of ciguatera for 1 week: the baby was unaffected at birth. Ciguatera was confirmed by mouse bioassay (Fenner et al., 1997).
2. Severe ciguatera poisoning occurred in another mother during the second trimester. The mother experienced increased fetal movements one hour after the poisonous meal, and had multiple ciguatera symptoms for 8 weeks. Ciguatera was suggested by immunoassay. The baby was unaffected at birth (Senecal and Osterloh, 1991).
3. A mother with ciguatera at term delivered an infant suffering from facial palsy and possible myotonia of the hands (Senecal and Osterloh, 1991). No long-term complications were described.

### Differential diagnosis

The diagnosis of ciguatera is usually one of clinical judgement. As such it requires careful assessment, as other illnesses and marine poisonings may have some similar symptoms. Diagnosis

needs a history of reef fish ingestion less than 24 hours previously, accompanied by one neurological symptom and one other symptom (Lewis and King, 1996). Similar symptoms may be caused by botulism, shellfish, scombroid, turtle intoxication (chelonitoxin), shark intoxication (carchatoxins), and sardine intoxication (clupeotoxin), with fatality rates being much higher in these groups (Champetier et al., 1997).

### Treatment

Intravenous mannitol (1 g/kg infused 30–60 min) given within 48 hours of the onset of symptoms can dramatically decrease the acute morbidity of ciguatera, without serious side effects (Palafox et al., 1988; Pearn et al., 1989; Stewart, 1991; Blythe et al., 1992; Palafox, 1992; Fenner et al., 1997). Treatment also appears to be safe and effective in cases 4–8 weeks after the onset of symptoms (Blythe et al., 1992; Fenner et al., 1997). However, animal experiments with mice using intraperitoneal and intravenous mannitol, both prior to and subsequent to intraperitoneal and intravenous ciguatoxin did not influence the signs of intoxication, or the time to death of the mice (Lewis et al., 1993; Purcell et al., 1999). Mannitol is the recommended therapeutic intervention where (i) ciguatera is confirmed or highly likely based on symptomology and the time to onset from eating a risk fish species, (ii) it is given before the start of the recovery phase, and (iii) the patient is adequately hydrated. Mannitol provides clearest clinical benefit in the more severe cases (typically times to onset of $< 6$ h), and a second infusion may provide additional benefit should there be a relapse after the first infusion.

### Fatalities

Fatalities from ciguatera are rare (Mebs, 1980; Lewis and King, 1996), with few accurately documented cases (Tonge, 1967; Bagnis, 1970; Bagnis et al., 1979). Although the authors have heard of unreported fatalities from ciguatera, there are few other published reports in the English literature. It has been suggested that the reason there are few fatalities is that the lethal effects of the cigua-toxins in fish could limit the levels of ciguatoxin concentrations carried by fish (Lewis, 1992).

## Related marine food poisonings

In a single outbreak on the East coast of Madagas-car, more than 500 people, 98 of whom died were poisoned by the flesh of a shark, *Carcharhinus amboinensis*. It is the first case of a severe outbreak caused by a shark, and it is the first case with a mortality rate of 20% (Habermehl *et al.*, 1994). Symptoms were similar to, and first diagnosed as ciguatera. Later testing showed this outbreak to be due to lipid soluble toxins, named carchatoxin-A and B (Boisier *et al.*, 1995). It remains to be determined if these toxins are related structurally and pharmacologically to known ciguatoxins.

Ciguatera can be distinguished from scombroid fish poisoning, which results mainly from con-sumption of Scombrid fish that contain unusually high levels of histamine and other spoilage-related products as a result of inappropriate storage or handling. Ciguatera also differs from tetrodotoxin intoxication, one of the most lethal seafood toxins associated with the consumption of puffer fish species (family *Tetraodontidae*). Interestingly, tetrodotoxin selectively blocks sodium channels in excitable membranes and antagonizes the action of ciguatoxin.

Another toxin potentially associated with cigua-tera is maitotoxin (MTX), a class of polyether toxins originally isolated from the gut content of the surgeonfish *Ctenochaetus striatus*, that is pro-duced by the dinoflagellate *G. toxicus* (Lewis *et al.*, 1994; Rakita, 1995). However, symptoms distinctive for MTX have not been characterized, despite the widespread production of MTX by *G. toxicus* (a few strains of which also produce ciguatoxins) and the fact that MTX and ciguatoxin have distinct pharmacology. Specifically, MTX acts on an unknown cell membrane target to in-crease intracellular $Ca^{2+}$ resulting in the release of hormones and neurotransmitters from secretory cells and nerve terminals (reviewed by Gusovsky and Daly, 1990). In addition, MTXs are at least 100-fold less potent than ciguatoxin when admin-istered by the oral route, while both have similar potency by the i.p. route ($0.1$–$0.25 \mu g/kg$ in mice).

Palytoxin is another class of highly toxic poly-hydroxy macromolecules, isolated originally from Zoanthid coelenterates, but now known also to be produced by the benthic dinoflagellate *Ostreopsis siamensis* (Usami *et al.*, 1995). Like ciguatoxin, palytoxin can accumulate in the marine food chain. While palytoxicoses are restricted to a relatively narrow range of species of tropical fish (e.g. certain Balistids, Scombrids, Clupeids (=clupeotoxism) and Monacanthids), incidences of human morbidity and mortality are not uncom-mon. Palytoxin produces a broad range of phar-macological effects that are due to the formation of non-selective channels (7–25 pS) associated with the $Na^+/K^+$-ATPase, which trigger a large influx of $Na^+$ and $Ca^{2+}$ into cells. The clinical signs of palytoxin poisoning include a spinal seizure-like syndrome with tonic contractions of all muscle groups, muscle spasms associated with markedly elevated levels of serum enzymes asso-ciated with tissue damage (e.g. creatinine phos-phokinase, lactic acid dehydrogenase and glutamic oxaloacetic transaminase), convulsions, extreme pain, myoglobinuria, respiratory distress, dyspnoea, and respiratory failure. Death can occur within 2–4 days of intoxication. The acute and severe nature of palytoxin poisoning distinguishes it from ciguatera (Kodama *et al.*, 1989), although mild forms of this intoxication may be more difficult to distinguish.

Finally, the flesh of some sharks is toxic to humans. In some instances this appears to be due to the presence of large amounts of trimethyl-amine oxide (Anthoni *et al.*, 1991). In other instances lipid-soluble toxins reminiscent of cig-uatoxins appear to be involved (Boisier *et al.*, 1995; Ramialiharisoa *et al.*, 1996). The structural properties of the shark and related Indian Ocean ciguatoxins are now under investigation.

## Ciguatoxins

The ciguatoxins are a family of complex, lipid-soluble, highly oxygenated, cyclic polyether mole-cules (Murata *et al.*, 1990: Lewis *et al.*, 1998).

Several ciguatoxins have been isolated from bio-detritus containing wild *G. toxicus* (Murata *et al.*, 1989, 1990; Holmes *et al.*, 1991; Legrand, 1992), from toxic strains of cultured dinoflagellate iso- lated from different parts of the world (Holmes *et al.*, 1991), or from various ciguateric fish. Using NMR techniques, the chemical structures of a number of Pacific ciguatoxins from fish and

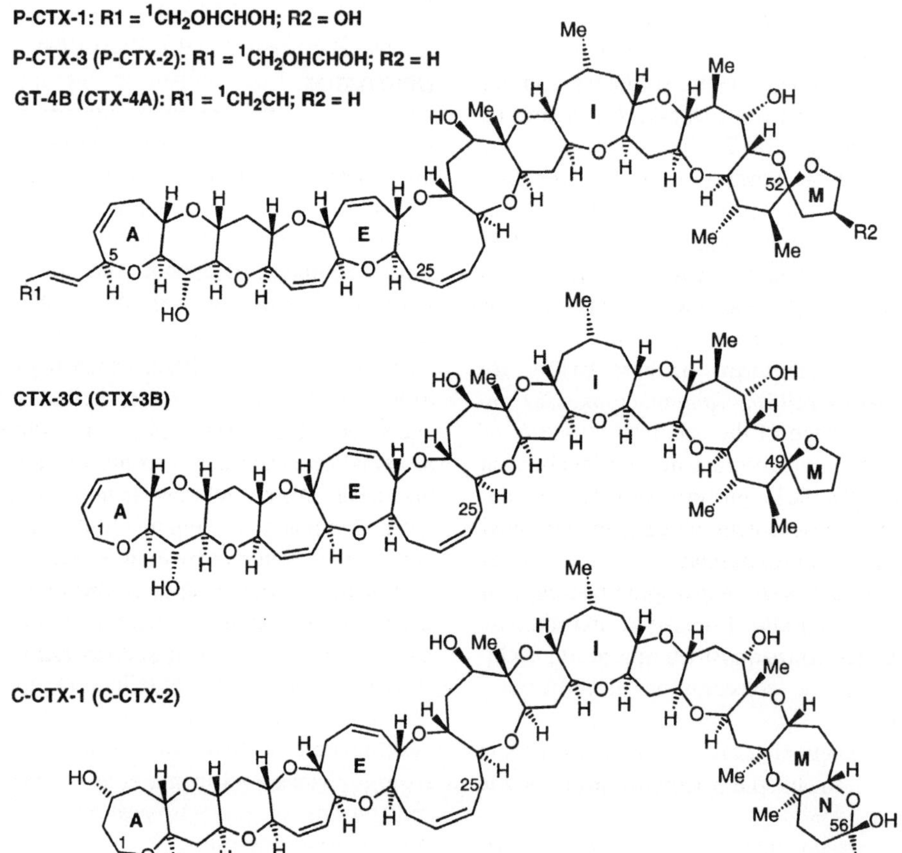

**Figure 20.1** Ciguatoxins from the Pacific Ocean and Caribbean Sea. Shown are P-CTX-1 (Murata *et al.*, 1990), P-CTX-3 (Lewis *et al.*, 1991), GT-4B (Murata *et al.*, 1990), P-CTX-3C (Satake *et al.*, 1993) and C-CTX-1 (Lewis *et al.*, 1998). Less energetically favourable epimers P-CTX-2 (52-epi P-CTX-3) (Lewis *et al.*, 1993), CTX-4A (= 52-epi GT-4B) (Satake *et al.*, 1997), P-CTX-3B (49-epi P-CTX-3C), and C-CTX-2 (56-epi C-CTX-1) (Lewis *et al.*, 1998) are indicated in parenthesis. 2,3-DihydroxyP-CTX-3C and 51-hydroxyP-CTX-3C have also been isolated from Pacific fish (Satake *et al.*, 1998). Brevetoxin (PbTx-2) is shown for comparison.

*G. toxicus* have been elucidated (Murata, 1989, 1990; Lewis *et al.*, 1991, 1993; Satake *et al.*, 1993, 1997, 1998). Recently, the structures of ciguatoxins, C-CTX-1 and C-CTX-2, from Caribbean fish, have been elucidated (Lewis *et al.*, 1998). The structures of known ciguatoxins are shown in Figure 20.1 and their origin and potency outlined in Table 20.2.

The ciguatoxins are the most potent sodium channel toxins known ($\sim$0.3 $\mu$g/kg either oral or i.p. to mice) (see Table 20.2). Despite this potency, ciguatoxins rarely accumulate in fish to levels that are lethal to humans. All the ciguatoxins isolated to date have a structural framework that is reminiscent of the brevetoxins (PbTx), another family of potent lipid-soluble polyether toxins produced by the marine dinoflagellate *Gymnodinium breve* (=*Ptychodiscus brevis)* that include PbTx-1 to PbTx-10 (Baden, 1989; Gawley *et al.*, 1992). From our knowledge of the chemical structure of ciguatoxins found at different trophic levels, it is evident that Pacific ciguatera (P-CTX-1), the dominant and most potent ciguatoxin extracted from the moray-eel *Gymnothorax javanicus*, arises from the acid-catalysed spiroisomerization and oxidative modification of P-CTX-4A produced by the dinoflagellate *G. toxicus* (Murata *et al.*, 1990;

Lewis and Holmes, 1993; (Satake *et al.*, 1998). The chemical structures of known ciguatoxins are compared with PbTx-2 in Figure 20.1.

# Effects of ciguatoxin on the voltage-sensitive sodium channel

Pharmacological studies have revealed that ciguatoxin acts on voltage-sensitive sodium channels (VSSCs). These ion channels are critical elements for the generation and propagation of electrical signals in most excitable cells, and are also present in some non-excitable cells, such as glial cells. Specifically, VSSCs mediate the rapid increase in membrane $Na^+$ conductance responsible for the depolarizing phase of action potentials in many excitable cells. These large membrane-spanning proteins are targeted by a suite of natural toxins that have either inhibitory (site 1) or excitatory (sites 2–5) actions (Figure 20.2). As a consequence of ciguatoxin binding to the VSSC, there is a hyperpolarizing shift in the voltage-dependence of activation of channel. This ciguatoxin-induced activation of sodium channels at the

**Table 20.2 Characteristics* of known ciguatoxins found in fish and *G. toxicus*.**

| Ciguatoxin | Origin | $[M + H]^+$ | Potency ($\mu$g/kg) |
|---|---|---|---|
| P-CTX-1 | Carnivore | 1111 | 0.25 |
| P-CTX-2 | Carnivore | 1095 | 2.3 |
| P-CTX-3 | Carnivore | 1095 | 0.9 |
| P-CTX-3C | *G. toxicus* | 1045 | 2 |
| 2,3-dihydroxyCTX-3C | Carnivore | 1057 | 1.8 |
| 51-hydroxyCTX-3C | Carnivore | 1039 | 0.27 |
| CTX-4A | *G. toxicus*, herbivore | 1061 | 2 |
| CTX-4B | G. toxicus, herbivore | 1061 | 4 |
| C-CTX-1 | Carnivore | 1141 | 3.6 |
| C-CTX-2 | Carnivore | 1141 | 1 |

*Protonated molecular mass ($[M + H]^+$) and intraperitoneal potency to mice are reported. It should be noted that while all ciguatoxins are believed to have their origin in dinoflagellate, many of the ciguatoxin metabolites are only found in fish.

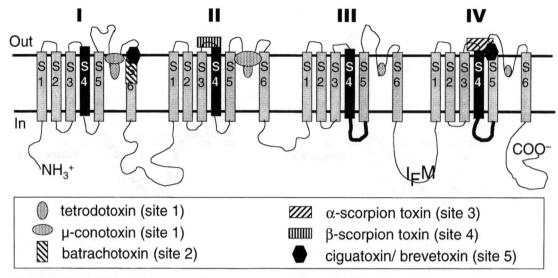

**Figure 20.2** Toxin binding sites 1–5 identified on the neuronal voltage-sensitive sodium channel. The sodium channel comprises the $\alpha$-subunit of about 240–280 kDa ($\sim$2000 amino acids) organized in four repeated homologous domains (I to IV), each containing six putative transmembrane spanning $\alpha$-helical segments (S1 to S6).

resting membrane potential is responsible for numerous $Na^+$-dependent effects (Molgo *et al.*, 1998). These effects include:

1. membrane depolarization and spontaneous and repetitive action potentials in excitable cells
2. altering the $Na^+$ gradient driving the $Na^+$–$Ca^{2+}$ exchanger, leading to an elevation in intracellular $Ca^{2+}$ concentration
3. repetitive, synchronous and asynchronous neurotransmitter release
4. transient increases and decreases in the quantal content of synaptic responses
5. spontaneous and tetanic muscle contractions, and positive and negative inotropic effects in cardiac musculature
6. impaired synaptic vesicle recycling that exhausts neurotransmitter available for release
7. swelling of axons, nerve terminals and perisynaptic Schwann cells (Molgo *et al.*, 1992).

The effects of ciguatoxin are typically observed at nanomolar concentrations. Although it is clear that ciguatoxin affects the biophysical properties of a fraction of VSSCs, the pharmacological properties of toxin-modified $Na^+$ channels remain largely unaffected (Benoit *et al.*, 1992, 1996).

P-CTX-1 (0.2 to 20 nM) affects both tetrodotoxin (TTX) sensitive and TTX-resistant voltage

sensitive sodium channels (VSSCs) (Strachan *et al.*, 1999) (Figure 20.3A and B, respectively). At TTX-sensitive sodium channels, P-CTX-1 causes a 13 mV hyperpolarizing shift in the voltage dependence of activation, a 22 mV hyperpolarizing shift in steady-state inactivation ($h_\infty$), and a TTX-sensitive leakage current. In contrast, the major effect of P-CTX-1 on TTX-resistant sodium channels was to increase the rate of recovery from sodium channel inactivation. A differential excitatory effect of ciguatoxin on TTX-sensitive and TTX-resistant sodium channels may contribute to the diversity of sensory neurological disturbances associated with ciguatera (Strachan *et al.*, 1999).

In single channel studies, 1–10 nM P-CTX-1 in the patch pipette markedly increased the open probability for single TTX-sensitive sodium channels in response to depolarizing voltage steps (Hogg *et al.*, 1998). In about half these patches P-CTX-1 caused single $Na^+$ channels to open spontaneously, even at membrane potentials hyperpolarized to $-160$ mV (Figure 20.3C). These changes were not associated with a change in the unitary conductance (10 pS) or reversal potential of the channel (Hogg *et al.*, 1998). Thus P-CTX-1 increases neuronal excitability by shifting the voltage dependence of activation of TTX-sensitive sodium channels to more negative

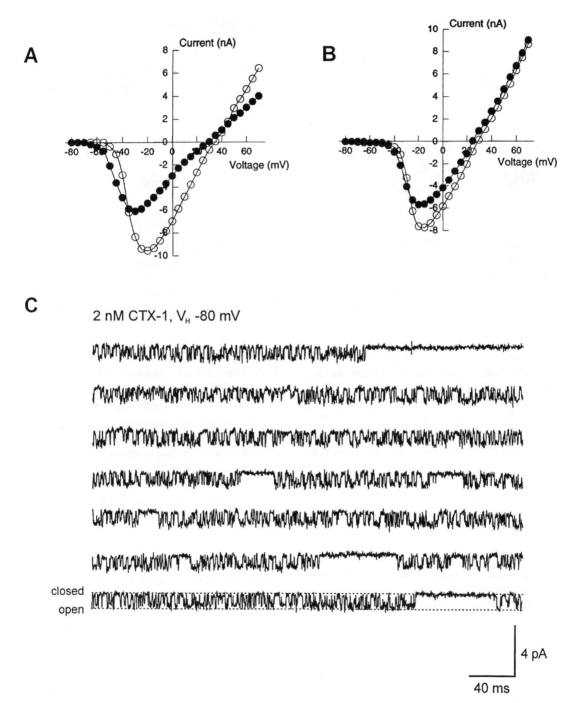

**Figure 20.3** Typical effects of P-CTX-1 on the voltage-dependence of activation of TTX-sensitive and TTX-resistant Na$^+$ currents. The peak Na$^+$ current at each voltage step was measured and plotted as a function of membrane potential for (A) TTX-sensitive and (B) TTX-resistant Na$^+$ currents in the absence (○) or presence of 5nMP-CTX-1(●). (Modified from Strachan *et al.*, 1999). (C) Spontaneous sodium channel openings obtained from a cell-attached membrane patch held at −80 mV in the presence of 2 nM P-CTX-1 under steady-state conditions. These sodium channels failed to stay closed, even at −160 mV. The inward currents in each of these records were ∼ 10 pS, and are shown as downward deflections. (Modified from Hogg *et al.*, 1998).

potentials, and by creating a population of channels that produce a persistent, non-inactivating $Na^+$ current. This latter effect most likely underlies the CTX-induced, TTX-sensitive leakage current seen in whole cell voltage clamp studies (Strachan et al., 1999).

In addition to having similar polyether structures (see Figure 20.1), ciguatoxins and brevetoxins both selectively target a common binding site on the neuronal VSSC protein (Poli et al., 1986, 1997; Baden, 1989; Lewis et al., 1991; Gawley et al., 1992; Pauillac et al., 1995). Brevetoxins bind with high affinity to neurotoxin receptor site 5 of the sodium channel, as revealed by direct binding studies using radioabelled [$^3$H]PbTx-3, and by binding assays that show non-competitive interactions between site 5 and a variety of toxin probes specific for sites 1–4 (Bidard et al., 1984; Poli et al., 1986; Sharkey et al., 1987; Cestele et al., 1996). Functional studies, such as increasing the potency of batrachotoxin-induced $Na^+$ influx into cells, further show that ciguatoxin does not act at as a competitor at sites 1–4 on the VSSC (Bidard et al., 1984). Using a photolabelled derivative of PbTx-3 and site-directed antibody mapping, the partial localization of the receptor site 5 of voltage-dependent $Na^+$ channels (from rat brain) has been suggested to be in the region of interaction of segments S6 and S5 of domains I and IV, respectively (Trainer et al., 1994) (see Figure 20.1).

Ciguatoxin causes oedema of the adaxonal Schwann cell cytoplasm in nerve fibres (Allsop et al., 1986) and significant slowing of both mixed and motor nerve conduction by prolonging sodium channel activation (Cameron et al., 1991). These electrophysiological disturbances can be blocked by intraperitoneal lignocaine (lidocaine) in mouse models, suggesting it might have a potential therapeutic application in the treatment of the neurological disturbance in acute ciguatera poisoning in humans (Cameron et al., 1993). However, the authors are not aware of clinical trials, or reports of clinical benefit from the use of lignocaine, although an orally active analogue, tocainide has been used occasionally with benefit (Lange et al., 1989). Some cases of intoxication, including one fatal case, have both peripheral and central nervous system involvement (Bagnis et al., 1977; Allsop et al., 1986).

# Testing for ciguateric fish

ELISA tests have been developed which reportedly detect ciguatera qualitatively and quantitatively in human fluids, as well as in contaminated fish tissue (Fleming et al., 1992). Also an MIA is a simple, rapid, sensitive, and specific detection method for CTX and its related polyethers, with no reported false negative results (Hokama et al., 1998a). Despite these encouraging reports, a validated test for ciguatera is not available commercially.

A number of sodium channel assays have also been developed to detect ciguatera. A neuroblastoma cell assay has the potential to be developed into a simple and sensitive method to detect sodium channel-specific marine toxins using a mitochondrial dehydrogenase activity end-point (Manger et al., 1993, 1995). Cells are sensitized to the action of ciguatoxin by the addition of veratridine (a partial agonist at site 2) and ouabain (an inhibitor of the $Na^+/K^+$ ATPase). Within 6 h, brevetoxins can be detected at $\geq 250$ pg and purified CTX-1 can be detected at subpicogram levels. A sensitive cell-based assay for brevetoxins, saxitoxins and ciguatoxins has also been reported that employs ac-fos-luciferase reporter gene stably expressed in cells (Fairey et al., 1997). [$^3$H]PbTx-3 binding to brain membrane can also be used to detect ciguatoxins in crude extracts (Poli et al., 1997) and can be developed into high-throughput assays. These sodium channel assays, and possibly antibody-based assays (Hokama et al., 1998b) have potential to replace animal testing for ciguatoxins, and warrant further validation to determine the potential of such assays to be developed into rapid screens for public health protection. Analytical methods are now being developed which have the required sensitivity, but are presently not cost-effective for routine screening (Lewis et al., 1999).

# Conclusions

Considerable progress has been made in determining the structures and modes of action of the principal toxins involved in ciguatera. The development of tests that detect the presence of ciguatoxin in fish prior to consumption are required to improve significantly the management of ciguatera, and to overcome present limitations of diagnosis and existing therapies. Differential diagnosis depends on clinical recognition of specific signs and symptoms, and is complicated by difficulties distinguishing ciguatera from other marine poisonings and other illnesses. Intravenous hyperosmolar D-mannitol has evolved as a unique remedy for acutely poisoned patients (Palafox *et al.*, 1988; Pearn *et al.*, 1989).

# References

Allsop, J. L., Martini, L., Lebris, H., Pollard, J., Walsh, J. and Hodgkinson, S. (1986). (Neurologic manifestations of ciguatera. 3 cases with a neurophysiologic study and examination of one nerve biopsy). *Rev Neurol (Paris)*, **142**, 590–7.

Anthoni, U., Christophersen, C., Gram, L., Nielsen, N. H. and Nielsen, P. (1991). Poisonings from flesh of the Greenland shark *Somniosus microcephalus* may be due to trimethylamine. *Toxicon*, **29**, 1205–12.

Arcila-Herrera, H., Castello-Navarrete, A., Mendoza-Ayora, J., Montero-Cervantes, L., Gonzalez-Franco, M. F. and Brito-Villanueva, W. O. (1998). (Ten cases of Ciguatera fish poisoning in Yucatan). *Rev Invest Clin.*, **50**, 149–52.

Baden, D. G. (1989). Brevetoxins: unique polyether dinoflagellate toxins. *FASEB J.*, **3**, 1807–17.

Bagnis, R. (1970). Concerning a fatal case of ciguatera poisoning in the Tuamotu Islands. *Clin Toxicol.*, **3**, 579–83.

Bagnis, R., Kuberski, T. and Laugier, S. (1979). Clinical observations on 3009 cases of ciguatera (fish poisoning) in the South Pacific. *Am J Trop Med Hyg.*, **28**, 1067–73.

Bagnis, R. A., Bronstein, J. A., Jouffe, G. *et al.* (1977). (Neurologic complications of ciguatera). *Bull Soc Pathol Exot Filiales*, **70**, 89–93.

Barton, E. D., Tanner, P., Turchen, S. G., Tunget, C. L., Manoguerra, A. and Clark, R. F. (1995). Ciguatera fish poisoning. A southern California epidemic. *West J Med.*, **163**, 31–5.

Benoit, E., Juzans, P., Legrand, A. M. and Molgo, J. (1996). Nodal swelling produced by ciguatoxin-induced selective activation of sodium channels in myelinated nerve fibers. *Neuroscience*, **71**, 1121–31.

Benoit, E. and Legrand, A. M. (1992). Purified ciguatoxin-induced modifications in excitability of myelinated nerve fibre. *Bull Soc Pathol Exot.*, **85**, 497–9.

Bidard, J. N., Vijverberg, H. P., Frelin, C. *et al.* (1984). Ciguatoxin is a novel type of Na⁺ channel toxin. *J Biol Chem.*, **259**, 8353–7.

Blythe, D. G., De Sylva, D. P., Fleming, L. E., Ayyar, R. A., Baden, D. G. and Shrank, K. (1992). Clinical experience with i.v. mannitol in the treatment of ciguatera. *Bull Soc Pathol Exot.*, **85**, 425–6.

Boisier, P., Ranaivoson, G., Rasolofonirina, N. *et al.* (1995). Fatal mass poisoning in Madagascar following ingestion of a shark (*Carcharhinus leucas*): clinical and epidemiological aspects and isolation of toxins. *Toxicon*, **33**, 1359–64.

Calvert, G. M., Hryhorczuk, D. O. and Leikin, J. B. (1987). Treatment of ciguatera fish poisoning with amitriptyline and nifedipine. *J Toxicol Clin Toxicol.*, **25**, 423–8.

Cameron, J. and Capra, M. F. (1993). The basis of the paradoxical disturbance of temperature perception in ciguatera poisoning. *J Toxicol Clin Toxicol.*, **31**, 571–9.

Cameron, J., Flowers, A. E. and Capra, M. F. (1991). Effects of ciguatoxin on nerve excitability in rats (Part I). *J Neurol Sci.*, **101**, 87–92.

Cameron, J., Flowers, A. E. and Capra, M. F. (1993). Modification of the peripheral nerve disturbance in ciguatera poisoning in rats with lidocaine. *Muscle Nerve*, **16**, 782–6.

Cestele, S., Sampieri, F., Rochat, H. and Gordon, D. (1996). Tetrodotoxin reverses brevetoxin allosteric inhibition of scorpion alpha-toxin binding on rat brain sodium channels. *J Biol Chem.*, **271**, 18329–32.

Champetier, D. R., Rasolofonirina, R. N., Ranaivoson, G., Razafimahefa, N., Rakotoson, J. D. and Rabeson, D. (1997). (Intoxication by marine animal venoms in Madagascar (ichthyosarcotoxism and chelonitoxism): recent epidemiological data). *Bull Soc Pathol Exot.*, **90**, 286–90.

DeFusco, D. J., O'Dowd, P., Hokama, Y. and Ott, B. R. (1993). Coma due to ciguatera poisoning in Rhode Island (see comments). *Am J Med.*, **95**, 240–3.

Fairey, E. R., Edmunds, J. S. and Ramsdell, J. S. (1997). A cell-based assay for brevetoxins, saxitoxins, and ciguatoxins using a stably expressed c-fos-luciferase reporter gene. *Anal Biochem.*, **251**, 129–32.

Fenner, P. J., Lewis, R. J., Williamson, J. A. and Williams, M. L. (1997). A Queensland family with ciguatera after eating coral trout. *Med J Aust.*, **166**, 473–5.

Fleming, L. E., Baden, D. G., Ayyar, R. A. *et al.* (1992). A pilot study of a new ELISA test for ciguatoxin in humans. *Bull Soc Pathol Exot.*, **85**, 508–9.

Gawley, R. E., Rein, K. S., Kinoshita, M. and Baden, D. G. (1992). Binding of brevetoxins and ciguatoxin to the voltage-sensitive sodium channel and conformational analysis of brevetoxin B. *Toxicon*, **30**, 780–5.

Geller, R. J. and Benowitz, N. L. (1992). Orthostatic hypotension in ciguatera fish poisoning. *Arch Intern Med.*, **152**, 2131–3.

Gillespie, N. C., Lewis, R. J., Pearn, J. H. *et al.* (1986). Ciguatera in Australia. Occurrence, clinical features, pathophysiology and management. *Med J Aust.*, **145**, 584–90.

Glaziou, P. and Martin, P. M. (1992). Study of factors that influence the clinical response to ciguatera fish poisoning. *Bull Soc Pathol Exot.*, **85**, 419–20.

Habermehl, G. G., Krebs, H. C., Rasoanaivo, P. and Ramialiharisoa, A. (1994). Severe ciguatera poisoning in Madagascar: a case report. *Toxicon*, **32**, 1539–42.

Hamburger, H. A. (1986). The neuro-ophthalmologic signs of ciguatera poisoning: a case report. *Ann Ophthalmol.*, **18**, 287–8.

Ho, A. M., Fraser, I. M. and Todd, E. C. (1986). Ciguatera poisoning: a report of three cases. *Ann Emerg Med.*, **15**, 1225–8.

Hogg, R. C., Lewis, R. J. and Adams, D. J. (1998). Ciguatoxin (CTX-1) modulates single tetrodotoxin-sensitive sodium channels in rat parasympathetic neurones. *Neurosci Lett.*, **252**, 103–6.

Hokama, Y., Nishimura, K., Takenaka, W. and Ebesu, J. S. (1998). Simplified solid-phase membrane immunobead assay (MIA) with monoclonal anti-ciguatoxin antibody (MAb-CTX) for detection of ciguatoxin and related polyether toxins. *J Nat Toxins*, **7**, 1–21.

Hokama, Y., Takenaka, W. E., Nishimura, K. L., Ebesu, J. S., Bourke, R. and Sullivan, P. K. (1998). A simple membrane immunobead assay for detecting ciguatoxin and related polyethers from human ciguatera intoxication and natural reef fishes. *J AOAC Int.*, **81**, 727–35.

Holmes, M. J., Lewis, R. J., Poli, M. A. and Gillespie, N. C. (1991). Strain dependent production of ciguatoxin precursors (gambiertoxins) by *Gambierdiscus toxicus* (Dinophyceae) in culture. *Toxicon*, **29**, 761–75.

Katz, A. R., Terrell-Perica, S. and Sasaki, D. M. (1993). Ciguatera on Kauai: investigation of factors associated with severity of illness. *Am J Trop Med Hyg.*, **49**, 448–54.

Kodama, A. M., Hokama, Y., Yasumoto, T., Fukui, M., Manea, S. J. and Sutherland, N. (1989). Clinical and laboratory findings implicating palytoxin as cause of ciguatera poisoning due to *Decapterus macrosoma* (mackerel). *Toxicon*, **27**, 1051–3.

Lange, W. R., Kreider, S. D., Hattwick, M. and Hobbs, J. (1988). Potential benefit of tocainide in the treatment of ciguatera: report of three cases. *Am J Med.*, **84**, 1087–8.

Lange, W. R., Lipkin, K. M. and Yang, G. C. (1989). Can ciguatera be a sexually transmitted disease? *J Toxicol Clin Toxicol.*, **27**, 193–7.

Legrand, A. M. (1992). Characterization of ciguatoxins from different fish species and wild *Gambierdiscus toxicus*. In *Proceedings of the Third International Conference on Ciguatera Fish Poisoning* (ed. Tosteson, T. R.). pp 25–32. Quebec: Polyscience Publications.

Legrand, A. M., Galonnier, M. and Bagnis, R. (1982).

Studies on the mode of action of ciguateric toxins. *Toxicon*, **20**, 311–5.

Levine, D. Z. (1995). Ciguatera: current concepts. *J Am Osteopath Assoc.*, **95**, 193–8.

Lewis, R. J. (1992). Ciguatoxins are potent ichthyotoxins. *Toxicon*, **30**, 207–11.

Lewis, R. J. (1992). Socioeconomic impacts and management ciguatera in the Pacific. *Bull Soc Pathol Exot.*, **85**, 427–34.

Lewis, R. J. and Holmes, M. J. (1993). Origin and transfer of toxins involved in ciguatera. *Comp Biochem Physiol C*, **106**, 615–28.

Lewis, R. J. and King, G. K. (1996). Ciguatera. In *Venomous and Poisonous Marine Animals: a Medical and Biological Handbook* (eds Williamson, J. A., Fenner, P. J., Burnett, J. W., Rifkin, J. F.) pp. 347–353. Sydney: NSW Uni Press.

Lewis, R. J., Sellin, M., Poli, M. A., Norton, R. S., MacLeod, J. K. and Sheil, M. M.(1991). Purification and characterization of ciguatoxins from moray eel (*Lycodontis javanicus*, Muraenidae). *Toxicon*, **29**, 1115–27.

Lewis, R. J., Norton, R. S., Brereton, I. M. and Eccles, C. D. (1993). Ciguatoxin-2 is a diastereomer of ciguatoxin-3. *Toxicon*, **31**, 637–43.

Lewis, R. J., Hoy, A. W. and Sellin, M. (1993). Ciguatera and mannitol: *in vivo* and i*n vitro* assessment in mice. *Toxicon*, **31**, 1039–50.

Lewis, R. J., Holmes, M. J., Alewood, P. F. and Jones, A. (1994). Ionspray mass spectrometry of ciguatoxin-1, maitotoxin-2 and -3, and related marine polyether toxins. *Nat Toxins*, **2**, 56–63.

Lewis, R. J., Vernoux, J. P. and Brereton, I. M. (1998). Structure of Caribbean ciguatoxin isolated from *Caranx latus*. *J Am Chem Soc.*, **120**, 5914–20.

Lewis, R. J., Jones, A. and Vernoux, J. P. (1999). HPLC/tandem electrospray mass spectrometry for the determination of Sub-ppb levels of Pacific and Caribbean ciguatoxins in crude extracts of fish. *Anal Chem.*, **71**, 247–50.

Manger, R. L., Leja, L. S., Lee, S. Y. *et al.* (1995). Detection of sodium channel toxins: directed cytotoxicity assays of purified ciguatoxins, brevetoxins, saxitoxins, and seafood extracts. *J AOAC Int.*, **78**, 521–7.

Manger, R. L., Leja, L. S., Lee, S. Y., Hungerford, J. M. and Wekell, M. M. (1993). Tetrazolium-based cell bioassay for neurotoxins active on voltage-sensitive sodium channels: semiautomated assay for saxitoxins, brevetoxins, and ciguatoxins. *Anal Biochem.*, **214**, 190–4.

Mebs, D. (1980). (Ciguatera (author's transl)). *Munch Med Wochenschr.*, **122**, 1413–4.

Molgo, J., Meunier, F. A., Dechraoui, M. Y., Benoit, E., Mattei, C. and Legrand, A. M. (1998). Sodium-dependent alterations of synaptic transmission mechanisms by brevetoxins and ciguatoxins. In *Harmful Microalgae* (eds Reguera, B., Blanco, J., Fernández, M. L.,

Wyatt, T.) pp. 594–597. Santiago De Compostella: Xunta de Galicia and Intergovernmental Oceanographic Commission of UNESCO.

Molgo, J., Benoit, E., Comella, J. X. and Legrand, A. M. (1992). Ciguatoxin: a tool for research on sodium-dependent mechanisms. In *Methods in Neuroscience, Neurotoxins*, vol. 8 (ed. Conn, P. M.) pp. 149–164. New York: Academic Press.

Murata, M., Legrand, A. M., Ishibashi, Y. and Yasumoto, T. (1989). Structures and configurations of ciguatoxin and its congener. *J Am Chem Soc*, **111**, 8929–31.

Murata, M., Legrand, A. M., Ishibashi, Y. and Yasumoto, T. (1990). Structures and configurations of ciguatoxin from the Moray eel *Gymnothorax-javanicus* and its likely precursor from the dinoflagellate *Gambierdiscus-toxicus*. *J Am Chem Soc.*, **112**, 4380–86.

Palafox, N. A. (1992). Review of the clinical use of intravenous mannitol with ciguatera fish poisoning from 1988 to 1992. *Bull Soc Pathol Exot.*, **85**, 423–4.

Palafox, N. A., Jain, L. G., Pinano, A. Z., Gulick, T. M., Williams, R. K. and Schatz, I. J. (1988). Successful treatment of ciguatera fish poisoning with intravenous mannitol. *JAMA*, **259**, 2740–2.

Pauillac, S., Bléhaut, J., Cruchet, P., Lotte, C. and Legrand, A. M. (1995). Recent advances in detection of ciguatoxins in French Polynesia. In *Harmful Algal Blooms* (eds Lassus, P., Arzul, G., Erard, E., Gentien, P., Marcaillou, C.) pp. 801–808. France: Lavoisier, Intercept Ltd.

Pearn, J., Harvey, P., De Ambrosis, W., Lewis, R. and McKay, R. (1982). Ciguatera and pregnancy (letter). *Med J Aust.*, **1**, 57–8.

Pearn, J. H., Lewis, R. J., Ruff, T. *et al.* (1989). Ciguatera and mannitol: experience with a new treatment regimen (see comments). *Med J Aust.*, **151**, 77–80.

Poli, M. A., Lewis, R. J., Dickey, R. W., Musser, S. M., Buckner, C. A. and Carpenter, L. G. (1997). Identification of Caribbean ciguatoxins as the cause of an outbreak of fish poisoning among U.S. soldiers in Haiti. *Toxicon*, **35**, 733–41.

Poli, M. A., Mende, T. J. and Baden, D. G. (1986). Brevetoxins, unique activators of voltage-sensitive sodium channels, bind to specific sites in rat brain synaptosomes. *Mol Pharmacol.*, **30**, 129–35.

Purcell, C. E., Capra, M. F. and Cameron, J. (1999). Action of mannitol in ciguatoxin-intoxicated rats. *Toxicon*, **37**, 67–76.

Quod, J. P. and Turquet, J. (1996). Ciguatera in Reunion Island (SW Indian Ocean): epidemiology and clinical patterns. *Toxicon*, **34**, 779–85.

Raikhlin-Eisenkraft, B., Finkelstein, Y. and Spanier, E. (1988). Ciguatera-like poisoning in the Mediterranean. *Vet Hum Toxicol.*, **30**, 582–3.

Rakita, R. M. (1995). Ciguatera poisoning. *J Travel Med.*, **2**, 252–4.

Ramialiharisoa, A., Rafenoherimanana, R., De Haro, L. and Jouglard, J. (1996). (Collective poisoning of ciguateric type after ingestion of shark in Madagascar. Data collected by the Antananarivo medical team (letter)). *Presse Med.*, **25**, 1350.

Sanner, B. M., Rawert, B., Henning, B. and Zidek,W. (1997). Ciguatera fish poisoning following travel to the tropics. *Z Gastroenterol.*, **35**, 327–30.

Satake, M., Ishibashi, Y., Legrand, A. M. and Yasumoto, T. (1997). Isolation and structure of ciguatoxin-4A, a new ciguatoxin precursor, from cultures of dinoflagellate *Gambierdiscus toxicus* and parrotfish *Scarus gibbus. Biosci Biotech Biochem.*, **60**, 2103–5.

Satake, M., Fukui, M., Legrand, A. M., Cruchet, P. and Yasumoto, T. (1998). Isolation and structures of new ciguatoxin analogs, 2,3-dihydroxyCTX3C and 51-hydroxyCTX3C, accumulated in tropical reef fish. *Tetrahedron Lett.*, **39**, 1197–8.

Satake, M., Murata, M. and Yasumoto, T. (1993). The structure of CTX3c, a ciguatoxin congener isolated from cultured *Gambierdiscus toxicus. Tetrahedron Lett.*, **34**, 1975–8.

Senecal, P. E. and Osterloh, J. D. (1991). Normal fetal outcome after maternal ciguateric toxin exposure in the second trimester. *J Toxicol Clin Toxicol.*, **29**, 473–8.

Sharkey, R. G., Jover, E., Couraud, F., Baden, D. G. and Catterall, W. A. (1987). Allosteric modulation of neurotoxin binding to voltage-sensitive sodium channels by *Ptychodiscus brevis* toxin 2. *Mol Pharmacol.*, **31**, 273–8.

Sozzi, G., Marotta, P., Aldeghi, D., Tredici, G. and Calvi, L. (1988). Polyneuropathy secondary to ciguatoxin poisoning. *Ital J Neurol Sci .*, **9**, 491–5.

Stewart, M. P. (1991). Ciguatera fish poisoning: treatment with intravenous mannitol. *Trop Doct.*, **21**, 54–5.

Stommel, E. W., Parsonnet, J. and Jenkyn, L. R. (1991). Polymyositis after ciguatera toxin exposure. *Arch Neurol.*, **48**, 874–7.

Stommel, E. W., Jenkyn, L. R. and Parsonnet, J. (1993). Another case of polymyositis after ciguatera toxin exposure (letter). *Arch Neurol.*, **50**, 571.

Strachan, L. C., Lewis, R. J. and Nicholson, G. M. (1999). Differential actions of pacific ciguatoxin-1 on sodium channel subtypes in mammalian sensory neurons. *J Pharmacol Exp Ther.*, **288**, 379–88.

Tonge, J. I., Battey, Y., Forbes, J. J. and Grant, E. M. (1967). Ciguatera poisoning: a report of two outbreaks and a probable fatal case in Queensland. *Med J Aust.*, **2**, 1088–90.

Trainer, V. L., Baden, D. G. and Catterall, W. A. (1994). Identification of peptide components of the brevetoxin receptor site of rat brain sodium channels. *J Biol Chem.*, **269**, 19904–9.

Usami, M., Satake, M., Ishida, S. *et al.* (1995). Palytoxin analogs from the dinoflagellate Ostreopsis siamensis. *J Am Chem Soc.*, **117**, 5389–90.

# Potential channel disorders

# Potential channelopathies:

### selected myotonic disorders – Schwartz Jampel syndrome (SJS), myotonic dystrophy (DM), myotonic dystrophy type-2 (DM-2), proximal myotonic myopathy (PROMM), and proximal myotonic dystrophy (PDM)

*Richard Moxley*

## Introduction

Schwartz Jampel syndrome (SJS), myotonic dystrophy (DM), myotonic dystrophy type-2 (DM-2), proximal myotonic myopathy (PROMM), and proximal myotonic dystrophy (PDM) are multisystem myotonic disorders. The exact molecular defects responsible for the muscle wasting and myotonia in these disorders remain a mystery. However, the presence of myotonia as a characteristic feature suggests that these diseases may be 'channelopathies'. Support for this speculation comes from reports that describe the beneficial effects of certain antimyotonia drugs in these disorders. Carbamazepine stabilizes electrical activity in nerve cells by reducing post-tetanic facilitation through its actions on sodium conductance. Carbamazepine reduces myotonia in SJS (Topaloglu *et al.*, 1993) and in DM (Sechi *et al.*, 1983). Mexiletine, a lidocaine derivative that acts on the sodium channel, controls myotonia in both sodium and chloride channelopathies as well as in DM (Kwiecinski *et al.*, 1992). This amelioration of myotonia by medications that influence channel function provides provisional support to the idea that SJS, DM and DM-related disorders are potential channelopathies.

This chapter begins with a brief discussion of SJS and concludes with a review of DM, DM-2, PROMM, and PDM. These diseases are reviewed as a group because of their remarkable clinical similarities and their possible genetic connections.

## Schwartz Jampel syndrome (chondrodystrophic myotonia)

The Schwartz Jampel Syndrome (SJS) is a rare disorder. Patients have stiffness and tightening in the muscles of the face (giving a pursed lips appearance), peculiar facies (sad rigid expression, small palpebral apertures–blepharophimosis, and low set ears), bony deformities, short neck, protuberant abdomen, sparse connective tissue, and joint contractures (Fontaine *et al.*, 1996; Brown *et al.*, 1997; Cook and Borkowski, 1997; Cormier-Daire *et al.*, 1997; Giedion *et al.*, 1997; Singh *et al.*, 1997; Superti-Furga *et al.*, 1998; al-Gazali *et al.*, 1999; Christova *et al.*, 1999). Facial features become more pronounced with age. Joint contractures usually involve elbows, wrists, and shoulders. Over time the shoulders become positioned forward with internal rotation of the arms. Osteoarticular abnormalities occur and may vary in severity (Fontaine *et al.*, 1996; Giedion *et al.*, 1997; al-Gazali *et al.*, 1999). Moderate bone dysplasia occurs usually in type 1A, and more pronounced dysplasia, recognizable at birth, occurs in type 1B and type 2. The most common type of SJS is type 1A. Symptoms appear within the first 3 years of life. Electromyography reveals continuous high frequency muscle fibre activity, myotonic runs and complex repetitive discharges. Action and muscle percussion myotonia are present.

There are three forms of SJS: types 1A and 1B, which link to chromosome 1p34-p36 (Fontaine *et al.*, 1996; Giedion *et al.*, 1997; al-Gazali *et al.*, 1999); and type 2, which does not link to this locus (Brown *et al.*, 1997). Table 21.1 summarizes their clinical, genetic, and electrodiagnostic characteristics. Table 21.2 summarizes the radiological features and treatment.

## Genetics

A brief mention of past description of dominant inheritance of SJS is necessary (Pascuzzi *et al.*, 1990). These cases probably represent sodium channelopathies (Rudel *et al.*, 1993). One report describes a severe form of sodium channel myotonia, myotonia permanens, caused by a mutation in the gene for the skeletal muscle sodium channel (Lereche *et al.*, 1993). The patients have muscle stiffness and facial features resembling SJS. Neurophysiological and genetic testing for sodium channel disease is useful in atypical cases of SJS.

Recent reports clearly establish that SJS is an autosomal recessive, genetically heterogeneous disorder (Fontaine *et al.*, 1996; Brown *et al.*, 1997; Giedion *et al.*, 1997). SJS type 1B and SJS type 2 are similar, and yet they have distinctly different genetic loci. Type 2 is the more severe. There is also a similarity between SJS type 2 and the Stuve-Wiedemann Syndrome (SWS) (Cormier-Daire, 1997; Superti-Furga *et al.*, 1998). Both SJS type 2 and SWS present in the neonatal period, have respiratory insufficiency, have feeding difficulties due to a reduced or absent swallowing reflex, and have episodic hyperthermia with decreased sweating. Both have a high frequency of death during infancy. The fundamental difference between the two is the absence of membrane irritability in SWS (Brown *et al.*, 1997; Superti-Furga *et al.*, 1998). The orthopaedic abnormalities are similar for both conditions. This observation indicates that contractures and bony defects in SJS do not develop solely as sequelae of continuous muscle fibre activity and myotonia. The cause for the episodic hyperthermia observed in SJS type 2 and SWS is unknown. The episodes of hyperthermia are not identical to the attacks in malignant hyperthermia, and there is no proven relationship between SJS type 2 and malignant hyperthermia. Genetic studies show no linkage to the ryanodine receptor gene locus on chromosome 19 or to the APOC II locus which is close by (Brown *et al.*, 1997).

## New clinical observations

There are relatively few new clinical observations. The most important is that there are two infantile onset forms, type1B linked to chromosome 1p34-p36, and type 2 not linked to this locus.

## Pathophysiology

The aetiology of the continuous muscle fibre activity and myotonia in the different types of SJS is unclear. Some reports indicate that the activity continues even in the presence of general anaesthesia and curare (Landau, 1952; Hofmann *et al.*, 1966), while other reports indicate that curare abolishes the myotonia and other discharges (Taylor *et al.*, 1972). One recent report describes multiplet discharges and long intermultiplet intervals that cannot be explained by abnormalities in the muscle membrane (Christova *et al.*, 1999). These investigators suggest that, at least in some cases of SJS, the abnormal muscle fibre activity is 'neuromyotonic'.

## Treatment

Ventilatory support and nasogastric or G-tube feeding are needed in severely affected infants. Control of episodic hyperthermia is necessary. Older children may develop respiratory problems, including obstructive sleep apnoea (Cook and Borkowski, 1997). Orthopaedic and radiological consultations are critical early in the course of treatment. Carbamazepine is useful to control the stiffness and myotonia (Topaloglu *et al.*, 1993).

**Table 21.1 Schwartz–Jampel syndrome (chondrodystrophic myotonia)**

| | Schwartz–Jampel syndrome type 1A | Schwartz–Jampel syndrome type 1B | Schwartz–Jampel syndrome type 2 |
|---|---|---|---|
| Inheritance | Autosomal recessive | Autosomal recessive | Autosomal recessive |
| Gene defect | Chromosome 1p34-p36; candidate genes include a receptor tyrosine Kinase (ERK) and collagen genes (Col 8A2 and Col 16A1) | Chromosome 1p34-p36; candidate genes same as type 1A; may be allelic to type 1A | Not linked to chromosome 1p34-36 or loci on chromosome 19 for malignant hyperthermia (ryanodine receptor gene); no established chromosomal localization |
| Onset of myotonia | Early childhood | Infancy or early childhood | Birth |
| Onset of bone dysplasia | Childhood | Birth | Birth |
| Clinical features | Decreased facial mobility; Blepharospasmus, blepharophimosis and microstomia with pursed lips; variably severe external rotation of legs with recurvatum of knees; eversion of ankles; muscle atrophy; flexion contractures; short stature; short neck; respiratory infections; high fevers; hypertrophy of base of tongue; occasional obstructive sleep apnoea; normal intelligence | Earlier onset of features noted for type 1A; more severe bone dysplasia | Neonatal hypomobility; feeding difficulty with reduced or absent swallowing reflex; episodic threatening hyperthermia; reduced sweating; contractures (fingers, elbows, knees); respiratory insufficiency; apnoeic episodes; myotonic in hands to percussion in newborn period becoming less prominent in infancy; death frequent in infancy |
| Electrophysiological findings | Continuous muscle activity (myotonia bursts, high frequency discharges of single motor units); multiplets with interpulse intervals varying from 2–12 ms; normal values for motor and sensory nerve conduction studies; muscle activity sometimes persists and other times disappears following curare | Continuous muscle activity; limited information about effects of curare; normal nerve conduction | Continuous muscle activity; myotonic discharges decrease in prominence later in infancy; some cases show disappearance of muscle discharges after curare; normal nerve conduction studies |

**Table 21.2 Schwartz-Jampel syndrome (chondrodystrophic myotonia) (continued)**

|  | *Schwartz-Jampel syndrome type 1A* | *Schwartz-Jampel syndrome type 1B* | *Schwartz-Jampel syndrome type 2* |
|---|---|---|---|
| Principal radiological findings | Mild epi-metaphyseal dysplasia with enlarged epiphyses at knees | Infancy: (short-limbed dysplasia with dumbbell-shaped femora); childhood: (spondylo-epi-metaphyseal dysplasia) | Infancy: (short-limbed dysplasia with bowing of legs); childhood: (under-tubulation of long bones) |
| Spine | Mild platyspondyly | Moderate platyspondyly; coronal clefts | Not characteristic |
| Pelvis | Narrow sciatic notch | Some flaring of iliac wings; presence of supra-acetabular notch | Not characteristic |
| Epiphyses | Moderately enlarged at knees and other long bones | Moderately enlarged at knees | Flattened at knees |
| Treatment | Careful monitoring of swallowing and breathing; orthopaedic consultations; carbamazepine; watch for hyperthermia; special care during general anaesthesia | Same as for SJS type 1A; often requires vigorous respiratory support – ventilator in infancy; feeding tube; death common in infancy or early childhood | Same as for SJS type 1B |

# Myotonic dystrophy (DM) and DM-related disorders (myotonic dystrophy type-2 (DM-2), proximal myotonic myopathy (PROMM), and proximal myotonic dystrophy (PDM))

This section discusses DM and DM-related disorders as a group. Following the discovery of the gene responsible for DM in 1992 (Brook *et al.*, 1992; Fu *et al.*, 1992; Mahadevan *et al.*, 1992) patients having symptoms similar to but distinct from DM have appeared. DNA testing of individuals suspected of having DM has identified patients with normal size of the DM gene. These individuals have, in many instances, been shown to have another, related, dominantly inherited, myotonic disorder. Many have posterior capsular cataracts, cardiac conduction disturbances, and endocrine abnormalities that resemble those observed with DM. In some patients the pattern of weakness, the severity of muscle wasting and myotonia, and the type of multisystem problems have differed from DM. However, it is a challenging task to identify the specific DM-related disorder affecting an individual in an isolated case. Each of these disorders has considerable variation in its phenotype. Mildly affected individuals may closely resemble each other. Examination of family members to establish the spectrum of disease manifestations is usually necessary to obtain a diagnosis. Ultimately, specific genetic testing will provide the diagnosis in isolated cases.

## Myotonic dystrophy

Myotonic dystrophy (DM) is an autosomal dominant, highly variable, multisytem disease (Harper, 1989; Moxley and Meola, 2000) that results from an unstable trinucleotide repeat (CTGn) expansion in the 3'-untranslated region of a gene on chromosome 19, which encodes a serine/threonine, cAMPdependent, protein kinase (DMPK) (Brook *et al.*, 1992; Fu *et al.*, 1992; Mahadevan *et al.*, 1992). Table 21.3 provides a summary of the clinical characteristics and treatment. Recent reviews discuss the clinical aspects and treatment for the congenital, childhood, and adult forms of DM in more detail (Harper 1989; Moxley and Meola, 2000). As a general rule, the larger the expansion of CTGn repeats in the DM gene, the earlier the onset of more severe symptoms. This rule serves as the genetic basis for the phenomenon of anticipation, the earlier onset of more severe symptoms in successive generations within a family. Anticipation is common in DM.

## Genetics

Despite the discovery of the gene lesion in DM and the development of a standardized DNA test to establish the diagnosis, there is still a considerable gap in our knowledge of the genetic pathomechanism.

A dominantly-inherited loss-of-function of the DM gene causing a deficiency of DMPK which, in turn, produces the disease, is not the likely genetic pathomechanism (Timchenko, 1999). This 'haploinsufficiency' model of the disease has received thorough testing with a variety of animal models, but none of the strains have developed typical DM. One interesting transgenic mouse model has observed myopathic changes and myotonia, mainly in oxidative muscle fibres (Mankodi *et al.*, 2000). This raises the possibility that changes in type I fibres may be an early feature of the muscle manifestations of DM.

The highly variable clinical manifestations of DM are likely due to a complex molecular pathogenesis, which includes deficiency of the DMPK protein, a transdominant misregulation of RNA homeostasis, and haploinsufficiency of neighbouring genes (a downstream homeobox gene SIX5/DMAHP; and an upstream gene DMWD/N59) (Alwazzan *et al.*, 1999; Eriksson *et al.*, 1999; Gennarelli *et al.*, 1999; Korade-Mirnics *et al.*, 1999; Tachi *et al.*, 1999; Timchenko, 1999; Winchester *et al.*, 1999; Gourdon *et al.*, 2000).

## New clinical observations

While it remains clear that more severe manifestations of DM develop as the size of the abnormal CTGn repeat increases (Livingston and Moxley, 1994; Jaspert *et al.*, 1995; Wong *et al.*, 1995;

**Table 21.3 Characteristics and treatment for myotonic dystrophy (DM) and myotonic dystrophy type 2 (DM-2)**

| Clinical features | Myotonic dystrophy (DM) | Myotonic dystrophy type-2 (DM2) |
|---|---|---|
| Inheritance | Dominant | Dominant |
| Gene defect | Chromosome 19; CTG expansion affecting a protein kinase; repeat size ranges from 50 to > 2000; normal 5–37 repeats | Chromosome 3q; normal size of CTG repeat in DM gene on chromosome 19 |
| Age of onset | Broad range of ages (infancy to adult life) | Childhood to adult life |
| Myopathy | Face, eyes, forearm, hands, and legs; generalized weakness and hypotonia in cases beginning in infancy | Mild to moderate weakness of finger flexors, foot dorsiflexors, toe extensors – milder than DM; mild weakness of neck and hip flexors and hip extensors; minimal facial weakness; occasional calf hypetrophy; only mild wasting |
| Myotonia | Primarily affects hand and forearm muscles, and tongue; occasionally affects respiratory muscles and smooth muscle, such as intestine or uterus | Myotonia mild in degree compared to DM; percussion myotonia is more common than action myotonia (e.g. grip myotonia) |
| Provocative stimuli | Myotonia worsened by rest and cold | Myotonia worsened by rest and cold |
| Creatine kinase | Normal or 2–5 × above normal | Normal or 2–5 × above normal |
| Muscle biopsy | Increased central nuclei, atrophy of type 1 fibres; ring binder and subsarcolemmal masses | Findings similar to those in DM |
| Other medical problems | Baldness; early onset cataracts; heart block; tachyarrhythmias; respiratory insufficiency; sleep apnoea; hypersomnia; mental retardation and talipes in infant-childhood forms; gastrointestinal dysfunction; hearing deficits; neuropsychological deficits; white matter changes on MR of head; testicular atrophy; insulin resistance | Cataracts; occasional balding; atrial and ventricular arrhythmias; hyperhydrosis; occasional hypersomnia; occasional hearing deficits |
| Therapy for symptoms | Bracing; cataract removal; monitoring for arrhythmias and respiratory insufficiency; pacemaker; antimyotonia therapy (mexiletine); avoid depolarizing muscle relaxants, opiates, and barbiturates, with surgery for all of these myotonic disorders | Cataract removal; monitoring for cardiac arrhythmias |

Gennarelli *et al.*, 1996; Gharehbaghi-Schnell *et al.*, 1998; Hamshere *et al.*, 1999; Moxley and Meola, 2000), there are clinical observations that do not fit easily into this phenotype/genotype hypothesis.

CTG repeat enlargement in leukocyte DNA does not predict reliably the severity of symptoms in specific patients, especially the non-skeletal muscle symptoms. Cardiac conduction disturbances, especially heart block and tachyarrhythmias, are common in DM (Harper, 1989; Babuty *et al.*, 1999; Lazarus *et al.*, 1999; Moxley and Meola, 2000). Two recent reports have found no correlation between abnormalities in ECG/electrophysiologic-pacing and the degree of expansion of the CTG repeat (Babuty *et al.*, 1999; Lazarus *et al.*, 1999). The range of CTG repeat expansions extends from 62 to 1335 repeats in the group with inducible atrial arrhythmias, while repeat sizes range from 100 to 1670 repeats in patients with no inducible atrial arrhythmia (Lazarus *et al.*, 1999).

Sleep disturbance (Harper, 1989; Ono *et al.*, 1998; Giubilei *et al.*, 1999; Phillips *et al.*, 1999; Moxley and Meola, 2000), cognitive problems, and white matter changes on MRI (Glantz *et al.*, 1988; Harper, 1989; Huber *et al.*, 1989; Chang *et al.*, 1998; Akiguchi *et al.*, 1999; Meola *et al.*, 1999; Moxley and Meola, 2000) are not uncommon in DM. The cause for sleep disturbances may, in part, relate to a loss of catecholaminergic neurons in the medullary reticular formation (Ono *et al.*, 1998) and to a loss of volume in the anterior portion of the corpus callosum (Giubilei *et al.*, 1999), but is not clearly related to the size of CTG repeat expansion in leukocyte DNA. One study examining proton spectroscopic changes in 14 patients with DM has shown a correlation between increased CTG repeat size and more advanced alteration on proton spectroscopy (Chang *et al.*, 1998). Another study has demonstrated a mild correlation between severity of cognitive impairment and CTG repeat enlargement (Perini *et al.*, 1999). However, a study of five patients with congenital DM has failed to show a correlation between either the clinical or imaging changes and the degree of repeat expansion (Martinello *et al.*, 1999). A large scale investigation of 20 DM patients that used measurements of neuropsychological function, PET scanning, and MR imaging of the brain has found a significant correlation between impaired visual-spatial functioning and a decrease in cerebral blood flow in frontal and anterior temporal regions in DM patients (Meola *et al.*, 1999). No significant correlation is seen between the alterations in brain function and either the findings on MR of the brain or in the size of the CTG repeat enlargement (Meola *et al.*, 1999).

The degree of CTG repeat expansion in skeletal muscle does not provide a clear association with the severity of muscle weakness. Recent findings demonstrate that the degree of CTG repeat expansion is similar in specimens obtained from very weak and only mildly weakened muscles from the same patient (Hedberg *et al.*, 1999). This observation strongly suggests that the degree of repeat expansion in muscle is not likely to account for the variable involvement of specific skeletal muscles in DM patients.

Hypomotility of the pharyngo-oesophageal muscles is another common complication of DM (Harper, 1989; Lecointe-Besancon *et al.*, 1999; Modolell *et al.*, 1999). The abnormalities in pharyngo-oesophageal function do not correlate with the severity of muscle weakness on clinical examination or with the degree of CTG repeat enlargement (Modolell *et al.*, 1999). It may be that it is myotonia in the muscles of swallowing that has an overriding influence on function compared to weakness in these muscles.

## Pathophysiology

The pathophysiology responsible for the muscle wasting and weakness in DM remains a mystery. One recent report suggests that a deficiency of DMPK leads to dysregulation of intracellular calcium metabolism (Ueda *et al.*, 1999). Other investigations have proposed alternatively that the weakness may result from atrophy and reduction in the number of type 2 muscle fibres (Tohgi *et al.*, 1994) or from involvement of type 1 oxidative muscle fibres (Mankodi *et al.*, 2000). There is also evidence that muscle wasting and weakness results in part from a deficiency in muscle anabolism. This deficiency results from decreases in growth hormone (Harper, 1989; Gomez *et al.*, 1994; Moxley, 1994), insulin-like growth factor-1 (Moxley, 1994; Vlachopapadopoulou *et al.*, 1995), DHEAS (Sugino *et al.*, 1998; Tsuji *et al.*, 1999), and testosterone (Griggs *et al.*, 1989; Harper, 1989), accompanied by an associated tissue specific insulin resistance (Livingston and Moxley, 1994; Moxley, 1994; Moxley and Meola, 2000). Continued investigation of these and other hormonal alterations are necessary to establish their role in the pathophysiology.

The pathophysiology of myotonia in DM is also not well defined. There is evidence of an alteration in the function of small conductance potassium channels (SK channels; slow potassium channels) in DM (Renaud *et al.*, 1986; Behrens *et al.*, 1994; Vergara and Ramirez, 1997; Bond *et al.*, 1999). SK channels are potassium selective, voltage independent, and become activated by increases in the level of intracellular calcium, such as occurs during an action potential (Bond *et al.*, 1999). The SK channels generate a long-lasting hyperpolarization with a time course that reflects the decay of intracellular calcium. Activation of SK channels cause membrane hyperpolarization and inhibit firing of the cell.

Apamin-sensitive SK channels are present in cultured myotubes, fetal muscle and completely denervated muscle, but they are absent in normal adult skeletal muscle and in muscle from patients with anterior horn cell diseases (Renaud *et al.*, 1986; Bond *et al.*, 1999). Apamin-sensitive SK channels are present in skeletal muscle samples from patients with DM (Renaud *et al.*, 1986). SK channels appear to influence myotonia in DM since the application of the bee venom toxin, apamin, which blocks SK channels, diminishes or abolishes the myotonia in patients (Behrens *et al.*, 1994).

Studies in resealed muscle fibre patches from patients with DM indicate that there is also an alteration in the function of the sodium channel (Franke *et al.*, 1990). Potassium conductance was normal and chloride conductance varied from values in the normal range to moderately low values. However, no consistent alteration in chloride conductance appeared, and the majority of patches from the DM patients revealed an increased frequency of late openings of the sodium channel. The cause for these late openings of the sodium channel and how they may contribute to the myotonia in DM requires further investigation.

## Treatment and prognosis

Supportive treatment is the cornerstone of care in DM. Recent reviews summarize the different aspects of treatment (Harper, 1989; Moxley and Meola, 2000). Two other recent reports have summarized the usual causes of death for DM patients who lived in Canada (Mathieu *et al.*, 1999) and in the Netherlands (de Die-Smulders *et al.*, 1998). Both reports emphasize that the majority of patients die from respiratory insufficiency/pneumonia or cardiac arrhythmias. One report has mentioned that there is an increase in the frequency of tumours in DM (Mathieu *et al.*, 1999).

## Therapeutic trials

Therapeutic trials in DM of testosterone (Griggs *et al.*, 1989), growth hormone (Moxley, 1994), and IGF-1 (Vlachopapadopoulou *et al.*, 1995) have led to some encouraging results. However, other than the use of testosterone as replacement therapy for testosterone deficiency in individual DM patients, the therapeutic use of these hormones remains experimental. At present the high cost of growth hormone and IGF-1, their relative lack of availability, and their risk of enhancing the growth of covert neoplasms, are problems that discourage their use in therapeutic trials.

There is also encouraging news about another potential anabolic treatment, DHEAS. Dehydroepiandrosterone sulphate (DHEAS) is a potentially anabolic adrenal hormone that is markedly reduced in patients with DM (Carter and Steinbeck, 1985). A recent open trial of treatment with DHEAS describes improvement in muscle strength and a reduction in myotonia following daily intravenous treatment with 200 mg of DHEAS (Sugino *et al.*, 1998; Tsuji *et al.*, 1999). Other studies are in progress using oral DHEAS to evaluate its safety and efficacy. For the present DHEAS is a hopeful therapeutic agent, but it is an investigational treatment that requires a large scale randomized, double-blind study to establish its efficacy in DM.

Other therapeutic trials are also in progress. One involves the use of troglitazone, an insulin enhancing thiozolidinedione derivative (Moxley, personal observations). This trial gives troglitazone 600 mg daily for 4 months. It has two major goals: to determine if troglitazone reverses the insulin resistance that typically occurs in patients with DM (Livingston and Moxley, 1994) and, to assess if there is an associated improvement in muscle strength or function. Preliminary results indicate that troglitazone leads to an improvement in insulin action, but no clear improvement in strength has occurred after four months of treatment (Moxley, personal observations).

Recent reports have also suggested that exercise may have a therapeutic role in DM. Open trials of supervised exercise of respiratory (Abe *et al.*, 1998) as well as limb muscles (Lindeman *et al.*, 1995; Tollback *et al.*, 1999) have reported a reduction of symptoms and increased endurance. More research, including controlled randomized trials, is necessary to evaluate the benefits and risks of specific types of exercise training in DM.

## Myotonic dystrophy type 2 (DM-2)

Myotonic dystrophy type 2 is an autosomal dominant, multisystem disease, linked to chromosome 3q, with many clinical similarities to myotonic dystrophy (DM) and proximal myotonic myopathy (PROMM) (Ranum *et al.*, 1998; Day *et al.*, 1999). Day and colleagues have identified this disorder by studying one large five-generation family in Minnesota with 25 affected members. Symptoms usually begin distally in the hands and dorsiflexors of the feet, but some patients have accompanying proximal weakness, especially the neck flexors. The face is relatively spared. Overall the severity of weakness, muscle wasting, and myotonia are less prominent than in DM. Respiratory failure is not a significant problem, although cardiac arrhythmias occur. Excessive sweating is a frequent complaint and muscle pain is also common. Out of 25 affected individuals, grip myotonia occurred in five while percussion myotonia was present in 14. The character of the myotonia was more like that in PROMM than DM. Detailed *in vitro* studies of isolated muscle fibres or sealed portions of fibres have not yet occurred. Whether the electrophysiological findings in DM-2 are comparable to those seen in PROMM (Ricker *et al.*, 1994) or resemble DM more closely remains to be established. More clinical studies are also necessary to define the natural history of DM-2. Table 21.3 outlines the major genetic and clinical features of DM-2.

## Proximal myotonic myopathy (PROMM)

Proximal myotonic myopathy is an autosomal dominant, multisystem, disorder, initially described in 1994 (Ricker *et al.*, 1994; Thornton *et al.*, 1994) that is similar to but distinct from DM (Ricker *et al.*, 1994, 1995, 1999; Thornton *et al.*, 1994; Gomez *et al.*, 1996; Meola *et al.*, 1996; Moxley, 1996; Sander *et al.*, 1996; Hund *et al.*, 1997; Moxley *et al.*, 1998; von zur Muhlen *et al.*, 1998; Newman *et al.*, 1999; Phillips *et al.*, 1998; Ricker, 1999; Gourdon *et al.*, 2000; Sansone *et al.*, 2000). The core diagnostic criteria for PROMM are: weakness that is predominantly proximal; myotonia on electromyography; cataracts (slit lamp examination demonstrates posterior, subcapsular, iridescent, lens opacities resembling the cataracts in DM) with an onset before 50 years of age; autosomal dominant inheritance (at least two generations) with large kindreds having male-to-male transmission; and, a normal size of the CTG repeat in the DM gene.

Table 21.4 outlines the clinical characteristics and treatment of this disorder. Two recent reviews give more details and list the many associated supportive findings (Moxley *et al.*, 1998; Ricker, 1999).

## Genetics

The genetic basis for PROMM is heterogeneous. Many cases in Germany show linkage to the DM-2 locus on chromosome 3q (Ricker *et al*, 1999) while other PROMM families show no linkage (Meola *et al.*, 1999; Wieser *et al.*, 2000).

## New clinical observations

Recent investigations demonstrate that the hormonal changes during pregnancy (Newman *et al.*, 1999) and acquired hypothyroidism (Sansone *et al.*, 2000) can cause a marked worsening of the symptoms of PROMM. The symptoms provoked by pregnancy seem to be more reversible than those resulting from hypothyroidism.

Brain manifestations occur in PROMM. These include white matter alterations (Hund *et al.*, 1997) and disturbances in brain function (Meola *et al.*, 1999). A recent report describes alterations in visual-spatial function and decreased cerebral blood flow in frontal cortex in PROMM (Meola *et al.*, 1999). Similar abnormalities occur in DM patients. The PROMM and DM patients in this study do not have white matter changes associated with their alterations in visual-spatial function and cerebral blood flow. More studies are necessary to define the spectrum of brain manifestations in PROMM and to identify if there is a difference in the manifestation in kindreds linked to chromosome 3q and those who are not.

**Table 21.4 Characteristics and treatment for proximal myotonic myopathy (PROMM) and proximal myotonic dystrophy (PDM)**

| Clinical features | Proximal Myotonic Myopathy (PROMM) | Proximal Myotonic dystrophy (PDM) |
|---|---|---|
| Inheritance | Dominant | Dominant |
| Gene Defect | Many families linked to chromosome 3q region close to DM-2; normal size of CTG repeat in DM gene | Linked to chromosome 3q close to DM-2 locus; normal size of CTG repeat in DM gene |
| Age of Onset | Teens to late adult life | Teens to adult life |
| Myopathy | Mild weakness of thighs, hips, neck flexors; occasional calf muscle hypertrophy | Muscle wasting and weakness prominent in scapulohumeral muscles, pelvofemoral muscles, and neck flexors; mild facial weakness; heel and toe walk are normal |
| Myotonia | Mainly in hands and thighs; varies, frequently hard to detect; pain occurs sometimes with and without myotonia | No clinical myotonia; myotonic discharges on electromyography |
| Provocative Stimuli | Myotonia is worsened by rest, but varies in severity, occasionally being absent on clinical exam | No established provocative factors |
| Creatine Kinase | Normal or 2-3X above normal | Normal or 2-3X above normal |
| Muscle Biopsy | Increased variation in fibre diameter; increased central nuclei; subsarcolemmal masses; occasional atrophic angular fibers; occasional atrophic fibers of both fibre types | Profound dystrophic changes in atrophic muscles (e.g. quadriceps femorus muscle); internal nuclei in hypertrophic fibres; increased fibrous tissue; biopsy of mildly affected muscles shows changes like PROMM |
| Other Medical Problems | Cataracts; cardiac arrhythmias; muscle and chest pains; tremor, hypogonadism; cognitive impairment; white matter changes on MR of head; insulin resistance | Cataracts; occasional diabetes; gonadal insufficiency; hearing deficits |
| Therapy of Symptoms | Cataract removal; occasional need for pacemaker; antimyotonia therapy often not necessary (phenytoin, mexiletine, acetazolamide); monitor carefully during and after surgery for muscle rigidity and rhabdomyolysis | Cataract removal; supportive treatment; treat hypogonadism, diabetes; hearing aids |

## Pathophysiology

The cause of the weakness and the aetiology of muscle pain in PROMM are both unclear. The explanation of the myotonia is also a puzzle. *In vitro* studies of isolated muscle fibres reveal that low extracellular potassium and increased extracellular insulin concentrations worsen the myotonia, while an elevation of extracellular potassium re-

duces myotonia (Ricker *et al.*, 1994). This response is opposite from the usual effects that low and high extracellular potassium have on chloride or sodium channel myotonia. Elevations of extracellular potassium typically exacerbate myotonia in these disorders. Apamin, the bee venom toxin which blocks SK channels, has an ameliorative effect on the myotonia in DM (Behrens *et al.*, 1994), but it exerts no beneficial effect on the myotonia in

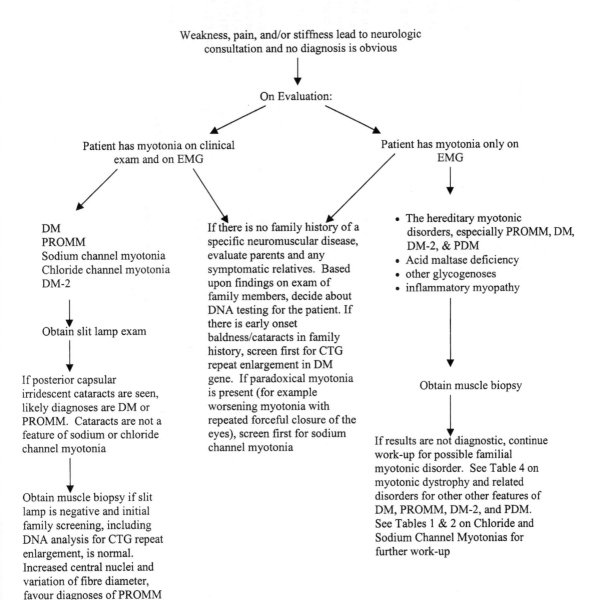

**Figure 21.1** Diagnostic approach to myotonic disorders in adult life

PROMM (Ricker *et al.*, 1994). These observations suggest that the mechanism for myotonia in PROMM may differ from that in chloride and sodium channelopathies. One report describes a worsening of the myotonia in PROMM after heating of the muscles (Sander *et al.*, 1996). Whether this finding and the unexpected lessening of myotonia with an elevation in extracellular potassium indicate a difference in the involvement of certain ion channels in PROMM compared to other myotonic disorders requires further investigation.

## Treatment

Table 21.4 and recent reviews (Moxley *et al.*, 1998; Ricker, 1999) provide a good overview of treatment.

## Proximal myotonic dystrophy (PDM)

A recent report describes a family from Bjorko Island off the west coast of Finland with an autosomal dominant, multisystem disorder, having an adult onset and progressive proximal greater than distal muscle wasting (Udd *et al.*, 1997). The affected individuals in this family have no clinical signs of myotonia, but myotonia is present in many muscles on electromyography (Udd *et al.*, 1997). Early onset cataracts, hypogonadism in males, and hearing loss are common. The investigators have termed this disorder, proximal myotonic dystrophy (PDM). The symptoms in PDM also occur in PROMM, and recent studies show linkage of PDM to the DM-2 locus on chromosome 3q (Meola *et al.*, 1999; Krahe *et al.*, 1999). As is the case with PROMM, it is not clear whether PDM is an allelic disorder to DM-2 or whether it has a genetic locus that is very close to that for DM-2. As additional families become apparent, our knowledge of the natural history of this disorder will increase. It is likely that another previously described family may also have PDM (Abbruzzese *et al.*, 1996). Once DNA testing becomes available for PDM it will help us define the spectrum of its manifestations.

Table 21.4 summarizes the clinical characteristics of PDM.

## Approach to the diagnosis of myotonic disorders

Figure 21.1 provides a general approach to diagnosis in the adult with myotonia. This approach is not all inclusive. Myotonic dystrophy and PROMM have such variable clinical presentations that a more lengthy review of presenting symptoms is necessary to cover the range of possibilities. There are recent reviews that discuss DM (Moxley and Meola, 2000) and PROMM (Moxley *et al.*, 1998; Ricker, 1999) which give more information to refine your diagnostic approach.

## References

Abbruzzese, C., Krahe, R., Liguori, M. *et al.* (1996). Myotonic dystrophy phenotype without expansion of (CTG)n repeat: an entity distinct from proximal myotonic myopathy (PROMM)? *J Neurol.*, **243**, 715–21.

Abe, K., Matsuo, Y., Kadekawa, J., Inoue, S. and Yanagihara, T. (1998). Respiratory training for patients with myotonic dystrophy. *Neurology*, **51**, 641–2.

Akiguchi, I., Nakano, S., Shiino, A. *et al.* (1999). Brain proton magnetic resonance spectroscopy and brain atrophy in myotonic dystrophy. *Arch Neurol.*, **56**, 325–30.

al-Gazali, L. I., Varghese, M., Varady, E., Al, T. J., Scorer, J. and Bakalinova, D. (1999). Neonatal Schwartz-Jampel syndrome: a common autosomal recessive syndrome in the United Arab Emirates. *J Med Genet.*, **33**, 203–11.

Alwazzan, M., Newman, E., Hamshere, M. G. and Brook, J. D. (1999). Myotonic dystrophy is associated with a reduced level of RNA from the DMWD allele adjacent to the expanded repeat. *Hum Mol Genet.*, **8**, 1491–7.

Babuty, D., Fauchier, L., Tena-Carbi, D. *et al.* (1999). Is it possible to identify infrahissian cardiac conduction abnormalities in myotonic dystrophy by non-invasive methods? *Heart*, **82**, 634–7.

Behrens, M. I., Jalil, P., Serani, A., Vergara, F. and Alvarez, O. (1994). Possible role of apamin-sensitive $K^+$ channels in myotonic dystrophy. *Muscle Nerve*, 1264–70.

Bond, C. T., Maylie, J. and Adelman, J. P. (1999). Small-conductance calcium-activated potassium channels. (Review; 52 refs). *Ann NY Acad Sci.*, **868**, 370–8.

Brook, J. D., McCurrach, M. E., Harley, H. G. *et al.* (1992). Molecular basis of myotonic dystrophy: Expansion of a trinucleotide (CTG) repeat at the 3' end of a transcript encoding a protein kinase family member. *Cell*, **68**, 799–808.

Brown, K. A., al-Gazali, L. I., Moynihan, L. M., Lench, N. J., Markham, A. F. and Mueller, R. F. (1997). Genetic heterogeneity in Schwartz-Jampel syndrome: two families with neonatal Schwartz-Jampel syndrome do not map to human chromosome 1p34-p36.1. *J Med Genet.*, **34**, 685–7.

Carter, J. N. and Steinbeck, K. S. (1985). Reduced adrenal androgens in patients with myotonic dystrophy. *J Clin Endocrinol Metab.*, **60**, 611–4.

Chang, L., Ernst, T., Osborn, D., Seltzer, W., Leonido-Yee, M. and Poland, R.E. (1998). Proton spectroscopy in myotonic dystrophy: correlations with CTG repeats (see comments). *Arch Neurol.*, **55**, 305–11.

Christova, L. G., Alexandrov, A. S. and Ishpekova, B. A. (1999). Single motor unit activity pattern in patients with Schwartz-Jampel syndrome (letter). *J Neurol Neurosurg Psychiatr.*, **66**, 252–3.

Cook, S. P. and Borkowski, W. J. (1997). Obstructive sleep apnea in Schwartz-Jampel syndrome. *Arch Otolaryngol Head Neck Surg.*, **123**, 1348–50.

Cormier-Daire, V., Superti-Furga, A., Munnich, A. et al. (1997). Clinical homogeneity of the Stuve-Wiedemann syndrome and overlap with the Schwartz-Jampel syndrome type 2. *Am J Med Genet.*, **78**, 146–9.

Day, J. W., Roelofs, R., Leroy, B., Pech, I., Benzow, K. and Ranum, L. P. (1999). Clinical and genetic characteristics of a five-generation family with a novel form of myotonic dystrophy (DM2). *Neuromusc Dis.*, **9**, 19–27.

de Die-Smulders, C. E. M., Howeler, C. J., Thijs, C. et al. (1998). Age and causes of death in adult-onset myotonic dystrophy. *Brain*, **121**, 1557–63.

Eriksson, M., Ansved, T., Edstrom, L., Anvret, M. and Carey, N. (1999). Simultaneous analysis of expression of the three myotonic dystrophy locus genes in adult skeletal muscle samples: the CTG expansion correlates inversely with DMPK and 59 expression levels, but not DMAHP levels. *Hum Mol Genet.*, **8**, 1053–60.

Franke, C., Hatt, H., Iaizzo, P. A. and Lehmann-Horn, F. (1990). Characteristics of sodium channels and chloride conductance in resealed muscle fibre segments from patients with myotonic dystrophy. *J Physiol.*, **425**, 391–405.

Fontaine, B., Nicole, S., Topaloglu, H. et al. (1996). Recessive Schwartz-Jampel syndrome (SJS): confirmation of linkage to chromosome 1p, evidence of genetic homogeneity and reduction of the SJS locus to a 3-cM interval. *Hum Genet.*, **98**, 380–5.

Fu, Y. H., Pizzuti, A., Fenwick, R. G. et al. (1992). An unstable triplet repeat in a gene related to myotonic muscular dystrophy. *Science*, 1256–8.

Gennarelli, M., Novelli, G., Andreasi, B. F. et al. (1996). Prediction of myotonic dystrophy clinical severity based on the number of intragenic [CTG]n trinucleotide repeats. *Am J Med Genet.*, **65**, 342–7.

Gennarelli, M., Pavoni, M., Amicucci, P., et al. (1999). Reduction of the DM-associated homeo domain protein (DMAHP) mRNA in different brain areas of myotonic dystrophy patients. *Neuromusc Dis.*, **9**, 215–9.

Gharehbaghi-Schnell, E. B., Finsterer, J., Korschineck, I., Mamoli, B. and Binder, B. R. (1998). Genotype-phenotype correlation in myotonic dystrophy. *Clin Genet.*, **53**, 20–26.

Giedion, A., Boltshauser, E., Briner, J. et al. (1997). Heterogeneity in Schwartz-Jampel chondrodystrophic myotonia. *Eur J Pediatr.*, **156**, 214–23.

Giubilei, F., Antonini, G., Bastianello, S. et al. (1999). Excessive daytime sleepiness in myotonic dystrophy. *J Neurol Sci.*, **164**, 60–3.

Glantz, R. H., Wright, R. B., Huckman, M. S., Garron, D. C. and Siegel, I. M. (1988). Central nervous system magnetic resonance imaging findings in myotonic dystrophy. *Arch Neurol.*, **45**, 36–7.

Gomez, J., Cervera, C., Fernandez, J. et al. (1996). Proximal myotonic myopathy report of three families. *Neuromusc Dis.*, (Suppl.), S46.

Gomez, S. M., Fernandez, R. M., Fernandez, C. M., Navarro, M. A., Martinez, M. A. and Soler, R. J. (1994). Study on growth hormone and insulin secretion in myotonic dystrophy. *Clin Invest.*, **72**, 508–11.

Gourdon, G., Devillers, M., Junien, C., Thornton, C. A., Roses, A. and Ashizawa, T. (2001). The 2nd MDA/AFM International Myotonic Dystrophy Consortium Conference (IDMC-2). *Neuromusc Dis.*, in press.

Griggs, R. C., Pandya, S., Florence, J. M. et al. (1989). Randomized controlled trial of testosterone in myotonic dystrophy. *Neurology*, **39**, 219–22.

Hamshere, M. G., Harley, H., Harper, P., Brook, J. D. and Brookfield, J. F. (1999). Myotonic dystrophy: the correlation of (CTG) repeat length in leucocytes with age at onset is significant only for patients with small expansions. *J Med Genet.*, **36**, 59–61.

Harper, P. S. (1989). *Myotonic Dystrophy*. London: W.B. Saunders Company.

Hedberg, B., Anvret, M. and Ansved, T. (1999). CTG-repeat length in distal and proximal muscles of symptomatic and nonsymptomatic patients with myotonic dystrophy: relation to muscle strength and degree of histopathological abnormalities. *Eur J Neurol.*, **6**, 341–6.

Hofmann, W. W., Alston, W. and Rowe, G. (1966). A study of individual neuromuscular junctions in myotonia. *Electroencephalogr Clin Neurophysiol.*, **21**, 521–37.

Huber, S. J., Kissel, J. T., Shuttleworth, E. C., Chakeres, D. W., Clapp, L. E. and Brogan, M. A. (1989). Magnetic resonance imaging and clinical correlates of intellectual impairment in myotonic dystrophy (see comments). *Arch Neurol.*, **46**, 536–40.

Hund, E., Jansen, O., Koch, M. C. et al. (1997). Proximal myotonic myopathy with MRI white matter abnormalities of the brain. *Neurology*, **48**, 33–7.

Jaspert, A., Fahsold, R., Grehl, H. and Claus, D. (1995).

Myotonic dystrophy: correlation of clinical symptoms with the size of the CTG trinucleotide repeat. *J Neurol.*, **242**, 99–104.

Korade-Mirnics, Z., Tarleton, J., Servidei, S. *et al.* (1999). Myotonic dystrophy: tissue-specific effect of somatic CTG expansions on allele-specific DMAHP/SIX5 expression. *Hum Mol Genet.*, **8**, 1017–23.

Krahe, R., Meola, G., Ptacek, L., Lee, D. and Udd, B. (1999). Dominant Multi-Systemic Proximal Myotonic Myopathic Syndromes: Clinical and Genetic Heterogeneity in Three Families. *The 2nd MDA/AFM International Myotonic Dystrophy Conference (IDMC-2)*, 39.

Kwiecinski, H., Ryniewicz, B. and Ostrzycke, A. (1992). Treatment of myotonia with antiarrhythmic drugs. *Acta Neurol Scand.*, **86**, 371–5.

Landau, W. M. (1952). The essential mechanism in myotonia: an electromyographic study. *Neurology, 2*, 369–88.

Lazarus, A., Varin, J., Ounnoughene, Z. *et al.* (1999). Relationships among electrophysiological findings and clinical status, heart function, and extent of DNA mutation in myotonic dystrophy. *Circulation*, **99**, 1041–6.

Lecointe-Besancon, I., Leroy, F., Devroede, G. *et al.* (1999). A comparative study of esophageal and anorectal motility in myotonic dystrophy. *Dig Dis Sci.*, **44**, 1090–9.

Lerche, H., Heine, R., Pika, U., George, A. L. J., Mitrovic, N., Browatzki, M. *et al.* (1993). Human sodium channel myotonia: slowed channel inactivation due to substitutions for a glycine within the III–IV linker. *Journal of Physiology*, **470**, 13–22.

Lindeman, E., Leffers, P., Spaans, F. *et al.* (1995). Strength training in patients with myotonic dystrophy and hereditary motor and sensory neuropathy: a randomized clinical trial. *Arch Phys Med Rehab.*, **76**, 612–20.

Livingston, J. N. and Moxley III, R. T. (1994). Myotonic dystrophy: Phenotype-genotype and insulin resistance. *Diabetes Rev.*, **2**, 29–42.

Mahadevan, M., Tsilfidis, C., Sabourin, L. *et al.* (1992). Myotonic dystrophy mutation: an unstable CTG repeat in the 3' untranslated region of the gene. *Science*, **255**, 1253–5.

Mankodi, A. K., Logigian, E. L., Orimo, S., Callahan, L. and Thornton, C. A. (2000). Transgenic model of myotonic dystrophy. *Neurology*, **54**, (Suppl. 3), A458.

Martinello, F., Piazza, A., Pastorello, E., Angelini, C. and Trevisan, C. P. (1999). Clinical and neuroimaging study of central nervous system in congenital myotonic dystrophy. *J Neurol.*, **246**, 186–92.

Mathieu, J., Allard, P., Potvin, L., Prevost, C. and Begin, P. (1999). A 10-year study of mortality in a cohort of patients with myotonic dystrophy. *Neurology*, **52**, 1658–62.

Meola, G., Sansone, V., Radice, S., Skradski, S. and Ptacek, L. (1996). A family with an unusual myotonic and myopathic phenotype and no CTG expansion (proximal myotonic myopathy syndrome): a challenge for future molecular studies. *Neuromusc Dis.*, **6**, 143–50.

Meola, G., Sansone, V., Perani, D. *et al.* (1999). Cognitive, brain MRI and PET studies in proximal myotonic myopathy and myotonic dystrophy. *Neurology*, **53**, 1042–50.

Meola, G., Udd, B., Sansone, V., Ptacek, L., Lee, D. and Krahe, R. (1999). Dominant Multi-System Proximal Myotonic Myopathic Syndromes: Clinical and Genetic Heterogeneity in Three Families. *Neurology*, **52**, (suppl. 2), A95.

Modolell, I., Mearin, F., Baudet, J. S., Gamez, J., Cervera, C. and Malagelada, J. R. (1999). Pharyngo-Esophageal Motility Disturbances in Patients with Myotonic Dystrophy. *Scand J Gastroenterol.*, **34**, 878–82.

Moxley III, R. T. and Meola, G. (2000). Myotonic Dystrophy. In *Monographs in Clinical Neuroscience: Neuromuscular Disease* (ed. Deymeer, F.). Basel: Karger.

Moxley, R. T. (1994). Potential for growth factor treatment of muscle disease. (Review; 36 refs). *Curr Opn Neurol.*, **7**, 427–34.

Moxley, R. T. (1996). Proximal myotonic myopathy: mini-review of a recently delineated clinical disorder. (Review; 27 refs). *Neuromusc Dis.*, **6**, 87–93.

Moxley, R. T., Udd, B. and Ricker, K. (1998). 54th ENMC International Workshop: PROMM (proximal myotonic myopathies) and other proximal myotonic syndromes. 10–12th October 1997, Naarden, The Netherlands. *Neuromusc Dis.*, **8**, 508–18.

Newman, B., Meola, G., O'Donovan, D. G., Schapira, A. H. and Kingston, H. (1999). Proximal myotonic myopathy (PROMM) presenting as myotonia during pregnancy. *Neuromusc Dis.*, **9**, 144–9.

Ono, S., Takahashi, K., Jinnai, K. *et al.* (1998). Loss of catecholaminergic neurons in the medullary reticular formation in myotonic dystrophy. *Neurology*, **51**, 1121–4.

Pascuzzi, R. M., Gratianne, R., Azzarelli, B. and Kincaid, J. C. (1990). Schwartz-Jampel syndrome with dominant inheritance. *Muscle Nerve*, **13**, 1152–63.

Perini, G., Menegazzo, E., Ermani, M. *et al.* (1999). Cognitive Impairment and (CTG)n Expansion in Myotonic Dystrophy Patients. *Biol Psychiatr.*, **46**, 425–31.

Phillips, M. F., Rogers, M. T., Barnetson, R. *et al.* (1998). PROMM: the expanding phenotype. A family with proximal myopathy, myotonia and deafness. *Neuromusc Dis.*, **8**, 439–46.

Phillips, M. F., Steer, H. M., Soldan, J. R., Wiles, C. M. and Harper, P. S. (1999). Daytime somnolence in myotonic dystrophy. *J Neurol.*, **246**, 275–82.

Ranum, L. P., Rasmussen, P. F., Benzow, K. A., Koob, M. D. and Day, J. W. (1998). Genetic mapping of a second myotonic dystrophy locus. *Nat Genet.*, **19**, 196–8.

Renaud, J. F., Desnuelle, C., Schmid-Antomarchi, H., Hugues, M., Serratrice, G., Lazdunski, M. (1986). Expression of apamin receptor in muscles of patients with myotonic muscular dystrophy. *Nature*, **319**, 678–80.

Ricker, K., Koch, M. C., Lehmann-Horn, F. *et al.* (1994). Proximal myotonic myopathy: a new dominant disorder with myotonia, muscle weakness, and cataracts. *Neurology*, **44**, 1448–52.

Ricker, K., Koch, M. C., Lehmann-Horn, F. *et al.* (1995). Proximal myotonic myopathy. Clinical features of a multisystem disorder similar to myotonic dystrophy. *Arch Neurol.*, **52**, 25–31.

Ricker, K., Grimm, T., Koch, M. C. *et al.* (1999). Linkage of proximal myotonic myopathy to chromosome 3q (see comments). *Neurology*, **52**, 170–1.

Ricker, K. (1999). Myotonic dystrophy and proximal myotonic myopathy. (Review; 26 refs). *J Neurol.*, **246**, 334–8.

Rudel, R., Ricker, K. and Lehmann-Horn, F. (1993). Genotype-phenotype correlations in human skeletal muscle sodium channel diseases. *Arch Neurol.*, **50**, 1241–8.

Sander, H. W., Tavoulareas, G. P. and Chokroverty, S. (1996). Heat-sensitive myotonia in proximal myotonic myopathy. *Neurology*, **47**, 956–62.

Sansone, V., Griggs, R. C. and Moxley III, R. T. (2000). Hypothyroidism Unmasking Proximal Myotonic Myopathy (PROMM). *Neuromusc Dis.*, **10**, 165–72.

Sechi, G. P., Traccis, S., Durelli, L., Monaco, F. and Mutani, R. (1983). Carbamazepine versus diphenylhydantoin in the treatment of myotonia. *Eur Neurol.*, **22**, 113–8.

Singh, B., Biary, N., Jamil, A. A. and al-Shahwan, S. A. (1997). Schwartz-Jampel syndrome: evidence of central nervous system dysfunction. *J Child Neurol.*, **12**, 214–7.

Sugino, M., Ohsawa, N., Ito, T. *et al.* (1998). A pilot study of dehydroepiandrosterone sulfate in myotonic dystrophy. *Neurology*, **51**, 586–9.

Superti-Furga, A., Tenconi, R., Clementi, M. *et al.* (1998). Schwartz-Jampel syndrome type 2 and Stuve-Wiedemann syndrome: a case for 'lumping'. *Am J Med Genet.*, **78**, 150–4.

Tachi, N., Ohya, K. and Chiba, S. (1999). Expression of the Myotonic Dystrophy Locus-Associated Homeodomain Protein in Congenital Myotonic Dystrophy. *J Child Neurol.*, **14**, 471–2(Abstr).

Taylor, R. G., Layzer, R. B., Davis, H. S. and Fowler, W. M. (1972). Continuous muscle fiber activity in the Schwartz-Jampel Syndrome. *Electroencephalogr Clin Neurophysiol.*, **33**, 497–509.

Thornton, C. A., Griggs, R. C. and Moxley, R. T. (1994). Myotonic dystrophy with no trinucleotide repeat expansion (see comments). *Ann Neurol.*, **35**, 269–72.

Timchenko, L. T. (1999). Myotonic dystrophy: the role of RNA CUG triplet repeats. (Review; 34 refs). *Am J Hum Genet.*, **64**, 360–4.

Tohgi, H., Kawamorita, A., Utsugisawa, K., Yamagata, M. and Sano, M. (1994). Muscle histopathology in myotonic dystrophy in relation to age and muscular weakness. *Muscle Nerve*, **17**, 1037–43.

Tollback, A., Eriksson, S., Wredenberg, A. *et al.* (1999). Effects of high resistance training in patients with myotonic dystrophy. *Scand J Rehab Med.*, **31**, 9–16.

Topaloglu, H., Serdaroglu, A., Okan, M., Gucuyener, K. and Topcu, M. (1993). Improvement of myotonia with carbamazepine in three cases with the Schwartz-Jampel syndrome. *Neuropediatrics*, **24**, 232–4.

Tsuji, K., Furutama, D., Tagami, M. and Ohsawa, N. (1999). Specific binding and effects of dehydroepiandrosterone sulfate (DHEA-S) on skeletal muscle cells: possible implication for DHEA-S replacement therapy in patients with myotonic dystrophy. *Life Sci.*, **65**, 17–26.

Udd, B., Krahe, R., Wallgren-Pettersson, C., Falck, B. and Kalimo, H. (1997). Proximal myotonic dystrophy – a family with autosomal dominant muscular dystrophy, cataracts, hearing loss and hypogonadism: heterogeneity of proximal myotonic syndromes? *Neuromusc Dis.*, **7**, 217–28.

Ueda, H., Shimokawa, M., Yamamoto, M. *et al.* (1999). Decreased expression of myotonic dystrophy protein kinase and disorganization of sarcoplasmic reticulum in skeletal muscle of myotonic dystrophy. *J Neurol Sci.*, **162**, 38–50.

Vergara, C. and Ramirez, B. U. (1997). Age-dependent expression of apamin-sensitive calcium-activated potassium channels in fast and slow rat skeletal muscle. *Exp Neurol.*, **146**, 282–5.

Vlachopapadopoulou, E., Zachwieja, J. J., Gertner, J. M. *et al.* (1995). Metabolic and clinical response to recombinant human insulin-like growth factor I in myotonic dystrophy – a clinical research center study. *J Clin Endocrinol Metab.*, **80**, 3715–23.

von zur Muhlen F., Klass, C., Kreuzer, H., Mall, G., Giese, A. and Reimers, C. D. (1998). Cardiac involvement in proximal myotonic myopathy. *Heart*, **79**, 619–21.

Wieser, T., Bonsch, D., Eger, K., Schulte-Mattler, W. and Zierz, S. (2000). A family with PROMM not linked to the recently mapped PROMM locus DM-2. *Neuromusc Dis.*, **10**, 141–3.

Winchester, C. L., Ferrier, R. K., Sermoni, A., Clark, B. J. and Johnson, K. J. (1999). Characterization of the expression of DMPK and SIX5 in the human eye and implications for pathogenesis in myotonic dystrophy. *Hum Mol Genet.*, **8**, 481–92.

Wong, L. J., Ashizawa, T., Monckton, D. G., Caskey, C. T. and Richards, C. S. (1995). Somatic heterogeneity of the CTG repeat in myotonic dystrophy is age and size dependent. *Am J Hum Genet.*, **56**, 114–22.

*Valeria Sansone*

## Introduction

Cardiac dysrhythmias are uncommon in periodic paralysis. The striking alteration in potassium metabolism that occurs during an attack of paralysis usually spares cardiac and respiratory muscles. However, electrocardiogram monitoring during an attack of periodic paralysis, shows that ECG does alter. Hypokalaemia prolongs ventricular repolarization, often with prominent U waves (Figure 22.1a). Hyperkalaemia produces a sequence of changes usually beginning with narrowing and peaking of the T waves (Figure 22.1b). These ECG changes are not usually accompanied by any cardiac symptoms. The ECG abnormalities that are associated with severe hyperkalaemia, namely AV conduction disturbances, diminution in P-wave amplitude, widening of the QRS interval, and asystole, do not normally occur during an attack of hyperkalaemic periodic paralysis.

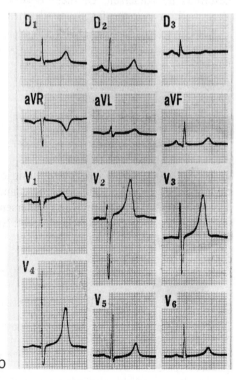

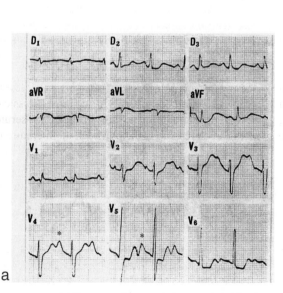

a

b

**Figure 22.1** (a) Electrocardiogram during hypokalaemia (2.1 mEq/L). Note the prominent U waves (*); (b) Electrocardiogram during hyperkalaemia (5.8 mEq/L).

However, there have been reports of isolated cases of periodic paralysis with associated cardiac arrhythmias (Klein *et al.*, 1963; Resnick *et al.*, 1969; Levitt *et al.*, 1972; Lisak *et al.*, 1972; Stubbs, 1976; Kramer *et al.*, 1979; Yoshimura *et al.*, 1983; Gould *et al.*, 1985; Fukuda *et al.*, 1988; Miller *et al.*, 1989; Baquero *et al.*, 1995). These reports prompted cardiac screening in all cases of periodic paralysis, especially in those cases of uncertain diagnosis in whom potassium and glucose-insulin loads are necessary to trigger the attack of paralysis.

The most striking cardiac dysrhythmia associated with periodic paralysis occurs in a distinctive syndrome that was first described by Andersen *et al.* in 1971 and later named *Andersen's syndrome* (AS) by Tawil and coworkers (1994). Some of the earlier reports (Klein *et al.*, 1963) of periodic paralysis with severe cardiac arrhythmias may have been additional cases of Andersen's syndrome (Rowland, 1994). However, no mention is made in these additional reports of the multiple developmental abnormalities also described by Andersen. Of these developmental abnormalities it is the facial peculiarities, which especially allow an early diagnosis of AS and hence recognition of the severe systemic manifestations associated with this syndrome.

# Andersen's syndrome

Andersen's syndrome is a rare neuromuscular disorder comprising less than 5% of all periodic paralysis. It is characterized by the triad of periodic paralysis, cardiac abnormalities, and both facial and skeletal dysmorphisms (Andersen *et al.*, 1971; Tawil *et al.*, 1994; Rowland, 1994; Sansone *et al.*, 1997; Djurhuus *et al.*, 1998; Canun *et al.*, 1999). Most cases show autosomal dominant inheritance, but sporadic cases have been described.

The diagnosis of Andersen's syndrome is a clinical one which relies on the presence of the clinical triad. However, affected family members of a patient with the full triad of AS may show a partial expression of the syndrome with absence of periodic paralysis or cardiac abnormalities in some. Cardiac involvement varies from asympto-matic ECG abnormalities like a prolonged QTc interval to isolated potentially fatal ventricular arrhythmias (Sansone *et al.*, 1997). Facial and skeletal abnormalities may often be difficult to detect. As the genetic basis for this syndrome is unknown, the diagnosis of Andersen's syndrome is still a clinical one.

## Neuromuscular manifestations

Attacks of periodic paralysis may be the presenting feature of AS but, in some cases, they have remained unrecognized until the onset of more severe cardiac symptoms. Attacks do not always have an identifiable trigger. The attacks do not neatly fit into either the hyperkalaemic or hypokalaemic category. In the initial case report of AS, the periodic paralysis is described as normokalaemic, since during the attack serum potassium levels remained normal. A glucose-load at that time did not cause a paralysis (Andersen *et al.*, 1971). In a follow-up study of this patient, attacks of paralysis were occasionally associated with hypokalaemia, and could be provoked by glucose ingestion (Djurhuus *et al.*, 1998). Tawil *et al.* (1994) described a case of AS presenting with episodic weakness associated with attacks of hyperkalaemia.

Sansone *et al.* (1997) described 11 patients from five unrelated families with Andersen's syndrome. Two patients had the hyperkalaemic periodic paralysis, three had the hypokalaemic periodic paralysis and the remaining six had attacks during which serum potassium levels remained normal. Although in most classical forms of periodic paralysis, changes in serum potassium are usually unequivocal, the literature is replete with cases of 'normokalaemic' or biphasic periodic paralysis (responding to both hypokalaemic and hyperkalaemic challenges) (Layzer *et al.*, 1967; Rowland and Lisak, 1972; Lewis *et al.*, 1979). Similarly, in some cases of AS a bipolar pattern has been observed with some attacks of paralysis being associated with hyperkalaemia and others with hypokalaemia, even within the same family tree. Thyrotoxic periodic paralysis has not been reported in AS patients. Canun *et al.* (1999) described two members of a typical AS family who had hyperthyroidism but they did not have periodic paralysis or cardiac arrhythmias so that the thyroid disorder seems to be unrelated to AS.

A persistent myopathy is usually present in patients with typical AS. Muscles may be of normal bulk or show minimal signs of proximal atrophy. There is often a moderate degree of weakness in a limb-girdle distribution, especially in the lower limbs, between attacks. Deep tendon reflexes are always absent during the attack but may be normal or, more often, brisk between attacks. Grip, percussion or lingual myotonia is usually absent even in those patients with hyperkalaemic periodic paralysis. Needle EMG is usually normal. Muscle biopsy shows tubular aggregates in most cases. In the original case described by Andersen, the muscle biopsy showed fibre-type disproportion without tubular aggregates (Djurhuus et al., 1998). In two patients with typical AS a 3-minute standard exercise test showed a progressive decline of 40% in the compound action potential amplitude after exercise, similar to what is seen in hyperkalaemic and hypokalaemic periodic paralysis (McManis et al., 1986; Katz et al.,1999).

## Cardiac involvement

Cardiac involvement in Andersen's syndrome can be severe. Syncopal episodes, bouts of symptomatic ventricular arrhythmia and cardiac arrest may be the presenting manifestations of the syndrome. A prolonged QTc interval may be present in asymptomatic family members as an isolated finding in otherwise typical AS kindreds. This has been suggested as the minimal diagnostic sign for AS (Sansone et al., 1997). More recently, Canun et al. (1999) found a long QTc in only three of eight affected family members of a typical AS kindred, again emphasizing the variable expression of the classical triad and variability in the severity of the cardiac manifestations. Echocardiography is usually normal in these patients. Three patients have required a pacemaker; other patients are on class 1 antiarrhythmic drugs or beta-blockers with careful monitoring of their ECG and serum potassium levels. Variations in potassium

levels risk precipitating potentially fatal ventricular arrhythmia in these patients.

## Facial and skeletal abnormalities

None of the patients described so far with AS have the severe dysmorphic features originally described by Andersen et al. (1971). However, all patients have distinct skeletal and facial features in common (Tawil et al., 1994; Sansone et al., 1997; Canun et al., 1999). It is the recognition of the characteristic face that permits an early diagnosis and allows one to anticipate the severe, but usually treatable, cardiac manifestations of the syndrome. In her initial description, Andersen described a short boy, with scaphocephaly, soft and hard palate defects, mandibular hypoplasia, hypertelorism and mandibular hypoplasia. Clinodactyly was also present. Subsequent reports have further delineated the facial and skeletal abnormalities that may be present in AS with a variable picture, ranging from clinodactyly alone to fullblown facial anomalies (Djurhuus et al., 1998; Canun et al., 1999). Table 22.1 summarizes these findings.

## Other neurological manifestations associated with AS

Fetal distress with poor Apgar scores and low birthweight have been reported in three of the patients with AS described so far. Motor milestones were initially delayed in two of these patients, but there are no reports of intellectual delay or of impaired intelligence. A computed cranial tomography in one case, which did have fetal distress, showed cortical atrophy (Canun et al., 1999). Normal magnetic resonance imaging was found in two patients with AS who had experienced fetal distress with delayed motor milestones. Fetal distress may account for some of the pyramidal signs found in some patients with AS.

In two patients with AS associated with a prolonged QTc interval, tonic clonic seizures have been described during bouts of ventricular tachycardia. However, it is difficult to interpret this finding as a sign of central nervous system invol-

| Table 22.1 Facial anomalies of patients with AS |
| --- |

*Face*
- Forehead: usually broad
- Eyes: may have downslanting palpebral fissures, more often bilateral ptosis and hypertelorism
- Ears: usually low-set
- Nose: usually broad
- Mouth: usually malar hypoplasia, more rarely cleft or high-arched palate and absent uvula
- Mandible: usually micrognathia
- Teeth: hypoplasia, aplasia and malposition of teeth

*Neck*
- Usually broad

*Hands*
- Usually clinodactyly or syndactyly, abnormal digit length, more rarely flattening of palmar creases

*Skeletal system*
- Usually thoracolumbar scoliosis, more rarely thoracic kyphosis

vement in AS *per se*, because focal or generalized seizures have also been reported in patients with congenital long QT syndrome having normal EEG (Horn *et al.*, 1986; Sundaram *et al.*, 1986). Treatment of seizures with traditional antiepileptic drugs like carbamazepine has worsened the cardiac arrhythmias in these patients, whereas treatment of the long QT syndrome has resolved the associated epileptic fits, suggesting that the origin of the loss of consciousness is cardiac and not neurogenic.

## Genetics

Linkage analysis in three large informative AS kindreds excluded linkage to the hyperkalaemic periodic paralysis locus on chromosome 17 and the long QT1, QT2, QT3 and QT4 syndrome loci (Keating *et al.*, 1991; Schwartz *et al.*, 1993; Martin *et al.*, 1995; Marks *et al.*, 1995a, b; Wang *et al.*, 1996). Kindreds were not large enough to perform linkage analysis to the calcium channel gene but mutational analysis ruled out the known calcium channel gene mutations (Fontaine *et al.*, 1994; Fouad *et al.*, 1997).

The coexistence of abnormalities of cardiac and skeletal muscle membrane excitability in AS, which involves different isoforms of the major ion channel proteins, suggests that the underlying pathogenic mechanism alters the function of more than one specific channel. This could occur as a result of a defective regulatory protein common to both tissues (Sperelakis, 1994). Alternatively, the genetic lesion may involve more than one gene (Lehmann-Horn *et al.*, 1990; Basson *et al.*, 1994, 1995).

## Treatment strategies

The risk–benefit ratio of treating the attacks of sudden weakness, the fixed limb-girdle myopathy, and especially the ventricular tachyarrhythmias, should be considered before beginning therapy in patients with AS. This is important because the antiarrhythmic agents may not only provoke or exacerbate the arrhythmia but also aggravate muscle weakness and increase the frequency of paralytic attacks. The mechanism of this paradoxical response is unclear but may be related to the anticholinergic action of some of the class 1 antiarrhythmic drugs usually used in the treatment of the cardiac abnormality. Treatment in AS is still empirical because a difficult balance must be struck between controlling the severity of cardiac arrhythmia and the severity and frequency of episodic weakness, while maximizing the quality of life of these patients. While the arrhythmias may be life threatening, frequent attacks of episodic weakness leading to severe fixed myopathy may also greatly limit the patient's everyday activities.

## Cardiac abnormalities

Management of cardiac dysrhythmias is best achieved in partnership between cardiologists and neurologists. In this way treatments which may help the dysrhythmia, such as raising potassium levels, can be monitored in case they aggravate attacks of periodic paralysis or worsen the fixed weakness. Sympathetic beta-blockers and class 1 (Na-channel blockers) or class IV (Ca-channel blockers) antiarrhythmic drugs have been used with partial success. The response to these treatments is often transitory and unpredictable and several patients have had to be switched from beta-blockers to antiarrhythmic drugs. Pacemaker implantation may be advisable in some cases.

## Periodic paralysis

Sodium-channel blockers (tocainide or mexiletine) and calcium-channel blockers (verapamil) have been used to reduce the frequency and severity of paralytic attacks in some patients with AS (Katz et al., 1999). The response is unpredictable. In most patients with AS a minimal dose of 600 mg daily of potassium chloride tablet intake is recommended. Careful serum potassium level monitoring and attention to minimal signs of gastrointestinal irritation allows long-term treatment. Usually the patients can detect the onset of the attack hours or days before it occurs so that treatment in these cases can be periodical and more direct. In most cases this approach has resulted in a reduction of the frequency of attacks, which are usually aborted by such treatment. Spironolactone, an aldosterone antagonist which raises potassium serum levels, was tried with partial success in the patient initially described by Andersen who had hypokalaemic-associated periodic paralysis (Djurhuus et al., 1998). During an attack of hypokalaemic periodic paralysis there is a decrease in intracellular muscle potassium concentration (Djurhuus et al., 1998) and this has prompted treatment with a Na/K-ATPase stimulating drug, terbutaline. Treatment with terbutaline

7.5 mg b.i.d. as a retarded formulation resulted in partial control of the attacks of weakness (Djurhuus et al., 1998). The response to acetazolamide is unpredictable, but no deleterious effect on cardiac conduction has been reported so far. Acetazolamide may be the first drug of choice in patients with AS and long QTc interval associated with epileptic fits, since as well as possible benefit in reducing attacks of periodic paralysis it is an anticonvulsant (Resor and Resor, 1990; Reiss and Oles, 1996). Dietary modification with a low-carbohydrate, low-sodium diet may decrease the severity of attacks in AS but does not eliminate them.

## Limb-girdle myopathy

Treatment options for the limb-girdle myopathy present in some patients with periodic paralysis are limited. Dichlorphenamide has been tried in one patient with AS. A reduction in the severity of attacks of weakness has been observed but follow-up data are needed to evaluate whether dichlorphenamide and, indeed other drugs used to control attacks of period paralysis, are effective in preventing persistent weakness.

## Facial and skeletal abnormalities

Cleft palate, syndactyly, marked thoracolumbar scoliosis and the palpebral ptosis are amenable to surgical treatment if appropriate. There have been no reports so far of anaesthetic complications during surgery, but normal precautions, as might apply to any neuromuscular disorder, would seem appropriate.

## Case report

I.F. is a 19-year-old girl who has been seeing a cardiologist since the age of 4 years.

Pregnancy had been uneventful but a mild psychomotor delay was observed at birth. Apgar scores were 7 at 1 minute and 8 at 5 minutes. Hypotrophy of the anterior and posterior compartments of the left thigh and leg was noted at birth as well as syndactyly of the second and third toes and clinodactyly of the fifth fingers. At 4 years of age she had a cardiac arrest. Bidirectional ventricular tachycardia was diagnosed and she was treated with beta-blockers with initial benefit. Syncopal episodes occurred again at age 10 years. At that time she experienced her first episode of generalized muscle weakness. She is unable to identify any triggering event. Her father, a 49 year-old man, having experienced the same episodes of sudden weakness in young adulthood and being a specialized nurse, has measured serum potassium levels during the attacks. Serum potassium was 3.3 mEq/L in most episodes. He started his daughter on potassium tablets, periodically checking serum potassium levels. At 15 years of age she was referred to us by the cardiologist because of a new episode of generalized muscle weakness. Physical examination revealed short stature (< third percentile for age), low-set ears, broad nose, clinodactyly of the fifth fingers, syndactyly of the second and third toes, scoliosis, and hypotrophy of the anterior and posterior compartments of the left leg (Figure 22.2a). Mild psychomotor delay was evident. Shoulder and pelvic girdle atrophy and weakness (MRC grade 4) were present, accounting for a positive Gower's manoeuvre, bilateral scapular winging, compensatory hyperlordosis and back-kneeing. There was no clinical myotonia. Her muscle stretch reflexes were increased and plantar responses were upgoing. Sensation was normal. Brain and spinal cord MRI were unremarkable. Needle EMG examination showed no evidence of myotonia. Muscle biopsy showed features of a mild chronic myopathy with tubular aggregates.

Follow-up 4 years later shows a bright girl of normal height who is overweight. Bilateral ptosis is evident (Figure 22.2b). She is currently taking 600 mg tablets of potassium chloride five times a day. Serum potassium levels are, on average 3.7 mEq/L. She is able to predict an episode of muscle weakness one or two days before the attack. This usually occurs before menses so that she increases potassium intake by one or two tablets and partially controls her attack. She may, however, experience fatiguability, during which time potassium levels have been found below normal (3.3 mEq/L). Attacks of muscle weakness resolve after 2 days. On examination there is a slight progression of her proximal muscle weak-

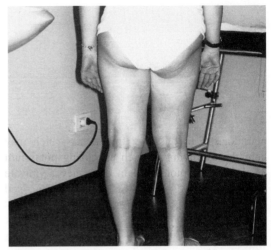

a

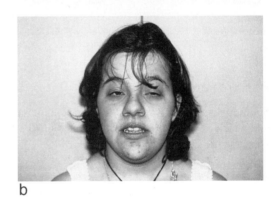

b

**Figure 22.2** I.F, a 19-year-old girl with AS. (a) Atrophy of the left leg and thigh. A thoracolumbar scoliosis is present and the hips are slightly slanted. (b) Note the characteristic face: broad forehead, severe bilateral ptosis, hypertelorism, broad nose, prognathism.

ness (from grade 4 MRC to grade 3+ in the lower limbs). From a cardiac point of view the girl is on beta-blockers (propranolol, 160 mg daily) and antiarrhythmic drugs (propaphenone 150 mg t.i.d.) with a good control of her cardiac ventricular arrhythmias (QTc 360 ms) (Figure 22.3).

The father experienced episodes of sudden muscle weakness associated with a decrease in serum potassium levels at the age of 13 years. A glucose challenge on initial evaluation provoked weakness with a fall in potassium levels to 3.1 mEq/L. No further episodes of weakness have occurred since

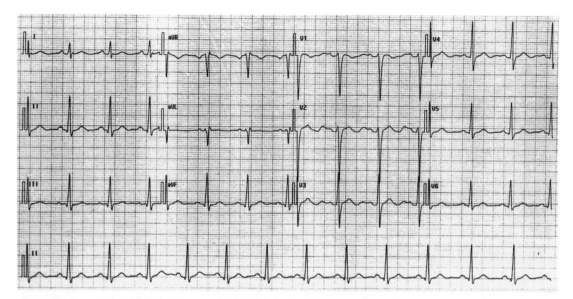

**Figure 22.3** Electrocardiogram of patient with AS described in the case report as I.F. Sinus rhythm 78 beats per minute; PQ = 0.16 seconds; no significant abnormalities in repolarization (QTc = 0.36 seconds). Treatment is indicated in the text.

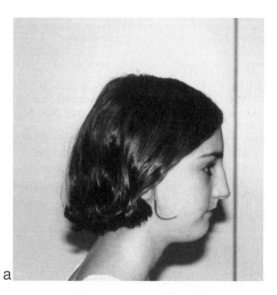

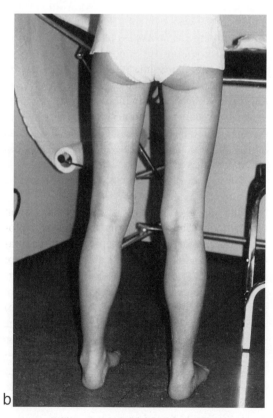

a                                                                    b

**Figure 22.4** (a) 12-year-old sister of I.F. Note micrognathia and low-set ears. (b) A mild degree of proximal atrophy is seen.

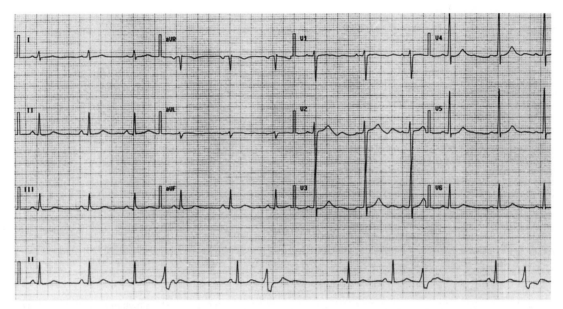

**Figure 22.5** Electrocardiogram of proband's sister (patient indicated in Figure 22.4). Sinus rhythm 67 beats per minute. PQ = 0.16 seconds. Note single, monomorphic ventricular extrasystoles. No significant abnormalities in repolarization (QTc = 0.38 seconds). No treatment yet.

then. Neurological exam, after 4-year follow up is normal except for a decrease in deep tendon reflexes. Physical examination is unchanged and shows short stature, broad neck, broad nose, prognathism, clinodactyly of second finger of both hands and simple syndactyly of the second and third toes of his feet

The 12 year-old sister has never experienced episodes of muscle weakness. Cardiac monitoring revealed a long QT interval on initial examination 4 years ago. The patient was initially asymptomatic except for occasional episodes of palpitation. Minor facial and skeletal abnormalities were found on initial examination. Follow up 4 years later is unchanged except for mild proximal atrophy in the shoulder and pelvic girdle (Figure 22.4b). The girl is also experiencing muscle cramps and episodes of mild generalized weakness after exercise. During these episodes potassium levels have been found to be above normal (5.2 mEq/L). She is also experiencing more frequent episodes of palpitations. Her ECG has worsened (Figure 22.5) and so she will require further cardiological intervention.

# References

Andersen, E. D., Krasilnikoff, P. A. and Overvad, H. (1971). Intermittent muscular weakness, extrasystoles, and multiple developmental abnormalities: A new syndrome? *Acta Pediat Scand.*, **60**, 559–64.

Baquero, J. L., Ayala, R. A., Wang, J. *et al.* (1995). Hyperkalemic periodic paralysis with cardiac dysrhythmia: a novel sodium channel mutation? *Ann Neurol.*, **37**, 408–11.

Basson, C. T., Cowley, G. S., Solomon, S. D. *et al.* (1994). The clinical and genetic spectrum of the Holt-Oram syndrome (Heart-Hand syndrome). *New Engl J Med.*, **330**, 885–91.

Basson, C. T., Solomon, S. D., Weissman, B. *et al.* (1995). Genetic heterogeneity of Heart-Hand syndromes. *Circulation*, **91**, 1326–9.

Canun, S., Perez, N. and Beirana, L. G. (1999). Andersen syndrome autosomal dominant in three generations. *Am J Med Genet.*, **85**, 147–56.

Djurhuus, M. S., Kliitgaard, N. A. H., Jensen, B. M., Andersen, P. E. and Schroder, H. D. (1998). Multiple anomalies, hypokalemic paralysis and partial symptomatic relief by terbutaline. *Acta Paediatr.*, **87**, 475–7.

Fontaine, B., Vale-Santos, J., Jurkat-Rott, K. *et al.* (1994). Mapping the hypokalemic periodic paralysis (HypoPP) locus to chromosome 1q31-32 in three European families. *Nat Gen.*, **6**, 267–72.

Fouad, G., Dalakas, M., Servidei, S. *et al.* (1997). Genotype-phenotype correlations of DHP receptor alpha1-subunit gene mutations causing hypokalemic periodic paralysis. *Neuromusc Dis.*, **7**, 33–8.

Fukuda, K., Ogawa, S., Yokozuka, H., Handa, S. and Nakamura, Y. (1988). Long-standing bidirectional tachycardia in a patient with hypokalemic periodic paralysis. *J Electrocardiol.*, **21**, 71–6.

Gould, R. J., Steeg, C. N., Eastwood, A. B., Penn, A. S., Rowland, L. P. and DeVivo, D. C. (1985). Potentially fatal cardiac dysrhythmia and hyperkalemic periodic paralysis. *Neurology*, **35**,1208–12.

Horn, C. A., Beekman, R. H., Dick, M. 2nd and Lacina, S. J. (1986). The congenital long QT syndrome. An unusual cause of childhood seizures. *Am J Dis Child.*, **140**, 659–61.

Katz, J. S., Wolfe, G. I., Iannaccone, S., Bryan, W. W. and Barohn, R. J. (1999). The exercise test in Andersen syndrome. *Arch Neurol.*, **56**, 352–6.

Keating, M., Atkinson, D., Dunn, C. *et al.* (1991). Linkage of a cardiac arrhythmia, the long QT syndrome, and the Harvey ras-1 gene. *Science*, **252**, 704–6.

Klein, R., Ganelin, R., Marks, J. F., Usher, P. and Richards, C. (1963). Periodic paralysis with cardiac arrhythmia. *J Pediatr.*, **62**, 371–85.

Kramer, L. D., Cole, J. P., Messenger, J. C. and Ellestad, M. H. (1979). Cardiac dysfunction in a patient with familial hypokalemic periodic paralysis. *Chest*, **75**, 189–92.

Layzer, R. B., Lovelace, R. E. and Rowland, L. P. (1967). Hyperkalemic periodic paralysis. *Arch Neurol.*, **16**, 455–72.

Lehmann-Horn, F., Iaizzo, P. A., Franke, C. *et al.* (1990). Schwartz-Jampel syndrome: II. Na$^+$ channel defect causes myotonia. *Muscle Nerve*, **13**, 528–35.

Levitt, L. P., Rose, L. I. and Dawson, D. (1972). Hypokalemic periodic paralysis with arrhythmia. *N Engl J Med.*, **286**, 253–4.

Lewis, E. D., Griggs, R. C. and Moxley, R.T. (1979). Regulation of plasma potassium in hyperkalemic periodic paralysis. *Neurology*, **29**, 1131–7.

Lisak, R. P., Lebeau, J., Tucker, S. H. and Rowland, L. P. (1972). Hyperkalemic periodic paralysis and cardiac arrhythmia. *Neurology*, **22**, 810–5.

Marks, M. L., Trippel, D. L. and Keating, M. (1995a). Long QT syndrome associated with syndactyly identified in females. *Am J Cardiol.*, **76**, 744–5.

Marks, M. L., Whisler, S. L., Clericuzio, C. and Keating, M. (1995b). A new form of long QT syndrome associated with syndactyly. *J Am Coll Cardiol.*, **25**, 59–64.

Martin, A. B., Perry, J. C., Robinson, J. L. *et al.* (1995). Calculation of QTc duration and variability in the presence of sinus arrhythmia. *Am J Cardiol.*, **75**, 950–2.

McManis, P. G., Lambert, E. H. and Daube, J. R.(1986). The exercise test in periodic paralysis. *Muscle Nerve*, **9**, 704–10.

Miller, D., delCastillo, J. and Tsang, T. K. (1989). Severe hypokalemia in thyrotoxic periodic paralysis. *Am J Emerg Med.*, **7**, 584–87.

Reiss, W. G. and Oles, K. S. (1996). Acetazolamide in the treatment of seizures. *Ann Pharmacother.*, **30**, 514–9.

Resnick, J. S., Dorman, J. D. and Engel, W. K. (1969). Thyrotoxic periodic paralysis. *Am J Med.*, **47**, 831–5.

Resor, S. R. Jr and Resor, L. D. (1990). Chronic acetazolamide monotherapy in the treatment of juvenile myoclonic epilepsy. *Neurology*, **40**, 1677–81.

Rowland, L. P. (1994). Andersen's syndrome? or Klein-Lisak-Andersen syndrome? (letter). *Ann Neurol.*, **35**, 252–3.

Rowland, L. P. and Lisak, R. P. (1972). Periodic paralysis: K levels during arrhythmia (letter). *N Engl J Med.*, **287**, 50.

Sansone, V., Griggs, R. C., Meola, G. *et al.* (1997). Andersen syndrome: a distinct periodic paralysis. *Ann Neurol.*, **42**, 305–12.

Schwartz, P. J., Moss, A. J., Vincent, G. M. and Crampton, R. S. (1993). Diagnostic criteria for the long QT syndrome: an update. *Circulation*, **88**, 782–4.

Sperelakis, N. (1994). Regulation of calcium slow channels of heart by cyclic nucleotides and effects of ischemia. *Adv Pharmacol.*, **31**, 1–24.

Stubbs, W. A. (1976). Bidirectional ventricular tachycardia in familial hypokalemic periodic paralysis. *Proc Roy Soc Med.*, **69**, 223–4.

Sundaram, M. B., McMeekin, J. D. and Gulamhusein, S. (1986). Cardiac tachyarrhythmias in hereditary long QT syndromes presenting as a seizure disorder. *Can J Neurol Sci.*, **13**, 262–3.

Tawil, R., Ptacek, L. J., Pavlakis, S. G. *et al.* (1994). Andersen's syndrome: potassium sensitive periodic paralysis, ventricular ectopy, and dysmorphic features. *Ann Neurol.*, **35**, 326–30.

Wang, Q., Curran, M. E., Splawski, I. *et al.* (1996). Positional cloning of a novel potassium channel gene: KVLQT1 mutations cause cardiac arrhythmias. *Nat Gen.*, **12**, 17–23.

Yoshimura, T., Kaneuji, M., Okuno, T. *et al.* (1983). Periodic paralysis with cardiac arrhythmia. *Eur J Pediatr.*, **140**, 338–43.

*Michael Rose and Robert C Griggs*

We stated in our preface that one principle aim of this book was to widen the appreciation of the role of channel disorders in neurology both currently and potentially. For some of the currently known channelopathies the channel dysfunction is fundamental to the pathophysiology of the disease, while for other neurological diseases such as migraine, an ion channel disorder may form just one part of the pathophysiological jigsaw. It is instructive to highlight the common strands that occur in the disease expression of many channelopathies. Recognition of these commonalities may allow one to suspect a channelopathy as a potential cause of other diseases, syndromes or symptoms.

## Channelopathy should be considered as a cause of intermittent neurological symptoms

One common theme for many channelopathies is the intermittent nature of the symptoms induced thus leading to terms such as paroxysmal, periodic or episodic to describe them. The symptoms may last for minutes, hours or days. Traditional neurology teaching tells us that symptoms with this time course should be regarded as vascular, epileptic, metabolic or demyelinating in aetiology. Readers of this book will realize that we should now introduce channelopathy as an alternative pathophysiology in these circumstances. For example, the short-lived symptoms of alternating hemiparesis of childhood (Bourgeois *et al.*, 1993) have been hard to fully explain on a vascular, epileptic or metabolic basis and would be a good candidate for being a channelopathy. Vascular pathology includes migraine and at times the differential

diagnosis for intermittent symptoms invokes debate as to whether they are migrainous or epileptic in nature. The appreciation that disorders of channel function may underlie both migraine and epilepsy adds a twist to such discussions. A similar aetiological debate has raged as to whether paroxysmal nocturnal motor movements are best classified as a form of paroxysmal dyskinesia or frontal epilepsy, a debate that becomes circular when one appreciates that both nocturnal frontal lobe epilepsy (Chapter 16) and paroxysmal dyskinesia (Chapter 17) share a common aetiology as channelopathies.

## Symptoms of channelopathy are mostly but not always 'positive' symptoms

The range of symptoms induced by channel disorders are most often positive symptoms: myotonia (Chapter 9), myokymia (Chapter 14), epilepsy (Chapter 16), dyskinesia (Chapter 17), hyperekplexia (Chapter 18), migraine (Chapter 19), and dysasthetic sensory symptoms (Chapter 20). However, negative symptoms: paralysis (Chapter 10) and myasthenia (Chapter 13) can occur. In some cases a mild defect of a given channel causes a positive symptom such as myotonia while a more severe defect in the same sodium channel causes the negative symptom of paralysis. Positive symptoms can arise from a channel defect that results in loss of inhibitory function, e.g. impaired neuronal potassium channel function as seen in neuromyotonia, while in other cases the positive symptoms arise from a channel defect that exerts a direct excitatory effect, e.g. marine toxin induced sodium channel dysfunction that leads to positive sensory symptoms of burning and parasthesia (Chapter 20).

## Channelopathies share common triggers

Another common theme amongst channelopathies is that symptoms often have specific triggers, and that different channelopathies may share common triggers. Thus episodic ataxia type 1 (Chapter 15) and paroxysmal kinesigenic dyskinesia (Chapter 17) are both triggered by the initiation of movement. Rest after exercise is a common trigger for both hypokalaemic and hyperkalaemic periodic paralysis. Dietary intake can be a trigger for hypokalaemic periodic paralysis (carbohydrate load) or hyperkalaemic periodic paralysis (potassium load) (Chapter 10). Stress and fatigue appear as frequent triggers in channelopathies, e.g. migraine, episodic ataxia, paroxysmal dyskinesia.

## The symptoms of channelopathies often overlap

Although the clinical descriptions of the different channelopathies identifies a core set of symptoms that define particular diseases, in many cases one finds symptoms that overlap those of other channelopathies. Thus we see that epilepsy has been described in cases of episodic ataxia (Chapter 15) and paroxysmal dyskinesia (Chapter 17). Dyskinesia has been described in cases of episodic ataxia. Ataxia can be a prominent symptom in some migraine attacks. This overlap may also be seen in the family histories of patients with a known channelopathy since there is the impression that there is an excess family history of migraine and epilepsy in such cases.

## The symptoms of channelopathy may dissociate

Symptoms that are normally grouped together as part of a given channelopathy syndrome can occur separately. Thus, for example, there are patients who have a KCNA1 gene mutation associated with episodic ataxia Type I but who only manifest as having myokymia (personal observation). If such dissociation of symptoms is a wider phenomenon then it suggests that any patient with a single symptom normally seen as part of a channelopathy could in fact have an ion channel disorder as the cause of that symptom. This hypothesis would greatly expand the scope for potential channelopathies.

## Channelopathies may lead to fixed neurological deficit

Although we have remarked on the intermittent symptoms that occur with most channelopathies the initial paroxysmal or episodic symptoms can give way to fixed deficits. Such examples include episodic ataxia where to begin with there is no inter-ictal cerebellar abnormality but subsequently cerebellar atrophy and persistent ataxia and cerebellar dysarthria can emerge (Chapter 15). Cerebellar atrophy and persistent ataxia can also occur in a proportion of those with familial hemiplegic migraine (Chapter 19). Patients with periodic paralysis usually develop fixed progressive muscle weakness and fixed weakness can also occur in some cases of myasthenia gravis. One of the challenges for the future is to obtain a better

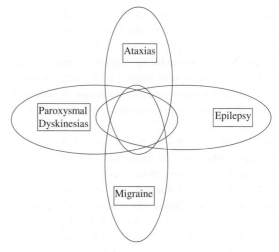

**Figure 23.1** This diagram illustrates the overlapping relationship of many channelopathy symptoms. (With the permission of Kailash Bhatia.)

understanding of how initial episodic symptoms give rise to fixed neurological deficits. We also need to determine whether treatment of the initial episodic syndromes, even if these are infrequent or tolerable without treatment, may prevent longer-term complications.

## Channelopathies may occur at any age

Many of the genetically determined channelopathies show autosomal dominant pattern of inheritance but with variable penetrance. Typically, presentation of such channelopathies (e.g. periodic paralysis, episodic ataxia and paroxysmal dyskinesias) is in the teens or early adulthood. However, some genetically determined, and of course all acquired channelopathies, can have a late onset of presentation. The changing expression of channel genes with development may account for some of these late onset presentations (Chapter 6). Some channelopathies, e.g. benign familial neonatal convulsions (Chapter 16) may only be present during a restricted period of life due to the reduced expression of mutant foetal channel gene subunits.

## Channelopathies may share similar treatment responses

Several of the channelopathies show similar treatment responses. Indeed, the appreciation that episodic ataxia type 2 was likely to be a channelopathy arose by serendipity when a patient with this disease was treated with acetazolamide for a misdiagnosed periodic paralysis. It was only then that the acetazolamide responsiveness of episodic ataxia type 2 was appreciated (Griggs *et al.*, 1978). Until recently the mechanism by which acetazolamide benefited channelopathies was unclear but now it has been demonstrated to influence channel function in an animal model (Tricarico *et al.*, 2000). The response of channelopathies to acetazolamide has led some physicians to propose that acetazolamide responsiveness may be supporting evidence for a diagnosis of a channelopathy. Acetazolamide was one of the earliest anti-epilepsy drugs and, like acetazolamide, most

of the other anti-epilepsy drugs have channel modulating properties. Some channelopathies such as pain syndromes, episodic ataxia, neuromyotonia and myotonia, may respond to carbamazepine, phenytoin and other anti-convulsants.

## How generalizable are genetically determined channelopathies?

The existence of known channelopathies in, for example, rare genetic forms of migraine and epilepsy does raise the important and interesting question as to how generalizable the mechanism of channelopathy might be to those people who have non-hereditary forms of epilepsy and migraine. Screening of the general population of those with migraine and epilepsy for the known relevant channel gene mutations has been undertaken with only a minority showing positive results (Chapters 16 and 19). However, could it be that unknown mutations in those genes or polymorphisms in a variety of channel genes might contribute to polygenic susceptibility to epilepsy or migraine?

## Gentically determined channelopathies may have their acquired counterpart

While it is possible that some sporadic cases of channelopathy may be genetically determined many may be acquired cases. It is interesting to note that many of the genetically determined channelopathies appear to have their acquired channelopathy counterpart. Thus, for example, myokymia can occur as part of a genetic abnormality in the KCNA1 gene, as seen in episodic ataxia Type I. It can also be seen as part of an auto-immune disorder affecting the same potassium channel, as seen in Isaac's syndrome or neuromyotonia. Similarly, we see that genetic disorders of ligand-gated acetylcholine receptor channel cause congenital myasthenia, while an auto-immune disorder of the same channel causes myasthenia gravis. How many other acquired neurological symptoms resembling channelopathy might be on an autoimmune basis? While on the subject of autoimmune channelopathy Angela Vincent (Chapter 13) raises a fascinating mechanism for congenital channelopathy. The presence in a mother of foetal-specific antibodies to channels may result in foetal abnormalities while the mother remains unaffected. This opens a whole Pandora's box of possibilities for acquired congenital channelopathies and indeed disease generally.

## Confirming a channelopathy?

Thus on the basis of a characteristic syndrome, whether partial or complete, or intermittent symptoms not explicable by traditional aetiologies, one might harbor the suspicion that a patient has a channelopathy. One's suspicions would be strengthened by the presence of a family history but sporadic cases may arise in genetic as well as acquired aetiologies. If the patient has what appears to be one of the traditional channelopathy syndromes screening for the common gene mutations for that disorder may provide confirmation of the diagnosis. However, the absence of a gene mutation on such screening does not exclude the diagnosis even if it were genetic and certainly would not be helpful in acquired cases. For some of the acquired channelopathies antibody screening is possible, such as for ACh receptor or calcium channel in cases of myasthenia gravis and lambert Eaton myasthenia, respectively, or potassium channel in cases of myokymia. Particularly for peripheral channelopathies, one has the option of direct investigation of the symptoms by way of neurophysiology studies, which may confirm features consistent with a channelopathy. Such confirmation is not possible for central nervous system symptoms and it is the sporadic suspected channelopathies of the CNS that are the hardest to confirm clinically. In view of the shared response of some channelopathies to acetazolamide some clinicians take recourse to therapeutic trials of this drug in order to strengthen a diagnosis of a suspected channelopathy. However, the results of such treatment trials may be difficult to interpret and attempts to make such trials less susceptible to placebo effect by giving blinded treatment are often confounded by the side effects of acetazolamide.

## Future treatment prospects for channelopathies

The chapters in this book have emphasized the enormous diversity of ion channel function and ion channel characteristics, which allow extreme fine-tuning of nervous system characteristics. Such diversity of ion channel functions could be advantageous in terms of fine-tuning pharmacological treatments for channel disorders (Chapters 3 and 7). This scenario is analogous to that applying to receptor specific pharmacological targeting. Treatment could be directly targeted at restoring the abnormal channel function or else it may be directed at altering the function of alternative channels that might compensate for the aberrant channel function. An example of the latter approach has been the attempts to use the potassium channel modulating drug 3,4-diaminopyridine in multiple sclerosis (Bever et al., 1996). Because some of the channelopathies are rare enough not to figure in the economics of drug research and development it is likely that potential channel modulating drugs for these conditions will have to come from the growth areas of pharmacology research into the epilepsies, migraine and pain syndromes, as well from research into non-neurological channelopathies such as cardiac dysrhymias.

## References

Bever, C.T. Jr., Anderson, P.A., Leslie, J., Panitch, H.S., Dhib-Jalbut, S., Khan, O.A., Milo, R., Hebel, J.R., Conway, K.L., Katz, E. and Johnson, K.P. (1996). Treatment with oral 3,4-diaminopyridine improves leg strength in multiple sclerosis patients. *Neurology* **47**, 1457–1462.

Bourgeois, M., Aicardi, J. and Goutieres, F. (1993). Alternating hemiplegia of childhood. *Journal of Pediatrics* **122**, 673–679.

Griggs, R.C., Moxley, R.T., Lafrance, R.A. and McQuillen, J. (1978). Hereditary paroxysmal ataxia: response to acetazolamide. *Neurology* **28**, 1259–1264.

Tricarico, D., Barbieri, M. and Conte Camerino, D. (2000). Acetazolamide opens the muscular $K_{Ca2+}$ channel: a novel mechanism of action that may explain the therapeutic effect of the drug in hypokalemic periodic paralysis. *Ann. Neurol.* **48**, 304–312.

# Index